PAIN MANAGEMENT:
THEORY AND PRACTICE

CONTEMPORARY NEUROLOGY SERIES AVAILABLE:

PAIN MANAGEMENT: THEORY AND PRACTICE

Editors

RUSSELL K. PORTENOY, M.D.
Director, Analgesic Studies, Pain Service
Associate Attending Neurologist
Memorial Sloan-Kettering Cancer Center
and
Associate Professor of Neurology
Cornell University Medical College
New York, New York

RONALD M. KANNER, M.D.
Chairman, Department of Neurology
Long Island Jewish Medical Center
New Hyde Park, New York
and
Professor of Neurology
Albert Einstein College of Medicine
Bronx, New York

F.A. DAVIS COMPANY • Philadelphia

F.A. Davis Company
1915 Arch Street
Philadelphia, PA 19103

Printed in the United States of America

Last digit indicates print number: 10 9 8 7 6 5 4 3 2 1

Medical Editor: Robert W. Reinhardt
Medical Developmental Editor: Bernice M. Wissler
Production Editor: Roberta Massey
Cover Designer: Steven Ross Morrone

As new scientific information becomes available through basic and clinical research, recommended treatments and drug therapies undergo changes. The authors and publisher have done everything possible to make this book accurate, up to date, and in accord with accepted standards at the time of publication. The authors, editors, and publisher are not responsible for errors or omissions or for consequences from application of the book, and make no warranty, expressed or implied, in regard to the contents of the book. Any practice described in this book should be applied by the reader in accordance with professional standards of care used in regard to the unique circumstances that may apply in each situation. The reader is advised always to check product information (package inserts) for changes and new information regarding dose and contraindications before administering any drug. Caution is especially urged when using new or infrequently ordered drugs.

Library of Congress Cataloging-in-Publication Data

Portenoy, Russell K., 1955–.
    Pain management : theory and practice / Russell K. Portenoy, Ronald M. Kanner.
      p.   cm. — (Contemporary neurology series ; 48)
    Includes bibliographical references and index.
    ISBN 0-8036-0171-9 (alk. paper)
    1. Pain—Treatment.   I. Kanner, Ronald, 1947– . II. Title. III. Series.
    [DNLM: 1. Pain—therapy. 2. Palliative Care. W1 CO769N v.48 1996 / WL 704 P843p 1996]
  RB127.P67   1996
  DNLM/DLC
  for Library of Congress
                                     95-52200
                                        CIP

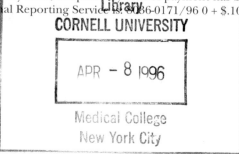

PREFACE

The broad purview of pain research and therapy brings together diverse areas within the basic sciences and clinical medicine and facilitates the connections between the laboratory and bedside. The neurobiology and clinical science of pain and its management are all progressing rapidly, and the information now accumulating will undoubtedly yield new scientific linkages and opportunities for improved patient care.

The development of *Pain Management: Theory and Practice* was guided by this concept of pain research and therapy as a bridge within and across disciplines. Although we could not exhaustively review all the information available about pain in a volume this size, we aimed to describe, as fully as possible, the expanding knowledge about nociception, pain syndromes, and analgesic therapies. We hope that we have done so in a way that highlights their relevance to clinical management.

We include a chapter on basic mechanisms that briefly describes both established and new data about nociception and the pathologic changes in the nervous system that may sustain clinical pain. In this chapter, we underscore the gradual shift from neurophysiology, which was the historical approach to the study of pain, to the modern focus on the interactions between neurophysiological responses and neuropharmacology. Each of the subsequent chapters on pain syndromes explores in more depth the relationships between these mechanisms and painful disease. This is a fascinating area of neuroscience and interested readers are referred to the references on basic mechanisms included in each of these chapters.

The authors who collaborated with us demonstrate the interdisciplinary nature of chronic pain syndromes and their management. The editors and Dr. Kathleen Foley, all neurologists, describe syndromes that are particularly relevant to neurology: headache, back pain, neuropathic pains, and cancer pain. Painful disorders of joints are discussed by Dr. Milton L. Cohen and Dr. Peter M. Brooks, both rheumatologists. Another rheumatologist, Dr. Frederick Wolfe, describes the challenging syndromes of fibromyalgia and myofascial pain. Anesthesiology (Dr. Ian R. Sutton and Dr. Michael J. Cousins), neurosurgery (Dr. Ronald R. Tasker), physiatry (Dr. Michael J. Brennan), and psychology (Dr. Justin M. Nash and Dr. Dennis C. Turk) are all represented among the chapters that describe common treatment approaches.

Our emphasis on treatment in this volume is purposeful. As suggested by the chapter on pain epidemiology, chronic pain is evaluated and managed inadequately in varied clinical settings. Treatment can improve if clinicians focus on the problem and apply currently available information. All clinicians can perform a comprehensive pain assessment, which can guide an appropriate therapeutic strategy. We devote a chapter to this assessment to emphasize its importance. Many analgesic techniques, including the broad range of pharmacologic therapies, can be implemented by primary care providers. We hope that the extensive coverage of pain therapy in *Pain Management: Theory and Practice* empowers clinicians to take a more active role in treating painful disorders and obtaining expert care for patients when this is needed.

The editors would like to thank all the contributing authors for the exceptional quality of their contributions and their forbearance during the development of this book. We are also deeply grateful to Marilyn Herleth and Ellen Cooper, whose editorial suggestions, encouragement, and support were invaluable. We also owe much gratitude to Bernice Wissler of F.A. Davis for her editorial help and to Dr. Sid Gilman for his encouragement and expert editing. Their assistance greatly improved the quality of this work.

Russell K. Portenoy, M.D.
Ronald M. Kanner, M.D.

CONTRIBUTORS

Michael J. Brennan, M.D.
Medical Director
Rehabilitation Center of Fairfield County
Chief, Section of Physical Medicine and Rehabilitation
Bridgeport Hospital
Bridgeport, Connecticut

Peter M. Brooks, M.B., B.S., M.D., F.R.A.C.P., F.A.C.R.M., F.A.F.P.H.M.
Professor and Head of Department of Medicine
University of New South Wales
St. Vincent's Hospital
Sydney, New South Wales, Australia

Milton L. Cohen, M.B., B.S., M.D., F.R.A.C.P.
Head, Department of Rheumatology and Pain Clinic
Senior Lecturer in Medicine
University of New South Wales
St. Vincent's Hospital
Sydney, New South Wales, Australia

Michael J. Cousins, A.M., M.B., B.S., M.D. (Sydney), F.R.C.A., F.A.N.Z.C.A.
Professor and Head
Department of Anaesthesia and Pain Management
University of Sydney
Royal North Shore Hospital
St. Leonards, New South Wales, Australia

Kathleen M. Foley, M.D.
Chief, Pain Service
Attending Neurologist
Department of Neurology
Memorial Sloan-Kettering Cancer Center
Professor of Neurology, Neuroscience and Clinical Pharmacology
Cornell University Medical College
New York, New York

Ronald M. Kanner, M.D.
Chairman, Department of Neurology
Long Island Jewish Medical Center
New Hyde Park, New York
Professor of Neurology
Albert Einstein College of Medicine
Bronx, New York

Justin M. Nash, Ph.D.
Division of Behavioral Medicine
Miriam Hospital
Assistant Professor
Department of Psychiatry
Brown University
Providence, Rhode Island

Russell K. Portenoy, M.D.
Director, Analgesic Studies, Pain Service
Associate Attending Neurologist
Department of Neurology
Memorial Sloan-Kettering Cancer Center
Associate Professor of Neurology
Cornell University Medical College
New York, New York

Ian R. Sutton, M.D., F.R.C.P.C.
Department of Anesthesia
University of Manitoba
Health Sciences Center
Winnipeg, Manitoba, Canada

Ronald R. Tasker, M.D., F.R.C.S.(C.)
Professor, Department of Surgery
University of Toronto
Division of Neurosurgery
The Toronto Hospital
Western Division
Toronto, Ontario, Canada

Dennis C. Turk, Ph.D.
Professor, Psychiatry, Anesthesiology, and Behavioral Science
Director, Pain Evaluation and Treatment Institute
University of Pittsburgh School of Medicine
Pittsburgh, Pennsylvania

Frederick Wolfe, M.D.
Clinical Professor of Internal Medicine and Family and Community Medicine
University of Kansas School of Medicine—Wichita
Director, Arthritis Research and Clinical Centers
Wichita, Kansas

CONTENTS

PART 1

Introduction

CHAPTER 1

DEFINITION AND ASSESSMENT OF PAIN

Russell K. Portenoy, M.D.
Ronald M. Kanner, M.D.

The characteristics and impact of pain vary greatly from patient to patient. Effective management depends on a comprehensive assessment that clarifies the pathogenesis and etiology and evaluates the degree to which the symptom itself or its associated manifestations undermine function and quality of life. This process is facilitated by the use of a standard nomenclature and an appreciation for the clinical characteristics that are most relevant to patient care.

DEFINITION OF PAIN

Pain has been defined by the International Association for the Study of Pain (IASP) as "an unpleasant sensory and emotional experience which we primarily associate with tissue damage or describe in terms of such damage, or both."[26] This definition incorporates two extremely important observations: First, the report of pain reflects both a sensory experience and the individual's affective and cognitive responses. Regardless of the clinical setting, the clinician must consider both the potential contribution of psychosocial factors in precipitating or sustaining the pain and the potential impact of the pain on physical and psychosocial functioning (see Chapter 15). One heuristic conceptualization[23,24] describes pain as a three-level hierarchy, which includes a sensory-discriminative component (location, intensity, quality, and other sensory aspects), a motivational-affective component (emotional responses), and a cognitive-evaluative component (meaning and implications).

Second, the IASP definition indicates that the relationship between pain and tissue damage is neither uniform nor constant. Based on the findings of the pain assessment, the clinician may infer that the pain is either proportionate or disproportionate to the tissue injury evident on examination. For

3

example, pain is often less than expected when tissue injury occurs at times of high stress, such as during battle.[4,5] There may even be a delay in pain onset following commonplace traumatic injuries such as cuts and bruises.[25] In contrast, patients with chronic nonmalignant pain syndromes often complain of pain that exceeds demonstrable tissue injury.[37]

Nociception and Pain

The relationship between tissue damage and pain can be clarified by exploring the differences among nociception, pain, and suffering (Fig. 1–1).[21] *Nociception* is the term applied to the activity induced in neural pathways by potentially tissue-damaging stimuli. In experimental settings, nociception can be measured by an observable response in nervous tissue or by a variety of reflex behaviors.[6] In the clinical setting, however, the degree of nociception can be inferred only by the overt evidence of tissue damage.

Pain is the conscious experience of nociception and, like other perceptions, is only partly determined by stimulus-induced activation of afferent neural pathways. Factors other than nociception influence the perception of pain and in some patients become the major determinants of the pain complaint. In some cases, these factors are inferred to be organic, such as the disturbances of somatosensory processing that become independent of associated tissue damage and result in neuropathic pains (e.g., painful polyneuropathy, trigeminal neuralgia, and central pain). In other cases, they are inferred to be psychologic.

A comprehensive assessment must characterize the range of factors that may be contributing to the pain or pain-related distress.

The existence of tissue damage should not be viewed as presumptive evidence that other processes (neuropathic or psychologic) are absent, and, similarly, the inference that psychologic factors contribute to the pain should not be viewed as evidence against the existence of a physical lesion. Perhaps most important, the inability to discern tissue damage sufficient to explain the pain should not be taken as proof of a psychologic causation (see Chapter 15).

The clinician is usually best served by the assumption that all pain is truly experienced, even when a causative lesion cannot be demonstrated. Although it is commonplace for clinicians to discuss whether or not a pain is "real," this is an intellectual trap that is usually counterproductive and may establish an adversarial relationship between patients and physicians. Although factitious pain (complaints of pain when pain is not experienced, either due to purely intentional malingering or psychiatric disorder) occurs, it is rare in clinical practice. In almost all cases, the clinically relevant issue is whether pain can be best understood as a disturbance of physical functioning, psychologic functioning, or both. From the information acquired through this assessment, the clinician should be able to elaborate a reasonable understanding of the nociceptive, neuropathic, and psychologic factors that may contribute to the pain and on this basis develop an appropriate multimodality treatment approach.

Pain and Suffering

Suffering is a more global construct intricately related to the experience of pain.[21] Like pain itself, suffering is both inherently subjective and multidimensional (see Fig. 1–1). Efforts to define suffering have char-

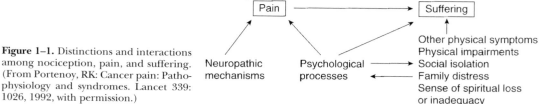

Figure 1–1. Distinctions and interactions among nociception, pain, and suffering. (From Portenoy, RK: Cancer pain: Pathophysiology and syndromes. Lancet 339: 1026, 1992, with permission.)

acterized it as a perceived threat to the patient as person[9] or as "total pain."[38] It may also be likened to overall impairment in quality of life.[31]

Suffering may result from any of numerous aversive perceptions. Pain, loss of physical function, social isolation, familial dissolution, and financial concerns all have impact. Current psychiatric disturbance, such as depression, anxiety, and premorbid character pathology, may also compound the problem. In some cases, spiritual issues (e.g., the meaning of one's life, past mistakes, lack of religious feeling) may be relevant to the larger experience.

The nomenclature applied to these concepts may depend on the clinical context. The terms "suffering" and "quality of life" are commonly used in the setting of cancer, AIDS, or other progressive medical diseases. Specific references to "function" (ability to work, engage in meaningful social interactions, contribute to family life, or experience pleasure) are more commonly described in the literature pertaining to chronic nonmalignant pain. Despite these differences, all terms highlight the impact of pain and other factors on the overall ability to participate in normal life and find joy in the process.

Comprehensive pain assessment must address issues related to suffering. Just as it has been observed that the treatment of tissue injury alone may not reduce pain that is sustained by other, nonnociceptive factors, it is also apparent that a therapeutic approach focused solely on pain may not meaningfully benefit a patient whose suffering is caused by other disturbances.[8]

Definitions of Related Terms

The nomenclature that has evolved to describe pain-related phenomena is often misused, hampering communication among professionals involved in the investigation or management of pain. Formal definitions of these phenomena have been developed by the Subcommittee on Taxonomy of the International Association for the Study of Pain, as follows:[26]

Dysesthesia is a general term used to denote the experience of an abnormal noxious sensation. The term includes both spontaneous perceptions and those induced by a stimulus, which may itself be noxious or nonnoxious. The "abnormal" criterion in this definition is most important. It suggests an unpleasant experience that is recognized by the patient as distinct from usual perceptions. Thus, a pricking pain from a pinprick is not labeled a dysesthesia, whereas unpleasant electrical sensations that persist after the pin is removed from the skin could be labeled in this way. A related term, *paresthesia,* has been defined as an abnormal nonpainful sensation, whether spontaneous or evoked.

Hyperpathia is a particularly unpleasant dysesthesia characterized by an exaggerated pain response to a noxious or nonnoxious stimulus. This response may demonstrate delayed onset, aftersensation, faulty localization, or emotional overreaction. The response may occur only after repeated stimuli and may have an explosive quality.

Allodynia refers to the phenomenon in which a nonnoxious stimulus is perceived as painful. Allodynia is typically considered to be a subtype of dysesthesia. It may also be labeled as hyperpathic if the pain response is particularly exaggerated.

Hyperalgesia is defined as an increased pain response to a noxious stimulus. As commonly used, hyperalgesia connotes less perversion of the pain perception than does dysesthesia. In contrast to dysesthesia, which suggests an unusual, or even bizarre, twist on normal experience, the hyperalgesic response is usually recognized by the patient as within the realm of normal perceptions, albeit greater in intensity than would be expected.

Hypalgesia denotes relatively diminished sensitivity to a noxious stimulus. Again, the perception can be related to normal experience by the patient.

Hyperesthesia and *hypesthesia* are used to describe an increase or decrease, respectively, in the sensitivity to nonnoxious stimulation. The perception is again qualitatively normal, but increased or decreased in intensity compared to homologous regions of the body or common experience.

CHARACTERISTICS OF PAIN

The complexity of this nomenclature reflects the extraordinary variability of pain complaints in the clinical setting. This variability, particularly as it presents among populations with chronic pain, can be addressed only if the assessment provides an understanding of the nature and impact of the pain.[20] The assessment begins with a detailed evaluation of the pain complaint itself (Table 1–1).

Temporal Aspects

The distinction between acute pain and chronic pain is highly salient (Table 1–2). *Acute* pain may be defined as pain of recent onset that ends or is anticipated to end during a period of days to weeks. When due to tissue injury, pain of this type has an essential biologic function, providing a warning of potential damage and impelling the organism to protect and rest the affected part.[44]

Acute pain may be accompanied by anxiety and the systemic signs of sympathetic hyperactivity ("fight or flight" response).[12] The latter signs include elevation of systolic and diastolic blood pressure; increase in pulse; mydriasis; diaphoresis; and a rise in alveolar ventilation, oxygen consumption, and, at times, respiratory rate. Gastrointestinal motility is decreased and muscle tension is increased, particularly in the region of the noxious stimulus.

These associated manifestations have a complex and poorly understood relationship with the characteristics of the pain and the events surrounding its onset. An acute pain that is moderate in intensity, slow in onset, and anticipated by the patient is far less likely to be associated with anxiety and sympathetic hyperactivity than a pain that is severe, abrupt in onset, and potentially indicative of a new medical crisis.

Pain that persists or recurs frequently is ultimately considered *chronic*, a perception that may require a profound shift in therapeutic strategy. For example, efforts to treat the underlying cause and provide rest and comfort, which are mainstay approaches for the management of acute pain, may be replaced in many cases by efforts to restore function and support coping. Despite the observation that this shift in therapeutic approach is guided by more than pain duration alone, definitions of "chronic" pain are typically based solely on a time criterion. Early definitions stated that pain should be considered chronic if it persists more than 3 or 6 months. A more recent definition[7] is an improvement but still focuses on the temporal factor: Pain is chronic if it persists for a month beyond the usual course of an acute illness or a reasonable duration for an injury to heal, if it is associated with a chronic pathologic process, or if it recurs at intervals for months or years.

Table 1–1. **PAIN CHARACTERISTICS**

Characteristic	Potential Descriptors
Temporal	Acute vs recurrent vs chronic Onset, duration, daily variation, course
Intensity	Pain "on average," pain "at its worst," pain "at its least," pain "right now"
Topography	Focal vs multifocal Focal vs referred Superficial vs deep
Exacerbating/relieving factors	Volitional ("incident pain") vs nonvolitional
Inferred pathophysiology	Nociceptive pain vs neuropathic pain vs psychogenic pain vs idiopathic pain
Syndrome	Examples: Reflex sympathetic dystrophy, thalamic pain, trigeminal neuralgia
Etiology	Examples: trauma (may cause reflex sympathetic dystrophy), stroke (may cause thalamic pain), aberrant arterial loop (may cause trigeminal neuralgia).

Table 1–2. **DIFFERENCES BETWEEN ACUTE PAIN AND CHRONIC PAIN**

	Acute Pain	**Chronic Pain**
Temporal features	Recent, well-defined onset; expected to end in days or weeks	Remote, ill-defined onset; duration unpredictable
Biologic function	Essential warning; impels rest and avoidance of further harm	None apparent
Intensity	Variable	Variable
Associated affect	Anxiety common when severe or cause is unknown	Irritability or depression
Associated pain-related behaviors	Pain behaviors common (such as moaning, splinting, rubbing, etc.) when severe or cause is unknown	May or may not give any indication of pain
Associated features	May have signs of sympathetic hyperactivity when severe	May have vegetative signs, such as lassitude, anorexia, weight loss, insomnia, loss of libido
Types and examples	Monophasic (such as postoperative, traumatic, and burned) Recurrent (such as headache, sickle cell anemia, hemophilia, inflammatory bowel disease)	Due to progressive medical diseases (such as cancer and AIDS) Due to nonprogressive or slowly progressive diseases (such as osteoporosis, osteoarthritis, and many neuropathic pains) Pain determined by psychologic factors

These definitions notwithstanding, the decision to shift therapy from an acute pain model to one more appropriate to chronic pain always involves consideration of the etiology and accompanying physical or psychosocial impairments. For example, some patients with nonmalignant pain for 1 or 2 months manifest the types of illness behaviors (such as physical inactivity, inability to work, social isolation, loss of interest in avocations, or overuse of medical resources)[27,28] that immediately suggest "chronic" pain in need of a management strategy that emphasizes functional restoration. In contrast, some patients with painful illnesses (rheumatoid arthritis, sickle cell disease) may be labeled chronic even when treatments are more similar to those used in acute pain. Thus, the terms "acute" and "chronic" should be viewed as imprecise labels that generally indicate a time criterion but may or may not reflect the important clinical issues.

A simple classification of pain patterns illustrates the remarkable clinical diversity subsumed by these labels:

Acute monophasic pains are short lived or are anticipated to be short lived, given the natural history of the underlying pathologic process. Those that require clinical intervention are typically associated with surgery, major trauma, and burns.

Recurrent acute pains include headaches, dysmenorrhea, and pains associated with sickle cell anemia, inflammatory bowel disease, and some arthritides or musculoskeletal disorders (e.g., hemophilic arthropathy).

Chronic pain associated with cancer is the model of pain associated with progressive medical disease.[15] The extremely large number of acute and chronic pain syndromes that have been identified in this population[11,14,32] highlights its heterogeneity. Cancer pain is a major health problem characterized by widespread undertreatment despite the availability of highly effective treatments.[46,47]

Chronic pain due to progressive medical diseases other than cancer is similarly prevalent and includes painful syndromes related to AIDS, sickle cell anemia, hemophilia, and some connective tissue diseases. Although these chronic pains vary in presentation, etiology, and impact, they share with cancer pain a fundamental relationship with the activity of the underlying disease.

Chronic pain associated with nonprogressive or slowly progressive diseases characterizes numerous musculoskeletal pain syndromes (e.g., treatment-refractory osteoporosis and spondylolisthesis) and neuropathic pain syndromes (e.g., postherpetic neuralgia, painful polyneuropathy, central pain, and reflex sympathetic dystrophy). The underlying lesion may also be prominent in the pathogenesis of these pains, but the relative stability of these problems may allow a more focused effort at rehabilitation.

Chronic idiopathic pain broadly encompasses pains that have no identifiable underlying lesion or appear to be excessive for the observable pathology. Some patients with this type of pain present physical and psychosocial findings that strongly suggest the existence of an organic lesion that is yet to be discovered, whereas others present findings that suggest the existence of predominating psychologic determinants for the pain.

Temporal features of the pain other than duration, such as onset, daily variation, and course, may also be clinically relevant. The onset of the pain may be insidious and poorly remembered or abrupt and recalled in fine detail. As part of the assessment, the patient should be asked to recall both the initiating event for the pain and any subsequent period that may denote a major change in the underlying pathogenesis. For example, the change in character of a post-traumatic pain from aching and throbbing to burning may be the herald of reflex sympathetic dystrophy.

The daily pattern of the pain may be predictable or unpredictable. Some pains have a diurnal variation. The pain of rheumatoid arthritis, for example, is usually worse in the morning and eases as the day progresses, whereas pain from osteoarthritis follows the opposite pattern. Headaches related to brain tumor are classically worse on awakening, whereas tension headaches may be present all day or worsen as the day progresses. Many patients with chronic pain of other types report that pain worsens at night. The causes of these different patterns are unknown.

Most patients experience pain that fluctuates on a daily basis in a pattern that is more unpredictable. Pain that is continuous or nearly so is commonly punctuated by intermittent episodes of acute severe pain. In the cancer pain population, this phenomenon is generally termed *breakthrough* pain and is reported by almost two-thirds of those with chronic pain.[34] Pain exacerbations may be brief or prolonged; some are spontaneous and others are associated with an identifiable precipitant, such as change in weather, stress, activity, or some other factor. When brief and precipitated by a voluntary action, such as movement, these superimposed acute pains are termed *incident* pains. From the clinical perspective, it is useful to obtain a detailed history that explores the importance of specific provocative or alleviating factors in the occurrence of these acute pains. This information may be important for diagnosis or therapy.

Pain Intensity

Measurement of pain severity is basic information that may have profound therapeutic implications. To be valid and reliable, a measurement scale should be used, and both the time frame and clinical context should be defined.[10] With chronic pain, it may be useful to inquire about the past month and obtain separate measurements for pain "in general," pain "at its worst," and pain "at its least." A measurement of pain "right now" sometimes offers a useful perspective on these other descriptors. Patients with acute pain are usually asked to describe pain "right now" and may also be asked to indicate the average intensity during the past day, or part thereof, to provide an indication of the course of the pain.

Valid pain measurement can be performed using simple scales or more sophisticated multidimensional measures. In clinical practice, the specific approach is probably less important than its systematic application repeatedly over time. The clinician should select a method and incorporate its use into the clinical routine, obtaining the measurement in the same manner each time.

The simplest scale is a categorical verbal rating scale (e.g., "Is your pain mild, moderate, or severe?"). Almost as simple is a numerical scale ("On a scale of zero to ten, in which zero is no pain and ten is the worst pain imaginable, how severe is your pain?"). Either of these scales can be applied at the bedside, where patients can be asked to respond to a verbal query or to a written question. The patient can be asked to use an identical scale at home as part of a pain diary that records the intensity of pain throughout the day. This can be a very useful technique in clarifying the relationship between pain and activity, the effects of pain treatments, and the daily temporal pattern of the pain.

A visual analog scale (VAS) is another simple and valid approach to pain measurement.[3,13] The most common form of this scale uses a 10-cm line anchored at one end by the descriptor "no pain" or "least possible pain" and anchored at the other end by "worst possible pain" (Fig. 1–2). The patient marks the line at the point that best describes the pain intensity and the distance from the left end to this mark is taken as the numeric measure of pain intensity. Although verbal pain reports do not increase along the scale in linear fashion,[45] these types of measurements are closely linked. Some studies have observed that the VAS is more sensitive than other scales to changes in pain intensity over time.[35] This finding has not been uniform, however, and some patients find the VAS more difficult to understand than a verbal rating scale or a numeric scale.

Multidimensional pain scales have been developed to quantitate the sensory and affective components of pain.[16,24] They are longer and are generally used in clinical research.

Exacerbating and Relieving Factors

It is often useful to record the patient's perception of factors that exacerbate or palliate pain on a daily basis. In some cases, this information can be directly applied in treatment. Information about the effects of activ-

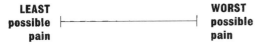

Figure 1–2. Example of a visual analog scale for pain intensity.

ity or stress, for example, is incorporated into cognitive and behavioral therapies for chronic pain (see Chapter 15).

Some exacerbating or relieving factors suggest an etiology or pathophysiology for the pain and may, therefore, have diagnostic value. For example, pain on weight bearing suggests a structural (nociceptive) musculoskeletal lesion, and allodynia in a region of normal-appearing skin may suggest a neuropathic mechanism. Back pain due to disk disease is almost invariably relieved by recumbency, whereas pain associated with vertebral metastasis may be worsened by this maneuver.

Topographic Characteristics

The location of pain also has important implications for diagnosis and therapy. Most patients have little difficulty describing the body topography of the pain. For those who do, body maps may be useful.[22] As part of this assessment, the patient should also be asked whether the pain is superficial or deep. Those who have difficulty with these descriptors can be asked whether they can liken the pain to a "muscle cramp" or a "sunburn."

Pains may be focal (i.e., experienced at one site), multifocal, or generalized. This distinction is clinically relevant and may indicate or contraindicate specific therapies (e.g., nerve blocks).

Pains that are experienced at a site remote from the presumed causative lesion are termed "referred pains."[43] Some patterns are very characteristic, such as cardiac pain radiating to the left shoulder and arm, pancreatic pain referring to the back, and renal colic referring to the inguinal region. More complex and overlapping patterns have been described for muscular, skeletal, and visceral structures.[17–19,36]

Referred pain from neurologic lesions presents a particularly complex problem. An injured nerve may produce focal pain immediately superficial to the site of injury (e.g., median nerve entrapment in the carpal tunnel presenting as aching in the wrist), or it may refer pain anywhere along the course of the nerve (e.g., stabbing pain in the toe as the first sign of sciatic neuropathy). In some cases, the pain may not respect a single nerve or dermatome; for example, patients with median nerve entrapment at the wrist may feel a diffuse aching in the upper arm.[40]

Injury to a nerve plexus can produce pains with varying distributions. Most commonly, the pain is segmental (e.g., tumor involvement of the brachial plexus often presents with symptoms of a C-8 radiculopathy), but it may involve multiple dermatomes. Pain may also occur focally anywhere in the distribution of the injured neural structure (e.g., brachial plexopathy can mimic local pathology in the elbow). Failure to recognize these pain referral patterns can lead to unnecessary delay in diagnosis; for example, the average time from the onset of pain to the diagnosis of a Pancoast tumor is 7 to 12 months.

Lesions affecting the nerve root itself may cause focal midline back pain or pain referred into the corresponding dermatome. The pain can radiate along the entire extent of the nerve or be localized to any site distal to the lesion. The clinician must recognize that the aching toe pain that heralds a sciatic mononeuropathy in one patient can indicate an L-5 or S-1 radiculopathy in another. Either of these lesions may also present as localized pain in the ipsilateral buttock, posterior thigh, popliteal fossa, posterolateral leg, or foot. Although concomitant back pain is suggestive of a root lesion, it is not specific, and painful radiculopathy can occur entirely without back pain.

Polyneuropathy usually produces pain in a different pattern. Dysesthesias, often described as burning, begin in the feet and may gradually ascend to involve the distal legs. With progression of the disorder, these sensations may involve the hands bilaterally. Muscle cramps, usually in the legs, are commonly noted in association with this pain.

The topography of neuropathic pain accompanying lesions of the central nervous system is equally variable. Pain related to a lesion of the spinal cord may be experienced as dysesthesias in one or more extremities or the torso. In some patients, these lesions cause symmetric pain in the feet and distal legs that can mimic painful polyneuropathy. Segmental pain may be caused by a coexistent lesion of a root at the level of the injury or a lesion of the root entry zone by the intramedullary process itself.

Rarely, medullary lesions become complicated by "crossed" dysesthesias affecting ipsilateral face and contralateral body; this pattern is pathognomonic for a lesion in this location. A more rostral lesion can cause chronic pain in the entire contralateral hemibody or a localized site. Although the experience of pain in a classic distribution can be useful in localizing a central nervous system lesion, the underlying lesion may be difficult to discern when pain is limited to a more discrete region.

Syndromic Characteristics

A constellation of symptoms and signs may define a discrete pain syndrome.[26] Recognition of the syndrome may suggest the need for additional evaluation, indicate specific treatments, or allow accurate prognostication.

Syndrome identification may also suggest a presumptive etiology for the pain. This is particularly evident in the cancer pain population (see Chapter 9).[11,14,32] For example, the syndrome of unilateral occipital pain, which radiates to the ipsilateral neck or shoulder and is associated with subtle dysfunction of cranial nerves IX, X, or XI, is highly specific for neoplastic invasion of the jugular foramen at the base of the skull (see Chapter 9). This pattern, like other typical cranial neuropathies, suggests the need for specific imaging of the skull base.

Syndrome recognition extends to the constellation of affective and behavioral disturbances that may accompany chronic pain and either suggests a predominating psychologic pathogenesis for the pain or, at least, indicates substantial psychosocial and behavioral dysfunction that must be addressed therapeutically. The nomenclature applied to these patients is ill-defined and tends to vary with the discipline of the practitioner. Pain specialists tend to use the nonspecific term "chronic nonmalignant pain syndrome" or any of a series of site-specific terms (e.g., atypical facial pain, failed low back syndrome, chronic tension headache, or chronic pelvic pain of unknown etiology). These imprecise labels all imply that pain has become associated with a high degree of disability.

Etiologic Considerations

Definition of the underlying organic processes that may be contributing to the pain is central to the comprehensive pain assessment. This information may clarify the nature of the disease, indicate prognosis, or suggest the use of specific therapies. For example, an appropriate medical evaluation of patients with cancer or other chronic medical illnesses (e.g., arthritis or inflammatory bowel disease) can elucidate the extent or activity of disease and thereby guide the use of primary therapy.

The search for an underlying etiology must be placed in the context of the patient's illness. Laboratory and radiographic procedures are usually appropriate as part of the assessment of patients with acute pain and patients with chronic pain that has not been adequately evaluated previously, has recently changed, or is now occurring in association with an evolving medical disease (e.g., cancer). In contrast, repeated testing of other patients with chronic pain rarely yields useful results and may divert attention from symptom control and functional restoration. In some cases, it may reinforce somatic preoccupation and illness behavior. If further evaluation is unlikely to change the diagnosis or the treatment, it is usually more salutary to concentrate on treatment.

Pathophysiologic Characteristics

Clinical observation and extrapolation of data from animal models suggest that the presentation and therapeutic response of a pain syndrome may be determined by factors linked to the underlying mechanism of the pain.[2,29] Although the classification that can be derived from these observations is empirical and obviously oversimplifies complex pathophysiologic processes (see Chapter 2), it has become widely accepted because of its clinical utility. According to this scheme, the predominating pathophysiology of pain can be broadly divided into nociceptive, neuropathic, and idiopathic categories.

Nociceptive pain can be defined as pain that is believed to be commensurate with the presumed degree of ongoing activation of peripheral nociceptors (primary afferent neurons that respond selectively to noxious stimuli). The nervous system is believed to be fundamentally intact, and the complaints of pain are viewed as an appropriate response to tissue damage.

Nociceptive pains related to ongoing activation of somatic primary afferents are also termed *somatic pains.* These pains are typically described as aching, squeezing, stabbing, or throbbing. Arthritis and some types of cancer pain (e.g., bone pain) exemplify somatic nociceptive pains.

Nociceptive pains related to activation of the primary afferent neurons that innervate viscera are also labeled *visceral pains.* When the underlying lesion involves obstruction of hollow viscus, the pains are often described as cramping or gnawing, as having a crescendo-decrescendo temporal pattern, and as being referred to common cutaneous sites (e.g., pancreas to back, gallbladder to shoulder). When organ capsules are involved, the pain is more often described as aching, stabbing, or throbbing.

Neuropathic pain can be defined as pain that is perceived to be sustained by aberrant somatosensory processing in the peripheral or central nervous system. Broad subtypes have been defined, again on the basis of empirically derived clinical criteria that do not reflect the true complexity of the pathologic mechanisms involved. These subgroups include deafferentation pains, sympathetically maintained pains, and a group that can be termed painful peripheral neuropathic pains (see Chapter 5).[30]

Idiopathic pain can be defined as pain that persists in the absence of an identifiable organic substrate or that is believed to be excessive for the organic processes extant. As discussed previously, a subgroup of patients with idiopathic pain presents positive evidence of a predominating psychologic contribution to the pain. These pains are appropriately described as psychogenic or labeled with a specific psychiatric diagnosis.[1]

Implicit in these descriptions of inferred pathophysiology is the importance currently ascribed to information about the quality of pain. Although no descriptor or set of descriptors is specific for a given mechanism, a link between the reported characteristics of the pain and the underlying mechanism is supported by clinical observations.[16] For example, pains inferred to have a neuropathic mechanism are often described as burning, lancinating, or electrical. It must be recognized, however, that these phenomena are neither empirically established nor specific. Burning pain also occurs after first-degree skin burns (sunburn), a syndrome that is best considered a somatic nociceptive pain.

These pathophysiologic constructs have important therapeutic implications. The response to opioids, for example, appears to be relatively better during treatment of pains perpetuated in large part by nociception than pains that are sustained by neuropathic mechanisms.[2,33] Nonnociceptive pains are also generally believed to be less responsive than nociceptive pains to techniques that isolate the painful part from the central nervous system; cordotomy, for example, has been reported to be far less effective in patients with deafferentation pain than those with pain related to nociceptive lesions (see Chapter 13).[39]

A recent effort to extend the utility of pathophysiologic constructs has attempted to integrate some type of medical-physical classification with a psychosocial and behavioral classification. Specifically, a so-called polydiagnostic approach has been proposed[42] that uses a system for psychosocial and behavioral classification based on empirically derived groupings that categorize patients into three broad types ("dysfunctional," "interpersonally distressed," and "adaptive copers").[20,41] Once classified into one of these groups, a medical-physical classification is added, such as the comprehensive taxonomy developed by the International Association for the Study of Pain.[26]

The objective of the latter model is to develop a classification that is derived from valid measures and combines psychosocial and biomedical models. It avoids the over-generalization of findings from one group of selected patients with pain (such as those referred to a multidisciplinary pain management program) to inherently dissimilar groups. Although the model has yet to be validated in clinical practice, it illustrates the complexity of the heterogeneous populations that seek treatment for pain and affirms the need to assess on a case-by-case basis the various organic and psychologic processes that contribute to pain and its impact.

ASSESSMENT OF PAIN-RELATED DISTURBANCES

To fashion an appropriate therapeutic strategy, the assessment must address the affective and functional concomitants of pain. This is particularly true for chronic pain. For example, a strategy in which analgesic drugs are administered by a single physician is clearly appropriate for most patients with a well-defined cancer-related pain and little disturbance in mood or function, but it is not appropriate for the patient with a chronic pain syndrome characterized by depression, physical inactivity, social isolation, and family distress. Identification of the latter problems can guide a multimodality therapeutic approach that would likely involve more than one clinician. A constellation of problems such as these may suggest the utility of referral to a traditional multidisciplinary pain management program.

The assessment of pain-related disturbances focuses on physical capabilities and the degree of psychologic and social dysfunction associated with the pain (Table 1–3). For those with acute pain, the expectations for function may be very limited, and the assessment may be concerned only with the impact of psychologic factors on the ability to manage the pain. For those with persistent pain, however, a detailed evaluation of these associated disturbances is needed.

At its most basic level, functional impairment refers to the specific activities that the patient is no longer able to perform as a result of the pain or its treatment. Specific queries might evaluate work, avocations, housekeeping tasks, activities of daily living, and sexual function. Current abilities should be assessed in terms of prior function and expectations for the future. It is useful to distinguish the effects of physical impairments (such as paresis) from the consequences of unrelieved pain or pain therapy.

The psychologic assessment may address the interaction among pain, pain-related disability, and a spectrum of psychologic concerns, including coping and distress, personality, and both present and past psychiatric disorders. In some settings, such as the traditional multidisciplinary pain program, the prevalence and importance of these psychologic issues is such that all patients routinely undergo an assessment by a psycholo-

Table 1–3. **SPECTRUM OF PAIN-RELATED DISTURBANCES THAT SHOULD BE EVALUATED AS PART OF THE COMPREHENSIVE PAIN ASSESSMENT**

	Potential Areas of Interest
Physical functioning	Specific impairments (e.g., paresis) Physical symptoms other than pain Ability to perform activities of daily living "Up time," walking distance, ability to lift Sleep quality, appetite, weight
Psychologic functioning	Psychologic symptoms Past and present psychiatric disorders Coping style, adaptation Psychologic reactions to illness in the past Personality variables Pain-reinforcing contingencies ("secondary gain")
Social functioning	Family disturbances Social isolation Intimacy Involvement in litigation or compensation systems
Role functioning	Ability to work Ability to perform housekeeping tasks Intactness of parenting role Ability to engage in avocations
Other considerations	History of drug use (prescription, over-the-counter, and illicit) Past history of chronic pain Family history of chronic disease, chronic pain, psychiatric disease, substance abuse

gist or psychiatrist who specializes in this area. In routine practice, it is the clinician's responsibility to perform an evaluation that is sufficient to guide a therapeutic program and identify those in need of psychiatric referral. If a significant psychiatric disorder such as major depression, anxiety disorder, panic disorder, somatization, or severe personality disorder is suspected, referral for psychiatric evaluation and specialized treatment is warranted. Lesser degrees of dysfunction should be addressed in treatment by the primary clinician.

The experience of pain often has a profound impact on members of the family and others in the patient's environment. In some families, the patient's chronic pain is used as an interpersonal device, with maladaptive consequences. Other patients exist in a home or work environment replete with obvious behavioral contingencies that have the unintentional effect of maintaining pain or

pain-related disability. These factors can be identified during the pain assessment, then addressed as part of the therapeutic program.

Families may also be a source of great support for patients who are attempting to cope with pain and continue to function. Families that offer assistance without reinforcing pain behaviors can be a resource used to further treatment goals.

Other Relevant Medical History

Previous reactions to nonpainful or painful diseases may be informative, particularly if the history includes periods of prolonged or chronic illness in the patient. Specific queries should address lifestyle changes and use of medical resources: Did the patient change jobs, become more dependent on family members, use physician or hospital services maladaptively, or seek long-term disability? What were the emotional responses to illness in the past?

Specific questioning may reveal a history of painful disorders, including recurrent back pain, dysmenorrhea, abdominal pain, headaches, or facial pain. Detailed information about the physical and psychosocial impairments associated with these pains, the degree of disability manifested as a result, and the outcomes of treatment efforts can be extremely valuable in understanding the current pain problem.

For patients with chronic pain, review of the relevant medical history should be complemented by acquisition of medical records. These records may be useful in clarifying the full range of physical and psychologic problems presented by the patient. In some cases, they provide the only means to reach an accurate diagnosis. For example, the diagnosis of somatization disorder may become apparent only after the information included in the medical records from other physicians becomes available.

The history of prior drug use is an essential part of the assessment. This history should address all types of drug use, including prescription drugs, over-the-counter remedies, and both licit and illicit recreational drugs. The characteristics and outcome of previous therapeutic trials may strongly influence future therapeutic decisions, and each trial should be assessed in terms of the adequacy of the dose and duration and the reasons for failure. An inadequate trial cannot be used to judge the efficacy of a drug or class of drugs.

Reports of "allergy" must also be carefully assessed so that a history of side effects can be distinguished from true hypersensitivity reactions. Nausea and constipation are commonly reported as "allergic" reactions to codeine, and "allergy" to pentazocine (a mixed agonist-antagonist opioid) reported by a patient who is physically dependent on another opioid may actually be withdrawal. If side effects that limited a past trial could potentially be managed better (perhaps through changes in dosing or specific concurrent treatments), the possibility of a future trial with the drug should be considered.

A history of substance abuse is extremely important, and deliberate questioning may be required to obtain sufficient detail. The history should clarify the use of specific drugs (including alcohol) and determine whether this use is remote, recent, or ongoing.

Medical and Neurologic Examination

All patients with acute or chronic pain require a complete medical and neurologic examination, and many require regular reexamination. The purpose of this examination is to clarify the relationship between the pain and the underlying anatomic or physiologic disturbances or, at least, to delineate clinical hypotheses about this relationship that can then be evaluated through appropriate radiographic or laboratory means. This information may provide an opportunity for primary therapy of the underlying disease (which can have analgesic consequences), suggest additional problems in need of treatment, or alter prognosis.

The need for repeated medical and neurologic evaluation is evident when pain is associated with an evolving medical disease, such as cancer, arthritis, or AIDS. The need is generally less clear-cut in patients with static lesions (such as postherpetic neuralgia) and those with idiopathic pain or pain previously determined to have a predominating psychologic pathogenesis. Like the decision to pursue additional radiographic studies, the need for repeated examination is based on a critical assessment of the information at hand. If the pain is adequately explained and symptoms have been relatively stable, repeated examination may unnecessarily divert attention from therapeutic goals. If, however, the nature of the pathology is not yet clear or symptoms have recently changed, the need for assessment becomes compelling.

Examination of the painful site must be detailed and include, if appropriate, assessment of function as well as structure. Inspection of the patient's movements, facial expression, and demeanor may also provide clues to the underlying pathogenesis of the pain or its behavioral concomitants.

FORMULATION OF A TREATMENT PLAN

It is useful to conceptualize the goal of the comprehensive assessment of the patient as the formulation of a pain-oriented problem list. The assessment yields detailed information about the nature of the pain and its relationship to other organic and psychologic disturbances that contribute to the patient's disability or suffering. The problem list can be used to prioritize the range of concerns presented by the patient and address each in turn through the development of a multimodality treatment program. For some patients, comfort is the major issue, and the treatment approach is properly directed to the implementation of analgesic therapies. For other patients, functional restoration is as important as comfort, and perhaps more attainable, and the treatment program may focus on rehabilitative therapies. If the problem list reflects a high level of disability, the clinician may readily perceive that the most efficient method of implementing a multimodality therapeutic strategy involves referral to a multidisciplinary pain management program.

The establishment of realistic goals is essential in the formulation of the problem list and the therapeutic program to address it. The patient's expectations commonly diverge from those of the clinician, and a fundamental objective of the early treatment period is to redefine the patient's agenda so that it is in keeping with the opportunities presented by treatment. For example, a patient may seek complete pain relief and initially perceive partial analgesia as failure. Because complete relief is uncommon among those with chronic pain, the patient's expectation is countertherapeutic.

Many patients with pain-related disability believe that comfort is the only appropriate goal of treatment and that successful pain relief will immediately result in functional improvement. This expectation conflicts with the rehabilitative model adopted by most multidisciplinary pain management programs, which focus on function at least as intensively as comfort. Successful participation in these programs depends on the patient's willingness to engage in treatments directed primarily at physical and psychosocial rehabilitation. Individual clinicians who manage such patients must similarly redirect the goals to these functional concerns. It may be useful to formulate a succession of small, intermediate goals for functional gains and keep the larger goals in the future, at least initially.

Case History

A case description provides a useful illustration of the principles of pain assessment.

PATIENT DESCRIPTION

A 41-year-old man seeks treatment of foot pain that has been present for 6 months and began 4 weeks after routine resection of a traumatic neuroma from the interdigital nerve between the third and fourth metatarsal bones (Morton's metatarsalgia). The pain is diffuse in the foot and is described as severe burning, which is increased by activity, contact, and stress. The pain has been steadily worsening, and the patient has been unable to work for more than 3 months. He reports increasing difficulty in performing household activities, depressed mood, loss of interest in all activities, severe sleep disturbance characterized by frequent awakenings, and progressive lassitude. He states that his wife has been supportive but admits that their sexual relationship ceased several months earlier. He has applied for disability.

The patient has been evaluated by other physicians and has been offered diagnoses of plantar fasciitis, reflex sympathetic dystrophy, and recurrent neuroma. He has undergone magnetic resonance imaging of the foot and electrodiagnostic studies, neither of which has been revealing. A family physician noted that he appeared depressed and prescribed fluoxetine. He has also received trials of various nonsteroidal anti-inflammatory drugs and is presently using both an anxiolytic and an opioid on an "as needed" basis.

On examination, the distal foot is cooler and slightly edematous compared with its counterpart. Movement of all the toes is impaired, and mild sensory loss along the distal half of the plantar surface is found. Early joint ankylosis and muscle wasting of the distal leg and foot are also evident.

COMMENT

The patient presents with a chronic pain syndrome, which is probably organically related to a neuropathic mechanism. The associated autonomic features suggest, but do not establish, the diagnosis of a reflex sympathetic dystrophy, which itself suggests sympathetically maintained pain (see Chapter 5). Some nociceptive component may also originate from associated joint and soft tissue changes, but these do not appear sufficient to explain the pain. There is substantial evidence of a coexisting psychiatric disorder, and it is possible that some component of the pain is determined by psychologic factors.

The pain complaint itself is one of several salient problems. The level of disability associated with the pain is very high. The patient cannot work and has lost his usual role within the family. His relationship with his spouse has deteriorated and, as noted, there is evidence of major depression. Efforts at treatment have been desultory, and his use of medications has limited guidance and may be contributing to his poor function.

From this assessment, a problem list can be formulated that includes (1) pain related to potentially treatable neuropathic, nociceptive, and psychologic pathophysiologies; (2) major depression; and (3) several of the most troubling areas of compromised function. This formulation can then be applied to the development of a multimodality treatment strategy including some treatments focused specifically on the pain and others targeted to the other features of the illness. Referral to a multidisciplinary pain management program can be considered if one is available and the patient has the necessary resources. If directed by the primary clinician, a treatment program can be organized through liaisons developed with a psychologist (or other mental health care provider), a physiatrist, and an anesthesiologist with training in pain management.

Management of the pain may begin with a trial of sympathetic nerve blocks, which are directed at the presumptive diagnosis of reflex sympathetic dystrophy. A program of physical therapy, perhaps combined with other physical medicine approaches, can be initiated concurrently. A variety of approaches can be used to stabilize drug therapy and offer sequential trials of analgesics, if needed after the nerve blocks. A change to an analgesic antidepressant may be implemented immediately to address both the pain and the depression (see Chapter 10). Ongoing psychotherapy can be incorporated into the overall approach to further address mood and function. The detailed assessment guides the selection of the many potential therapies that can be used to improve both pain and functional impairments.

SUMMARY

Pain is a complex and heterogeneous phenomenon, inherently containing a sensory component and a reactive psychosocial component. Chronic pain may complicate a progressive medical disease, persist despite stable disease or total resolution of an injury in the past, or occur in the absence of explanatory organic processes. Unlike acute pain, persistent pain appears to fulfill no adaptive biologic function and, for many patients, becomes the primary disease process itself.

Pain is a perception, which must be distinguished from both nociception (the activity in the sensorineural pathways sensitive to noxious stimuli) and the more global construct of suffering (impairment in quality of life). These distinctions help clarify the range of issues that must be assessed if the major goals of pain management, usually broadly conceptualized as both comfort and function, are to be addressed therapeutically.

The management of chronic pain begins with a comprehensive assessment, which characterizes the pain complaint and the impact of the pain on functioning. This assessment should characterize the pain in terms of its sensory qualities, such as its temporal features, intensity, and location, and in terms of its etiology, associated syndrome and inferred pathophysiology.

Although the pathophysiology of pain cannot be confirmed in patients, inferences about the predominating types of mechanisms have proved to be clinically useful. Based on the clinical evaluation, various components of the pain syndrome can be labeled nociceptive, neuropathic, psychogenic, or idiopathic. These distinctions may help guide further assessment or treatment.

Evaluation of the impact of the pain on function must reflect a broad range of concerns. These concerns include aversive changes in physical, psychologic, or social functioning. Together, these changes clarify the degree of global disability associated with the pain. The optimal therapeutic approach is strongly influenced by the nature and severity of this pain-related disability. Whereas patients who have pain and little associated disability may be appropriately managed by primary analgesic approaches often administered by a single clinician, the highly disabled patient with chronic pain may benefit substantively only by the administration of a multimodality approach that emphasizes functional restoration and is implemented by a team in a multidisciplinary pain management program.

REFERENCES

1. American Psychiatric Association Task Force on Nomenclature and Statistics: Diagnostic and Statistical Manual of Mental Disorders, (DSM III), ed 3. American Psychiatric Association, Washington, DC, 1980.
2. Arner S, and Myerson BA: Lack of analgesic effect of opioids on neuropathic and idiopathic forms of pain. Pain 33:11–23, 1988.
3. Banos JE, Bosch F, Canellas M, et al: Acceptability of visual analogue scales in a clinical setting: A comparison with verbal rating scales in postoperative pain. Methods Find Exp Clin Pharmacol 11: 123–127, 1989.
4. Beecher HK: Pain in men wounded in battle. Ann Surg 123:96–105, 1946.
5. Beecher HK: Relationship of significance of wound to pain experienced. JAMA 161:1609–1613, 1956.
6. Besson J-M, and Chaouch A: Peripheral and spinal mechanisms of nociception. Physiol Rev 67:67–185, 1987.
7. Bonica JJ: Definitions and taxonomy of pain. In Bonica JJ (ed): The Management of Pain. Lea & Febiger, Philadelphia, 1990, pp 18–27.
8. Carlsson AM: Assessment of chronic pain. II. Problems in the selection of relevant questionnaire items for classification of pain and evaluation and prediction of therapeutic effects. Pain 19:173–184, 1984.
9. Cassel EJ: The nature of suffering and the goals of medicine. N Engl J Med 306:639–645, 1982.
10. Chapman CR, Casey KL, Dubner R, et al: Pain measurement: An overview. Pain 22:1–31, 1985.
11. Cherny NC, and Portenoy RK: Cancer pain: Principles of assessment and syndromes. In Wall PD, and Melzack R (eds): Textbook of Pain, ed 3. Churchill Livingstone, Edinburgh, 1994, pp 787–824.
12. Engel, BT: Some physiological correlates of hunger and pain. J Exp Psychol 57:389–396, 1959.
13. Fishman B, Pasternak S, Wallenstein SL, et al: The Memorial Pain Assessment Card. A valid instrument for the evaluation of cancer pain. Cancer 60: 1151–1181, 1987.
14. Foley KM: Pain syndromes in patients with cancer. Med Clin North Am 71:169–184, 1987.
15. Gonzales GR, Elliott KJ, Portenoy RK, et al: The impact of a comprehensive evaluation in the management of cancer pain. Pain 47:141–144, 1991.
16. Gracely RH, and Kwilosz DM: The Descriptor Differential Scale: Applying psychophysical principles to clinical pain assessment. Pain 35:279–288, 1988.

17. Head H: On disturbances of sensation with especial reference to the pain of visceral diseases. Brain 16:1–133, 1893.
18. Inman VT, and Saunders JB: Referred pain from skeletal structures. J Nerv Ment Dis 99:660–667, 1944.
19. Kellgren JH: On the distribution of pain arising from deep somatic structures with charts of segmental pain areas. Clin Sci 4:35–46, 1939.
20. Kerns RD, Turk DC, and Rudy TE: The West Haven Yale Multidimensional Pain Inventory (WHYMPI). Pain 23:345–356, 1985.
21. Loeser JD: Definition, etiology and neurological assessment of pain originating in the nervous system following deafferentation. In Bonica JJ, Lindblom U, and Iggo A (eds): Advances in Pain Research and Therapy, Vol 5. Raven Press, New York, 1983, pp 701–711.
22. Margoles MS: The pain chart: Spatial properties of pain. In Melzack RM (ed): Pain Measurement and Assessment. New York: Raven Press, 1983, pp 215–231.
23. Melzack R: Neurophysiological foundations of pain. In Sternbach RA (ed): The Psychology of Pain. Raven Press, New York, 1986, pp 1–25.
24. Melzack R, and Casey KL: Sensory, motivational and central control determinants of pain: A new conceptual model. In Kenshalo D (ed): The Skin Senses. Charles C. Thomas, Springfield, IL, 1968, pp 423–439.
25. Melzack R, Wall PD, and Ty TC: Acute pain in an emergency clinic: Latency of onset and descriptor patterns related to different injuries. Pain 14:33–43, 1982.
26. Mersky H, and Bogduk N (eds): Classification of Chronic Pain, ed 2. IASP Press, Seattle, 1994.
27. Pilowsky I, Chapman CR, and Bonica JJ: Pain, depression, and illness behavior in a pain clinic population. Pain 4:183–192, 1977.
28. Pilowsky I, and Spence ND: Pain and illness behavior: A comparative study. J Psychosom Res 20:131–134, 1976.
29. Portenoy RK: Mechanisms of clinical pain: Observations and speculations. In Portenoy RK (ed): Neurologic Clinics, Vol 7, No. 2, Pain: Mechanisms and Syndromes. WB Saunders, Philadelphia, 1989, pp 205–230.
30. Portenoy RK: Issues in the management of neuropathic pain. In Basbaum A, Besson J-M (eds): Towards a New Pharmacotherapy of Pain. John Wiley & Sons, New York, 1991, pp 393–416.
31. Portenoy RK: Pain and quality of life: Theoretical aspects. In Osoba D (ed): Quality of Life in Cancer Patients. CRC Press, Boca Raton, FL, 1991, pp 279–292.
32. Portenoy RK: Cancer pain: Pathophysiology and syndromes. Lancet 339:1026–1031, 1992.
33. Portenoy RK, Foley KM, and Inturrisi CE: The nature of opioid responsiveness and its implications for neuropathic pain: New hypotheses derived from studies of opioid infusions. Pain 43:273–286, 1990.
34. Portenoy RK, and Hagen NA: Breakthrough pain: Definition, prevalence and characteristics. Pain 41:273–282, 1990.
35. Price DD: Psychological and neural mechanisms of pain. Raven Press, New York, 1988, pp 28–38.

36. Procacci P, and Zoppi M: Pathophysiology and clinical aspects of visceral and referred pain. In Bonica JJ, Lindblom U, and Iggo A (eds): Advances in Pain Research and Therapy, Vol 5. Raven Press, New York, 1983, pp 643–658.

37. Rosomoff HL, Fishbain DA, Goldberg M, et al: Physical findings in patients with chronic intractable benign pain of the neck and/or back. Pain 37:279–287, 1989.

38. Saunders C: The philosophy of terminal care. In Saunders C (ed): The management of terminal malignant disease. Edward Arnold, London, 1984, pp 232–241.

39. Tasker RR, and Dostrovsky JO: Deafferentation and central pain. In Wall PD, Melzack R (eds): Textbook of Pain, ed 2. Churchill Livingstone, Edinburgh, 1989, pp 154–180.

40. Torebjork HE, Ochoa JL, and Schady W: Referred pain from intraneural stimulation of muscle fascicles in the median nerve. Pain 18:145–156, 1984.

41. Turk DC, and Rudy TE: Toward an empirically derived taxonomy of chronic pain patients: Integra-

tion of psychological assessment data. J Consult Clin Psychol 56:233–238, 1988.

42. Turk DC, and Rudy TE: The robustness of an empirically derived taxonomy of chronic pain patients. Pain 43:27–35, 1990.

43. Vecchiet L, Albe-Fessard DA, Lindblom U (eds): New Trends in Referred Pain and Hyperalgesia. Elsevier, New York, 1993.

44. Wall PD: On the relation of injury to pain. Pain 6: 253–264, 1979.

45. Wallenstein SL: The VAS Relief scale and other analgesic measures: Carryover effect in parallel and crossover studies. In Max M, Portenoy RK, and Laska E (eds): Advances in Pain Research and Therapy, Vol 18: The Design of Analgesic Clinical Trials. Raven Press, New York, 1991, pp 97–103.

46. World Health Organization: Cancer pain relief. World Health Organization, Geneva, 1986.

47. World Health Organization: Cancer pain relief and palliative care. World Health Organization, Geneva, 1990.

CHAPTER 2

BASIC MECHANISMS

Russell K. Portenoy, M.D.

Extraordinary advances in pain-related research have yielded insights into both the physiology of the neural systems that respond to noxious stimuli and the diverse perturbations in these systems that may underlie clinical pain. This knowledge provides a useful foundation for the assessment and management of patients with painful disorders.

NEURAL SUBSTRATE OF PAIN TRANSMISSION

Nociceptors

Nociceptors can be defined as primary afferent neurons that have the capacity to distinguish between noxious and innocuous events.[164] The axons from these neurons are generally lightly myelinated (A-delta fibers) or unmyelinated (C fibers). Those nociceptors innervating skin have been best characterized.

A-delta nociceptors have been identified in numerous species, including man. The best studied units, which have been termed *high-threshold mechanoreceptors* by some investigators,[66,163] usually respond to intense heat as well as noxious mechanical stimuli and, consequently, are better classified as mechano-heat nociceptors.[144] Silent in the absence of stimulation, some of these units discharge only when noxious stimulation is applied, and others respond to innocuous stimuli but increase their firing rates with a tissue-damaging stimulus.[163] Sensitization following exposure to noxious stimuli may occur.[66] There is ample evidence that these nociceptors are involved both in the perception of pain following noxious mechanical and heat stimuli and in the development of hyperalgesia following tissue injury.

Unmyelinated primary afferent neurons that respond to noxious thermal, mechanical, and chemical stimuli (so-called C poly-modal nociceptors or C fiber mechano-heat nociceptors) have also been identified in humans and are clearly involved in pain perception.[191,192,196] Some of these polymodal nociceptors discharge with nonnoxious stimuli and increase their firing rate as stimulus intensity increases; others discharge only with potentially tissue-damaging stimulation.[18,111] Sensitization after a noxious stimulus has also been demonstrated.[130]

Other types of cutaneous nociceptors have been described. Electrophysiologic studies have identified A-delta fibers with response characteristics identical to that of the C poly-modal nociceptors, unmyelinated units responsive only to high-threshold mechanical stimulation, and both A-delta and C fiber units responsive to intense cold.[18,111,112] Recent studies further suggest that some classes of nociceptors are responsive to noxious stimuli only after they become conditioned by prolonged injury or inflammation.[107,178]

Primary afferent fibers responsive to noxious stimulation also have been identified in the viscera[34] and other somatic tissues, including muscle,[108] joints,[43,178] cornea,[19] and tooth pulp and periodontium.[180] Nociceptive information from the heart is mediated by nerves that travel with sympathetic pathways; this has been demonstrated by both the failure of experimental vagotomy to diminish responses to noxious stimulation[28] and the prompt abolition of angina by section of the sympathetic trunk.[206] Although lung parenchyma and visceral pleura are insensitive to noxious stimulation, nociceptive afferents, at least some of which traverse the vagus nerve, innervate the larynx, airways, and so-called J receptors[147,158]; parietal pleura is innervated by somatic nociceptors in the intercostal nerves. Intra-abdominal and pelvic viscera are similarly innervated by nociceptors that are carried in sympathetic or parasympathetic nerves.[33,67,109,150] The stimuli that activate visceral nociceptors vary with the type of nociceptor and the specific tissue innervated.

Termination of Primary Afferent Neurons

Most afferent input enters the spinal cord through the dorsal root. There is evidence that fibers segregate by size as they approach the cord, with those of smaller diameter moving laterally.[184] A lesion placed selectively in the lateral aspect of the root can produce segmental analgesia.[183] Ventral roots also carry a significant afferent input, most of which is carried by unmyelinated axons that transmit nociceptive information.[40,42] Afferent fibers in the ventral root may account for the failure of dorsal rhizotomy for pain in some cases.

A-delta nociceptors have been found to terminate primarily in lamina I, the outer aspect of lamina II, and deeper in lamina V.[125] A few collaterals cross to the contralateral dorsal horn. C fiber nociceptors also terminate predominantly in the most superficial layers of the dorsal horn.[152] Specific nociceptive input to the trigeminal nuclei has a similar distribution and may be limited to the caudal aspect of the nuclear complex.[128] Visceral afferents, which have extensive rostral-caudal collaterals, probably terminate in a distribution similar to somatic afferents.[149]

The pharmacology of primary nociceptive afferents is extremely complex (Table 2–1).[56,217] Approximately one-third of small dorsal root ganglion cells, a proportion of which are presumably nociceptive, contain neuropeptides,[91] and many neurons contain more than one.[46] Among the best studied of these peptides is substance P, which appears to be an important transmitter for C fiber nociceptors.[84,117,152,215] Numerous other peptides are also involved in the function of these primary afferent neurons, and other types of messenger compounds also play a role, including excitatory amino acids and nucleotides.[56]

The role of excitatory amino acids (EAA) and their receptors in pain perception and pathophysiology is currently undergoing intensive investigation. Activation of dorsal horn nociceptive neurons appears to be mediated, in part, by rapid excitatory effects produced by glutamate and aspartate, which act at N-methyl-D-aspartate (NMDA) receptor sites and other EAA receptor sites. Recent studies have implicated the NMDA receptor in several important pain-related phenomena, including (1) neuronal "wind-up" (progressive increase in the discharge of dorsal horn neurons following repetitive frequency activation of nociceptive affer-

Table 2–1. **PARTIAL LIST OF COMPOUNDS INVOLVED IN THE NEURAL CIRCUITRY OF THE DORSAL HORN OF THE SPINAL CORD***

	Primary Afferents	Intrinsic Neurons	Descending Fibers
Peptides			
Atrial natriuretic factor	+	−	+
Angiotensin II	+	NE	NE
Bombesin/gastrin-releasing peptide	+	+	NE
Brain natriuretic peptide	−	−	+
Cholecystokinin	+	+	+
Calcitonin gene-related peptide	+	−	−
Corticotropin-releasing factor	+	+	+
Endothelin	+	+	NE
Galanin	+	+	+
Growth hormone–releasing factor	+	NE	NE
Neuropeptide Y	+	+	+
Neurotensin	−	+	+
Oxytocin	+	−	+
Prodynorphin opioid peptides†	+	+	+
Proenkephalin opioid peptides†	+	+	+
Pro-opiomelanocortin peptides†	+	−	+
Somatostatin	+	+	+
Tachykinins‡	+	+	+
Thyrotropin-releasing hormone	−	+	+
Vasoactive intestinal peptide	+	+	NE
Vasopressin	+	+	+
Excitatory amino acids			
Aspartate	+	NE	+
Glutamate	+	NE	+
Inhibitory amino acids			
GABA	NE	+	NE
Glycine	NE	+	+
Monoamines			
Serotonin	NE	+	+
Norepinephrine	−	−	+
Epinephrine	−	−	+
Dopamine	NE	+	+
Histamine	−	−	+
Miscellaneous			
Acetylcholine	NE	+	+
Adenosine 5′-triphosphate	+	NE	NE

*All these compounds may be involved in nociception, although the amount of supporting evidence varies: + = present; − = absent; NE = not established.

†Numerous distinct compounds exist, which vary in distribution.

‡Among the several distinct compounds is substance P, which is widely regarded as an important primary afferent neurotransmitter involved in nociception.

ents),[19] (2) hyperexcitability of dorsal horn nociceptive neurons produced by high-intensity stimulation of small-diameter primary afferents,[213] and (3) hyperexcitability of nociceptive neurons caused by peripheral inflammation.[78]

NMDA receptor activation is mediated by nitric oxide (NO), the production of which is controlled by a specific enzyme, nitric oxide synthase. NMDA receptor antagonists and NO synthase antagonists reduce both the aforementioned pain-related experimental phenomena and nociceptive responses in animals. NMDA receptor antagonists are currently in clinical trials.

Two classes of cells in the dorsal horn receive input from nociceptive afferents. Nociceptive-specific neurons respond exclusively to noxious stimuli, whereas so-called wide-dynamic-range cells can be activated by both innocuous and noxious stimulation.[38,212] Both types of cells respond to noxious stimulation, many in a graded fashion to increasing intensity of the noxious stimulus.[111,144]

Wide-dynamic-range cells receive fine afferents from muscle and the viscera, as well as skin.[34,68] Virtually all visceral afferents converge upon neurons that also receive cutaneous input, an observation relevant to the phenomenon of referred pain. For example, high-intensity activation of cardiac sympathetic fibers excites spinothalamic tract neurons that also respond to stimulation applied to the inner aspect of the forearm, a common referral site for the pain of myocardial ischemia.[21] These observations support the hypothesis that at least some types of referred pain result from convergent input onto projection neurons from visceral and somatic structures (see following).

Dorsal Horn Processing

The dorsal horn and the homologous region in the trigeminal complex are processing structures in which primary afferent neurons, interneurons, and descending supraspinal systems interact to modulate incoming activity before relaying it to higher centers of the nervous system.[217] The pharmacology of these interacting systems is extraordinarily complex (see Table 2–1).

Dense opioid receptor binding occurs in the superficial layers of the dorsal horn, and both enkephalin terminals and enkephalinergic cells are found in this region, as well as in deeper laminae.[73] In the substantia gelatinosa, enkephalin is found in stalk and islet cells[73] and is presumably involved in local inhibitory circuits. Opioid mechanisms may underlie both presynaptic inhibition of the primary afferent nociceptor[216] and postsynaptic inhibition of transmission cells.[110,176] Presynaptic inhibition by dynorphin, which may originate either from a subpopulation of primary afferents or from interneurons, has also been proposed.[9]

Neurotensin may also be involved in local inhibitory circuits in the dorsal horn. This peptide, which originates exclusively in central nervous system neurons, is concentrated in the superficial dorsal horn.[53] Intrathecal neurotensin is antinociceptive in mice,[98] and there is evidence that this compound may excite interneurons that presynaptically inhibit the primary afferent nociceptor.[185]

Interneurons that contain γ-aminobutyric acid (GABA), a ubiquitous inhibitory neurotransmitter,[161] may also play a role in nociception, but studies of this compound have not been conclusive.[29,90,124] An antinociceptive role for GABA at the level of the dorsal horn is supported by the analgesic efficacy of intrathecal baclofen[210] and the prolonged inhibition of functionally identified nociceptive dorsal horn neurons produced by intravenous baclofen.[89] Baclofen is a ligand for one of the two identified subtypes of GABA receptor,[25] the GABA-B receptor. The GABA-B receptor is concentrated in superficial laminae of the dorsal horn[169] and, with the GABA-A receptor, has been localized on A-delta and C primary afferent fibers.[47] This localization suggests that GABA segmentally inhibits transmission of nociceptive input, perhaps presynaptically. GABA may also be involved in tonically active inhibitory circuits that prevent innocuous stimuli from activating nociceptive systems.

Descending pathways that terminate in the dorsal horn influence the transmission of incoming nociceptive activity. Multiple bulbospinal pathways contribute to the spinal processing of nociception. The best-characterized of these are serotonergic and noradrenergic, but a dopaminergic pathway is probably involved as well.[1,10,27,80] Descending peptidergic pathways have also been identified; these contain cholecystokinin, thyrotropin-releasing hormone, enkephalin, substance P, and oxytocin. Many of these putative neurotransmitters co-localize to the same terminals or cells of origin.[26]

Ascending Pathways

The segmental and suprasegmental connections that originate with the second-order nociceptive neurons in the dorsal horn are complex (Table 2–2).[211] Numerous ascending pathways interact with many brainstem sites and terminate in multiple thalamic nuclei.

The vast majority of spinothalamic tract neurons sends myelinated axons to the contralateral thalamus via the anterolateral quadrant of the spinal cord. The importance of this region in human nociception is evident from the observation that anterolateral cordotomy produces contralateral analgesia below the lesion.[187]

Clinical[154] and experimental[209] evidence supports a spinothalamic projection that ascends uncrossed in the spinal cord. In the lumbosacral enlargement of the monkey spinal cord, for example, 5 percent of the cells projecting to lateral thalamus and 10 percent of those terminating in medial thalamus are ipsilateral.[209] This ipsilateral projection may explain the observation that pain often returns after successful cordotomy.[44]

It is often assumed that the spinothalamic tract ascends for several segments before decussating. This conclusion is founded on the observation that the analgesia produced by cordotomy begins several segments below the level of the lesion. The anatomic correlate of this observation, however, has never been demonstrated in humans, and alternative explanations, such as rostral movement of the primary afferent itself before it synapses with projection cells, are also possible. Similarly, the common assumption that the spinothalamic tract divides into a lateral portion that transmits information about pain and temperature and a medial portion that subserves touch is also an unproven hypothesis, which is contradicted by the experimental demonstration of a heterogeneous distribution for fibers in this tract.[7,209]

Axons from spinothalamic tract cells terminate in both medial and lateral thalamus. Some branch and synapse in both regions and some send collaterals to brainstem structures en route.[71] These collaterals have been identified in both the periaqueductal gray and medullary reticular formation,[119,136] a potential anatomic substrate for the activation of endogenous brainstem pain-modulating systems by incoming nociceptive input (see following).

Other polysynaptic pathways originate from dorsal horn projection neurons and ultimately supply information to thalamic nuclei. Spinobulbar projections accompany spinothalamic fibers in the anterolateral quadrant. Most of these fibers terminate in the medullary reticular formation (spino-

Table 2–2. **SEGMENTAL AND SUPRASEGMENTAL NOCICEPTIVE OUTPUT FROM THE DORSAL HORN.***

Segmental	Direct interlaminar and intralaminar connections
	Connections to local interneurons
	Propriospinal connections
	Connections to the ventral horn
	Intersegmental connections
	Contralateral connections
Suprasegmental	To the thalamus
	To the brainstem reticular formation
	To other midbrain areas
	To lower brainstem and cervical cord

*Conceptually, the ascending pathways may be divided into a "neospinothalamic" tract that terminates in lateral thalamic nuclei and multiple "paleospinothalamic" tracts that terminate in medial thalamic structures.

reticular tract) or in the midbrain (spino-mesencephalic tract).[138] Many of the neurons of origin for these tracts are nociceptive,[141] and the brainstem regions to which they project are likely involved in pain transmission and modulation. As noted, these pathways may subserve the affective, motivational, and autonomic responses to pain, rather than the discriminative aspects.[139,168] They may also have an important role in the activation of endogenous pain-modulating systems.

Thalamus and Subcortical Nuclei in Nociception

In the primate, the spinothalamic tract terminates principally in four distinct nuclear regions: the ventrobasal complex; the posterior nuclei; parts of the intralaminar complex, chiefly the central lateral nucleus and adjacent portion of the medial dorsal nucleus; and the nucleus submedius.[24,137] Nociceptive-specific neurons and wide-dynamic-range neurons that respond to noxious stimuli have been identified in these nuclei.[32,77,100] Cells in the pontomedullary and mesencephalic reticular formation that receive input from nociceptive neurons in the dorsal horn project to many medial thalamic structures.[54,119] Some of these projections may also relay through the ventrobasal complex.[79]

The complex inflow to the thalamus from projection neurons in the spinal gray and trigeminal complex can be conceptualized as a laterally placed portion terminating primarily in the ventral posterior and posterior nuclear group, and a more medial portion terminating in medial thalamic structures. The former has been termed the "neospinothalamic" tract, and the latter, which comprises both a direct pathway and those neurons relayed through brainstem structures, has been termed the "paleospinothalamic" tracts. This division has been postulated to represent the anatomic substrate for the sensory-discriminative and affective-motivational aspects of the pain experience, respectively.[139]

Recent studies have also begun to elucidate a role for other subcortical nuclei in the processing of nociceptive information. For example, nociceptive neurons in the parabrachial area of the pons have been shown to project to regions of the amygdala.[15] The parabrachial area of the pons receives a dense projection from lamina I of the dorsal horn, and it has been postulated that this spino (trigemino) pontoamygdaloid tract may be involved in the affective and autonomic concomitants of pain perception.[16] Similarly, nociceptive projections have been identified from the spinal cord to the hypothalamus.

Cortical Involvement in Pain Transmission

The involvement of cortex in nociception was doubted by early investigators,[86] who noted the relative preservation of pain and temperature sensibility in patients with cerebral wounds. Pain sensation was often attributed to thalamic processing alone. This notion, however, cannot account for a number of clinical observations. For example, profound cutaneous analgesia can occasionally follow a traumatic lesion in the cortex.[131] Central pain has been observed after cortical lesions,[62] and pain can accompany electrical stimulation of exposed cortex[162] and focal seizures.[195] Finally, electrophysiologic studies have demonstrated both nociceptive-specific and wide-dynamic-range cortical neurons.[105]

NEUROPHYSIOLOGIC CHANGES UNDERLYING CLINICAL PAIN

The simplest way to account for the experience of acute and chronic pain is by persistent activation of the neural pathways that subserve acute nociception. Unfortunately, it is intuitively evident that this model fails to explain many types of acute pain and all those chronic pains driven primarily by pathophysiologic changes in the afferent pathways themselves or by psychologic factors. In addition, the extraordinary plasticity of the nervous system, which can be demonstrated experimentally after short-lived stimuli,[55] suggests that even those pains that can be directly related to persistent noxious stimuli may actually involve fundamental changes in the peripheral and central neural pathways subserving nociception. Moreover, these specific changes undoubtedly vary with the type of inciting event and other characteristics of the pain syndrome. These observations indicate that elucidation of the mechanisms involved in clinical pain states must extend beyond examination of the nociceptive system to the diverse phenomena that occur in response to prolonged injury. The process has begun,[57] but the information currently available is rudimentary.

Nociceptive Pain

The clinical inference that pain is "nociceptive" implies that ongoing activation of the nociceptive system is the predominating factor sustaining the pain (see Chapter 1). Processes associated with the inflammatory response are certainly involved in the pathogenesis of many types of acute and chronic nociceptive pain. Although the pain-related pathophysiology of acute inflammation has been the object of intense investigation during the past two decades, very little is known yet of the relationship between chronic pain and inflammation.

After a tissue-damaging stimulus, local vasodilatation and exudation of plasma occur. These phenomena are produced both by the action of local inflammatory cells and by antidromic stimulation of C polymodal nociceptors, which release substance P and other substances from peripheral nerve terminals.[205] The inflammatory response caused by a tissue-damaging stimulus is reduced by proximal nerve lesions or the administration of capsaicin,[88] suggesting that this neurogenic inflammation may be important even when evident tissue damage occurs.

Many endogenous substances involved in the inflammatory response, including serotonin, histamine, substance P, and bradykinin, are noxious when applied to the base of a blister in a human subject.[103] Pain can also be elicited in humans by intraperitoneal and intra-arterial injections of bradykinin[126] and by intra-arterial injections of substance P.[167] Direct activation of nociceptive afferents can be produced by the subcutaneous injection of inflammatory compounds, such as histamine, serotonin, bradykinin, acetylcholine, and potassium.[102] Prostaglandins, which are generated in regions of tissue injury through the metabolism of arachidonic acid, do not themselves activate nociceptors but produce lowered thresholds to noxious stimulation.[60,61,93]

Sensitization of nociceptors, which is clinically associated with hyperalgesia, can be induced by the direct and indirect actions of many substances released by injured tissue, inflammatory cells, and nerve endings. In addition to the prostaglandins, these substances include serotonin, adenosine, leukotrienes, bradykinin, norepinephrine, interleukin, and nerve growth factor.[120]

Chronic inflammation predominates as the major feature of the tissue-level changes that evolve after injury. As noted, it can be speculated that this process is involved in the development of chronic nociceptive pain, such as that accompanying arthritis. The mechanisms underlying the transition from acute to chronic inflammation, and the impact that this transition may have on nociception and pain, are poorly understood.

Neuropathic Pain

Inflammation may or may not play a role in sustaining so-called neuropathic pain. Injury to peripheral tissues (neural or nonneural) can induce aberrant somatosensory processing at varying levels of the nervous system. Presumably, neuropathic pain, or at least some types of neuropathic pain, occurs when these pathophysiologic changes become independent of the inciting event and sustain a chronic pain state.

The development of chronic neuropathic pain may involve any number of interacting pathophysiologic processes in the peripheral or central nervous system (Fig. 2–1).[48] Not surprisingly, the spectrum of neuropathic pain syndromes that may result is extremely large (see Chapter 5). On the basis of clinical observation, some of these syndromes are presumed to involve a predominating peripheral "generator" that sustains the pain, whereas others appear to depend on sympathetic efferent function (sympathetically maintained pain) or on a sustaining central mechanism.[166]

Complex neurophysiologic and neuroanatomic changes have been identified as potential mediators of neuropathic pains. For

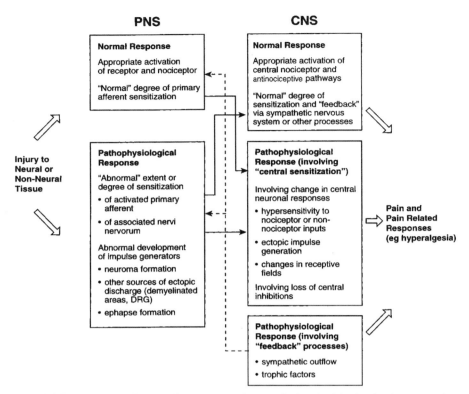

Figure 2–1. Model demonstrating the complex processes that may be involved in the development of neuropathic pain states. PNS = peripheral nervous system; CNS = central nervous system; DRG = dorsal root ganglion.

example, axonal injury results in changes that evolve during weeks to months. Multiple nerve sprouts from each axon grow during the first week. Those entering a nearby Schwann cell tube continue to grow toward the periphery, whereas others from the same axon disappear. Without a Schwann cell tube, however, these sprouting axons form a neuroma.[49] Thus, neuroma formation after injury may be minimal or profuse, depending on the degree of damage to supporting perineural structures. Small, so-called "neuromas-in-continuity" may also occur within damaged or grafted nerve if most but not all axons find the structures needed to guide growth.

Nerve sprouts from damaged axons generate spontaneous activity. This activity peaks in several weeks but thereafter continues at a lower level.[177,200] Unlike normal axons, neuromas are exquisitely sensitive to mechanical distortion,[177] which is clinically associated with tenderness and the appearance of a Tinel's sign. Chemical sensitivity is

also a feature,[200] and increased spontaneous activity may occur with ischemia, increased extracellular potassium concentration, or exposure to α-adrenergic agonists.[106]

After time, ephapses may develop between nerve sprouts in the region of damaged nerve, allowing the spread of impulses from one axon to another.[179] This "cross-talk" can also occur between demyelinated axons in the absence of sprouting or neuroma formation.[173] Activation of nociceptors via ephaptic transmission from sympathetic nerves or low-threshold afferents may also be important in some types of chronic neuropathic pain.

Ectopic discharges also occur in the dorsal root ganglia after damage to peripheral nerve,[199] and the concentration of neurotransmitters secreted by primary afferents diminishes in the dorsal horn.[8] After some time, transganglionic degeneration of central nerve terminals can occur.[45]

Peripheral nerve injury can produce dramatic changes in the response characteristics of central neurons.[213] For example, denervated dorsal horn neurons can develop expanded receptive fields[50] and become responsive to stimuli delivered near the deafferented region. These changes, combined with others, may be relevant to several important clinical phenomena, such as hyperalgesia and "spreading" pain or neurologic deficits.

The morphologic and biochemical changes associated with experimental dorsal rhizotomy are relevant to some types of neuropathic pain. Dorsal root fibers sprout from ganglia near the injured root,[97] and the activity of dorsal horn neurons increases.[6] This finding has been confirmed in the human spinal cord.[129]

Spontaneous epileptiform-like activity in the spinal cord, thalamus, and cortex may occur following injury to the peripheral or central nervous systems.[4,118,190,211,213] Presumably, this phenomenon relates to multiple potential mechanisms, which may involve central sensitization of neurons, loss of central inhibition, or abnormal "feedback" processes such as sympathetic or trophic responses[14] (see Fig. 2–1).

Mechanisms of Common Pain-Related Phenomena: Hyperalgesia and Referred Pain

The complexity of the peripheral and central neural processes described previously can be illustrated by the phenomena of hyperalgesia and referred pain. These phenomena provide useful examples of the types of relationships that may exist between neurophysiologic disturbances and clinical events.

Hyperalgesia following tissue injury has been divided into *primary* and *secondary* types.[123] Primary hyperalgesia occurs within the site of injury, and secondary hyperalgesia occurs in the region adjacent to it. Studies of primary hyperalgesia have demonstrated that it can be produced by multiple mechanisms, which may vary between hairy and nonhairy skin and between thermal and mechanical stimuli.[143,144]

Some studies have correlated sensitization of nociceptors and primary hyperalgesia.[193]

Any pain associated with tissue injury, therefore, may include hyperalgesia in the injured region that is due to nociceptor sensitization.

Secondary hyperalgesia in a region of skin adjacent to an injury is a poorly understood phenomenon, with psychophysical characteristics different from those of primary hyperalgesia. Recent studies suggest that both peripheral and central neural mechanisms are involved.[78,143,190,212,213]

Some types of neuropathic pain demonstrate hyperalgesia that may have mechanisms distinct from those associated with the hyperalgesia that follows injury to nonneural tissue. The peripheral processes may involve abnormal nociceptor sensitization, and the central processes may involve hyperexcitable neurons that are activated by nonnociceptive myelinated afferents or by nociceptors.[14,30] Hyperalgesia that follows central nervous system lesions is not understood but presumably involves central processes only.

Thus, the phenomenon of hyperalgesia, which can appear clinically similar in patients with different syndromes, may actually represent the end result of one or more distinct processes, the pathophysiology of which may reside predominantly in the periphery or in the central nervous system. Pain syndromes with identical phenomenology may or may not have mechanisms in common. This complexity complicates efforts to identify therapies that can be targeted to specific syndromes on the basis of pathophysiology.

The neural mechanisms underlying referred pain are similarly complex. Pain can be referred from a nociceptive focus in muscle, nerve, or viscera. Referred pain of any type may be accompanied by tenderness, which may be superficial or deep.

Referral sites for pain associated with damaged muscle have been evaluated experimentally in humans[104] and empirically by careful observation of patients with myofascial pain syndromes related to trigger points in muscle.[194] The pathophysiology of this referral is unknown. In an interesting observation that may be relevant to these processes, stimulation of motor fascicles of the median nerve at the wrist produced widespread referral of pain to multiple sites in the arm.[193] The latter finding suggests that primary peripheral nerve pathology may lead to pain that is experienced as if produced by a lesion deep in muscle. Referred pain associated with muscle injury can be accompanied by adjacent cutaneous hyperalgesia.

Referred pains associated with visceral lesions are highly variable. These pains can also be associated with cutaneous hyperalgesia, and trigger points or reflex spasm may occur in the muscles near the site of referred pain. Injection of these tender areas may change the pain experience. For example, patients with cardiac abnormalities whose angina was referred to the chest wall reported that injection of myalgic points changed the quality of the pain to a substernal aching more reminiscent of true anginal pain.[170]

As discussed previously, considerable evidence supports a "convergence-projection theory" of referred pain.[175] This theory proposes that noxious stimuli transmitted by one set of nociceptors can increase activity in central nervous system neurons that also receive input from another set of nociceptors, leading to misinterpretation by higher neural centers. Convergence of visceral and cutaneous afferents onto projection neurons in the dorsal horn has been confirmed experimentally.[21,148]

Referred pain may also be explained by branching of primary nociceptors, such that one neuron innervates both somatic and visceral structures. Such branching of sensory fibers in spinal nerves has been demonstrated,[113] and nociceptors have been identified with receptive fields in both skin and muscle.

NEURAL SUBSTRATE OF PAIN MODULATION

Presumably, the experience of acute or chronic pain represents a balance between afferent processes that subserve nociception and the activity in endogenous pain-modulating pathways. The observation that endogenous neural systems influence pain perception was developed by Melzack and Wall[140] into the heuristic "gate control" model, in which it was postulated that the activity of projection neurons in the dorsal horn of the spinal cord is modulated by both segmental and supraspinal influences. Although the details of this theory have been criticized[153] and the model refined in response,[198] the existence of multiple, anatomically distinct, segmental and suprasegmental systems subserving analgesia is now established.

Endorphins and Their Receptors

Elucidation of pain-modulating systems was spurred by the discovery of endogenous opioids (or endorphins) and their receptors two decades ago.[94,96,165,182,188] Endorphins comprise three groups of peptides, all of which are pharmacologically related to morphine (Table 2–3).[1,58] Each group originates from its own precursor molecule.

Peptides derived from the precursor molecule pro-opiomelanocortin are concentrated in the pituitary gland but also have been found in the brain, primarily the hypothalamus.[22] The amino acid sequence of the precursor contains within it sequences of a variety of active products, including adrenocorticotropic hormone, beta lipotropin, melanocyte-stimulating hormone, and beta endorphin. Specific peptidases cleave the various active compounds in concentrations that vary from tissue to tissue.

Proenkephalin contains the amino acid sequences of several active peptides, including met-enkephalin and leu-enkephalin.[76] The distribution of these peptides is extremely broad and includes structures at every level of the neuraxis, as well as adrenal medulla and gastrointestinal tract.[95]

The precursor molecule, prodynorphin, is parent to at least three peptides, all of which contain the sequence of leu-enkephalin, alpha and beta neoendorphin, dynorphin A, and dynorphin B. These compounds have been found in the gastrointestinal tract, posterior pituitary, and brain.[204]

Endogenous opioid compounds bind to specific receptors. Multiple receptor subtypes have been identified,[74] adding greatly to the complexity of these systems. Three types of receptors are generally believed to be involved in analgesia: mu, delta, and kappa.[1] Studies have demonstrated the existence of two subtypes of the mu receptor, two subtypes of the delta receptor, and at

Table 2–3. **ENDORPHINS AND THEIR PRECURSORS**

Precursor Molecule	Locations	Peptides
Pro-opiomelanocortin	Pituitary Hypothalamus	Beta endorphin Adrenocorticotropic hormone Beta lipotropin Melanocyte-stimulating hormone
Proenkephalin	Spinal cord Brain (multiple structures) Adrenal medulla Gastrointestinal tract	Met-enkephalin Leu-enkephalin
Prodynorphin	Spinal cord Brain (multiple structures) Pituitary Gastrointestinal tract	Dynorphin A Alpha and beta neoendorphin Leu-enkephalin

least three subtypes of the kappa receptor.[159,160] Of the endogenous opioids, the enkephalins are most active at mu and delta receptors and the dynorphins are most selective for kappa and mu sites.[1,36,159]

Activation of the different opioid receptor subtypes yields varying effects. For example, studies that have used irreversible blockade of the mu-1 receptor[159] have demonstrated that supraspinal analgesia and prolactin release are mediated by mu-1, whereas sedation, growth hormone release, and inhibition of gastrointestinal motility act through mu-2.

The delta receptor mediates enkephalin-induced antinociception and appears to be relatively selective for analgesic systems operating on a spinal level.[127] This finding has raised the possibility that specific delta agonists may be useful clinically in patients who are appropriate candidates for spinal administration of opioids.[151]

Activation of the kappa receptor by the compound ketocyclazocine produces miosis, depressed flexor reflex, and sedation in the spinal dog.[132] Kappa agonists do not alter pulse rate, temperature, or respiratory rate, or suppress the abstinence syndrome induced by the abrupt discontinuation of morphine in animals made physically dependent.[72] Many kappa-selective compounds produce agitation in animals, presaging the relatively high incidence of psychotomimetic effects associated with the clinical use of the currently available kappa agonist drugs (see Chapter 11).

Function of the Endorphins

The widespread distribution of the endorphins, their prominent role in antinociception, and their close association with systems known to regulate homeostasis and response to stress indicate that these substances have multiple functions linked to basic survival mechanisms.[92,146] The affective and motivational changes that can be induced by the exogenous opioids also suggest that the endorphins play a role in emotion and higher integrative functions.[142]

Endorphins are clearly important in analgesia. Enkephalin and beta endorphin are analgesic in both animals and humans,[151] and inhibitors of the enzymes that degrade enkephalin have been shown to be antinociceptive in animal models.[174] A role for the endorphins in the mediation of some types of clinical pain is suggested by the observation that naloxone, the specific opioid antagonist, can produce hyperalgesia in postoperative patients[121] and reverse the analgesia provided by some forms of transcutaneous nerve stimulation.[35]

Mechanisms of Endorphin Analgesia

The discovery of stimulation-produced analgesia in animals began to clarify some of the mechanisms involved in the endogenous, opioid-mediated analgesia system.

Electrical stimulation of specific sites in the thalamus, hypothalamus, midbrain, and medulla causes a dramatic reduction in the nociceptive responses of animals.[31,136] This analgesia can be reversed by naloxone[3] and duplicated by microinjection of morphine in the same loci.[70,155] In some cases, animals rendered analgesic through brain stimulation are cross-tolerant to systemic morphine.[133] These observations provide strong evidence that the sites involved in stimulation-produced analgesia also mediate endorphinergic systems.

The best-characterized endorphinergic pain-modulatory system links the midbrain periaqueductal gray matter, the rostroventral medulla, and the trigeminal nucleus caudalis or spinal dorsal horn.[10] Endogenous opioids and opioid receptors are found in all of these regions. Stimulation or microinjection of morphine in the periaqueductal gray produces profound behavioral analgesia in animals.[3,219] This region receives descending afferents from the hypothalamus, frontal and insular cortex, and amygdala; it receives ascending afferents from medullary nuclei, including the locus coeruleus, and sites in the pontomedullary reticular formation.[13]

The outflow from the periaqueductal gray includes an important excitatory connection to the rostral ventromedial medulla,[12,155] with which it is reciprocally connected. Activation of the rostroventral medulla inhibits dorsal horn neurons and produces analgesia in animals.[63,64] A lesion in this region blocks the inhibitory effect on spinal cord neurons of stimulation in the periaqueductal gray[12] and diminishes the analgesic effect of systemic morphine.[218] Thus, the rostroventral medulla appears to be a relay for descending antinociceptive activity, which originates in the periaqueductal gray and exerts its effects by inhibiting transmission neurons in the dorsal horn and trigeminal nucleus caudalis.

Axons from the rostroventral medulla travel through the dorsolateral funiculus of the spinal cord. A lesion in this pathway reduces the effects both of analgesia produced by stimulation of rostral sites and of systemic morphine.[11] The latter observation indicates that the action of systemic morphine probably depends on activation of both supraspinal descending pathways that traverse the dorsolateral funiculus and local enkephalinergic inhibitory systems in the dorsal horns.[220]

Other Pain Modulating Systems

A variety of other established and putative neurotransmitters are involved in endogenous pain-modulating pathways[56] (see Table 2–1). The biogenic amines—serotonin and norepinephrine, for example—appear to play an important role in the function of the endorphinergic system described previously. Depletion of serotonin blocks the analgesic effect of systemic opioids, and both serotonin depletion and administration of serotonin antagonists reduce the analgesia produced by brain stimulation or microinjection of morphine into brainstem sites.[2,81,214] These observations suggest that both endogenous and exogenous opioids increase the activity in a pathway descending from the periaqueductal gray to the rostroventral medulla, which in turn activates a descending serotonergic pathway that terminates in the dorsal horn. The precise mechanisms by which these opioid neurons interact with these other pathways are unknown, but recent studies suggest that a combination of actions in so-called "on" cells and "off" cells is involved.[65] In the spinal cord itself, there is both indirect and direct evidence that the release of serotonin activates local enkephalinergic interneurons, which in turn inhibit pain transmission neurons.[156]

Iontophoretic application of norepinephrine reduces the firing of nociceptive neurons in the dorsal horn.[87] Intrathecal administration of an α-adrenergic antagonist, phentolamine, reduces the antinociception produced by activation of periaqueductal gray neurons,[214] and this effect is additive to that produced by a serotonin blocker. The latter observation indicates that independent descending pain-modulating systems are mediated by the biogenic amines.[101] Activation of these pathways is probably the salient analgesic mechanism of some adjuvant analgesics, such as tricyclic antidepressants (see Chapter 10).

A large number of other putative transmitters have been implicated in pain modulation (see Table 2–1). In addition to its local segmental effects (see previously), neurotensin may have antinociceptive actions at rostral levels of the nervous system. For example, neurotensin administration into the ventricles or cisterns produces analgesia in animals,[41] an effect that appears to be independent of the endorphins. In one study, this effect was mitigated by thyrotropin-releasing hormone,[157] suggesting a role for the latter peptide in antinociception. Other studies have linked central cholinergic pathways[20,83] and GABAergic pathways[29,90,210] to nociceptive processing. Systemic or intrathecal cholecystokinin attenuates morphine analgesia,[59] and the cholecystokinin antagonist proglumide potentiates the effects of morphine and the analgesia produced by either endorphin administration or stress.[201–203] Other evidence supports a role for vasopressin,[17] prolactin,[172] and histamine.[23] Vasoactive intestinal peptide, oxytocin, and somatostatin have also been identified within neurons that are suspected to be important in pain-modulating systems,[56] and clinical reports suggest that somatostatin and calcitonin are analgesic in humans[69,145] (see Chapter 10).

ACTIVATION OF PAIN-MODULATING SYSTEMS

The identification of multiple endogenous pain-modulating systems has been accomplished using experimental techniques, such as microinjection of drugs and single-cell recording, that are far removed from the physiologic functioning of the systems under study. Relatively little is known about the complex and dynamic factors that mediate these processes in the clinical setting. In addition to analgesic drugs, which presumably operate via activation of endogenous pain-modulating systems, many other events may be involved in the moment-to-moment functioning of endogenous analgesia.[135] For example, stimulation of afferent neural pathways can also activate pain-modulating pathways. Physiologically, this mechanism is probably involved in the salutary effects of rubbing an injured limb, massaging a strained muscle, or stroking the abdominal wall to alleviate visceral pain. The most notable therapeutic outgrowth has been the development of transcutaneous electrical nerve stimulation (TENS). Other so-called neurostimulatory techniques comprise acupuncture, percutaneous nerve stimulation, dorsal column stimulation, and deep brain stimulation.

The specific mechanisms and neurochemical substrates of the endogenous analgesia systems activated by afferent stimulation are unknown. Activation of an endogenous analgesia system by peripheral stimulation may occur at one or more of three levels: peripheral, spinal (segmental), and supraspinal. Peripheral stimulation can produce both transient slowing of conduction velocity in the nerve or diminished response to subsequent stimuli,[99] although the importance of this effect in routine TENS is questionable.

At a spinal level, peripheral stimulation is believed to activate segmental inhibitory processes, as conceptualized by the gate control theory.[140] Inhibition of dorsal horn cells has been demonstrated following electrical stimulation of skin within their receptive fields, peripheral afferents with input to these cells, or dorsal columns.[82] Moreover, peripheral stimulation at low frequency (e.g., acupuncture or so-called acupuncture-like TENS) has been demonstrated to involve mediation by endorphins, a mechanism different from high-frequency stimulation.[134] The involvement of supraspinal mechanisms in the analgesia produced by peripheral stimulation is suggested by the inhibition of antinociceptive stimulation in animals by systemic, but not intrathecal, administration of serotonin depletors[37] and the loss of this effect with spinal cord transection.[181]

A supraspinal mechanism is also responsible for the analgesia that can occur after noxious cutaneous stimulation. Nociceptive dorsal horn and trigeminal neurons can be inhibited by a painful stimulus applied to an unrelated region of the body, a phenomenon termed *diffuse noxious inhibitory control*.[51,114–116] This inhibition is eliminated by spinal cord transection, confirming its supraspinal origin, and is believed to involve both a serotonergic and enkephalinergic mechanism.[52,114–116] A similar phenomenon has been confirmed in humans.[208] These data suggest that endogenous analgesic pathways may function physiologically to mitigate the effects of an incoming nociceptive barrage in what is essentially a negative feedback loop.

Diffuse noxious inhibitory controls are related to the broader paradigm of stress-induced analgesia. A variety of environmental stressors are capable of producing potent analgesia in animals.[85] Some of the effective stressors yield an analgesia that is reversible with naloxone, whereas others presumably activate nonendorphinergic pain-modulating systems.[85,135] A naloxone-reversible, stress-induced experimental analgesia has also been demonstrated in humans.[207]

The multiplicity of pain-modulating systems and the variety of stimuli sufficient to activate one or more suggest that these systems serve important physiologic functions. Data in humans are meager, however, and the basal activity of these systems (i.e., ongoing activity during the pain-free condition) and their role in clinical pain remain poorly understood. The inability to alter experimental pain thresholds by the administration of naloxone suggests that the tonic activation of the endorphinergic systems is not great.[75] Individual differences may be important, however[122]; for example, a naloxone-induced change in pain thresholds has been demonstrated in a group of subjects with relatively high baseline thresholds.[197] The basal functioning of the nonopioid pain-modulating systems in pain-free states is entirely unknown.

The experimental demonstration of diffuse noxious inhibitory controls in humans[208] suggests the involvement of endogenous pain-modulating systems in the experience of pain associated with acute injury. Other evidence is provided by the inverse relationship between endorphin in cerebrospinal fluid (CSF) and pain in patients undergoing myelography for presumed discogenic disease,[39] the relatively low levels of CSF endorphin among postoperative patients,[171] and the inverse relationship between preoperative CSF endorphin and postoperative meperidine levels achieved by on-demand analgesia.[186]

The function of the endogenous pain-modulating systems in chronic pain states is least understood of all. CSF endorphin has been reported to be lower in patients with neuropathic pain than in those with painless organic disease,[189] and patients with organic pain have been found to have lower CSF endorphin than those with psychogenic pain.[5] A group of patients with chronic pain had CSF endorphin concentration intermediate between normal controls and the very low levels measured in a group of postoperative patients.[171] These observations suggest that

the endorphinergic pain-modulating systems may be involved in at least some types of chronic pain states in humans. The specific mechanisms are unknown, as are the effects produced by other antinociceptive systems in clinical disorders.

SUMMARY

During the past three decades, knowledge of normal systems of nociception and pain modulation has increased rapidly. Studies have also begun to elucidate the pathologic changes in these systems that could be responsible for chronic pain states in humans.

Nociceptors, which comprise a variety of lightly myelinated and unmyelinated primary afferent neurons, innervate virtually all peripheral tissues. Although these neurons have varying response characteristics, all signal a response to a potentially tissue-damaging stimulus. The central processes of these neurons synapse on second-order neurons in the dorsal horn of the spinal cord, which is a site of complex nociceptive processing. The complex neurochemistry of this region involves neurotransmitters and neuromodulators that originate from the primary afferent (such as substance P and the excitatory amino acids), interneurons (such as neurotensin), and descending pathways (such as serotonin and norepinephrine).

Multiple ascending nociceptive pathways include a direct spinothalamic pathway and multiple polysynaptic pathways that interact with brainstem sites and other regions, such as the amygdala. Nociceptive processing occurs in both medial and lateral thalamic nuclei and the cortex. The areas of the brain that receive this input may account for the conscious perception of the discriminative aspects of the pain and the affective, motivational, and autonomic changes that accompany it.

Endorphinergic and nonendorphinergic pain-modulating systems interact in segmental and suprasegmental systems. The endorphins, which comprise multiple peptides that are cleaved from one of three distinct precursor molecules, are found at all levels of the neuraxis and interact with three major types of receptors, each of which has distinct subtypes. The best-characterized nonendorphinergic systems descend from the lower brainstem and use monoamines (both serotonin and norepinephrine) as neurotransmitters. Many other neurotransmitters are involved in these systems. The functioning of these systems in healthy individuals and in those with acute or chronic pain is poorly understood.

Some types of acute and chronic pain may occur as a result of ongoing activation of the intact nociceptive system and others involve pathologic changes in these systems. Presumably, a process like chronic inflammation could sustain activity in intact nociceptors or lead to enhanced activity through processes that sensitize these neurons and their central connections. Although numerous processes induced by nerve injury could potentially be involved in the development of other types of chronic pain, little is known about the mechanisms involved.

REFERENCES

1. Akil H, and Lewis JW (eds): Neurotransmitters and Pain Control. Karger, Basel, 1987.
2. Akil H, and Liebeskind JC: Monoaminergic mechanisms of stimulation-produced analgesia. Brain Res 94:279–296, 1975.
3. Akil H, Mayer D, and Liebeskind JC: Antagonism of stimulation-produced analgesia by naloxone, a narcotic antagonist. Science 191:961–962, 1976.
4. Albe-Fessard D, and Lombard MC: Use of an animal model to evaluate the origin of and protection against deafferentation pain. In Bonica JJ, Lindblom U, and Iggo A (eds): Advances in Pain Research and Therapy, Vol 5. Raven Press, New York, 1983, pp 691–700.
5. Almay BGL, Johansson F, Von Knorring L, et al: Endorphins in chronic pain. I. Differences in CSF endorphin levels between organic and psychogenic pain syndromes. Pain 5:153–162, 1978.
6. Anderson LS, Black RG, Abraham J, et al: Neuronal hyperactivity in experimental trigeminal deafferentation. J Neurosurg 35:444–452, 1971.
7. Applebaum AE, Leonard RB, Kenshalo DR, et al: Nuclei in which functionally identified spinothalmic tract neurons terminate. J Comp Neurol 188:575–687, 1979.
8. Barbut DP, Polak JM, and Wall PD: Substance P in spinal cord dorsal horn decreases following peripheral nerve injury. Brain Res 205:289–298, 1981.
9. Basbaum AI: Functional analysis of the cytochemistry of the spinal dorsal horn. In Fields HL, Dubner R, and Cervero F (eds): Advances in Pain Research and Therapy, Vol 9. Raven Press, New York, 1985, pp 149–175.
10. Basbaum AI, and Fields HL: Endogenous pain control systems: Brainstem spinal pathways and endorphin circuitry. Annu Rev Neurosci 7:309–338, 1984.
11. Basbaum AI, Marley NJE, O'Keefe J, et al: Reversal of morphine and stimulus-produced analgesia by subtotal spinal cord lesions. Pain 3:43–56, 1977.
12. Behbehani MM, and Fields HL: Evidence that an excitatory connection between the periaqueductal gray and nucleus raphe magnus mediates stimulation produced analgesia. Brain Res 170:85–93, 1979.
13. Beitz AJ: The organization of afferent projections to the midbrain periaqueductal grey of the rat. Neuroscience 7:133–159, 1982.
14. Bennett GJ: Neuropathic pain. In Wall PD, Melzack R (eds): Textbook of Pain, ed 3. Churchill Livingstone, Edinburgh, 1994, pp 201–224.
15. Bernard JF, Alden M, and Besson J-M: The organization of the efferent projections from the pontine parabrachial area to the amygdaloid complex: A phaseolus vulgaris leukoagglutin (PHA-L) study in the rat. J Comp Neurol 329:201–229, 1993.
16. Bernard JF, and Besson J-M: The spino (trigemino)-pontoamygdaloid pathway: Electrophysiological evidence for involvement in pain processes. J Neurophysiol 63:473–490, 1990.
17. Berson BS, Berntson GG, Zipf W, et al: Vasopressin-induced antinociception: An investigation into its physiological and hormonal basis. Endocrinology 113:337–343, 1983.
18. Bessou P, and Perl ER: Response of cutaneous sensory units with unmyelinated fibers to noxious stimuli. J Neurophysiol 32:1025–1043, 1969.
19. Beuerman RW, and Tenelian DL: Corneal pain evoked by thermal stimulation. Pain 7:1–14, 1979.
20. Bhargava HN, and Way EL: Acetylcholinesterase inhibition and morphine effects in morphine tolerant and dependent mice. J Pharmacol Exp Ther 183:31–40, 1972.
21. Blair RW, Weber RN, and Foreman RD: Characteristics of primate spinothalamic tract neurons receiving viscerosomatic convergent inputs in the T3–T5 segments. J Neurophysiol 46:797–811, 1981.
22. Bloom FE, Battenberg E, and Rossier JEA: Endorphins are located in the intermediate and anterior lobes of the pituitary gland, not in the neurophysiophysis. Life Sci 20:43–48, 1977.
23. Bluhm R, Zsigmond EK, and Winnie AP: Potentiation of opioid analgesia by H, and H2 antagonists. Life Sci 31:1229–1232, 1982.
24. Boivie J: An anatomical reinvestigation of the termination of the spinothalamic tract in the monkey. J Comp Neurol 186:343–370, 1979.
25. Bowery NG: Baclofen—10 years on. Trends Pharmacol Sci 3:400–403, 1982.
26. Bowker RM, Steinbusch HWM, and Coulter JD: Serotonergic and peptidergic projections to the spinal cord demonstrated by a combined retrograde HRP histochemical and immunocytochemical staining method. Brain Res 211:412–417, 1981.
27. Bowker RM, Westlund KN, Sullivan MC, et al: Organization of descending serotonergic projections to the spinal cord. Prog Brain Res 57:239–265, 1982.
28. Brown AM: Excitation of afferent cardiac sympathetic nerve fibers during myocardial ischemia. J Physiol (Lond) 190:35–53, 1967.
29. Buckett WR: Induction of analgesia and morphine potentiation by irreversible inhibitors of GABA-transaminase. Br J Pharmacol 68:129–130, 1980.
30. Campbell JN, Raja SN, Meyer RA, et al: Myelinated afferents signal the hyperalgesia associated with nerve injury. Pain 32:89–94, 1988.

31. Carr KD, and Uysal S: Evidence of a supraspinal opioid analgesic mechanism engaged by lateral hypothalamic electrical stimulation. Brain Res 335:55–62, 1985.

32. Casey KL, and Morrow TJ: Ventral posterior thalamic neurons differentially responsive to noxious stimulation of the awake monkey. Science 221:675–677, 1983.

33. Cervero F: Afferent activity evoked by natural stimulation of the biliary system in the ferret. Pain 13:137–151, 1982.

34. Cervero F: Sensory innervation of the viscera: Peripheral basis of visceral pain. Physiol Rev 74:95–138, 1994.

35. Chapman RN, and Benedetti I: Analgesia following transcutaneous electrical stimulation and its partial reversal by a narcotic antagonist. Life Sci 21:1645–1648, 1977.

36. Chavkin C, James IF, and Goldstein A: Dynorphin is a specific endogenous ligand of the kappa opioid receptor. Science 215:413–415, 1982.

37. Cheng RSS, and Pomeranz B: Electroacupuncture analgesia could be mediated by at least two pain-relieving mechanisms: Endorphin and non-endorphin systems. Life Sci 25:1957–1962, 1979.

38. Christenson BN, and Perl ER: Spinal neurons specifically excited by noxious or thermal stimuli: Marginal zone of the dorsal horn. J Neurophysiol 33: 293–307, 1970.

39. Cleeland CS, Shacham S, Dahl JL, et al: CSF β-endorphin and the severity of pain. Neurology 34: 378–380, 1984.

40. Clifton GL, Coggeshall RE, Vance WH, et al: Receptive fields of unmyelinated ventral root afferent fibers in the cat. J Physiol (Lond) 256:573–600, 1976.

41. Clineschmidt BV, and McGuffin JC: Neurotensin administered intracisternally inhibits responsiveness of mice to noxious stimuli. Eur J Pharmacol 46:395–396, 1977.

42. Coggeshall RE: Afferent fibers in the ventral root. Neurosurgery 4:443–448, 1979.

43. Coggeshall RE, Hong RAP, Langford LA, et al: Discharge characteristics of five medial articular afferents at rest and during passive moments of inflamed knee joints. Brain Res 272:185–188, 1983.

44. Cowie RA, and Hitchcock ER: The late results of anterolateral cordotomy for pain relief. Acta Neurochir (Wien) 64:39–50, 1982.

45. Csillik N, and Knyihar E: Biodynamic plasticity in the rolando substance. Prog Neurobiol 10:203–230, 1978.

46. Dahlsgard CJ, Vincent S, Hokfelt T, et al: Immunohistochemical evidence for coexistence of cholecystokinin and substance P-like peptides in primary sensory neurons. Neurosci Abstr 8:474, 1982.

47. Desarmenien M, Feltz PO, Occhipinti GSF, et al: Coexistence of GABA A and GABA B receptors on A and C primary afferents. Br J Pharmacol 81:327–333, 1984.

48. Devor M: Mechanisms of neuropathic pain following peripheral injury. In Basbaum A, and Besson J-M (eds): Towards a New Pharmacotherapy of Pain. John Wiley & Sons, Chichester, 1991, pp 417–440.

49. Devor M, and Govrin-Lippmann R: Selective regeneration of sensory fibers following nerve crush injury. Exp Neurol 65:300–315, 1979.

50. Devor M, and Wall PD: Effect of peripheral nerve injury on the receptive fields of cells in the cat's spinal cord. J Comp Neurol 199:277–291, 1981.

51. Dickenson AH, LeBars D, and Besson JM: Diffuse noxious inhibitory controls (DNIC). Effects of trigeminal nucleus caudalis neurons in the rat. Brain Res 200:293–301, 1980.

52. Dickenson AH, LeBars D, and Besson JM: Diffuse noxious inhibitory controls (DNIC) in the rat with or without P-CPA pretreatment. Brain Res 216:313–321, 1981.

53. Difiglia MAN, and Leeman SE: Ultrastructural localization of immunoreactive neurotensin in the monkey superficial dorsal horn. J Comp Neurol 225:1–13, 1984.

54. Dostrovsky JO, and Guilbaud G: Nociceptive responses in the medial thalamus of the normal and arthritic rat. Pain 40:93–104, 1990.

55. Dubner R: Neuronal plasticity and pain following peripheral tissue inflammation or nerve injury. In Bond MR, Charlton JE, Woolf CJ (eds): Proceedings of the VIth World Congress on Pain. Elsevier, Amsterdam, 1991, pp 263–276.

56. Duggan AW, and Weihe E: Central transmission of impulses in nociceptors: Events in the superficial dorsal horn. In Basbaum AI, and Besson J-M (eds): Toward a New Pharmacotherapy of Pain. John Wiley and Sons, Chichester, 1991, pp 35–67.

57. Elliott K: Taxonomy and mechanisms of neuropathic pain. Semin Neurol 14:195–205, 1994.

58. Evans CJ, Hammond DL, and Fredrickson RCA: The opioid peptides. In Pasternak GW (ed): The Opiate Receptors. Humana Press, Clifton, NJ, 1988, pp 23–71.

59. Farris PL, Komisaruk BR, Watkins LR, et al: Evidence for the neuropeptide cholecystokinin as an antagonist of opiate analgesia. Science 219:310–312, 1983.

60. Ferreira SH: Prostaglandin, aspirin-like drugs and analgesia. Nature 240:200–203, 1972.

61. Ferreira SH, Corenzetti BB, and Correa FMA: Central and peripheral antialgesic action of aspirin-like drugs. Eur J Pharmacol 53:29–48, 1978.

62. Fields HL, and Adams JE: Pain after cortical injury relieved by electrical stimulation of the internal capsule. Brain 97:169–178, 1974.

63. Fields HL, Basbaum AI, Clanton CH, et al: Nucleus raphe magnus inhibition of spinal cord dorsal horn neurons. Brain Res 126:441–453, 1977.

64. Fields HL, Clanton CH, and Anderson SD: Somatosensory properties of spinoreticular neurons in the cat. Brain Res 120:49–66, 1977.

65. Fields HL, Heinricher MM, and Mason P: Neurotransmitters in nociceptive modulatory circuits. Annu Rev Neurosci 14:219–245, 1991.

66. Fitzgerald M, and Lynn B: The sensitization of high threshold mechanoreceptors with myelinated axons by repeated heating. J Physiol (Lond) 365:549–563, 1977.

67. Floyd K, and Lawrenson G: Mechanosensitive afferents in the cat's pelvic nerve. J Physiol (Lond) 290: 51–52, 1979.

68. Foreman RD, Schmidt RF, and Willis WD: Effects of mechanical and chemical stimulation of fine muscle afferents upon primate spinothalamic tract cells. J Physiol (Lond) 286:215–231, 1979.

69. Fraioli F, Fabbri A, Gnessi L, et al: Calcitonin and analgesia. In Benedetti C, Chapman CR, and Moricca G (eds): Advances in Pain Research and Therapy, Vol 7. Raven Press, New York, 1984, pp 237–250.

70. Gebhart GF, Sandkuhler J, and Thalhammer ZM: Inhibition in spinal cord of nociceptive information by electrical stimulation and morphine microinjection at identical sets in midbrain of the cat. J Neurophysiol 51:75–89, 1984.

71. Giesler GJ, Yezierski RP, Gerhart KD, et al: Spinothalamic tract neurons that project to medial and/or lateral thalamic nuclei: Evidence for a physiologically novel population of spinal cord neurons. J Neurophysiol 46:1285–1308, 1981.

72. Gilbert PE, and Martin WR: The effects of morphine and nalorphine-like drugs in the non-dependent, morphine-dependent, and cyclazocine-dependent chronic spinal dog. J Pharmacol Exp Ther 198:66–82, 1976.

73. Glazer EJ, and Basbaum AI: Immunohistochemical localization of leucine-enkephalin in the spinal cord of the cat: Enkephalin-containing marginal neurons and pain modulation. J Comp Neurol 196:377–389, 1981.

74. Goodman RR, and Pasternak GW: Multiple opiate receptors. In Kuhar M, and Pasternak G (eds): Analgesics: Neurochemical, Behavioral and Clinical Perspectives. Raven Press, New York, 1984, pp 67–96.

75. Grevert P, and Goldstein A: Endorphins: Naloxone fails to alter experimental pain or mood in humans. Science 199:1093–1095, 1978.

76. Gubler U, Kilpatrick DL, Seeburg PH, et al: Detection and partial characteristics of proenkephalin mRNA. Proc Natl Acad Sci USA 78:5484–5487, 1981.

77. Guilbaud G, Calice D, Besson JM, et al: Single unit activities in ventral posterior and posterior group thalamic nuclei during nociceptive and non-nociceptive stimulations in the cat. Arch Ital Biol 115:38–58, 1977.

78. Haley JE, Sullivan AF, and Dickenson AH: Evidence for spinal N-methyl-D-aspartate receptor involvement in prolonged chemical nociception in the rat. Brain Res 518:218–226, 1990.

79. Hamilton BL: Projections of the nuclei of the periaqueductal gray matter in the cat. J Comp Neurol 152:45–58, 1973.

80. Hammond DL: Control systems for afferent nociceptive processing: The descending inhibitory pathways. In Yaksh TL (ed): Functional Organization of Spinal Afferent Processing. Plenum Press, New York, 1985, pp 363–390.

81. Hammond DL, and Yaksh TL: Antagonism of stimulation-produced antinociception by intrathecal administration of methysergide or phentolamine. Brain Res 298:329–337, 1984.

82. Handwerker HO, Iggo A, and Zimmermann M: Segmental and suprasegmental action on dorsal horn neurons responding to noxious and non-noxious skin stimuli. Pain 1:147–165, 1975.

83. Harris LS, Dewey WL, Howes JF, et al: Narcotic-antagonist analgesics: Interactions with cholinergic systems. J Pharmacol Exp Ther 169:17–22, 1969.

84. Hayes AG, and Tyers MB: Effects of capsaicin on nociceptive heat, pressure and chemical thresholds and on substance P levels in the rat. Brain Res 189:561–564, 1980.

85. Hayes RL, Bennett GJ, Newlon PG, et al: Behavioral and physiological studies of non-narcotic analgesia in the rat elicited by certain environmental stimuli. Brain Res 155:69–90, 1978.

86. Head H, and Holmes G: Sensory disturbances from cerebral lesions. Brain 34:102–254, 1911.

87. Headley PM, Duggan AW, and Griersmith BT: Selective reduction by noradrenaline and 5-hydroxytryptamine of nociceptive responses of cat dorsal horn neurons. Brain Res 145:185–189, 1978.

88. Helme RD, and Andrews PV: The effect of nerve lesions on the inflammatory response to injury. J Neurosci Res 13:453–459, 1985.

89. Henry JL: Pharmacological studies on the prolonged depressant effects of baclofen on lumbar dorsal horn units in the cat. Neuropharmacology 21:1085–1093, 1982.

90. Hill RC, Mauer R, Buescher HH, et al: Analgesic properties of the GABA-mimetic THIP. Eur J Pharmacol 69:221–224, 1981.

91. Hokfelt T, Johansson O, Ljungdahl A, et al: Peptidergic neurons. Nature 284:515–521, 1980.

92. Holaday JW: Cardiovascular effects of endogenous opiate systems. Annu Rev Pharm Toxicol 23:541–594, 1983.

93. Horton EW: Action of prostaglandin E1 on tissues which respond to bradykinin. Nature 200:892–893, 1963.

94. Hughes J: Isolation of endogenous compound from the brain with pharmacological properties similar to morphine. Brain Res 88:295–308, 1975.

95. Hughes J, Kosterlitz HW, and Smith TW: The distribution of methionine-enkephalin and leucine-enkephaline in the brain and peripheral tissues. Br J Pharm 61:639–647, 1977.

96. Hughes J, Smith TW, Kosterlitz HW, et al: Identification of two related pentapeptides from the brain with potent opiate agonist activity. Nature 258:577–579, 1975.

97. Hulsebosch CE, and Coggeshall RE: Sprouting unmyelinated dorsal root axons in response to spinal or dorsal root injury. In Bonica JJ, Lindblom U, and Iggo A (eds): Advances in Pain Research and Therapy, Vol 5. Raven Press, New York, 1983, pp 125–129.

98. Hylden JLK, and Wilcox GL: Antinociceptive action of intrathecal neurotensin in mice. Peptides 4:517–520, 1983.

99. Ignelzi RJ, and Nquisi JK: Excitability changes in periphreal nerve fibers after repetitive electrical stimulation. J Neurosurg 51:824–833, 1979.

100. Ishijima B, Yoshimasu N, Fukushima T, et al: Nociceptive neurons in human thalamus. Confinia Neurol 37:99–106, 1975.

101. Jensen TS, and Yaksh TL: Effects of an intrathecal dopamine agonist, apomorphine, on thermal and chemical evoked noxious responses in rats. Brain Res 296:285–293, 1984.

102. Juan H, and Lembeck F: Action of peptides and other algesic agents on paravascular pain receptors of the isolated perfused rabbit ear. Naunyn Schmiedebergs Arch Exp Pathol Pharmakol 283:151–164, 1974.

103. Keele CA, and Armstrong D: Substances Producing Pain and Itch. Edward Arnold, London, 1964.

104. Kellgren JH: Observations on referred pain arising from muscle. Clin Sci 3:175–190, 1937.

105. Kenshalo DR, and Isensee O: Responses of primate SI cortical neurons to noxious stimuli. J Neurophysiol 50:1479–1496, 1983.

106. Korenman EMD, and Devor M: Ectopic adrenergic sensitivity in damaged peripheral nerve axons in the rat. Exp Neurol 72:63–81, 1981.

107. Kress M, Koltzenburg M, Reeh PW, et al: Responsiveness and functional attributes of electrically localized terminals of cutaneous C-fibres in vivo and in vitro. J Neurol 68:581–595, 1992.

108. Kumazawa T, and Mizumura K: Thin-fiber receptors responding to mechanical, chemical, and thermal stimulation in the skeletal muscle of the dog. J Physiol (Lond) 273:179–194, 1977.

109. Kumazawa T, and Mizumura K: Mechanical and thermal responses of polymodal receptors recorded from the superior spermatic nerve of dogs. J Physiol (Lond) 299:233–245, 1980.

110. LaMotte CC, and deLanerolle NC: Human spinal neurons: Innervation by both substance P and enkephalin. Neuroscience 6:713–723, 1981.

111. LaMotte RH, and Campbell JN: Comparison of responses of warm and nociceptive C fiber afferents in monkey with human judgements of thermal pain. J Neurophysiol 41:409–528, 1978.

112. LaMotte RH, and Thalhamamer JG: Response properties of high threshold cutaneous cold receptors in the primate. Brain Res 244:279–287, 1982.

113. Langford LA, and Coggeshall RE: Branching of sensory axons in the peripheral nerve of the rat. J Comp Neurol 203:745–750, 1981.

114. LeBars D, Chitour D, Kraus E, et al: Effect of naloxone upon diffuse noxious inhibitory controls (DNIC) in the rat. Brain Res 204:387–402, 1981.

115. LeBars D, Dickenson AH, and Besson JM: Diffuse noxious inhibitory controls (DNIC) I. Effects on dorsal horn convergent neurones in the rat. Pain 6:282–304, 1979.

116. LeBars D, Dickenson AH, and Besson JM: Diffuse noxious inhibitory controls (DNIC) II. Lack of effect on non-convergent neurons, supraspinal involvement and theoretical implications. Pain 6:305–327, 1979.

117. Lembeck F, Folkers K, and Donnerer J: Analgesic effect of antagonists of substance P. Biochem Biophys Res Commun 103:1318–1321, 1981.

118. Lenz FA: The thalamus and central pain syndromes: Human and animal studies. In Casey KI (ed): Pain and Central Nervous System Disease: The Central Pain Syndrome. Raven Press, New York, 1991, pp 171–182.

119. Levante A, Cesaro P, and Albe-Fessard D: Electrophysiological and anatomical demonstration of a bulbar relayed pathway towards the CM-CL in the rat. Neurosci Lett 38:139–144, 1983.

120. Levine J, and Taiwo Y: Inflammatory pain. In Wall PD, and Melzack R (eds): Textbook of Pain, ed 3. Churchill Livingstone, Edinburgh, 1994, pp 45–56.

121. Levine JD, Gordon NC, and Fields HL: Naloxone dose-dependently produces analgesia and hyperalgesia in post-operative pain. Nature 278:740–741, 1979.

122. Levine JD, Gordon NC, Jones RT, et al: The narcotic antagonist naloxone enhances clinical pain. Nature 272:826–827, 1978.

123. Lewis T: Pain. Macmillian, New York, 1942.

124. Liebman JM, and Pastor G: Antinociceptive effects of baclofen and muscimol upon intraventricular administration. Eur J Pharmacol 61:225–230, 1980.

125. Light AR, and Perl ER: Spinal termination of functionally identified primary afferent neurons with slowly conducting myelinated fibers. J Comp Neurol 186:133–150, 1979.

126. Lim RKS, Miller DG, Guzman F, et al: Pain and analgesia evaluated by intraperitoneal bradykinin-evoked pain method in man. Clin Pharmacol Ther 8:521–542, 1967.

127. Ling GSF, and Pasternak GW: Different opioid receptors mediate spinal and supraspinal opioid analgesia in the mouse. Neurology (Suppl 2)33: 148, 1983.

128. Lisney SJW: Observations on facial nociception in a monkey after destruction of the rostral part of the trigeminal sensory nuclear complex. Pain 21:129–135, 1985.

129. Loeser JD, Ward AA, and White LE: Chronic deafferentation of human spinal cord neurons. J Neurosurg 29:48–50, 1986.

130. Lynn B: The heat sensitization of polymodal nociceptors in the rabbit and its independence of the local blood flow. J Physiol (Lond) 287:493–507, 1979.

131. Marshall J: Sensory disturbances in cortical wounds with special reference to pain. J Neurol Neurosurg Psychiatry 14:187–204, 1951.

132. Martin WR, Eades CG, Thompson JA, et al: The effects of morphine and nalorphine-like drugs in the non-dependent and morphine dependent chronic spinal dog. J Pharmacol Exp Ther 197:517–532, 1976.

133. Mayer DJ, and Hayes RL: Stimulation-produced analgesia: Development of tolerance and cross-tolerance to morphine. Science 188:941–943, 1976.

134. Mayer DJ, Price DD, and Rafil A: Antagonism of acupuncture analgesia by the narcotic antagonist naloxone. Brain Res 121:368–372, 1977.

135. Mayer DJ, and Watkins LR: Multiple endogenous opiate and non-opiate analgesic systems. In Kruger L, and Liebeskind JC (eds): Advances in Pain Research and Therapy, Vol 6. Raven Press, New York, 1984, pp 253–276.

136. Mayer DJ, Wolfe TL, Akil H, et al: Analgesia from electrical stimulation in the brainstem of the rat. Science 174:1351–1354, 1971.

137. Mehler WR: Some neurological species differences—a posteriori. Ann NY Acad Sci 167:424–468, 1969.

138. Mehler WR, Feferman ME, and Nauta WJH: Ascending axon degeneration following anterolateral cordotomy: An experimental study in the monkey. Brain 83:718–751, 1960.

139. Melzack R: Neurophysiological foundation of pain. In Sternbach RA (ed): The Psychology of Pain. Raven Press, New York, 1986, pp 1–24.

140. Melzack R, and Wall PD: Pain mechanisms: A new theory. Science 150:971–979, 1965.

141. Menetrey D, Chaouch A, and Besson JM: Location and properties of dorsal horn neurons at origin of spinoreticular tract in lumbar enlargement of the rat. J Neurophysiol 44:862–877, 1980.

142. Metz J, Busch DA, and Weltzer HY: Clinical, electrophysiological and biochemical effects of des-tyrosine-endorphin in psychiatric patients. Ann NY Acad Sci 398:496–509, 1982.

143. Meyer RA, and Campbell JN: Myelinated nociceptive afferents account for the hyperalgesia that follows a burn to the hand. Science 213:1527–1529, 1981.

144. Meyer RA, Campbell JN, and Raja SN: Peripheral neural mechanisms of nociception. In Wall PD, and Melzack R (eds): Textbook of Pain, ed 3. Churchill Livingstone, Edinburgh, 1994, pp 13–44.

145. Meynadier J, Chrubasik DM, and Wunsch E: Intrathecal somatostatin in terminally ill patients. A report of two cases. Pain 23:9–12, 1985.

146. Millan MJ, and Herz A: The endocrinology of the opiates. Int Rev Neurobiol 26:1–83, 1985.

147. Mills JE, Sellic H, and Widdicombe JG: Activity in lung irritant receptors in pulmonary microembolism, anaphylaxis, and drug-induced bronchoconstrictions. J Physiol (Lond) 203:337–357, 1969.

148. Milne RJ, Foreman RD, and Giesler WWD: Convergence of cutaneous and pelvic visceral nociceptive inputs onto primate spinothalamic neurons. Pain 11:163–183, 1981.

149. Morgan C, Nadelhaft I, and deGrat WC: The distribution of visceral primary afferents from the pelvic nerve to Lissauer's tract and the spinal grey matter and its relationship to the sacral parasympathetic nucleus. J Comp Neurol 201:415–440, 1981.

150. Morrison JFB: The afferent innervation of the gastrointestinal tract. In Brooks FB, and Eves PW (eds): Nerves in the Gut. CB Slack, Thorofare, NJ, 1977, pp 297–322.

151. Moulin DE, Max MD, Kaiko RF, et al: The analgesic efficiency of intrathecal D-Ala2-D-Leu5-enkephalin in cancer patients with chronic pain. Pain 23:213–221, 1985.

152. Nagy JI, Hunt SP, Iversen LL, et al: Biochemical and anatomical observations on the degeneration of peptide-containing primary afferent neurons after neonatal capsaicin. Neurosci 6:1923–1934, 1981.

153. Nathan PW: The gate-control theory of pain. A critical review. Brain 99:123–158, 1976.

154. Noordenbos W, and Wall PD: Diverse sensory functions with an almost totally divided spinal cord. A case of spinal cord transection with preservation of part of one anterolateral quadrant. Pain 2:185–195, 1976.

155. Oleson TD, Twombly DA, and Liebeskind JC: Effects of pain-attenuating brain stimulation and morphine on electrical activity in the raphe nuclei of the awake rat. Pain 4:211–230, 1978.

156. Oliveras JL, Hosobuchi Y, Redjeme F, et al: Opiate antagonist, naloxone, strongly reduces analgesia induced by stimulation of a raphe nucleus (centralis inferior). Brain Res 120:221–229, 1977.

157. Osbahr AJ, Nemeroff CB, Luttinger D, et al: Neurotensin-induced antinociception in mice: Antagonism by thyrotropin-releasing hormone. J Pharmacol Exp Ther 217:645–651, 1981.

158. Paintal AS: Mechanism of stimulation of type J pulmonary receptors. J Physiol (Lond) 203:511–532, 1969.

159. Pasternak GW: Opiate, enkephalin, and endorphin analgesia: Relations to a single subpopulation of opiate receptors. Neurology 31:1311–1315, 1981.

160. Pasternak GW, Carroll-Buatti M, and Spiegel K: The binding and analgesic properties of a sigma opiate, SKF 10, 047. J Pharmacol Exp Ther 219:192–198, 1981.

161. Patrick JT, McBride WJ, and Felten DL: Distribution of glycine, GABA, aspartate and glutamate in the rat spinal cord. Brain Res 10:415–418, 1983.

162. Penfield W, and Boldrey E: Somatic motor and sensory representation in the cerebral cortex of man as studied by electrical stimulation. Brain 60:389–443, 1937.

163. Perl ER: Myelinated afferent fibers innervating the primate skin and their response to noxious stimuli. J Physiol (Lond) 197:593–615, 1968.

164. Perl ER: Characterization of nociceptors and their activation of neurons in the superficial dorsal horn: First steps for the sensation of pain. In Kruger L, and Liebeskind JC (eds): Advances in Pain Research and Therapy, Vol 6. Raven Press, New York, 1984, pp 23–51.

165. Pert CB, and Snyder SH: Opiate receptor—its demonstration in nervous tissue. Science 179:1011–1014, 1973.

166. Portenoy RK: Issues in the management of neuropathic pain. In Basbaum A, and Besson J-M (eds): Towards a New Pharmacotherapy of Pain. John Wiley & Sons, Chichester, 1991, pp 393–416.

167. Potter GD, Guzman F, and Lim RKS: Visceral pain evoked by intra-arterial injection of substance P. Nature 193:983–984, 1962.

168. Price DD, and Dubner R: Neurons that subserve the sensory-discriminative aspects of pain. Pain 3:307–338, 1977.

169. Price GW, Wilkin GP, Turnbull MJ, et al: Are baclofen-sensitive GABA B receptors present on primary afferent terminals of the spinal cord? Nature 307:71–74, 1984.

170. Procacci P, and Zoppi M: Pathophysiology and clinical aspects of visceral and referred pain. In Bonica JJ, Lindblom U, and Iggo A (eds): Advances in Pain Research and Therapy, Vol. 5. Raven Press, New York, 1983, pp 643–658.

171. Puig MM, Laorden ML, Miralles FS, et al: Endorphin levels in cerebrospinal fluid of patients with postoperative and chronic pain. Anesthesiology 57:1–4, 1982.

172. Ramaswamy S, Pillai NP, and Bapna JS: Analgesic effect of prolactin: Possible mechanisms of action. Eur J Pharmacol 96:171–173, 1983.

173. Rasminsky M: Ectopic generation of impulses of cross-talk in spinal nerve roots of "dystrophic" mice. Ann Neurol 3:351–357, 1978.

174. Roques BP, Fournie-Zaluski MC, and Soroca EEA: The enkephalinase inhibitor thiorphan shows antinociceptive activity in mice. Nature 288:286–288, 1980.

175. Ruch TC: Pathophysiology of pain. In Ruch TC, and Patton HD (eds): Physiology and Biophysics. WB Saunders, Philadelphia, 1965, pp 345–363.

176. Ruda MA: Opiates and pain pathway: Demonstration of enkephalin synapses on dorsal horn projection neurons. Science 215:1523–1524, 1982.

177. Scadding JW: Development of ongoing activity, mechanosensitivity, and adrenalin sensitivity in severed peripheral nerve axons. Exp Neurol 73: 345–364, 1981.

178. Schaible H, and Schmidt RF: Effects of an experimental arthritis on the sensory properties of fine articular afferent units. J Neurophysiol 54:1109–1122, 1985.

179. Seltzer Z, and Devor M: Ephaptic transmission in chronically damaged peripheral nerves. Neurology 29:1061–1064, 1979.

180. Sessle BJ: Is the tooth pulp a "pure" source of noxious input? In Bonica JJ, Liebeskind JC, and Albe-Fessard DG (eds): Advances in Pain Research and Therapy, Vol 3. Raven Press, New York, 1979, pp 245–260.

181. Shimizu T, Koja T, Fujisaki T, et al: Effects of methysergide and naloxone on analgesia induced by peripheral electric stimulation in mice. Brain Res 108:463–467, 1981.

182. Simanton R, and Synder SH: Morphine-like peptides in mammalian brain: Isolation, structure elucidation and interactions with the opiate receptor. Proc Natl Acad Sci USA 73:2515–2519, 1976.

183. Sindou M, Fisher G, and Mansuy L: Posterior selective rhizotomy and selective posterior rhizidiotomy. Prog Neurol Surg 7:201–280, 1976.

184. Snyder RL: The organization of dorsal root entry zone in cats and monkeys. J Comp Neurol 174: 47–70, 1977.

185. Stanzione P, and Zieglagansberger W: Action of neurotensin on spinal cord neurons in the rat. Brain Res 268:111–118, 1983.

186. Tamsen A, Hartvig P, Dahlstrom B, et al: Endorphins and on-demand analgesia. Lancet 8:769–775, 1980.

187. Taren JA, Davis R, and Crosby EC: Target physiologic corroboration in sterotaxic cervical cordotomy. J Neurosurg 30:569–584, 1969.

188. Terenius L: Characteristics of the receptor for narcotic analgesics in the synaptic membrane fractions from rat brain. Acta Pharm Hung 33:377–384, 1973.

189. Terenius L, and Wahlstrom A: Endorphins and clinical pain: An overview. Adv Exp Med Biol 116: 261–277, 1979.

190. Thompson SWN, King AE, and Woolf CJ: Activity-dependent changes in rat ventral horn neurones in vitro; summation of prolonged afferent evoked postsynaptic depolarizations produce a d-APV sensitive windup. Eur J Neurosci 2:638–649, 1990.

191. Torebjork HE: Afferent C units responding to mechanical, thermal and chemical stimuli in human non-glabrous skin. Acta Physiol Scand 92:374–390, 1974.

192. Torebjork HE, and Hallin RG: Identification of afferent C units in intact human skin nerves. Brain Res 67:387–403, 1974.

193. Torebjork HE, Ochoa JL, and Schary W: Referred pain from intraneural stimulation of muscle fascicles in the median nerve. Pain 118:145–156, 1984.

194. Travell J, and Simons D: Myofascial Pain Syndrome. Williams & Wilkins, Baltimore, 1985.

195. Trevathan E, and Cascino GD: Partial epilepsy presenting as focal paroxymal pain. Neurology 38: 329–330, 1988.

196. Van Hees J, and Gybels JM: Pain related to single afferent C fibers from human skin. Brain Res 48:397–400, 1972.

197. Von Knorring L, Almay BGL, Johansson F, et al: Pain perception and endorphin levels in cerebrospinal fluid. Pain 5:359–365, 1978.

198. Wall PD: The gate control theory of pain mechanisms: A re-examination and re-statement. Brain 101:18, 1978.

199. Wall PD, and Devor M: The effect of peripheral nerve injury on dorsal root potentials and on transmission of afferent signals into the spinal cord. Brain Res 209:95–111, 1981.

200. Wall PD, and Gutnick M: Ongoing activity in peripheral nerves and the physiology and pharmacology of impulses originating in a neuroma. Exp Neurol 43:580–593, 1974.

201. Watkins LR, Kinscheck IB, Kaufman EFS, et al: Cholecystokinin antagonist selectively potentiates analgesia induced by endogenous opiates. Brain Res 327:181–190, 1985.

202. Watkins LR, Kinscheck IB, and Mayer DJ: Potentiation of morphine analgesia by the cholecystokinin antagonist proglumide. Brain Res 327: 169–180, 1985.

203. Watkins LR, Kinscheck IB, and Mayer DJ: Potentiation of opiate analgesia and apparent reversal of morphine tolerance by proglumide, a cholecystokinin antagonist. Science 224:395–396, 1985.

204. Watson SJ, Akil H, Ghazorossian VE, et al: Dynorphin immunocytochemical localization in brain and peripheral nervous system: preliminary studies. Proc Natl Acad Sci USA 78:1260–1263, 1981.

205. White DM, and Helme RD: Release of substance P from peripheral nerve terminals following electrical stimulation of the sciatic nerve. Brain Res 336: 27–31, 1985.

206. White JC, and Bland EF: The surgical relief of severe angina pectoris: Methods employed and results in 83 patients. Medicine 27:1–42, 1948.

207. Willer JC, Dehen H, and Cambier J: Stress-induced analgesia in humans: Endogenous opioids and naloxone-reversible depression of pain reflexes. Science 212:689–691, 1981.

208. Willer JC, Roby A, and LeBars D: Psychophysical and electrophysiological approaches to the pain-relieving effects of heterotopic nociceptive stimuli. Brain 107:1095–1112, 1984.

209. Willis WD, Kenshalo DR, and Leonard RB: The cells of origin of the primate spinothalamic tract. J Comp Neurol 188:543–574, 1979.

210. Wilson PR, and Yaksh TL: Baclofen is antinociceptive in the spinal intrathecal space of animals. Eur J Pharmacol 51:323–330, 1978.

211. Woolf CJ: The dorsal horn: State-dependent sensory processing and the generation of pain. In Wall PD, and Melzack R (eds): Textbook of Pain, ed 3. Churchill Livingstone, Edinburgh, 1994, pp 101–112.

212. Woolf CJ, and Fitzgerald M: The properties of neurons recorded in the superficial dorsal horn of the rat spinal cord. J Comp Neurol 221:313–328, 1983.

213. Woolf CJ, and Thompson SWN: The induction and maintenance of central sensitization is dependent on N-methyl-D-aspartic acid receptor activa-

tion; implications for the treatment of post-injury pain hypersensitivity states. Pain 44:293–299, 1991.

214. Yaksh TL: Direct evidence that spinal serotonin and noradrenaline terminals mediate the spinal antinociceptive effects of morphine in the periaqueductal grey. Brain Res 160:180–185, 1979.

215. Yaksh TL, Farb DH, Leeman SE, et al: Intrathecal capsaicin depletes substance P in the rat spinal cord and produces prolonged thermal analgesia. Science 206:481–483, 1979.

216. Yaksh TL, Jessell TM, Gamse R, et al: Intrathecal morphine inhibits substance P release from mammalian spinal cord in vivo. Nature 286:155–157, 1980.

217. Yaksh TL, and Malmberg AB: Central pharmacology of nociceptive transmission. In Wall PD, and Melzack R (eds): Textbook of Pain, ed 3. Churchill Livingstone, Edinburgh, 1994, pp 165–200.

218. Yaksh TL, Plant RL, and Rudy TA: Studies on the antagonism by raphe lesions of the antinociceptive action of systemic morphine. Eur J Pharmacol 41:399–408, 1977.

219. Yaksh TL, and Rudy TA: Narcotic analgesics: CNS sites and mechanisms of action as revealed by intracerebral injection techniques. Pain 4:299–359, 1978.

220. Yeung JC, and Rudy T: Multiplicative interaction between narcotic agonisms expressed at spinal and supraspinal sites of antinociceptive action as revealed by concurrent intrathecal and intracerebroventricular injections of morphine. J Pharmacol Exp Ther 215:633–642, 1980.

CHAPTER 3

THE SCOPE OF THE PROBLEM

Ronald M. Kanner, M.D.

In a time of diminishing health care resources, it is striking to note that more than 80 percent of health care dollars are spent on less than 20 percent of the general population.[69] Pain is the most common symptom for which patients seek medical help, and the small percentage of those with pain who enter the health care and disability systems have come to represent a "chronic pain and disability epidemic."[2] To clarify the scope of this problem, this chapter reviews the prevalence of painful disorders in the general population and specific medical settings and describes the socioeconomic impact of pain-related disability.

DIFFICULTIES WITH DATA INTERPRETATION

Interpretation of epidemiologic data requires an understanding of their limitations. Prevalence and incidence data are gathered from the general population by surveys of specific geographic areas, worker groups, or health care plans. Variability in selection criteria and response biases may make these data difficult to interpret.[16,20,48] Even when a specific pain syndrome is studied, the perceived prevalence may depend more on the investigators' defined limits of the syndrome than on the pain itself.[85] The epidemiologic literature on chronic pain is characterized by a lack of consensus about basic definitions and inconsistencies in measurement techniques.[30,61]

Response Biases

If a randomly selected population is asked to complete a pain-related questionnaire, individuals with pain are more likely to take an interest, and the results are skewed toward a higher prevalence. Only one study reviewed showed a 100 percent response rate,[12] and this was conducted by "instructed interviewers" in the People's Republic of China. Pain is more likely to be reported in an urban population than in a rural one,[12,39,64] and women tend to report slightly higher rates of symptoms than do men.[10] In a clinic population, however, women may outnumber men by 3:1, despite a nearly equal distribution of pain symptoms in the general population.[38] Gender differences may play a role in the type of pain syndromes suffered and in the intensity of the pain experienced, but such data must be interpreted cautiously.[67]

Interestingly, the type of survey (telephone versus mail) does not seem to have an important influence on response bias.[76] Postal surveys are the easiest to perform, but these have a relatively low response rate. One survey that reported a 93 percent response rate actually had only 27 percent responding to the first mailing, with three reminders and a phone call needed to bring the response rate up to actually 82 percent.[7] Although subjects who respond early have different demographic characteristics than those who reply late, these differences do not appear to skew the data significantly.[49]

Other factors, however, may introduce response bias. Educational levels, marital status, gender, and socioeconomic status have a strong influence on pain reporting.[44,65] Surveys of populations that differ from the general population on any of these factors may not yield generalizable results.[17] Similarly, worker surveys may not take into account subjects who are already disabled by pain and are out of the work force, thereby skewing pain prevalence downward. Worker surveys also tend to eliminate the very young and the very old.

Case Definitions

Another confounding factor is the lack of uniformity in assessing case definition. Case definition refers to the parameters used to identify an individual with pain. Obviously, results vary if the parameter is "any pain," pain of more than 1 week, constant pain for more than 1 month, or pain of sufficient severity and duration to interfere with employment or daily living. Inconsistencies in defining disability, handicap, and impairment further confuse the statistical issues.[80]

Time Frame

Point prevalence refers to pain at a given point in time, as opposed to pain during a specific period of time. The longer the period studied, the higher the prevalence. For example, a large population study in New Zealand[41] showed that 17.5 percent of responders had low back pain at the time of the study, 33.4 percent had pain in the prior week, 63.7 percent had it in the prior year, and the lifetime prevalence was 79 percent. Studies addressing point prevalence and period prevalence cannot be compared directly.

RESULTS OF GEOGRAPHIC SURVEYS

The Nuprin Report,[31] performed by a national polling company, was a random telephone sampling of 1254 Americans between 18 and 65 years of age. Of the subjects responding, 13 to 14 percent had suffered from headaches or back pain or both for more than 30 days in the prior year. The response rate to the survey was not stated, and true prevalence rates cannot be extrapolated accurately.

A Danish survey[74] used the obligatory reporting of "strong analgesic" use as a measure of the prevalence of severe pain. In a population area of 480,000, they found that 0.2 percent had used opioid analgesics for pain. The most common acute pain was backache (23 percent) or trauma (17 percent); headache was the most common recurrent problem (25 percent), and back pain was the most common chronic ailment (29 percent).

A Swedish postal survey of over 1000 residents age 18 to 84 years[7] revealed that 66 percent had suffered from "some pain," and 40 percent had "obvious pain" (pain of sufficient intensity to hamper activities of daily living). Thirty-one percent of the respondents reported back pain. Elderly patients were less likely to complete the forms and were less likely to report that pain hampered activities. Another survey, which used an interview format to evaluate nearly 1500 adults, observed that the majority had "life-disturbing" pain and that older subjects were more likely than younger subjects to have pain.[35] An English study reported that "chronic widespread pain" was present in 11.2 percent of a surveyed population.[14]

More meaningful numbers can be gathered by targeting specific symptoms. Back pain and headache are the most common chronic pain syndromes reported,[50,81] and back pain is the leading cause of long-term disability from work.[40] The lifetime prevalence of low back pain is reported to be 60 to 75 percent. One study reported a prevalence of only 13.8 percent, but this was due to a restrictive criterion of pain lasting more than 2 weeks.[20] A Finnish study of 8000 individuals over 30 years of age had a high response rate and demonstrated that 75 percent of respondents had at least one episode of low back pain and more than half had six or more episodes.[32] Of the subjects with pain, 60 percent reported some disability, but severe limitations were rare.

Although back pain is often thought to have a strong male preponderance, one study showed that 45 percent of unmarried women age 50 to 64 reported back pain on a questionnaire, compared to only 9 to 11 percent of educated, married men.[65] Overall, men and women are equally affected but, after age 60, women are more likely to complain of back pain.

Headache is the most common recurrent pain.[74] The lifetime prevalence of headache is close to 90 percent and, although only a small percentage of these subjects seek medical attention, these patients account for nearly a quarter of all neurologic consultations.[34] A large-scale telephone survey of more than 10,000 residents of Maryland[46] yielded a period prevalence of 63 percent for headaches in the prior 4 weeks. Five to ten percent of the population seek intermittent medical aid for the relief of disabling headache,[86] while the lifetime prevalence of severe or disabling headache is estimated at 20 percent in women and 11 percent in men.[23] Among patients presenting to a physician for nonpainful disease, a history of headache can be obtained in more than half of the patients.

Future epidemiologic studies in the general population should not simply address the prevalence or incidence of pain but should also stress the identification of groups at greatest risk for developing pain-related disability.[15]

RESULTS OF AGE-SPECIFIC SURVEYS

Pain in Children

The epidemiology of pain in children is of particular interest because of the possibility that it could illuminate the factors that predispose to chronic pain in adults. The degree and pattern in which pain syndromes cluster in families might allow the formulation of hypotheses concerning biologic or psychologic contributions to pathogenesis, much the way twin studies did in schizophrenia and geographic studies did in multiple sclerosis.[27] At present, however, the relationship between childhood pain and adult pain is unknown. For example, it is not clear how neglect or overindulgence might affect a child's pain behavior or what role physical or sexual abuse plays in the development of chronic pain.

Prevalence studies in children are subject to the same problems as those in adults, with the added difficulties caused by the need to define age-appropriate measures and time of recall.[27] Depending on the time frame used, estimates of the prevalence of headaches in adolescents have ranged from 11 to 82 percent.[19,62] Although the true prevalence of migraine in childhood is about 5 percent,[45] a far higher proportion of migraine patients give a history of headaches in childhood. About 3 percent of 7-year-olds and 11 percent of 14-year-olds relate a history of headaches.[70] Interestingly, the female predominance is present even in early childhood.[45]

Low back pain, the most common cause of prolonged disability in adults, is experienced by 30 percent of adolescents and may restrict the activities of one-third of those affected.[59] The highest prevalence is in the older teenage years.[3] Despite this high prevalence rate, however, very few children are seen clinically for back pain.[27]

Pain in the Elderly

Although it is usually assumed that old age brings with it painful disorders, this has not been confirmed by all systematic studies. A study of 3097 elderly people in rural Iowa revealed that 23.6 percent of women and 18.8 percent of men had experienced low back pain in the prior year; the prevalence decreased with advancing age, and 75 percent of those with pain stated that the pain had started before age 65.[42] Only about half of the patients with pain were using analgesics,[33] and one-quarter had a hospitalization for a pain-related problem. After their general physician, this group most often sought help from a chiropractor.

A questionnaire survey of 1119 patients older than 70 years of age observed that 28 percent of women and 17 percent of men reported abdominal pain of sufficient severity or duration to have influenced their well-being in the prior year.[33] These figures are similar to the prevalence rates for low back pain in this age group.

RESULTS OF WORKERS' SURVEYS

Surveys performed in specific work environments may elucidate those factors that contribute to the development of pain. Surprisingly, the overall prevalence of pain is not significantly different among various jobs: Miners report about the same prevalence of back pain as office workers,[47] and the prevalence rate of low back pain is similar in pharmaceutical workers, Finnish reindeer herders, manufacturing workers, and "sportsmen" (hunters and fishermen).[8,58,66,79]

Nonetheless, within any given group of workers, certain demographic and job factors can influence the reporting of pain.[6] The older members of the reindeer-herding group reported a lower prevalence of back pain than the younger herders, possibly because they were no longer required to do the strenuous parts of the job.[58] The pharmaceutical workers who reported the highest prevalence of pain had jobs comparable to those of the rest of the group, but they had chairs that were not ergonomically correct.[66]

The lifetime prevalence of back pain among chiropractors (the practitioners most frequently consulted for back pain) was found to be 87 percent,[56] and the vast majority of them felt that the height of their tables was the most important factor. Workers involved in heavy lifting may not have any greater prevalence of back pain than those involved in less physical jobs, but the severity of pain and disability among those affected may be greater.[78] Garment workers had a similar prevalence of back pain across various job descriptions, but knee pain caused more disability in machine operators who stressed the knee more.[73]

Workers who are dissatisfied with their jobs or who have a low level of education are more likely to report pain than workers who are more highly educated or satisfied.[44] Even people with higher levels of education may be reluctant to report pain to their superiors; 78 percent of the nurses who reported back pain on a questionnaire had not reported the problem to their supervisors.[9]

SURVEYS OF PAIN IN MEDICAL ILLNESS

General Hospital Admissions

Although pain is extraordinarily common among patients with diverse types of medical illness, it receives relatively little attention. Donovan[22] found that 353 of 454 hospitalized patients (greater than 75 percent) had been bothered by pain in the prior 24 hours. Although 58 percent described their pain as "excruciating," fewer than half had been asked about pain by a medical professional, and the patients who were ordered analgesics received about one-quarter of the maximum amount allowed. A survey of consecutive hospital admissions revealed that 157 (70 percent) of 224 nonsurgical admissions had nonprocedural pain on presentation, and 80 (34.8 percent) had pain as the chief complaint.[28] The latter survey observed that headache was the most common complaint, that women were more likely than men to report pain, and that pain assessment was poor. Another survey of 2415 nonsurgical patients disclosed a 21 percent prevalence of moderate to severe pain during the prior 24 hours, but analgesic use again was low.[1] Even with surgical patients, a group in which pain is almost universally expected, little medication use is the rule.[53]

In a study of hospitalized children age 4 to 14, the point prevalence of pain was 87 percent, with 19 percent reporting it as severe.[37] Only 38 percent of the children had received medications for their pain, and surgical patients were three times as likely as medical patients to receive analgesics for the same severity of pain. Another study revealed that no analgesics were ordered for 16 percent of the children in pain, and 39 percent of the children for whom opioid analgesics were ordered did not receive them.[52]

General Outpatient Clinics

In a general medical outpatient setting, pain was the presenting complaint in about one-third of the cases.[71] Most of these were musculoskeletal in nature.

Psychologic dysfunction in patients with chronic pain has received a great deal of attention, but the prevalence of pain in patients with psychiatric disease is less well-recognized. Marchesi[51] found that 51.9 percent of 160 depressed patients suffered from chronic headaches. Smith[72] found an increased incidence of depressive symptoms in patients with somatoform disorder and an increased incidence of hypochondriasis in patients with depression. Among 500 consecutive patients in a psychiatric clinic,[11] the prevalence of chronic pain was 60 percent in anxiety neurosis, 45 percent in depression, and 24.3 percent in hysteria. The prevalence was less than 3 percent in patients with psychosis. Depressed patients with pain tended to be older, and anxious patients were more likely to be receiving disability payments.

Patients With Cancer

One-third to one-half of all patients with cancer experience pain, and this number rises to 70 to 90 percent with advanced disease.[5,25,63] Children with cancer suffer from pain with about the same frequency as adults.[57] Pain in adults is most likely to be re-lated to a direct effect of the tumor, whereas pain in children with cancer is more likely to be due to treatment side effects.[5,57] Surveys in the cancer population have begun to define a distinctive group of cancer pain syndromes (see Chapter 9).

Patients With AIDS

Despite the attention paid to the immunologic and social issues in AIDS, there is a paucity of information on the painful syndromes that complicate the disease. In a retrospective chart review,[43] more than half of the medical records contained a mention of nonprocedural pain. This almost certainly underestimates the magnitude of the problem, because pain problems frequently go unmentioned in hospital charts when medical problems are pressing. The most common syndrome was chest pain, presumably due to the high prevalence of pneumocystis pneumonia. Painful peripheral neuropathy and joint pains were also common.[60]

DISABILITY SURVEYS

The terminology used for describing impairment and disability is vague and may be confusing.[30] *Impairment* is defined as any anatomic, physiologic, or psychologic abnormality or loss[80]; it is a medical assessment and is measureable. *Disability* is not a strict medical judgment and reflects the decisions of administrators as much as those of physicians. It is an assessment of the patient's actual or presumed ability to engage in specific activities.[2]

The proportion of disabled people of working age is estimated to be about 4.5 to 9 percent.[61] The number of people in the United States who are totally disabled is more than 8 million, or about 6 percent of the workforce.

In a biomedical model, physicians are trained to recognize certain types of pathology as causing impairment. Usually, there are clearly defined deficits that are attributable to an underlying pathology. When pain is the only complaint, however, there may be few explanatory physical findings, and disability may far exceed impairments.[82] A psychosocial-rehabilitation model is used to minimize the disability by using techniques that no longer seek a remedy for the pain but rather focus on the physical and psychologic functioning of the patient.[77]

Disability is a costly issue.[18,21] Back pain accounts for 25 percent of all compensation claims.[68] The 1981 Workers' Compensation bill for low back pain was $4.6 billion. In 1986, the total compensable cost was $11.1 billion,[83] with 31.5 percent representing medical costs and 67.2 percent, indemnity costs. The largest cost, however, is in lost work time.

It is difficult to predict which workers will become disabled from back pain, but it appears that psychologic, environmental, and work factors are more predictive than physical issues.[26] Indeed, back pain sufferers may have a psychologic profile that further predisposes them to disability. They describe their jobs as boring, repetitive, and dissatisfying,[4] and depression, hypochondriasis, and anxiety are commonly associated problems.

The possibility that compensation may play a role in perpetuating disability has received mixed support in the literature. In a comparison of compensation recipients and patients with pain who had settled their claims, compensation recipients showed more signs of emotional distress, had greater difficulty coping with pain, and reported that pain disrupted various aspects of their life to a greater degree.[29] Another study that compared groups of patients with low back pain who received no compensation, time-limited compensation, or unlimited social security disability benefits demonstrated that the third group had a higher percentage of physician-rated symptom dramatization and pain behavior and greater use of medication than the other two.[36] In both of these studies, the disabled group may have had more pain than the others, but this could not be documented. The concept of "litigation neurosis" is not well documented,[55] and it is possible that the role of compensation in chronic pain has been overstated.[24,54]

Attempts to recognize and eliminate the causes for disability have met with mixed results.[68] The immensity of the problem, as well as the inability of individual physicians to deal with it, has led to the development of the multidisciplinary pain clinic model.

Most pain clinics treat disabled patients and have rehabilitation, rather than pain relief alone, as their goal. Treatment in a multidisciplinary pain clinic can help some patients reduce the use of other services that may be more costly.[13,84] Some pain rehabilitation programs establish working relationships with businesses to decrease time away from work.[75]

SUMMARY

Population-based surveys have repeatedly demonstrated that chronic pain is an extremely prevalent condition. However, surveys are complicated by response biases, lack of uniformity in case definitions, and inconsistencies in time frame assessed.

Geographic studies have demonstrated that back pain and headache are the most common types of chronic pain. The lifetime prevalence of back pain is reported to be 60 to 75 percent, and it is the leading cause of long-term disability. More than 10 percent of the population may suffer from "chronic widespread pain," and older patients are more likely to suffer from pain than are younger subjects.

Results of pain surveys in workers reveal that the overall prevalence of pain is not significantly different among various jobs and that job satisfaction and level of education may have more to do with pain-related disability than do the specific tasks involved in the job.

Data from hospital admissions suggest that the majority of patients suffer from pain, and their pain is generally undertreated. The problem of undertreatment may be even more pervasive in hospitalized children.

Pain-related disability is an extremely costly issue. The current compensation system may perpetuate disability in some patients.

REFERENCES

1. Abbot FV, Gray DK, Sewitch J, et al: The prevalence of pain in hospitalized patients and resolution over six months. Pain 50(1):15–28, 1992.
2. Aronoff GM: Chronic pain and the disability epidemic. Clin J Pain 7:330–338, 1991.

3. Balague F, Dutoit G, and Waldburger M: Low back pain in schoolchildren. Scand J Rehab Med 20: 175–179, 1988.

4. Bergenudd H, and Nilsson B: Back pain in middle age; occupational workload and psychologic factors: An epidemiologic survey. Spine 13(1):58–60, 1988.

5. Bonica JJ: Treatment of cancer pain: Current status and future needs. In Fields HL, Dubner R, and Cervero F (eds): Advances in Pain Research and Therapy, Vol 9. Proceedings of the Fourth World Congress on Pain. Raven Press, New York, 1985, pp 589–616.

6. Borenstein, D: Low back pain: Epidemiology, etiology, diagnostic evaluation, and therapy. Curr Opin Rheumatol 3(2):207–217, 1991.

7. Brattberg G, Thorslund M, and Wikman A: The prevalence of pain in a general population. The results of a postal survey in a county of Sweden. Pain 37:215–222, 1989.

8. Burchfiel CM, Boice JA, Stafford BA, et al: Prevalence of back pain and joint problems in a manufacturing company. J Occup Med 34(2):129–134, 1992.

9. Cato C, Olson DK, and Studer M: Incidence, prevalence, and variables associated with low back pain in staff nurses. AORN J 37(8):321–327, 1989.

10. Celentano DD, Linet MS, and Stewart WF: Gender differences in the experience of headache. Soc Sci Med 30(12):1289–1295, 1990.

11. Chaturvedi SK: Prevalence of chronic pain in psychiatric patients. Pain 29:231–237, 1987.

12. Cheng XM, Ziegler DK, Li SC, et al: A prevalence survey of "incapacitating headache" in the People's Republic of China. Neurology 36(6):831–834, 1986.

13. Cicala RS, and Wright H: Outpatient treatment of patients with chronic pain: An analysis of cost savings. Clin J Pain 5(3):223–226, 1989.

14. Croft P, Rigby AS, Boswell R, et al: The prevalence of chronic widespread pain in the general population. J Rheumatol 20(4):710–713, 1993.

15. Crombie IK, Davies HTO, and Macrae WA: The epidemiology of chronic pain: Time for new directions. Pain 57:1–3, 1994.

16. Crook J, Rideout E, and Browne G: The prevalence of pain complaints in a general population. Pain 18(3):299–314, 1984.

17. Crook J, Tunks E, Rideout E, et al: Epidemiologic comparison of persistent pain sufferers in a specialty pain clinic and in the community. Arch Phys Med Rehabil 67:451–455, 1986.

18. de Girolamo G: Epidemiology and social costs of low back pain and fibromyalgia. Clin J Pain 7(1): S1–S7, 1991.

19. Deubner DC: An epidemiologic study of migraine and headache in 10–20 year olds. Headache 17:173–180, 1977.

20. Deyo RA, and Tsui Wu-Y J: Descriptive epidemiology of low-back pain and its related medical care in the United States. Spine 12(3):264–268, 1987.

21. Deyo RA, Cherkin D, Conrad D, et al: Cost, controversy, crisis: Low back pain and the health of the public. Annu Rev Public Health 12:141–156, 1991.

22. Donovan M, Dillon P, and McGuire L: Incidence and characteristics of pain in a sample of medical-surgical inpatients. Pain 30(1):69–78, 1987.

23. Duckro PN, Tait RC, and Margolis RB: Prevalence

of very severe headache in a large US metropolitan area. Cephalalgia 9(3):199–205, 1989.

24. Dworkin RH: Compensation in chronic pain patients: Cause or consequence? Pain 43(3):387–388, 1990.

25. Foley KM: Pain syndromes in patients with cancer. In Bonica JJ, and Ventafridda V (eds): Advances in Pain Research and Therapy, Vol 2. Raven Press, New York, 1979, pp 59–75.

26. Frymoyer JW: Predicting disability from low back pain. Clin Orthop 279:101–109, 1992.

27. Goodman JE, and McGrath PJ: The epidemiology of pain in children and adolescents: A review. Pain 46:247–264, 1991.

28. Gu X, and Belgrade MJ: Pain in hospitalized patients with medical illnesses. Journal of Pain and Symptom Management 8(1):17–21, 1993.

29. Guest GH, and Drummond PD: Effect of compensation on emotional state and disability in chronic back pain (see comments). Comment in: Pain 48(2):121–123, 1992.

30. Harper AC, Harper DA, Lambert LJ, et al: Symptoms of impairment, disability and handicap in low back pain: A taxonomy. Pain 50:189–195, 1992.

31. Harris L and Associates: Nuprin Pain Report. New York, 1985.

32. Heliovaara M, Sievers K, Impivaaro O, et al: Descriptive epidemiology and public health aspects of low back pain. Ann Med 21(5):327–333, 1989.

33. Helling DK, Lemke JH, Semla TP, et al: Medication use characteristics in the elderly: The Iowa 65+ Rural Health Study. J Am Geriatr Soc 35(1):4–12, 1987.

34. Hopkins A, Menken M, and DeFriese G: A record of patient encounters in neurological practice in the United Kingdom. J Neurol Neurosurg Psychiatry 52(4):436–438, 1989.

35. James FR, Large RG, Bushnell JA, et al: Epidemiology of pain in New Zealand. Pain 44(3):279–283, 1991.

36. Jamison RN, Matt DA, and Parris WC: Effects of time-limited vs unlimited compensation on pain behavior and treatment outcome in low back pain patients. J Psychosomat Res 32(3):277–283, 1988.

37. Johnston CC, Abbott FV, Gray-Donald K, et al: A survey of pain in hospitalized patients aged 4–14 years. Clin J Pain 8(2):154–163, 1992.

38. Kent G: Prevalence vs incidence of the mandibular pain dysfunction syndrome: Implications for epidemiological research. Comm Dent Oral Epidemiol 13(2):113–116, 1985.

39. Khan AA: The prevalence of myofascial pain dysfunction in a lower socio-economic group in Zimbabwe. Comm Dent Health (2):189–192, 1990.

40. Klein BP, Jensen RC, and Sanderson LM: Assessment of workers' compensation claims for back strain/sprains. J Chron Dis:38(8):691–702, 1985.

41. Laslett M, Crothers C, Beattie P, et al: The frequency and incidence of low back pain/sciatica in an urban population. N Z Med J 104(921):424–426, 1991.

42. Lavsky-Shulan M, Wallace RB, Kohout FJ, et al: Prevalence and functional correlates of low back pain in the elderly: The Iowa 65+ Rural Health Study. J Am Geriatr Soc 33(1):23–28, 1985.

43. Lebovits AH, Lefkowitz M, McCarthy D, et al: The prevalence and management of pain in patients

with AIDS: A review of 134 cases. Clin J Pain 5(3):245–248, 1989.

44. Leigh JP, and Sheetz RM: Prevalence of back pain among fulltime United States workers. Br J Ind Med 46(9):651–657, 1989.
45. Linet MS, Stewart WF, Celentano DD, et al: An epidemiologic study of headache among adolescents and young adults. JAMA 261(15):2211–2216, 1989.
46. Linet MS, and Stewart WF: Migraine headache: Epidemiologic perspectives. Epidemiol Rev 6:107–139, 1984.
47. Lloyd MH, Gauld S, and Soutar CA: Epidemiologic study of back pain in miners and office workers. Spine 11(2):136–140, 1986.
48. Locker D, and Grushka M: Response trends and nonresponse bias in a mail survey of oral and facial pain. J Public Health Dent 48(1):20–25, 1988.
49. Locker D, and Grushka M: Prevalence of oral and facial pain and discomfort: Preliminary results of a mail survey. Community Dent and Oral Epidemiol 15(3):169–172, 1987.
50. Loeser JD, and Volinn E: Epidemiology of low back pain. Neurosurg Clin N Am 2(4):713–718, 1991.
51. Marchesi C, DeFerri A, Petrolini N, et al: Prevalence of migraine and muscle tension headache in depressive disorders. J Affect Disord 16(1):33–36, 1989.
52. Mather L, and Mackie J: The incidence of postoperative pain in children. Pain 15(3):271–282, 1983.
53. Melzack R, Abbott FV, Zackson W, et al: Pain on a surgical ward: A survey of the duration and intensity of pain and the effectiveness of medication. Pain 29(1):67–72, 1987.
54. Mendelson G: Compensation and chronic pain. Pain 48(2):125–130, 1992.
55. Mendelson G: Chronic pain, compensation and clinical knowledge. Theor Med 12(3):227–246, 1991.
56. Mior SA, and Diakow PR: Prevalence of back pain in chiropractors. J Manipulative Physiol Ther 10(6):305–309, 1987.
57. Miser AW, Dothage JA, Wesley RA, et al: The prevalence of pain in a pediatric and young adult cancer population. Pain 29(1):73–83, 1987.
58. Nayha S, Videman T, Laakso M, et al: Prevalence of back pain and joint problems in a manufacturing company. J Occup Med 34(2):129–134, 1992.
59. Olsen TL, Anderson RL, Dearwater SR, et al: The epidemiology of low back pain in an adolescent population. Am J Public Health 82(4):606–608, 1992.
60. O'Neill WM, and Sherrard JS: Pain in human immunodeficiency virus disease: A review. Pain 54:3–14, 1993.
61. Osterweis M, Kleinman A, and Mechanic D: The epidemiology of chronic pain and work disability. In Osterweis M, Kleinman A, and Mechanic D (eds): Pain and Disability. National Academy Press, Washington, DC, 1987.
62. Passchier J, and Orlebeke JF: Headaches and stress in schoolchildren: An epidemiological study. Cephalalgia 5:167–176, 1985.
63. Portenoy RK: Cancer pain. Epidemiology and syndromes. Cancer 63:2298–2307, 1989.
64. Rao MB, and Rao CB: Incidence of temporomandibular joint pain dysfunction syndrome in rural population. Int J Oral Surg 10(4):261–265, 1981.

65. Reisbord LS, and Greeland S: Factors associated with self-reported back-pain prevalence: A population-based study. J Chronic Dis 38(8):691–702, 1985.
66. Rotgoltz J, Derazne E, Froom P, et al: Prevalence of low back pain in employees of a pharmaceutical company. Isr J Med Sci 29(8–9):615–618, 1992.
67. Ruda MA: Gender and pain. Pain 53:1–2, 1993.
68. Shi L: A cost-benefit analysis of a California county's back injury prevention program. Public Health Rep 108(2):204–211, 1993.
69. Shortell SM, and Reinhardt S: Creating and executing health care policy in the 1990's. In Improving Health Policy and Management. Health Administration Press, Ann Arbor, 1992.
70. Sillanpaa M: Changes in the prevalence of migraine and other headaches during the first seven school years. Headache 23:15–19, 1983.
71. Skootsky SA, Jaeger B, and Oye RK: Prevalence of myofascial pain in general internal medicine practice. West J Med 151(2):157–160, 1989.
72. Smith GR: The epidemiology and treatment of depression when it coexists with somatoform disorders, somatization, or pain. Gen Hosp Psychiatry 14(4):265–272, 1992.
73. Sokas RK, Spiegelman D, and Wegman DH: Self-reported musculoskeletal complaints among garment workers. Am J Ind Med 15(2):197–206, 1989.
74. Sorensen HT, Rasmussen HH, Moller-Petersen JF, et al: Epidemiology of pain requiring strong analgesics outside hospital in a geographically defined population in Denmark. Dan Med Bull 39(5):464–467, 1992.
75. Steig RL: The cost-effectiveness of pain treatment: Who cares? Clin J Pain 6(4):301–304, 1990.
76. Sudman S, and Bradburn NM: Response effects in surveys. Aldine, Chicago, 1974.
77. Sullivan MD, and Loeser JD: The diagnosis of disability. Treating and rating disability in a pain clinic. Arch Intern Med 152:1829–1835, 1992.
78. Turnbull N, Dornan J, Fletcher B, et al: Prevalence of spinal pain among the staff of a district health authority. Occup Med 42(3):143–148, 1992.
79. Van der Linden SM, and Fahrer H: Occurrence of spinal pain syndromes in a group of apparently healthy and physically fit sportsmen (orienteers). Scand J Rheumatol 17(6):475–481, 1988.
80. Vasudevan S: Clinical perspectives on the relationship between pain and disability. Neurologic Clinics 7(2):429–435, 1989.
81. Von Korff M, Dworkin SF, LeResche L, et al: An epidemiologic comparison of pain complaints. Pain 32(2):173–183, 1988.
82. Waddell G: Occupational low-back pain, illness behavior, and disability. Spine 16(6):683–685, 1991.
83. Webster BS, and Snook SH: The cost of compensable back pain. J Occup Med 32 (1):13–15, 1990.
84. Weir R, Browne GB, Tunks E, et al: A profile of users of specialty pain clinic services: Predictors of use and cost estimates. J Clin Epidemiol 45(12):1399–1415, 1992.
85. Wolfe F, and Cathey MA: The epidemiology of tender points: A prospective study of 1520 patients. J Rheumatol 12(6):1164–1168, 1985.
86. Ziegler DK, Hassanein RS, and Couch J: Characteristics of life headache in a non-clinic population. Neurology 27:265–269, 1977.

PART 2

Pain Syndromes

CHAPTER 4

HEADACHE AND FACIAL PAIN

Ronald M. Kanner, M.D.

Headache is the most common recurrent pain complaint.[125] A British study[266] showed that approximately 80 percent of the general population had experienced headache during the prior year; about one-third used an analgesic during the prior 14 days, and one-third of the latter group reported at least one "very severe or almost intolerable headache" in the prior year. In another study, fewer than 10 percent of a non–clinic population denied having headache.[274]

Despite the high prevalence of headache, fewer than 10 percent of patients with headache seek medical attention, and an even smaller number are sent for neurologic consultation or further investigation.[120,123] This small fraction, however, still accounts for about 25 percent of patient visits to neurologists.[62,121] Structural intracranial pathology accounts for less than 1 percent of these visits,[122] so the vast majority of headache patients are managed medically and psychologically. Emphasis should be put on the word "managed," because headaches, like other chronic pain syndromes, are rarely cured.

CLASSIFICATION OF HEADACHES

The real need for classification is to aid in communication among clinicians and investigators.[1,53,236] Unfortunately, there is no unifying theory of etiology, pathogenesis, or diagnostic criteria and, consequently, a fully satisfactory classification does not exist.

In 1988, the Headache Classification Committee of the International Headache Society (IHS) published the "Classification and Diagnostic Criteria for Headache Disorders, Cranial Neuralgias, and Facial Pain."[52] They defined 13 categories of headache (Table 4–1).

This classification proposes a diagnosis for each type of headache and recognizes that most headache patients have more than one distinct type. Although these criteria, which are now widely accepted, facilitate accurate communication among investigators, the clinician need not be familiar with each of the categories. For reference purposes, the full classification is listed at the end of the chapter (see Appendix I).

Even the headaches that were thought to fit rigid criteria have been undergoing a blurring of boundaries. Traditionally, migraine headache has been divided into classic (with aura) and common (without aura). This division, however, may not reflect fundamentally different pathophysiologies.[194,270] Simi-

Table 4–1. IHS CLASSIFICATION AND DIAGNOSTIC CRITERIA FOR HEADACHE DISORDERS, CRANIAL NEURALGIAS, AND FACIAL PAIN

1. Migraine
2. Tension-type headache
3. Cluster headache and chronic paroxysmal hemicrania
4. Miscellaneous headaches unassociated with structural lesion
5. Headache associated with head trauma
6. Headache associated with vascular disorders
7. Headache associated with nonvascular intracranial disorder
8. Headache associated with substances or their withdrawal
9. Headache associated with noncephalic infection
10. Headache associated with metabolic disorder
11. Headache or facial pain associated with disorder of cranium, neck, eyes, ears, nose, sinuses, teeth, mouth, or other facial or cranial structures
12. Cranial neuralgias, nerve trunk pain, and deafferentation pain
13. Headache not classifiable

Source: Darof RB: Classification and diagnostic criteria for headache disorders, cranial neuralgias and facial pain. Headache Classification Committee of the International Headache Society. Cephalalgia 8 (suppl 7): 1–96, 1988, with permission.

larly, a clear line may not divide migraine from tension headaches.[8,171]

NOCICEPTION IN HEADACHE

In most headache syndromes, the nociceptive substrate, if it exists, remains unclear. The scalp, extracranial vessels, periosteum, sinuses, meninges, and large intracranial vessels are innervated by nociceptors. The tentorium cerebelli and some of the supratentorial structures are innervated by the trigeminal nerve. Pathologic processes that affect these structures tend to refer pain to the eye and forehead. Retro-orbital pain is often referred from the cavernous sinus, the tentorium, or the carotid artery. Infratentorial structures are innervated mainly by the glossopharyngeal and vagus nerves. Brain parenchyma is not pain-sensitive, and the pain associated with space-occupying lesions localizes to the appropriate side in only half the cases.

CLINICAL APPROACH TO THE PATIENT WITH HEADACHE

Accurate diagnosis depends on a directed clinical history, physical examination, and judicious use of ancillary tests. The assessment has three main goals:
1. To identify rapidly the small subset who have intracranial disease or headache as part of a systemic illness
2. To classify accurately the nonstructural headache syndromes and the individual headache attacks
3. To institute diagnosis-specific therapy

Ninety percent of headache diagnoses are made on the basis of the history (Table 4–2); another 5 to 6 percent are elucidated by the physical examination or ancillary tests, and the rest cannot be diagnosed. Salient historical data include temporal characteristics, localization and quality of pain, exacerbating and relieving factors, associated symptoms, family history, history of other pain syndromes, and present medical history. These data usually establish the headache syndrome and determine whether the current episode is a part of that syndrome.[51] Neuroimaging (magnetic resonance imaging [MRI] or computed tomography [CT]) is

Table 4–2. **HEADACHE CHARACTERISTICS**

	Migraine	Tension	Cluster	TMJ	TIC	AFP	TA	Tumor
Age at onset	15–25	Variable	20–30	20–40	>50	20–40	>60	Any
Childhood history	Common	15%	No	No	No	No	No	No
Family history	Yes	±	No	No	No	No	No	No
Sex distribution	F>M	F>M	M>F	F>M	F>M	F>M	±	M = F
Aura	+Classic	No	No	No	No	No	No	No
Pain character	Throbbing	Aching	Stabbing	Aching	Lancinating	Dull	Ache	Ache
Pain distribution	± Unilateral	Diffuse	Retro-orbital	Ear	Trigeminal	Diffuse	Temporal	Variable
Pain duration	Hr–days	Hr–constant	20–40 min	Variable	Seconds	Constant	Constant	Worse AM
Associated symptoms	Nausea Photophobia Phonophobia	Depression	Horner's Lacrimation Coryza	Jaw click Tenderness	None	Depression	Malaise High ESR	Focality

Key: TMJ = temporomandibular joint dysfunction; TIC = tic douloureux; AFP = atypical facial pain; TA = temporal arteritis; ESR = erythrocyte sedimentation rate.

rarely helpful in the management of patients with a clear headache history and a normal neurologic examination and may turn up an incidental lesion in a vanishingly small number of patients.[92]

On the basis of temporal characteristics, headache syndromes may be classified as acute, subacute, chronic recurrent, and chronic daily (Table 4–3).

ACUTE HEADACHE

Subarachnoid Hemorrhage

The sudden onset of an extremely severe headache is the hallmark of subarachnoid hemorrhage. Major subarachnoid hemorrhages may be preceded by a number of less severe headaches that are presumably signs of smaller hemorrhages ("sentinel hemorrhages") or expansion of an aneurysm.[136] The diagnosis of subarachnoid hemorrhage should be sus-

pected in any previously healthy patient who experiences one or several acute severe headaches. Such a patient should immediately undergo an unenhanced computed tomography (CT) scan, which shows subarachnoid blood in most patients with ruptured aneurysms.[265] If the scan is negative, lumbar puncture is usually needed to exclude the diagnosis. This is particularly important if the headache occurred more than four days before the examination; beyond this time, subarachnoid blood may no longer be demonstrable on CT.

The acute pain of subarachnoid hemorrhage is due to activation of meningeal nociceptors. Pain tends to be occipital and diffuse, with associated meningismus. The initial pain subsides with the standard early measures for subarachnoid hemorrhage, including bed rest. Small doses of opioid analgesics provide mild sedation and pain relief.

Cerebrovascular Disease

Headache is a common concomitant of cerebrovascular disease.[72,104,207] Edmeads found that 25 percent of 400 consecutive patients with transient ischemic attack or stroke had headache at the time of the event.[72] Clinical presentation or outcome was not specifically determined by the nature of the headache.[207]

Carotid artery dissection presents with pain referred to the eye and cheek. Fisher's review[86] indicated that pain usually precedes other manifestations including Horner's syndrome, visual disturbance, and hemispheric symptoms. Acute severe retro-orbital pain in a previously healthy person with no history of cluster headaches should prompt a search for structural carotid disease. Cluster headaches have a similar presentation (see following).

Acutely increased intracranial pressure is usually due to a rapidly enlarging intracranial mass or to sudden obstruction of cerebrospinal fluid (CSF) pathways. Pain is assumed to be due to stretching of the meninges, falx, and tentorium, and to distortion of the vessels at the base of the brain. Supratentorial expanding masses tend to refer pain to the anterior two-thirds of the head, and infratentorial masses tend to refer to the occiput. Acute obstruction of CSF flow

Table 4–3. **TEMPORAL CLASSIFICATION OF HEADACHES**

Acute headache syndromes include:
1. Subarachnoid hemorrhage
2. Occlusive cerebrovascular disease
3. Acutely increased or decreased intracranial pressure
4. Meningitis and encephalitis
5. Local infections and inflammations
6. Ocular causes
7. Any first episode of the syndromes listed below

Subacute headache syndromes include:
1. Expanding mass lesions
2. Headache with systemic disease
3. Increased intracranial pressure

Chronic recurrent headache syndromes include:
1. Migraine syndromes
2. Cluster
3. Chronic paroxysmal hemicrania
4. "Tension and tension-vascular"
5. Postconcussive headache
6. Facial pain syndromes
7. Miscellaneous syndromes

Chronic daily headache syndrome

produces a diffuse head pain. Pain increases with bending over, Valsalva maneuvers, and lying supine, presumably as a result of further increases in intracranial pressure. Therapy for the headache depends on identification and treatment of the underlying cause.

Acutely decreased intracranial pressure can occur after lumbar puncture or CSF leaks of other types. The headache occasionally occurs without clear evidence of dural tear. The headache is characteristically positional,[208] relieved by recumbency, and exacerbated by standing. The amount of time a patient remains recumbent after lumbar puncture apparently has little effect on the incidence of the headache.[45] One study[149] demonstrated an increased likelihood of postspinal headache in young women and patients with a history of travel sickness. Small needles, which produce a small hole in the dura, are less likely to result in headache than are large needles.

Most post–lumbar puncture headaches resolve spontaneously, within a few days.[84] Forced hydration may be of some benefit, and caffeine sodium benzoate (500 mg in 1 L of fluid) has been reported to provide complete relief.[89] In extreme cases, when continued drainage is suspected as the cause, epidural blood patches may be used.[96,198] In the latter procedure, 15 to 20 mL of autologous blood is injected into the epidural space. This should be done no sooner than 24 hr after the initial puncture to avoid the risk of contaminating the subarachnoid space with blood. The procedure is contraindicated in patients with blood dyscrasia, anticoagulant therapy, or local infection.

The headache of meningitis is associated with the other signs of meningeal irritation, such as stiff neck and Kernig's and Brudzinski's signs. In acute bacterial meningitis, the headache is overshadowed by the acute illness, with the rapid onset of obtundation. Treatment of the headache syndrome is subordinate to rapid treatment of the underlying bacterial infection. Despite adequate therapy, one-third of patients cured of bacterial meningitis go on to have persistent headaches.[32] These patients have no signs of continued infection or increased intracranial pressure. A small fraction of patients develop subdural collections that require drainage.

Viral meningitis may present as an acute headache with a paucity of other signs. The headache is more severe than would be expected from a febrile illness, and photophobia and pain on movement of the eyes may occur. Stiff neck is absent in a majority of cases. The most common causes are enteroviral infections with either echovirus or Coxsackievirus.[54] An erythematous rash is a common accompaniment and helps in establishing the diagnosis. Cerebrospinal fluid shows a lymphocytic pleocytosis, with slight elevations in protein and a normal glucose.

Human immununodeficiency virus (HIV) can also present with a picture of aseptic meningitis and headache.[79] This is usually an early manifestation of the disease and may occur before seroconversion.

Treatment of meningitis-related headache is symptomatic. Patients should be kept in quiet, dimly lit rooms and given a nonsteroidal anti-inflammatory drug or an opioid analgesic.

The headache associated with cerebritis or encephalitis is almost invariably associated with some alteration in mentation and/or focal neurologic signs. Otherwise, it is indistinguishable from the headache of aseptic meningitis. Herpes simplex is the most common cause and produces the only encephalitis that occurs sporadically throughout the year, in all regions of the world and in patients of all ages.[133] Herpes simplex virus has a predilection for the temporal lobes; this encephalitis is characterized by a rapidly progressive headache, personality changes, aphasia, or temporal lobe seizures.

Acute infection or inflammation of local structures (paranasal sinuses or other pain-sensitive structures) can present with headache. These syndromes usually have some localizing sign or symptom that points to the involved structure. The hallmarks are fever and focal tenderness; in severe cases, direct spread of the infection can cause oculomotor paresis or cranial neuropathies.

The clinical presentation associated with sinusitis is varied.[158] Acute frontal sinusitis usually presents with fever and frontal headache. Without effective treatment, obtundation may ensue. There is tenderness over the frontal sinuses and the patient appears systemically ill. The most common causative organisms are *Staphylococcus aureus* and *Streptococcus pneumoniae*. Maxillary sinusitis also presents with pain and tenderness localized to the area of the sinus. Cerebral symptoms are uncommon, and the diagnosis is easily made on plain radiographs, which show a fluid collection in the sinus.

Sphenoid or ethmoid sinusitis presents a difficult diagnostic problem. Headache is the most common presenting symptom, but it is poorly localized and may be multifocal. The diagnostic clues are hypesthesia or hyperesthesia in the ophthalmic or maxillary dermatomes, pus in the area of the middle or superior turbinate, and severe headache.[28] Predisposing factors include deep-sea diving and cocaine sniffing. In a series of 15 cases,[159] the six cases that were diagnosed quickly were treated with intravenous antibiotics and made an uneventful recovery; delay in the diagnosis of the other nine led to serious complications (cavernous sinus thrombosis or meningitis) and death. Early recognition is, therefore, essential, and suspected cases should be treated empirically with a high dose of penicillinase-resistant penicillin. If symptoms do not subside quickly, surgical drainage should be performed. Chronic sinusitis, occasionally a cause of headaches in children,[82] is discussed more fully later.

Noninfectious, inflammatory cranial syndromes can also present with headache. The Tolosa-Hunt syndrome presents as orbitofrontal pain associated with oculomotor palsies. It is a steroid-responsive, idiopathic, granulomatous inflammation that is usually diagnosed by the process of exclusion.[137] High-resolution CT[150] and, presumably, MRI demonstrate changes in the apex of the orbit or cavernous sinus in this condition.

Although ocular causes of headache are common complaints in office practice, the incidence of eye pathology as a cause of headache is low. Acute headache is a feature of angle-closure glaucoma, but most patients with chronically increased intraocular pressure (glaucoma) are asymptomatic. Acute glaucoma usually is due to narrowing of the angle between the pupil and the cornea; in 5 percent of patients it results from processes that block the outflow of aqueous humor.[262] In predisposed patients, pupillary dilatation may precipitate an acute increase in intraocular pressure, with severe orbital pain, headache, conjunctival injection, and visual disturbance.[262] It should be treated emergently

with the intravenous administration of mannitol (50 g in a 20 percent solution), an orally administered carbonic anhydrase inhibitor (Diamox, 250 mg QID), and pilocarpine (4 percent), applied topically; an ophthalmologic consultation should be obtained, and surgery is sometimes necessary.

SUBACUTE HEADACHE SYNDROMES

Expanding Mass Lesions

Expanding intracranial mass lesions produce pain by distorting pain-sensitive intracranial structures. The most common lesions are cerebral metastases from systemic cancers.[276] Head pain is diffuse, localizing to the side of the lesion in only half of cases.[200] Supratentorial tumors tend to refer pain anteriorly, sometimes to the orbit. Infratentorial tumors are likely to cause diffuse, occipital, or nuchal pain. Pain is intense in the early morning and may subside as the day goes on. This pattern may be due to increases in intracranial pressure that occur with recumbency and sleep-related CO_2 retention. Initially, the pain responds well to aspirin or acetaminophen, and the response to steroids is usually dramatic. The headache generally increases in severity over days to weeks.

Fewer than half the patients with expanding mass lesions complain of focal weakness, but a hemiparesis can be found in nearly two-thirds.[200] Similarly, cognitive deficits are not a common complaint, but subtle changes can be detected in more than half.

Pseudotumor Cerebri

Increased intracranial pressure without a space-occupying lesion presents as diffuse head pain, which is usually exacerbated by Valsalva maneuvers and bending forward. The pathogenesis of this pain is not clear. In healthy volunteers, intrathecal infusions that raise CSF pressure to over 600 mm do not evoke pain.[148]

Pseudotumor cerebri (benign intracranial hypertension) is primarily a disease of obese young women characterized by intense generalized headache.[130,231] Numerous predisposing factors have been identified.[231] The diagnosis is established in a patient with headache and papilledema by the finding of normal imaging studies and elevated CSF pressure without other CSF abnormalities. CT or MRI shows the ventricles to be normal or small, sometimes appearing "slitlike." In long-standing pseudotumor, an empty sella may be found.[88]

The pathogenesis of the increased intracranial pressure in pseudotumor is not understood. Decreased CSF reabsorption is the most widely held theory.[165]

Transient visual symptoms are common in patients with pseudotumor cerebri. Visual obscurations occur in 5 to 50 percent of patients, either on the basis of posterior cerebral artery compression or direct pressure on the optic nerves. Permanent visual loss is reported in 4 to 23 percent of cases,[242] with a significant correlation between transient visual obscurations and permanent visual loss,[231] but with no relationship between visual loss and duration of symptoms.[88]

Headache relief in patients with pseudotumor cerebri or other causes of diffusely increased CSF pressure (e.g., chronic meningitis of any cause) depends on lowering intracranial pressure. As CSF is removed, headache improves, but because CSF fluid is produced at a rate of 0.4 mL per minute, the amount removed is rapidly replaced. A large-bore spinal needle can produce in the dura a large hole that may create a fistula for continued drainage into the subcutaneous tissue and prolong the analgesic benefits of lumbar puncture. This approach, however, may be complicated by a low-pressure or "post–lumbar puncture" headache, as described earlier. Some patients with pseudotumor cerebri recover after repeated lumbar punctures.[2]

A variety of pharmacologic approaches have also been advocated for the treatment of pseudotumor cerebri. Hyperosmotic agents such as glycerol (15 to 60 mg per day) have been used, but weight gain may be an unwanted effect in an already obese population. Prednisone, in doses of 20 to 60 mg per day, will relieve the headache within a few days, but prolonged therapy is more problematic, and some studies have suggested that prolonged steroid therapy may actually cause pseudotumor. Although papilledema may resolve quickly, it often recurs when steroids are stopped.[46] Carbonic anhydrase inhibitor diuretics (acetazolamide) presumably slow production of CSF at the membrane level in the choroid plexus. Other diuretics such as furosemide have also been efficacious.[177]

In particularly refractory cases of pseudotumor cerebri, lumboperitoneal shunting may be used.[264] In one case, acute visual loss occurred after shunting, presumably from retinal hemorrhage. If papilledema does not resolve, the sheath of the optic nerve can be opened to prevent further visual loss.[242] Although vision is stabilized initially, it may deteriorate after months to years.[252]

Temporal Arteritis

Temporal arteritis is another serious acute or subacute cause of headache. This disorder usually occurs in the elderly; biopsy-proven cases in patients under the age of 60 are exceedingly rare.[23] Headache, usually aching and poorly localized, may be accompanied by temporal artery tenderness, jaw claudication, and constitutional symptoms.[125] Polymyalgia rheumatica is present in about half of cases.[4] Visual loss, which results from retinal artery occlusion, is the most common serious complication.[27] Inflammation in other extracranial arteries rarely may lead to occlusion or rupture.[161] Involvement of intracranial arteries is uncommon.

An elevated erythrocyte sedimentation rate (ESR) is a hallmark of temporal arteritis, but cases have been reported with only modest elevations of the ESR.[80] Pathologic examination of medium-sized arteries shows a chronic panarteritis, with multinucleated giant cells. Given the potential for sampling error, a negative biopsy does not exclude the diagnosis.[227]

Temporal arteritis usually subsides over a few years, but high doses of corticosteroids are needed initially. Prednisone should be started in doses of 60 to 100 mg per day, and this dose should be continued for 4 to 6 weeks. Symptoms usually subside within a few days, and the ESR declines during subsequent weeks. If there is both clinical and laboratory improvement, the dose can be lowered gradually.[22]

CHRONIC RECURRENT HEADACHE SYNDROMES

Migraine Syndromes

Dorland's[65] defines migraine as "an often familial symptom complex of periodic attacks of vascular headache, usually temporal and unilateral in onset, commonly associated with irritability, nausea, vomiting, constipation or diarrhea, and often photophobia; attacks are preceded by constriction of the cranial arteries, usually with resultant prodromal sensory (especially ocular) symptoms, and commence with the vasodilatation that follows."

The Ad Hoc Committee of 1962[1] recognized three migraine syndromes: *common migraine,* which is migraine without focal neurologic symptoms; *classic migraine,* which has sharply defined, transient visual and other sensory or motor prodromes, or both; and *hemiplegic migraine,* which is characterized by sensory and motor phenomena that persist during and after the headache.

The International Headache Society (IHS) classification defines migraine without aura (previously used terms were "common migraine" and "hemicrania simplex") as: "idiopathic, recurring headache disorder manifesting in attacks lasting 4–72 hours. Typical characteristics of headache are unilateral location, pulsating quality, moderate or severe intensity, aggravation by routine physical activity, and association with nausea, photo- and phonophobia." The symptoms that provide the best discrimination between migraine and other headache subtypes are photophobia, phonophobia, osmophobia, and gastrointestinal symptoms.[174,214] The diagnostic criteria are seen in Table 4–4.

This definition is useful but has one significant drawback. If at least five similar attacks are required to make the diagnosis, patients with infrequent headaches can go for years without a diagnosis, although they clearly have migraine. Despite this drawback, the criteria provide uniform terminology for international trials and a method for targeting a group of headache patients in need of care.[196]

PATHOPHYSIOLOGY

Migraine has been considered a "vascular" headache since the early work of Graham

Table 4–4. **IHS MIGRAINE CRITERIA**

A. At least 5 attacks fulfill B–D.
B. Headache attacks last 4–72 hours (untreated or unsuccessfully treated).
C. Headache has at least two of the following characteristics:
   1. Unilateral location.
   2. Pulsating quality.
   3. Moderate or severe intensity (inhibits or prohibits daily activities).
   4. Aggravation by walking stairs or similar routine physical activity.
D. During headache at least one of the following occurs:
   1. Nausea and/or vomiting.
   2. Photophobia and phonophobia.
E. At least one of the following is true:
   1. History, physical and neurologic examinations do not suggest one of the disorders listed in groups 5–11 (of Appendix).
   2. History and/or physical and/or neurologic examinations do suggest such disorder, but it is ruled out by appropriate investigations.
   3. Such disorder is present, but migraine attacks do not occur for the first time in close temporal relation to the disorder.

and Wolff.[106,108,263] The vascular theory held that an initial phase of vasoconstriction brought with it the cerebral symptoms of classic migraine (migraine with aura). This was followed by a vasodilatory phase that was accompanied by the typical, pounding headache of migraine. The appropriate changes in blood flow can be demonstrated in a classic migraine attack,[100,153,154,246] and the pain relief provided by vasoconstriction further supports a vascular hypothesis.

Alternative theories have also been proposed. According to one competing theory, the vascular changes are actually secondary to cerebral events.[152,156,197,202] This model states that a form of "spreading depression" is the primary phenomenon at the core of migraine and reflects a central neuronal disorder. The observation that pain may or may not accompany dilatation of extracranial arteries supports the need for such an alternative theory.

Olesen[195] proposes a "vascular-supraspinal-myogenic (VSM) model" for migraine, in which pain is determined by the sum of nociception from cephalic arteries and pericranial myofascial tissues. This nociception is primed by the release of vasoactive and algogenic substances, including prostaglandin, histamine, serotonin, and tyramine.

Considerable circumstantial evidence suggests that prostaglandins are involved in migraine pain. Prostaglandin E compounds are potent vasodilators, particularly in the extracranial arteries. Intravenous infusion of PGE_1 can cause migrainelike headaches (including visual symptoms and nausea), even in patients who do not suffer from migraine. Nonsteroidal anti-inflammatory drugs, which are potent prostaglandin inhibitors, are efficacious in aborting migraine.[124] Serotonin is a prostaglandin-releasing factor, and the roles of serotonin and prostaglandins in migraine may be interwoven.

Intravenous infusion of histamine produces severe headaches in nearly all migraineurs, but a similar response occurs in only 50 percent of tension headache sufferers and in no normal controls.[139] Changes in histamine also can be shown in tissues and blood of patients with migraine.[114] Nonetheless, antihistaminic agents are not uniformly successful in preventing or aborting migraine attacks,[13,166] and the role of histamine in the pathogenesis of migraine is unclear.

Serotonin, the best studied of the vasoactive substances in migraine, is a neurotransmitter in an endogenous pain suppression system.[7,19,213] Although it is a potent vasoconstrictor in the cerebral circulation,[164] central serotonergic mechanisms also could explain vasodilatation and head pain.[101] Free and platelet-bound serotonin levels drop during headaches,[12] and migraine headaches can be precipitated by drugs that release platelet serotonin. Antiserotonin drugs, such as methysergide, are effective in migraine prophylaxis.[49] Paradoxically, headache also can be relieved by serotonin.[10,31]

Although the data pertaining to serotonin in migraine pathophysiology are conflicting, changes in this neurotransmitter could potentially explain many of the phenomena that characterize this disorder. Raskin[213] has observed that dysmodulation of serotonin receptors in the myenteric plexus could account for gastrointestinal symptoms, that modulation of serotonin receptors by ovarian hormones could explain the changes seen with menses and pregnancy, that the decrease of receptors with aging could explain the tendency for migraine to improve with aging, and that the change in firing of serotonin neurons with sleep could explain the influence of sleep on migraine. Further studies are needed to clarify the role of this substance and its receptors in migraine.

CLINICAL PRESENTATION

Migraine is a chronic, recurrent headache syndrome. The frequency of attacks is variable; the modal number of attacks per month is four.[240] Untreated, headaches last from a few hours to a few days. Sleep often relieves an attack.[30] Although characteristically described as unilateral and pounding, Olesen[193] reported that only 44 percent of his 678 patients with migraine reported hemicranial pain; 36 percent were either holocephalic or bifrontal. Valsalva, head movement, and exercise exacerbate the pain, whereas pressure over the temporal or carotid artery usually alleviates it. Gastrointestinal symptoms, usually nausea and vomiting, are the most common accompaniments. Photophobia is the next most common complaint.

A parental history of migraine is five times more common in headache patients than in headache-free subjects.[272] The inheritance pattern, however, is unclear, and twin studies have yielded conflicting results.[163,275]

In a series of 500 migraine patients, Selby and Lance[240] found that 36 percent had visual disturbances. Other estimates are lower, and it is generally accepted that approximately 20 percent of migraine sufferers have some type of visual prodrome (classic migraine; migraine with aura). Photopsia (small areas of light) and scintillating scotomata are the most common visual symptoms. "Blurred vision" is a common and unexplained complaint. The aura of migraine lasts less than an hour and resolves entirely. Rare patients experience "prolonged aura," with visual disturbances, sensory changes, or hemiparesis lasting up to one week. In the old terminology, prolonged aura was called "complicated migraine." A number of these patients have small infarctions on CT scan.[17,35]

Ophthalmoplegic migraine[25,70] is a rare variant in which ophthalmoparesis accompanies a prolonged headache. The age range is about the same as it is for other forms of migraine, and this form is usually preceded by one of the more common forms. The differential diagnosis for this syndrome should include Tolosa-Hunt syndrome, carotid aneurysm, and other forms of painful ophthalmoplegia.

In "basilar migraine," the aura is referable to the brainstem and is characterized by a mixture of visual symptoms (often total blindness), dysarthria, vertigo, tinnitus, decreased hearing, double vision, ataxia, bilateral paresthesias, bilateral paresis, or decreased level of consciousness.[24] Although brainstem symptoms may occur in other forms of migraine, the diagnosis of basilar migraine is made when the events are very stereotyped, are followed by a headache, resolve spontaneously, and no other cause is found.

Many factors have been reported to precipitate headache in predisposed individuals,[187,188,206,241] but no single factor is causative across the broad range of migraine patients. The clearest example of this variability occurs with specific food sensitivities.[205] Occasional patients are sensitive to chocolate and will have headaches produced reliably with ingestion of small amounts; those who are not sensitive can eat chocolate without limit. This observation suggests that there is little basis for drastic changes in diet among most headache sufferers. Other common migraine precipitants include hormonal changes, hunger, sleep deprivation, and stress.

The course of the migraine syndrome is highly variable. The prevalence of migraine is approximately 6 percent among men and 15 to 17 percent among women.[253] Migraine occasionally begins in early childhood,[26] but most patients present in adolescence or early adult life.[228] Partially because migraine affects patients during their prime working years, the financial impact can be enormous and must take into account not only the direct expenses of medical care but lost wages as well.[57] Fewer than 10 percent of patients have onset after age 50.[58,169] Migraine attacks tend to become less frequent and less intense with advancing age and with menopause. At any point, but commonly after prolonged treatment, migraine may evolve into chronic daily headache.[176]

DIAGNOSTIC EVALUATION

Migraine is a clinical diagnosis, and imaging studies are needed only to exclude other diagnoses. When imaging studies are performed, abnormalities are commonly found. Even in migraine patients without focal neurologic deficits, CT reveals subclinical areas of infarction more often than in age-matched controls,[35] and MRI often shows white matter foci.[147] These lesions are usually felt to be clinically insignificant. Rarely, a stroke may present with clinical features of migraine and, occasionally, migraine may be a cause of stroke.[269]

In today's litigious climate, it is probably wise to perform a CT or MRI at the time of first presentation or if there has been a significant change in the character of the headache. As noted earlier, however, incidental tumors or AVMs turn up in fewer than 0.4 percent of migraine patients.[220] Conversely, a retrospective study showed that fewer than 6 percent of patients referred to a neurosurgeon for intracerebral lesions had presented with isolated headaches.[268]

Electroencephalograms are more often abnormal in migraine than they are in the general population,[102,116] but the findings have no diagnostic value. Patients with epilepsy, however, are more than twice as likely to develop migraine as are their relatives without epilepsy.[160] Furthermore, the prevalence of epilepsy in patients with migraine is far greater than that seen in the general population.[5] The explanation for this comorbidity may rest in a common "state of neuronal hyperexcitability."[160]

The association of arteriovenous malformation with migraine headache is not strong enough to warrant angiography in patients who do not have other signs or symptoms to suggest a lesion. In cases of ophthalmoplegic or basilar migraine, however, arteriography may be required to rule out a causative lesion.

Lumbar puncture is rarely indicated unless meningitis is suspected. Patients with uncomplicated migraine occasionally have a mild, mononuclear pleocytosis[55] in association with a headache; this finding is more common in patients with complicated migraine.

TREATMENT

The pharmacologic management of migraine pain is divided into abortive and prophylactic therapies.[20] Abortive measures attempt to limit the intensity and duration of a given episode, whereas prophylactic measures decrease the overall frequency and intensity of attacks.

Abortive Therapies. The ergot alkaloids are vasoconstrictors that were initially used in migraine on the basis of the theory that the pain was due to vasodilatation. Early studies confirmed that ergotamine could produce vasoconstriction in the external carotid artery and that this vasoconstriction was related to headache relief.[6] The vasoconstriction may be mediated through a direct effect on arterial serotonin receptors.[3]

Ergotamine, ergonovine, methylergonovine, and dihydroergotamine are the most commonly used ergots.[245] Ergotamine can be administered orally, rectally, sublingually, or by inhalant. *Ergonovine is given orally, and dihydroergotamine can be given intramuscularly or intravenously. They are most effective when given early in the attack. Sensitivity, both for pain relief and for side effects, varies widely among patients, and individual titration of dose is mandatory. An initial loading dose should be given at the first sign of a headache.

The vasoconstriction produced by ergots is not limited to the cranial circulation. Acroparesthesia, abdominal cramps, and diarrhea are common side effects. The most serious manifestation of ergotism, gangrene of the limbs, is very rare. Symptoms of preexisting angina and peripheral vascular disease may be worsened after treatment with ergot preparations, and these conditions contraindicate the use of these drugs. Cerebral and myocardial infarctions are rare adverse effects.[103] Dihydroergotamine has primarily venoconstrictor effects, with less influence than ergotamine on arterial circulation.[215]

Patients with severe, prolonged migraine attacks require parenteral therapy.[245] A combination of an antiemetic and dihydroergotamine (DHE) can be effective.[216] Metoclopramide (10 mg) is given initially, followed by DHE (0.5 mg). If nausea is severe or the headache ceases, no further DHE is given for 8 hours. The object is to determine the subnauseating dose of DHE, then repeat the combination of metoclopramide and DHE every 8 hours for 2 days. The patient can then be put on a prophylactic regimen.

Ergotamine can produce paradoxic responses, both acutely and chronically. With prolonged administration, tolerance and physical dependence can be a problem.[91,237] Frequent use can lead to rebound headache. Suspicion of this phenomenon necessitates withdrawal of ergot preparations.[233] Rebound phenomenon can also follow prolonged use of short-acting analgesics or sedative/hypnotics. Again, the difficult course of drug withdrawal is indicated, which often requires hospitalization, substitution of a longer-acting drug (e.g., phenobarbital for butalbital and methadone for codeine or oxycodone), and gradual tapering of the dose.

Sumatriptan is a recently tested 5-HT$_1$ receptor agonist that aborts acute migraine when administered orally in doses of 70 to 280 mg,[15] subcutaneously in doses of 6 to 8 mg,[254] and intranasally in doses of 20 mg.[85] One large study showed oral sumatriptan to be well tolerated and more effective than an oral ergotamine/caffeine product.[191] Nausea, vomiting, and a bitter taste are the most common side effects with oral dosing.

A nonsteroidal anti-inflammatory drug (NSAID) or an opioid can effectively abort acute attacks in some patients. For example, oral naproxen (375 mg) has been shown to abort acute headache.[208] Ketorolac is an NSAID with a parenteral formulation, and an intramuscular dose of 60 mg may be particularly useful when headache is complicated by nausea and vomiting. In more refractory cases, an opioid in a dose equivalent to 10 mg of parenteral morphine can be effective. Opioid-induced somnolence is an added benefit, because sleep itself can often break a migraine attack.

A neuroleptic may also be a useful abortive

*Because of problems with stability, the sublingual preparation is off the market; the suppository is widely available.

therapy. For example, a double-blind, placebo-controlled study of emergency room patients[131] demonstrated that prochlorperazine (Compazine), 10 mg intravenously, can be effective in acute migraine and severe tension headaches. Metoclopramide and chlorpromazine also have demonstrated efficacy as abortive therapy. Hydroxyzine, 100 mg intramuscularly, has been shown to provide analgesia similar to 8 mg of morphine and has an additive analgesic effect when combined with morphine.[21] Oral hydroxyzine is an effective antinauseant and tranquilizer but has no proven analgesic efficacy.

Migraine patients characteristically report feeling much better after a brief nap.[232] Although sleep deprivation is a well-recognized precipitant of migraine, "deep sleep deprivation" may decrease migraine frequency and severity.[98] A combination of sedative/hypnotic drugs and antiemetics can be used to abort an acute attack.[44] Thermal biofeedback and relaxation techniques can also be used to lessen the intensity of individual attacks in well-trained subjects.[42,116]

Prophylactic Therapies

Beta Blockers. β-Adrenergic blocking agents reduce the frequency and severity of migraine headaches and are the most widely used drugs for the treatment of recurrent migraine.[260] Beta blocking agents may modulate vascular tone,[248] platelet function,[113] central neural transmission,[64] and serotonergic activity. In accordance with the vascular theory of migraine, they could block the painful vasodilatory phase of the attack. These drugs also may inhibit peripheral release of serotonin from platelets, which has also been implicated in the pathogenesis of migraine.[132] Beta blockers inhibit central hyperactive catecholaminergic neurons.[213,238]

Propranolol has been extensively studied in the prophylaxis of migraine. Doses must be titrated from the usual starting dosage of 10 mg four times daily; many patients need as much as 320 mg a day. After initial titration of the dose, the drug may be given as infrequently as two or three times a day. If no relief is obtained after treatment with 320 mg daily for 3 to 4 weeks, a different type of prophylaxis should be tried. Other beta blockers, such as atenolol, metoprolol, timolol, and nadolol, are also efficacious but are less widely used.[203]

Beta blockers are contraindicated in congestive heart failure and asthma. Bradycardia, fatigue, and mild somnolence are common side effects and usually do not require discontinuation of the drug. If side effects are intolerable or the drug is ineffective, the dose must be tapered slowly, over a period of 2 to 3 weeks. Abrupt discontinuation in patients with cardiovascular disease may lead to angina or myocardial infarction.

Methysergide. Methysergide, a semisynthetic ergot alkaloid, is a potent peripheral antagonist of serotonin.[190] Although this compound presumably has a mechanism of action similar to other ergot drugs, it may be effective in some patients who have not responded well to routine ergot therapy.[64,66] Dosing is started at 1 mg two or three times a day and increased gradually to a maximum of 2 mg four times a day. Patients have been treated with as much as 14 mg a day, but side effects are very common at these levels. Even at routine therapeutic levels, 30 percent of patients experience side effects, most commonly nausea, muscle cramps, or abdominal pain.[216] Side effects are most commonly reported early in the course of therapy. The potential for vasoconstriction contraindicates use of the drug in patients with peripheral vascular or cardiovascular disease.

Prolonged use of methysergide may be associated with idiopathic fibrotic complications such as retroperitoneal fibrosis, pulmonary fibrosis, and endocardial fibrosis.[107] Fibrosis has been reported after more than 6 months of use, usually in doses of over 8 mg per day. If patients require long-term prophylactic therapy, drug holidays of 1 to 2 months should be provided after every few months of use.

Tricyclic Antidepressants. Epidemiologic studies have demonstrated a significant comorbidity between migraine and depression.[33] Amitriptyline decreases the frequency and intensity of attacks in patients with migraine.[47] Theoretically, this effect relates to inhibition of serotonin uptake in pain-modulating neural pathways.[14] Although side effects such as dry mouth and sedation are common, they are typically transitory and the risk of more serious cardiac side effects is low.[99] Dosing guidelines are similar to those applied during the treatment of other chronic pains (see Chapter 10).

Calcium Channel Blockers. Calcium channel blockers such as verapamil appear to decrease the frequency, but not the intensity, of recurrent migraine attacks.[108,183,249] Verapamil is given in divided doses or as a sustained-release product at doses of up to 360 mg per day.

Other Drugs. Clonidine had a brief period of interest as a prophylactic agent for migraines but has not proved to be effective.[43] Nonsteroidal anti-inflammatory drugs can be helpful, although some reports indicate that they decrease the severity but not the frequency of migraine attacks.[273] Chronic ergotamine administration is slightly less effective than methysergide but has fewer side effects and a similar mechanism of action.[18] It is contraindicated in patients with asthma or angina and in pregnancy. In a selected subgroup of patients, opioid analgesics can be used successfully with tolerable risks.[172]

Nonpharmacologic Dietary Modalities. At least 25 percent of patients with migraine can identify some type of dietary precipitant.[205] Foods containing tyramine, mainly aged cheeses, have been implicated in patients suffering from "dietary migraine."[247]

Ethyl alcohol and chocolate can also precipitate attacks, presumably because of the phenylalanine content. If an offending food is identified, it should be avoided, but there is little to justify rigorous dietary restrictions in the vast majority of migraine patients.

Psychologic Modalities. Personality features have been implicated in the manifestations of migraine, but no rigorously controlled studies have substantiated any particular psychologic factor.[115,201,204,261] While stress appears to play a role in migraine, and migraine patients appear to have a reaction to stress different from that of control subjects,[271] the role of stress is not straightforward. Some patients experience headache at the time of increased stress, and others develop pain shortly after it has subsided.

Relaxation techniques and cognitive/behavioral approaches, such as biofeedback, can decrease the frequency and severity of migraine attacks.[41,127] In any refractory headache syndrome, these and other behavioral techniques and therapies designed to reduce abnormal illness behavior should be considered.

Cluster Headache

There are many superannuated terms for cluster headaches. Those of historical interest include erythroprosopalgia of Bing, ciliary or migrainous neuralgia (Harris), erythromelalgia of the head, Horton's headache, histaminic cephalalgia, petrosal neuralgia (Gardner), sphenopalatine, vidian and Sluder's neuralgia, and hemicrania periodica neuraliformis.

Cluster is the only headache syndrome that is significantly more common in men than women, with a ratio of about 5 to 7:1. The average age of onset is slightly higher than in migraine and may be higher in women than in men. The frequency of attacks tends to decrease with advancing age.[75]

The description of cluster headache is stereotyped and distinct from migraine[142] (see IHS diagnostic criteria in Table 4–5). A

Table 4–5. **IHS CLUSTER HEADACHE CRITERIA**

A. At least 5 attacks fulfill B–D.

B. Severe unilateral orbital, supraorbital, and/or temporal pain lasts 15–180 minutes untreated.

C. Headache is associated with at least one of the following signs, which have to be present on the painful side:
  1. Conjunctival injection
  2. Lacrimation
  3. Nasal congestion
  4. Rhinorrhea
  5. Forehead and facial sweating
  6. Miosis
  7. Ptosis
  8. Eyelid edema

D. Frequency of attacks ranges from 1 every other day to 8 per day.

E. At least one of the following is true:
  1. History, physical and neurologic examinations do not suggest one of the disorders listed in groups 5–11 (of Appendix).
  2. History and/or physical and/or neurologic examinations do suggest such disorder, but it is ruled out by appropriate investigations
  3. Such disorder is present, but cluster headache does not occur for the first time in close temporal relation to the disorder.

cluster period typically lasts about 6 weeks. There can be pain-free intervals of many months between clusters. Many patients appear to cycle on a seasonal basis. About 10 percent of patients have chronic cluster, which, in most cases, has evolved over time from a classic pattern.[168] Headache usually occurs between once and several times daily during a cluster period. During each headache, the maximum intensity of the pain occurs within a few minutes and continues for 20 minutes to 1 to 2 hours. Pain is usually described as stabbing or piercing. The most common site is retro-orbital, but pain may radiate to the cheek or gums. The pain of the full attack is invariably unilateral and usually affects the same side; a few patients have attacks that alternate from one side to another. The facial location and unilaterality of the pain, along with its piercing character, are reminiscent of trigeminal neuralgia, and the two may be associated.[60] In contrast to migraine patients, who try to find a quiet place to go to sleep, cluster patients often pace, holding the affected side. Approximately half of cluster patients have predominantly nocturnal attacks, which typically follow a stereotyped time pattern, awakening the patient at the same time every night during the cluster.[144]

Cluster headache is usually accompanied by a partial Horner's syndrome, with ptosis and miosis. Most patients also develop hyperhidrosis with lacrimation and coryza.[73,168]

Cluster headaches are precipitated by vasodilatory substances during a cluster period. Clinically, the most common precipitating factor is alcohol. Histamine can routinely precipitate an attack,[11] but antihistaminic medications have been ineffective in controlling pain. Between clusters, precipitating factors are not effective.

PATHOGENESIS

The pathogenesis of cluster headache is unknown. It is unlikely that it is a primary vascular headache, based on the autonomic phenomena and rhythmicity. Kudrow[144] divides cluster into three clinicopathologic processes: the cluster period, attack provocation, and pain production. "Each process appears to be dependent on the one before: hence, pain pathways are triggered by an attack-provoking mechanism, which, in turn, may be stimulated only in an altered physiologic environment defined as the cluster period."

TREATMENT

Treatment strategies for cluster headache begin with the avoidance of precipitating factors during clusters. This includes alcohol and high altitudes. (Prophylactic ergotamines may be helpful with the latter.)

Treatment of an individual attack requires either rapid bioavailability of the drug administered or pretreatment if attacks are predictable. Abortive therapy with inhaled ergotamine can be effective if the inhalations are taken at the very onset of the headache.[9,76] Inhalation of high flow oxygen (7 to 10 L per minute) can also abort an attack.[87,143] Intranasal application of anesthetic agents also has been reported to be effective[126]; both lidocaine and cocaine have been used. It is unclear whether this relief represents sphenopalatine ganglion block or an effect on sensory afferents. In patients who know the time of onset of their daily headaches, 2 mg of ergotamine taken 1/2 hr before predicted onset can be effective, and in patients with nocturnal headaches, 2 mg of ergotamine at bedtime may be prophylactic.[144]

Most therapeutic regimens for cluster are prophylactic.[251] Methysergide is effective for the treatment of episodic cluster but relatively ineffective for chronic cluster. The drug is used as recommended for migraine. Because cluster is usually time-limited, the complications of long-term therapy are avoided.

Lithium is an effective agent for chronic cluster and can reduce the frequency and severity of episodic cluster in more than 70 percent of patients.[74] The mechanism of action of lithium in cluster is not known but is thought to be related to its effects on circadian rhythms. When breakthrough headaches occur, they often can be controlled with doses of ergotamine that do not provide relief without lithium therapy. The effective dosage of lithium varies widely,[167] from 300 to 1500 mg per day. Dosing should be initiated at 300 mg twice daily, then adjusted according to effects and side effects. Plasma concentrations should be maintained in the range of 0.9 to 1.1 mEq/L. At therapeutic levels, lithium can cause a mild tremor, gastrointestinal side effects, and polyuria. Intoxication, which is more likely to occur in patients given diuretics[234] or those who have become dehydrated for other reasons (e.g., diarrhea), produces encephalopathy and fasciculations.

Prednisone can abort a cluster episode rapidly[141] and is the drug of choice for breaking chronic cluster. The mechanism of action is not known. Dosing is usually started at 60 to 80 mg per day for a week and then tapered over the following week. If no response is obtained within 2 days, it is not likely to occur later, and the drug should be stopped. Prednisone can be used as a first-line drug while another prophylactic therapy, such as methysergide or lithium, is being started.

Small, uncontrolled studies have reported that calcium channel blocking agents can be effective in the management of cluster.[97,184] Verapamil is usually administered in dosages of 80 mg four times a day.

Anesthetic and ablative procedures have been proposed for refractory cases of cluster headache.[74,253,256] Injection of lidocaine and a steroid into the area of the greater occipital nerve has been reported to provide relief, whereas lidocaine alone has not.[135] There are anecdotal reports of ablative procedures directed at various branches of the trigeminal nerve or the nervus intermedius. Surgical intervention is reserved for a desperate last resort.

Chronic Paroxysmal Hemicrania

This uncommon disorder is characterized but sudden bouts of unilateral, intense pain. The pain is deep and piercing, lasts seconds to minutes, and is sometimes accompanied by ptosis, lacrimation, and nasal stuffiness. In this disorder, unlike cluster, women are more commonly affected than men. An excellent response to indomethacin is characteristic. A dosage of 25 to 50 mg three times a day can eliminate pain entirely.[219]

Although it resembles cluster headache in the location and quality of the pain, as well as the associated autonomic features, episodic paroxysmal hemicrania is distinguished by the greater frequency and shorter duration of individual headaches. Differentiation of these disorders is important because episodic paroxysmal hemicrania, like chronic paroxysmal hemicrania, invariably responds to treatment with indomethacin but not to standard cluster headache therapy.[145,192]

Tension Headache

Tension headache is the most common recurrent pain syndrome. It is not a clearly defined entity and represents a spectrum of headaches that ranges from those that are purely psychogenic to those that are clearly related to muscle spasm or cervical osteoarthritis. A common working definition, however, is "head pain devoid of migrainous characteristics."[217]

The IHS diagnostic criteria for episodic tension-type headache are listed in Table 4–6.

There may be significant overlap between tension and migraine headaches, with both groups occasionally experiencing visual symptoms, nausea, or throbbing.[68] This observation has encouraged the formulation of a unified theory of pathogenesis.

PATHOGENESIS

The IHS subdivides tension headaches according to whether there is "disorder of the pericranial muscles." This is probably not useful, unless there is clear underlying pathology. Electromyographic (EMG) evidence of increased muscle activity in tension headaches is not uniform and, when present, may represent either a cause or an effect of the headache. Migraine patients also have increased resting EMG activity.[134] Tender points in the scalp and neck, commonly considered as part of the tension headache syndrome, can be found in migraine sufferers with about the same frequency.[67,261] Relaxation techniques and biofeedback, which may be aimed at relieving muscle contraction, can be beneficial in those with no signs of increased muscle tension on EMG.[36] There is, therefore, no convincing evidence that muscle contraction is any more a causative factor in tension headaches than in other headache syndromes.

Table 4–6. **IHS TENSION HEADACHE CRITERIA**

A. At least 10 previous headache episodes fulfill criteria B–D listed below. Number of days with such headache is 180/year (15/month).

B. Headache lasts from 30 minutes to 7 days.

C. At least two of the following pain characteristics:
  1. Pressing/tightening (nonpulsating) quality.
  2. Mild or moderate intensity (may inhibit but does not prohibit activities).
  3. Bilateral location.
  4. No aggravation by walking stairs or similar routine physical activity.

D. Both of the following:
  1. No nausea or vomiting (anorexia may occur).
  2. Photophobia and phonophobia are absent, or one but not the other is present.

E. At least one of the following:
  1. History, physical, and neurologic examinations do not suggest one of the disorders listed in groups 5–11 (of Appendix).
  2. History and/or physical and/or neurologic examinations do suggest such disorder, but it is ruled out by appropriate investigations.
  3. Such disorder is present, but tension-type headache does not occur for the first time in close temporal relation to the disorder.

Disturbances of blood flow have been suggested in the pathogenesis of tension headache. Both tension headache and migraine headache attacks, however, can be precipitated by the intravenous infusion of histamine,[140] yet another vasodilator (alcohol) can relieve tension headaches. Xenon studies show increased cerebral blood flow in both tension headache and migraine patients.[185] Thus, vascular factors have not been shown to be significantly different in tension headaches versus migraine. Indeed, these data suggest that it may be useful to regard tension headaches and migraine as two points on a spectrum.[63,171]

Psychologic factors may also be involved in the pathophysiology of both tension headache and migraine. On the Minnesota Multiphasic Personality Inventory (MMPI), headache patients had relatively high scores for depression, anxiety, and hypochondriasis. This finding mirrors the results obtained from patients with other chronic pain syndromes.[146,180] MMPI data can differentiate headache patients from normals but cannot differentiate among headache types.[212] Studies of anxiety state have not shown clear-cut differences between headache patients and other pain populations.[117] Depressive symptoms are very common in patients with chronic tension headaches,[173] but there is no convincing evidence that depression is the cause, rather than the effect, of the pain. In short, evidence suggests that psychologic factors could be involved in the pathogenesis of tension headache, but the processes involved are poorly understood.

TREATMENT

Most patients with episodic tension headache effectively self-medicate with over-the-counter analgesics. Patients with frequent headaches may not be adequately helped, and, as discussed previously, repeated use of such drugs at short intervals could theoretically exacerbate the headache syndrome.[174,186]

Patients with very frequent episodic headache or chronic daily tension headache should be considered for a multimodality approach that integrates psychologic and pharmacologic treatments. Cognitive therapies may be useful in some patients. A recent randomized study showed that home-based cognitive/behavioral techniques were as effective as tricyclic antidepressants in decreasing headaches.[119] Relaxation techniques, using any format, can decrease the frequency and severity of recurrent attacks.[29] The technique may be as simple as progressive muscle relaxation or as complex as "alpha training." EMG or thermal biofeedback is used commonly to achieve a relaxed state.

Drug therapies for chronic tension headache begin with the tricyclic antidepressants. Amitriptyline was effective in a controlled trial[59] and is generally considered the first-line drug (see Chapter 10). Other drugs are considered in selected cases. Benzodiazepines, despite their sedating and "muscle relaxant" properties, have not been proved efficacious in the treatment of tension headache. Sedative/hypnotic drugs are usually ineffective in the long run.

Postconcussive Headache

The postconcussive syndrome is a neuropsychologic disorder characterized by dull, aching headaches, lightheadedness, vertigo, memory impairment, depression, and anxiety. Headache may appear anywhere from 1 day to many weeks after the trauma.[127] The results of imaging procedures are normal; EEG and evoked responses may be abnormal[223] but have no prognostic value. Although psychiatric manifestations are common, it is often unclear whether these changes may have predated the trauma.[181] The issue of secondary gain from insurance or litigation is believed to impede recovery, but settlement of claims does not necessarily resolve the problem.[259] Most cases resolve spontaneously but may take up to 6 months. After 6 months, spontaneous resolution is less common.[199] Patients should be treated with reassurance, without minimizing the complaints. A multimodality treatment approach may be useful.

Chronic Daily Headache

Many patients experience headache that is constantly present or has occurred for at least 1 hour every day for at least 6 months. The pain is characteristically bilateral or diffuse and tight or bandlike; radiation to the posterior neck is common. Features typical of migraine are usually absent but may occur with individual headaches. The onset is most commonly in the fourth and fifth decades, and women are more frequently affected than men.

Chronic daily headache usually evolves from migraine or episodic tension headaches. Frequent use of short-acting analgesics has been implicated in the conversion of episodic headaches into chronic daily headache.[63,175,243] Inpatient treatment protocols for these drug-induced chronic headaches have been described.[216,233] Following an inpatient withdrawal program, more than 50 percent of patients have persistent reduction in headache frequency and intensity.[63]

Patients most likely to obtain benefits are those who had migraine as the primary headache, duration of headache of less than 10 years, and a history of regular ergotamine use.

Miscellaneous Headache Syndromes

ICE CREAM HEADACHE

A brief headache may be felt deep within the head or frontotemporally after the ingestion of ice cream or a very cold drink. This pain is probably a vascular response to cold stimulation of the hard palate and the oropharynx.[219] It may be more common in patients with migraine than in normals. Pain subsides in less than 1 minute.

COITAL HEADACHE

A rare form of headache occurs just before or with orgasm. In some patients, the headache is explosive in nature. The first episode warrants an evaluation for subarachnoid hemorrhage. In other cases, pain begins as a dull ache during coitus and reaches a peak at orgasm. The mechanism of the headache is unclear, but it is probably vascular in nature and related to blood pressure changes.[151]

HANGOVER

Despite its very common occurrence, the etiology of hangover headache[218] is not known. It occurs long after alcohol has been cleared from the system and may represent a type of withdrawal syndrome. Metabolites such as acetaldehyde and pyruvate have been implicated but not proved. Liquors with high congener contents (cognac and other oak-aged products) appear to be more likely to yield hangover than clear, neutral spirits, such as vodka.

FACIAL PAIN

It is clinically useful to divide facial pain into three main categories:
1. *Nociceptive* pains are presumably due to ongoing tissue damage. Sinusitis is a common example.

2. *Neuropathic* pains comprise cranial neuralgias, postherpetic neuralgia, and miscellaneous pains.
3. *Idiopathic* pains include several recognized syndromes, such as atypical facial pain and burning mouth syndrome.

A subgroup of patients with idiopathic pain have sufficient evidence to establish a diagnosis of somatoform disorder—that is, pain due primarily to psychologic factors.

Nociceptive Syndromes

Inflammation or destruction of pain-sensitive structures in or around the face can cause chronic facial pain. The most obvious site is the paranasal sinuses. Acute bacterial sinusitis is a well-recognized cause of localized facial pain and tenderness. The relationship between chronic sinusitis and facial pain is less clear, however. Thickening of the sinus mucosa is a common incidental finding on MRI and is likely to be unrelated to facial pain. In most cases, "sinus pain" is probably a form of tension headache, and causative sinus pathology cannot be demonstrated.[239]

Facial pain is an unusual presentation for destructive lesions. Occasionally, intracranial or carotid tumors present as facial pain, generally in the form of a cranial neuralgia (see Chapter 9).

Neuropathic Pains

CRANIAL NEURALGIAS

Trigeminal Neuralgia. Trigeminal neuralgia is the most stereotyped of the facial pain syndromes. Pain is limited to one or more of the divisions of the trigeminal nerve, is lancinating in character, and lasts for only seconds. Patients are pain-free between paroxysms. About half of the patients have trigger points on the face or in the mouth.

The syndrome of trigeminal neuralgia can be divided into a primary form (without a clear cause on routine examination) and a symptomatic form (due to a defined lesion). In primary trigeminal neuralgia, there is no objective sensory loss and motor function is intact.[69] Neurologic dysfunction should suggest the diagnosis of symptomatic trigeminal neuralgia. Imaging studies, preferably MRI, are mandatory in these circumstances.

Primary trigeminal neuralgia is most common in the sixth and seventh decade. It is uncommon under the age of 40, and its appearance in the young should prompt a search for demyelinating disease.[34,155] Women are more commonly affected than men.

The pathophysiology of primary trigeminal neuralgia is unknown. One hypothesis suggests that a combination of peripheral and central neural mechanisms may be involved[37,162] (see Chapter 5). In most surgically treated cases, an aberrant loop of artery or vein has been observed to compress the nerve near its origin.[128] Microsurgical decompression of the nerve usually relieves the pain in these cases,[129] suggesting that the peripheral factor is important in the pathogenesis of the pain. Trigeminal neuralgia can occur without compression or other overt peripheral lesions, however, and cross-compression of the trigeminal root is found in 7 to 12 percent of autopsied patients without a history of trigeminal neuralgia.[138] Thus, the nature of the peripheral process, like the central processes that are presumed to be important, is not clear.

Symptomatic trigeminal neuralgia can be caused by any type of peripheral compressive lesion. For example, typical pain has been caused by tumors[182] and by vascular malformations.[48] Other causes of symptomatic trigeminal neuralgia include multiple sclerosis and herpes zoster. The theory that abnormal cavities in alveolar bone may be involved[221,222] has not been adequately substantiated.[105]

Medical Management. Many drugs may be useful in the management of lancinating neuralgias, including trigeminal neuralgia (see Chapter 10). Experience is greatest with the anticonvulsants. These drugs facilitate segmental inhibition and depress excitatory transmission in the spinal trigeminal nucleus.[93,94] Carbamazepine is generally the preferred drug. It should be started at low doses and titrated. Transient leukopenia is common, but persistent leukopenia is rare.[226] Aplastic anemia is an idiosyncratic reaction.[204] Two-thirds to three-quarters of patients have a very good initial response, but only about one-half remain pain-free for more than 2 years.[225] In some patients, a drug holiday may restore efficacy.

Patients who fail carbamazepine may respond to any of a large group of adjuvant analgesics, which include baclofen,[95] phenytoin, clonazepam, valproate, or pimozide; other drugs, such as mexiletine or a tricyclic antidepressant, which have not been evaluated specifically in this disorder, may be useful in selected patients (see Chapter 10). Occasional patients benefit from sequential trials of these agents until one is found with the most favorable spectrum of effects. Over time, many patients become refractory to medical treatment and surgical intervention must be considered.

Surgical Interventions. Microvascular decompression of the trigeminal nerve has been advocated on the basis of the hypothesis that an aberrant loop of artery or vein that cross-compresses the root of the trigeminal nerve is the causative lesion.[112,128,129] At surgery, such a lesion is found in more than 85 percent of cases. Initial success rates of more than 90 percent have been reported, with a very low rate of recurrence.[38,235]

Radiofrequency lesioning of a branch of the trigeminal nerve, which can be performed percutaneously, provides relief to some patients; the problem of trigeminal nerve dysfunction limits the use of the technique.[178,255,258] Although success rates may be as high as 80 percent, there is a 25 to 50 percent recurrence rate at 2 years.[50]

Retrogasserian chemical rhizotomy with glycerol, phenol, or another neurolytic solution can be performed percutaneously.[77,257] Glycerol instillation was reported also to be successful in 91.3 percent of 252 patients with primary trigeminal neuralgia.[61] There was a recurrence rate of 10.9 percent in the first 2 years, and the long-term recurrence rate was 36.9 percent. Hypalgesia occurred in about one-third of the patients, but none had a decrease in corneal sensation. Both chemical rhizotomy and radiofrequency lesioning have a higher incidence of recurrent pain than has microvascular decompression.

On the basis of the poorly validated theory that trigeminal neuralgia is the result of anaerobic infections of cavities in the alveolar bone, osteocavitation techniques have been performed.[222] The studies that have evaluated this technique are not well controlled and there is currently little support for the procedure.[105]

OTHER NEURALGIAS (SEE CHAPTER 5)

Glossopharyngeal neuralgia is a less common disorder than trigeminal neuralgia. Pain is sharp and stabbing and usually felt in the back of the throat or in the ear. Pain is exacerbated by swallowing and sometimes accompanied by syncope.[42] "Swallow syncope," presumably due to a vagal discharge, is most often seen in patients with recurrent tumors of the neck.[157] Medical treatment is the same as in trigeminal neuralgia,[78] and surgical interventions are performed rarely.

Geniculate neuralgia (neuralgia of the nervus intermedius) is an uncommon syndrome characterized by sharp pain deep within the ear. Local causes must be excluded, and then the treatment is as with other neuralgias. Surgical intervention has demonstrated vascular compressions and benign tumors. Decompression provides initial relief, but the recurrence rate is high.[211,230]

POSTHERPETIC NEURALGIA

The first (ophthalmic) division of the trigeminal nerve is a common site for herpetic eruptions. Postherpetic neuralgia is a frequent and challenging cause of head and facial pain, particularly in the elderly (see Chapter 5).

DEAFFERENTATION PAIN FOLLOWING DENTAL PROCEDURES

Tooth extraction or root canal work can lead to a phantom-tooth pain syndrome in 2 to 6 percent of patients.[39,170] Some evidence indicates that this disorder is more common in patients with a history of migraine or cluster headache.[244] Deafferentation pain in the face is often mistaken for ongoing dental pathology, leading to still more interventions and further damage. The clinical picture is highly variable. The management is similar to other deafferentation pains (see Chapter 5).

Idiopathic Pains

TEMPOROMANDIBULAR JOINT DYSFUNCTION

Temporomandibular joint (TMJ) dysfunction is one of the most frequently diagnosed causes of headache or facial pain. There is a great deal of controversy surrounding the limits of the syndrome. The IHS diagnostic criteria are listed in Table 4–7.

Clinically, TMJ syndrome is usually defined as pain around the joint or ear, with exacerbation on movement of the jaw and with evidence of abnormal noises and jaw deviation.[40,229] Some patients have a clearly identifiable abnormality in the joint or muscles, leading to pain. Many others have pain in the area without sufficient local pathology to explain the pain. It is often difficult to differentiate between these groups. If disease in the TMJ cannot be identified, the label "idiopathic pain" is appropriate.

The TMJ offers a number of sites for primary pain problems, and specific syndromes have been attributed to derangements in each of the components.[81] The joint is composed of the articulation of the mandibular condyle with the temporal bone. There is an articular meniscus in between, a synovial capsule surrounding, and masticatory muscles inserting around the joint. Attempts have been made to differentiate syndromes

Table 4–7. IHS TEMPOROMANDIBULAR JOINT (TMJ) SYNDROME CRITERIA

A. At least two of the following:
   1. Pain of the jaw precipitated by movement and/or clenching
   2. Decreased range of movement
   3. Noise during joint movements
   4. Tenderness of the joint capsule
B. Positive x ray and/or isotope scintigraphic findings.
C. Pain is mild to moderate and located at the temporomandibular joint and/or radiating from there.

---

according to "internal derangement" (meniscal problems), structural abnormalities of the bone, and myofascial pain/dysfunction. Patients with straightforward mechanical problems in the joint are easily managed by dentists and oral surgeons with appropriate splinting or other local devices.[16]

TMJ dysfunction is much more common in women than in men, and the onset is usually in the third or fourth decades of life. Prevalence seems to decrease with advancing age, making it unlikely that purely structural disease of the joint is a major factor in the pathogenesis of the pain. One of the more convincing theories about pain emanating from the TMJ is that of a "myofascial pain/dysfunction syndrome." Myofascial pain may affect any area of the body and is characterized by "pain in a zone of reference, trigger points in muscles, occasional associated symptoms, and the presence of contributing factors."[90] Patients with this syndrome present with limitation of jaw opening and/or jaw deviation, muscle tenderness to palpation, and, often, psychologic distress. Although muscle tenderness is part of the syndrome, EMG studies of activity in the masticatory muscles have provided conflicting results.[189,224]

ATYPICAL FACIAL PAIN

Atypical facial pain is a term used to denote facial pain syndromes that do not fit any of the established syndromes. Pain of this type is much more common in women than in men. The pain usually starts unilaterally but often becomes bilateral. Most patients experience pain that is deep and aching in nature and is nearly constant.[250]

Psychologic factors play an important role in atypical facial pain, though patients tend to deny it.[56,71] It is not clear, however, that psychologic dysfunction is any more prevalent than it is in any other chronic pain syndrome.

BURNING MOUTH SYNDROME

Burning mouth syndrome is an idiopathic pain syndrome that is most common in postmenopausal women.[109] It is characterized by a generalized feeling of burning throughout the mouth. Local factors, such as ill-fitting dentures, subclinical infections, reduced salivary gland function, and vitamin deficiencies can occasionally be found, but none is universally present. Psychologic dysfunction is extremely common, with depression, anxiety, and fear of cancer as the prevailing disorders,[110,111] but the etiologic importance of these disturbances is unknown.

SUMMARY

Headache is the most common presenting pain complaint in neurologists' offices. A guided history and physical examination, aided by the judicious selection of ancillary diagnostic tests, can identify rapidly the life-threatening syndromes of subarachnoid hemorrhage, cerebrovascular disease, expanding mass lesions, and temporal arteritis. Attention can then be paid to the accurate diagnosis of the more common recurrent headache syndromes and the institution of syndrome-specific treatment.

Migraine is the only recurrent headache syndrome whose therapy is based on inferred mechanisms of disease. Abortive therapies were first undertaken with the ergot preparations and are now evolving into more receptor-specific agents, such as the serotonin agonists. Prophylactic therapies with β-adrenergic blockers and calcium channel blockers also have their theoretic basis in presumed disease mechanisms.

The pathophysiology of tension headache, cluster, chronic paroxysmal hemicrania, postconcussive headache, and chronic daily headache are less well defined, and treatment is primarily symptomatic.

The truly idiopathic pain syndromes, such as burning mouth, atypical facial pain, and temporomandibular joint dysfunction, are probably best viewed as chronic pain problems of varied and ill-defined causes.

REFERENCES

1. The Ad Hoc Committee on Classification of Headache: Special Report. Arch Neurol 6:173–176, 1962.
2. Disturbances of Cerebrospinal Fluid Circulation. In Adams RD, and Victor M (eds): Principles of Neurology. McGraw-Hill, New York, 1989.
3. Aellig WH: Influence on pizotifen and ergotamine on the venoconstrictor effect of 5-hydroxytryptamine and noradrenaline in man. Eur J Clin Pharmacol 25:759–762, 1983.
4. Allen NB, and Studenski SA: Polymyalgia rheumatica and temporal arteritis. Med Clin North Am 70:369–384, 1986.
5. Andermann E, and Anderman FA: Migraine-epilepsy relationships: Epidemiological and genetic aspects. In Anderman FA, and Lugaresi E (eds): Migraine and Epilepsy. Butterworths, Boston, 1987,281–291.
6. Andersen AR, Tfelt-Hansen P, and Lassen NA: The effect of ergotamine and dihydroergotamine on cerebral blood flow in man. Stroke 18:120–123, 1987.
7. Andersen E, and Dafny N: An ascending serotonergic pain modulation pathway from the dorsal raphe nucleus to the parafascicularis nucleus of the thalamus. Brain Res 269:57–67, 1983.
8. Anderson CD, and Frank RD: Migraine and tension headache: Is there a difference? Headache 21:63–71, 1981.
9. Andersson P-G, and Jespersen L-T: Dihydroergotamine nasal spray in the treatment of attacks of cluster headache. A double-blind trial versus placebo. Cephalalgia 6(1):51–54, March 1986.
10. Anthony M: The biochemistry of migraine. In Rose FC (ed): Handbook of Clinical Neurology, Vol 48. Elsevier, Amsterdam, 1986, pp 85–105.
11. Anthony M, and Lance JW: Histamine and serotonin in cluster headache. Arch Neurol 25:225–231, 1971.
12. Anthony M, and Lance JW: The role of serotonin in migraine. In Pearce J (ed): Modern Topics in Migraine. Heinemann, London, 1975, pp 107–123.
13. Anthony M, Lord GDA, and Lance JW: Controlled trials of cimetidine in migraine and cluster headache. Headache 18:261–264, 1978.
14. Baldessarini RG: Drugs and the treatment of psychiatric disorders. In Goodman AG, and Gilman S (eds): The Pharmacological Basis of Therapeutics. Pergamon Press, New York, 1990, pp 404–414.
15. Banarjee M, and Findley LJ: Sumatriptan in the treatment of acute migraine with aura. Cephalalgia 12(1):39–44, Feb 1992.
16. Baragona PM, and Cohen HV: Long-term orthopedic appliance therapy. Dent Clin North Am 31(1):109–121, 1991.
17. Bardwell A, and Trott JA: Stroke in migraine as a consequence of propanolol. Headache 27:381–383, 1987.
18. Barrie MA, Fox WR, Weatherall M, et al: Analysis of symptoms of patients with headaches and their response to treatment with ergot derivatives. Q J Med 37:319–336, 1968.
19. Basbaum AI, and Fields LH: Endogenous pain control mechanisms. Review and hypothesis. Ann Neurol 4:451–462, 1978.
20. Baumel B: Migraine: A pharmacologic review with newer options and delivery modalities. Neurology 44(Suppl 3), S13–S17, 1994.
21. Beaver WT, and Feise G: Comparison of the analgesic effects of morphine, hydroxyzine and their combination in patients with post-operative pain. In Bonica JJ, Albe-Fessard D (eds): Advances in pain research and therapy, Vol 1. New York, Raven Press, 1976, pp 553–557.
22. Bengtsson BA, and Malmvall BE: Alternate-day corticosteroid regimen in maintenance therapy of giant cell arteritis. Surv Ophthalmol 20:247–260, 1976.

23. Bethlenfalvay NC, and Nusynowitz NL: Temporal arteritis: A rarity in the young adult. Arch Intern Med 114:487–489, 1964.
24. Bickerstaff ER: Basilar artery migraine. Lancet 1: 15–17, 1961.
25. Bickerstaff ER: Ophthalmoplegic migraine. Rev Neurol (Paris) 110:582–588, 1964.
26. Bille B: The development of pediatric headache research. Headache Q 1:39–42, 1990.
27. Birkhead NC, Wagener HP, and Schick RM: Treatment of temporal arteritis with adrenal corticosteroids: Results of 55 cases in which lesions were proven at biopsy. JAMA 163:821–827, 1957.
28. Birt D: Headaches and head pains associated with diseases of the ear, nose and throat. Med Clin North Am 62:523–531, 1978.
29. Blanchard EB, Applebaum KA, and Guarnieri P: A five year prospective follow-up on the treatment of chronic tension headache with biofeedback and/or relaxation. Headache 27:580–583, 1987.
30. Blau JN: Resolution of migraine attacks: Sleep and recovery phase. J Neurol Neurosurg Psychiatry 45: 223–226, 1982.
31. Blau JN, and Cummings JN: Methods of precipitating and preventing some migraine attacks. British Medical Journal 2:1242–1243, 1966.
32. Bohr V, Hansen B, Kjersem H, et al: Sequelae from bacterial meningitis and their relation to the clinical condition during acute illness, based on 667 questionnaire returns. Part II of a three part series. J Infect 7(2):102–110, Sept. 1983.
33. Breslau N, Merikangas K, and Bowden CL: Comorbidity of migraine and major affective disorders. Neurology 44(Suppl 7):S17–S22, 1994.
34. Brisman R: Trigeminal neuralgia and multiple sclerosis. Arch Neurol 44:379, 1987.
35. Broderick JP, and Swanson JW: Migraine-related strokes. Arch Neurol 44:868–871, 1987.
36. Bruhn P, Olesen J, and Melgaard B: Controlled trial of EMG feedback in muscle contraction headache. Ann Neurol 6:34–36, 1979.
37. Burchiel KJ: Abnormal impulse generation in focally demyelinated trigeminal roots. J Neurosurg 53:674, 1980.
38. Burchiel KJ, Clarke H, Haglund M, et al: Long-term efficacy of microvascular decompression in trigeminal neuralgia. J Neurosurg 69:35, 1988.
39. Campbell RL, Parks KW, and Dodds RN: Chronic facial pain associated with endodontic therapy. Oral Surg Oral Med Oral Pathol 69(3):287–290, 1990.
40. Cawson RA: Temporomandibular cephalalgia. In Vinken PJ, Bruyn GW, Klawans HL, et al (eds): Handbook of Clinical Neurology, Vol 48. Elsevier, Amsterdam, 1986, pp 413–416.
41. Chapman SL: A review and clinical perspective on the use of EMG and thermal biofeedback for chronic headache. Pain 27:1–43, 1986.
42. Chawla JC, and Falconer MA: Glossopharyngeal and vagal neuralgia. British Medical Journal 2:527, 1967.
43. Clonidine in migraine prophylaxis—now obsolete. Drug Therapy Bull 28(20):79–80, 1990.
44. Coddon D: Personal communication, Sept, 1991.
45. Cook NR, Davies MJ, and Beavis RE: Bedrest and postlumbar puncture headache—the effectiveness of 24 hours' recumbency in reducing the incidence of post lumbar puncture headache. Anesthesia (44):389–391, 1989.
46. Corbett JJ, Savino PJ, Thompson HS, et al: Visual loss in pseudotumor cerebri: Follow-up of 57 patients from 5 to 41 years and a profile of 14 patients with permanent severe visual loss. Arch Neurol 39:461–474, 1982.
47. Couch JR, Ziegler DK, and Hassanein R: Amitriptyline in the prophylaxis of migraine: Effectiveness and relationship of antimigraine and antidepressant effects. Neurology 26:121–127, 1976.
48. Cruccu G, et al: Idiopathic and symptomatic trigeminal pain. J Neurol Neurosurg Psychiatry 53(12): 1034–1042, 1990.
49. Curran DA, and Lance JW: Clinical trial of methysergide and other preparations in the management of migraine. J Neurol Neurosurg Psychiatry 27:463–469, 1964.
50. Dalessio DJ: Diagnosis and treatment of cranial neuralgias. Med Clin North Am 75(3):605–615, 1991.
51. Dalessio DJ: Diagnosing the severe headache. Neurology: 44 (Suppl 3), S6–S12, 1994.
52. Daroff RB: Classification and diagnostic criteria for headache disorders, cranial neuralgias and facial pain. Headache Classification Committee of the International Headache Society. Cephalalgia 8(Suppl 7):1–96, 1988.
53. Daroff RB: New headache classification. Surg Neurol 31(2):112, 1989.
54. Davies LE: Acute viral meningitis and encephalitis In: Kennedy PGE, and Johnson RT (eds). Infections of the Nervous System. Butterworths, London, 1987, Chapter 9.
55. Day TJ, and Knezevic W: Cerebrospinal fluid abnormalities associated with migraine. Med J Aust 141:459–461, 1984.
56. Delaney JF: Atypical facial pain as a defense against psychosis. Am J Psychiatry 133:1151, 1976.
57. de Lissovoy G, and Lazarus SS: The economic cost of migraine: Present state of knowledge. Neurology 44(Suppl 4):S56–S62, 1994.
58. Diamond S: Migraine headaches. Med Clin North Am 75(3):545–566, 1991.
59. Diamond S and Baltes BJ: Chronic tension headache treated with amitriptyline: A double-blind study. Headache 11(3):110–116, 1971.
60. Diamond S, Freitag FG, and Cohen JS: Cluster headache with trigeminal neuralgia. An uncommon association that may be more than coincidental. Postgrad Med 75(2):165–172, 1984.
61. Dieckmann G, Bockerman V, and Heyer C: Five-and-a-half years' experience with percutaneous retrogasserian glycerol rhizotomy in treatment of trigeminal neuralgia. Applied Neurophysiology 50: 401, 1987.
62. Diehr P, Wood RW, Barr V, et al: Acute headaches: Presenting symptoms and diagnostic rules to identify patients with tension and migraine headache. Journal of Chronic Diseases 34:147–158, 1981.
63. Diener HC, Dichgans J, Scholz E, et al: Analgesic-induced chronic headache: Long-term results of withdrawal therapy. J Neurol 236(1):9–14, 1989.
64. Diener HC, Scholz E, Dichgans J, et al: Central effects of drugs used in migraine prophylaxis evaluated by visual evoked potentials. Ann Neurol 25(2):125–130, 1989.

65. Dorland's Illustrated Medical Dictionary, ed 24. WB Saunders, Philadelphia, 1988.

66. Drummond PD: Effectiveness of methysergide in relation to clinical features of migraine. Headache 25:145–146, 1985.

67. Drummond PD: Scalp tenderness and sensitivity to pain in migraine and tension headache. Headache 27:45–50, 1987.

68. Drummond PD, and Lance JW: Clinical diagnosis and computer analysis of headache symptoms. J Neurol Neurosurg Psychiatry 47:128–133, 1984.

69. Dubner R, et al: Idiopathic trigeminal neuralgia: Sensory features and pain mechanisms. Pain 31:23, 1987.

70. Durkan GP, Troost BT, Slamovitz TL, et al: Recurrent painless oculomotor palsy in children: A variant of ophthalmoplegic migraine. Headache 21:58–62, 1981.

71. Dworkin SF, and Burgess JA: Orofacial pain of psychogenic origin: Current concepts and classification. J Am Dent Assoc 115(4):565–571, 1987.

72. Edmeads J: The headaches of ischemic cerebrovascular disease. Headache 19:345–349, 1979.

73. Ekbom, K: A clinical comparison of cluster headache and migraine. Acta Neurol Scand 46 (Suppl 41):1–44, 1970.

74. Ekbom K: Lithium for cluster headache: Review of the literature and preliminary results of long-term treatment. Headache 21:132–139, 1981.

75. Ekbom K, and De Olivarius B: Chronic migrainous neuralgia—diagnostic and therapeutic aspects. Headache 11:97–101, 1971.

76. Ekbom K, Krabbe AE, Paalzow G, et al: Optimal routes of administration of ergotamine tartrate in cluster headache patients. A pharmacokinetic study. Cephalalgia 3:15–20, 1983.

77. Ekbom K, Lindgren L, Nilsson-B Y, et al: Retro-Gasserian glycerol injection in the treatment of chronic cluster headache. Cephalalgia 7(1):21–27, 1987.

78. Ekbom KA, and Westerberg CE: Carbamazepine in glossopharyngeal neuralgia. Arch Neurol 14:595–596, 1966.

79. Elder GA, and Sever JL: AIDS and neurological disorders: An overview. Ann Neurol (3):S4–6, 1988.

80. Ellis ME, and Ralston S: The ESR in the diagnosis and management of the polymyalgia rheumatica/giant cell arteritis syndrome. Ann Rheum Dis 42:168–170, 1983.

81. Ettala-Ylitalo VM, Syrjanen S, and Halonen P: Functional disturbance of the masticatory system related to temporomandibular joint involvement by rheumatoid arthritis. J Oral Rehabil 14:415, 1987.

82. Faleck H, Rothner AD, and Erenberg G: Headache and subacute sinusitis in children and adolescents. Headache 28:96–98, 1988.

83. Featherstone HJ: Migraine and muscle contraction headaches: A continuum. Headache 25:194–198, 1985.

84. Fernandez E: Headache associated with low spinal fluid pressure. Headache 30(3):122–128, 1990.

85. Finnish Sumatriptan Group and the Cardiovascular Clinical Research Group: A placebo-controlled study of intranasal sumatriptan for the acute treatment of migraine. Eur Neurol 31(5):332–388, 1991.

86. Fisher CM: The headache and pain of spontaneous carotid dissection. Headache 22(2):60–65, 1982.

87. Fogan L: Treatment of cluster headache. A double-blind comparison of oxygen v air inhalation. Arch Neurol 42(4):362–363, 1985.

88. Foley KM, and Posner JB: Does pseudotumor cerebri cause the empty sella syndrome? Neurology 25:565–569, June 1975.

89. Ford CD, Ford DC, and Koenigsberg MD: A simple treatment of postlumbar-puncture headache. J Emerg Med 7(1):29–31, 1989.

90. Fricton JR: Clinical care for myofascial pain. Dent Clin North Am 31(1):1–28, 1991.

91. Friedman AP, Brazil P, and von Storch, TJC: Ergotamine tolerance in patients with migraine. JAMA 157:881–884, 1955.

92. Frishberg BM: The utility of neuroimaging in the evaluation of headache in patients with normal neurological examinations. Neurology 44(7):1191–1197, 1994.

93. Fromm GH: Pharmacological consideration of anticonvulsants. Headache 9:35, 1969.

94. Fromm GH: The pharmacology of trigeminal neuralgia. Clin Neuropharmacol 12:185, 1989.

95. Fromm GH, Terrence CF, and Chatta AS: Baclofen in the treatment of trigeminal neuralgia: Double-blind study and long-term follow-up. Ann Neurol 15:240, 1984.

96. Fry RA, and Perera A: Failure of repeated blood patch in the treatment of spinal headache. Anaesthesia 44(6):492, 1989.

97. Gabai IJ, and Spierings EL: Prophylactic treatment of cluster headache with verapamil. Headache 29(3):167–168, 1989.

98. Gans, cited in Sahota and Dexter Ref. #232.

99. Glassman AH, and Bigger JT: Cardiovascular effects of therapeutic doses of tricyclic antidepressants. Arch Gen Psychiatry 38(7):815–820, 1981.

100. Gloor P: Migraine and regional cerebral blood flow. Trends Neurosci 9:21, 1986.

101. Goadsby PJ, Piper RD, Lambert GA, et al: Effect of stimulation of nucleus raphe dorsalis on carotid blood flow. I. The monkey. Am J Physiol 248:R257–R262, 1985.

102. Goldensohn ES: Paroxysmal and other features of the electro-cephalogram in migraine. Research and Clinical Studies in Headache 4:118–128, 1976.

103. Goldfischer JD: Acute myocardial infarction secondary to ergot therapy. Report of a case and review of the literature. N Engl J Med 262:860–863, 1960.

104. Gorelick PB, Hier DB, Caplan LR, et al: Headache in acute cerebrovascular disease. Neurology 36(11):1445–1450, 1986.

105. Graff-Radford S: Are bony cavities exclusively associated with atypical facial pain and trigeminal neuralgia? Abstr West USA Pain Society, May, 1988.

106. Graham JR, and Wolff HG: Mechanisms of migraine headache and action of ergotamine tartrate. Archives of Neurology and Psychiatry 39:737–763, 1938.

107. Graham JR, Suby HI, LeCompte PR, et al: Fibrotic disorders associated with methysergide therapy for headache. N Engl J Med 274(7):359–368, 1966.

108. Greenberg DA: Calcium channel antagonists and the treatment of migraine. Clin Neuropharmacol 9(4):311–328, 1986. (Review)

109. Grushka M, and Sessle BJ: Burning mouth syndrome. Dent Clin North Am 35(1):171–184, 1991.

110. Grushka M, Sessle BJ, and Miller R; Pain and personality profiles in burning mouth syndrome. Pain 28(2):155–167, 1987.

111. Hammaren M, and Hugoson A: Clinical psychiatric assessment of patients with burning mouth syndrome resisting oral treatment. Swed Dent J 13(3):77–88, 1989.

112. Hardy DG, and Rhoton AJ Jr: Microsurgical relationships of the superior cerebellar artery and the trigeminal nerve. J Neurosurg 49:669, 1978.

113. Hedman C, Winther K, and Knudson JB: The difference between non-selective and beta 1-selective beta-blockers in their effect on platelet function in migraine patients. Acta Neurol Scand 74(6):475–478, 1986.

114. Heimart M, Pradalier A, Launay JM, et al: Whole blood and plasma histamine in common migraine. Cephalalgia 7(1):39–42, 1987.

115. Henryk-Gutt R, and Rees WL: Psychological aspects of migraine. J Psychosom Res 17:141–153, 1973.

116. Hockaday JM, and Whitty WM: Factors determining the electroencephalogram in migraine. A study of 560 patients according to clinical type of migraine. Brain 92:769–788, 1969.

117. Holm JE, Holroyd KA, Hursey KG, et al: The role of stress in recurrent tension headache. Headache 26:1960–1967, 1986.

118. Holmes DS, and Burish TG: Effectiveness of biofeedback for treating migraine and tension headaches: A review of the evidence. J Psychosom Res 27(6):515–532, 1983.

119. Holroyd KA, Nash JM, and Pingel JD: A comparison of pharmacological (amitriptyline HCl) and nonpharmacological (cognitive-behavioral) therapies for chronic tension headaches. J Consult Clin Psychol 59(3):387–393, 1991.

120. Hopkins A: A neurologist's approach to patients with headache. In Hopkins A (ed): Headache: Problems in Diagnosis and Management. WB Saunders, London, 1988, pp 39–76.

121. Hopkins A: Lessons for neurologists from the United Kingdom Third National Morbidity Survey. J Neurol Neurosurg Psychiatry 52(4):430–433, 1989.

122. Hopkins A, Menken M, and DeFriese G: A record of patient encounters in neurological practice in the United Kingdom. J Neurol Neurosurg Psychiatry 52(4):436–438, 1989.

123. Hopkins A, and Ziegler DK: Headache—the size of the problem. In Hopkins A (ed): Headache: Problems in Diagnosis and Management. WB Saunders, London, 1988, pp 1–8.

124. Horrobin DF: Prostaglandins and migraine. Headache 17:113–117, 1977.

125. Huston KA, Hunder GG, Lie JT, et al: Temporal arteritis: A 25 year epidemiologic, clinical and pathologic study. Ann Intern Med 88:162–167, 1978.

126. Jacobsen E: Progressive Relaxation. University of Chicago Press, Chicago, 1938.

127. Jacobson SA: The Post-traumatic Syndrome Following Head Injury. Charles C. Thomas, Springfield, IL, 1963.

128. Janetta PJ: Arterial compression of the trigeminal nerve at the pons in patients with trigeminal neuralgia. J Neurosurg 26:159, 1967.

129. Janetta PJ: Microsurgical management of trigeminal neuralgia. Arch Neurol 42:800, 1985.

130. Johnston I, and Paterson A: CSF Pressure and Circulation. Brain 97:301–312, 1974.

131. Jones J, Sklar D, Dougherty J, et al: Randomized double-blind trial of intravenous prochlorperazine for the treatment of acute headache. JAMA 261:1174–1176, 1989.

132. Joseph R, Steiner TJ, Schultz L, et al: Platelet activity and selective beta-blockade in migraine. Stroke 19(6):704–708, 1988.

133. Jubelt B, and Miller JR: Viral infections. In Rowland LP (ed): Merritt's Textbook of Neurology, ed. 8. Lea & Febiger, Philadelphia, 1988, p 114.

134. Kaganov JA, Bakal DA, and Dunn BE: The differential contribution of muscle contraction and migraine symptoms to problem headache in the general population. Headache 21:157–163, 1981.

135. Kittrelle JP, Grouse DS, and Seybold M: Cluster headache: Local anaesthetic abortive agents. Arch Neurol 42:496–498, 1985.

136. Klara PM, and George ED: Warning leaks and sentinel headaches associated with subarachnoid hemorrhage. Mil Med 147(8):660–662, 1982.

137. Kline LB: The Tolosa-Hunt syndrome. Surv Ophthalmol 27:79–95, 1982.

138. Klun B, and Prestor B: Microvascular relations of the trigeminal nerve: An anatomical study. Neurosurgery 19(4):535–539, 1986.

139. Krabbe AA, and Olesen J: Headache provocation by continuous intravenous infusion of histamine. Clinical results and receptor mechanisms. Pain (8)2:253–259, 1980.

140. Krabbe AA, and Olesen J: Effect of histamine on regional cerebral blood flow in man. Cephalalgia 2(1):15–18, 1982.

141. Kudrow L: Comparative results of prednisone, methysergide, and lithium therapy in cluster headache. In Greene, R (ed): Current Concepts in Migraine Research. Raven Press, New York, 1978, pp 159–163.

142. Kudrow L: Cluster Headache: Mechanisms and Management. Oxford University Press, New York, 1980.

143. Kudrow L: Response of cluster headaches to oxygen inhalation. Headache 21:1–4, 1981.

144. Kudrow L: Diagnosis and treatment of cluster headache. Med Clin North Am 75(3):579–594, 1991.

145. Kudrow L, Experanza P, and Vijayan N: Episodic paroxysmal hemicrania? Cephalalgia 7:197–201, 1987.

146. Kudrow L, and Sutkus BJ: MMPI pattern specificity in primary headache disorders. Headache 19:18–24, 1979.

147. Kuhn MJ, et al: cited in Prager JM, and Mikulis DJ: The radiology of headache. Med Clin North Am 75(3):525–544, 1991.

148. Kunkle EC, Ray BS, and Wolff HG: Experimental studies on headache: Analysis of the headache associated with changes in intracranial pressure. Arch Neurol Psychiatry 49:323–358, 1943.

149. Kuntz KM, Kokmen E, Stevens JC, et al: Post–lumbar puncture headaches: Experience in 501

consecutive procedures. Neurology 42:1884–1887, 1992.

150. Kwan ES, Wolpert SM, Hedges TR 3rd, et al: Tolosa-Hunt syndrome revisited: Not necessarily a diagnosis of exclusion. Am J Roentgenol 150(2): 413–418, Feb, 1988.

151. Lance JW: Headaches related to sexual activity. J Neurol Neurosurg Psychiatry 39:1226–1230, 1976.

152. Lauritzen M: Cortical spreading depression as a putative migraine mechanism. Trends Neurosci 10:8–13, 1987.

153. Lauritzen M, and Olesen J: Regional cerebral blood flow during migraine attacks by xenon-133 inhalation and emission tomography. Brain 107: 447–461, 1984.

154. Lauritzen M, Skyhoj Olsen T, et al: Regulation of regional cerebral blood flow during and between migraine attacks. Ann Neurol 14:569–572, 1983.

155. Lazar ML, and Kirkpatrick JB: Trigeminal neuralgia and multiple sclerosis: Demonstration of the plaque in an operative case. Neurosurgery 5:711, 1979.

156. Leao AAP: Spreading depression of activity in cerebral cortex. J Neurophysiol 7:359–390, 1944.

157. Levin B, and Posner JB: Swallow syncope. Report of a case and review of the literature. Neurology 22:1086–1093, 1972.

158. Levine HL: Otorhinolaryngologic causes of headache. Med Clin North Am 75:677–692, 1991.

159. Lew D, Southwick FS, Montgomery WW, et al: Sphenoid sinusitis: A review of 30 cases. N Engl J Med 309(19)1149–1154, 1983.

160. Lipton RB, Ottman R, Ehrenberg BL, et al: Comorbidy of migraine: The connection between migraine and epilepsy. Neurology 44(Suppl 7): S28–S32, 1994.

161. Lipton RB, Rosenbaum D, and Mehler MF: Giant cell arteritis causes recurrent posterior circulation transient ischemic attacks which respond to corticosteroid. Eur Neurol 27(2):97–100, 1987.

162. Loeser JD: Tic douloureux and atypical facial pain. In Wall PD, and Melzack R (eds): Textbook of Pain. Churchill Livingstone, Edinburgh, 1984, pp 426–434.

163. Lucas RN: Migraine in twins. J Psychosom Res 21:147–156, 1977.

164. MacKenzie ET, Edvinsson L, and Scatton B: Functional basis for a central serotonergic involvement in classic migraine: A speculative view. Cephalalgia 5:69–78, 1985.

165. Mann JD, Johnson RN, Butler AB, et al: Impairment of cerebrospinal fluid circulatory dynamics in pseudotumor cerebri and response to steroid treatment. Neurology 29:550, 1979.

166. Mansfield LE: The role of antihistamine therapy in vascular headaches. J Allergy Clin Immunol 86(4 pt 2):673–676, 1990.

167. Manzoni GC, Bono G, Lanfranchi M, et al: Lithium carbonate in cluster headache: Assessment of its short- and long-term therapeutic efficacy. Cephalalgia 3:109–114, 1983.

168. Manzoni GC, Terzano MG, and Bono G: Cluster headache—Clinical findings in 180 patients. Cephalalgia 3:21–30, 1983.

169. Manusov EG: Late-life migraine accompaniments: A case presentation and literature review. J Fam Pract 24(6):591–594, 1987.

170. Marbach JJ, Hulbrock J, Hohn C, et al: Incidence of phantom tooth pain: An atypical facial neuralgia. Oral Surg Oral Med Oral Pathol 53(2):190–193, 1982.

171. Marcus DA: Migraine and tension-type headaches: The questionable validity of current classification systems. Clin J Pain 8:32–36, 1992.

172. Markley HG: Chronic headache: Appropriate use of opiate analgesics. Neurology 44(Suppl 3) S18–S24, 1994.

173. Martin MJ: Tension headache: A psychiatric study. Headache 6:648–655, 1966.

174. Mathew NT: Drug-induced headache. Neurol Clin 8(4):903–912, 1990.

175. Mathew NT, Kurman R, and Perez F: Drug induced refractory headache: Clinical features and management. Headache 30(10):634–638, 1990.

176. Mathew NT, Stabits E, and Nigam MP: Transformation of episodic migraine into daily headache: Analysis of factors. Headache 22:66–68, 1982.

177. McCarthy KD, and Reed DJ: The effect of acetazolamide and furosemide on CSF production and choroid plexus carbonic anhydrase activity. J Pharmacol Exp Ther 189:194–201, 1974.

178. Meglio M, and Cioni B: Percutaneous procedures for trigeminal neuralgia: Microcompression versus radiofrequency thermocoagulation. Personal experience. Pain 38:9–16, 1989.

179. Merikangas KR, Dartigues MD, Whitaker A, et al: Diagnostic criteria for migraine. A validity study. Neurology 44(Suppl 4):11–16, 1994.

180. Merskey H, and Boyd D: Emotional adjustment and chronic pain. Pain 5:173–178, 1978.

181. Merskey H, and Woodforde JM: Psychiatric sequelae of minor head injury. Brain 95:521–528, 1972.

182. Metzer WS: Trigeminal neuralgia secondary to tumor with normal exam, responsive to carbamazepine. Headache 31(3):164–166, 1991.

183. Meyer JS: Calcium channel blockers in the prophylactic treatment of vascular headache. Ann Intern Med 102:395–397, 1985.

184. Meyer JS, and Hardenberg J: Clinical effectiveness of calcium entry blockers in prophylactic treatment of migraine and cluster headaches. Headache 23(6):266–277, 1983.

185. Meyer JS, Zetusky W, Jonsdottir M, et al: Cephalic hyperemia during migraine headaches. A prospective study. Headache 26:388–397, 1986.

186. Michultka DA, Blanchard EB, Applebaum KA, et al: The refractory headache patient—II. High medication consumption (analgesic rebound) headache. Behav Res Ther 27:411–420, 1989.

187. Moffett AM, Swash M, and Scott DF: Effect of chocolate in migraine: A double-blind study. J Neurol Neurosurg Psychiatry 37:445–448, 1974.

188. Monro J, Carini C, and Brostoff J: Migraine is a food-allergic disease. Lancet 2:719–721, 1984.

189. Moss RA, and Adams HE: Physiological reactions to stress in subjects with and without myofascial pain dysfunction symptoms. J Oral Rehab 11:219, 1984.

190. Muller-Schweinitzer E, and Weidmann H: Basic pharmacological properties. In Berde B, and

Schild HO (eds): Ergot Aklaloids and Related Compounds (Vol 49, Handbook of Experimental Pharmacology). Springer-Verlag, New York, 1978, pp 87–232.

191. Multi-national Oral Sumatriptan and Cafergot Comparative Study Group. A randomized, double-blind comparison of sumatriptan and cafergot in the acute treatment of migraine. Eur Neurol 31(5):314–322, 1991.

192. Newman LC, Gordon ML, Lipton RB, et al: Episodic paroxysmal hemicrania: Two new cases and a literature review. Neurology 42:964–966, 1992.

193. Olesen J: Some clinical features of acute migraine attack. An analysis of 750 patients. Headache 18: 268–271, 1978.

194. Olesen J: Are classical and common migraine different entities? Headache 25:213, 1985.

195. Olesen J: Clinical and pathophysiological observations in migraine and tension-type headache explained by integration of vascular, supraspinal and myofascial inputs. Pain (46):125–132, 1991.

196. Olesen J, and Lipton RB: Migraine classification and diagnosis. International Headache Society Criteria. Neurology 44(Suppl 4) S6–S10, 1994.

197. Olesen J, Tfelt-Hansen P, Henriksen L, et al: The common migraine attack may not be initiated by cerebral ischemia. Lancet 2:438–440, 1981.

198. Olesen KS: Epidural blood patch in the treatment of post–lumbar puncture headache. Pain 30(3): 293–301, Sept 1987 (Review).

199. Packard RC: Posttraumatic headache: Determining chronicity. Headache 33(3):133–134, 1993.

200. Patchell RA, and Posner JB: Neurologic complications of systemic cancer. Neurol Clin 3(4):729–750, Nov, 1985.

201. Pearce J: Migraine: A psychosomatic disorder. Headache 17:125–128, 1977.

202. Pearce JMS: Migraine: A cerebral disorder. Lancet 2:86–89, 1984.

203. Peatfield RC, Fozard JR, and Rose FC: Drug treatment of migraine. In Rose FC (ed): Handbook of Clinical Neurology, Vol 48. Elsevier, Amsterdam, 1986, pp 173–216.

204. Pellock JM, and Willmore J: A rational guide to routine blood monitoring in patients receiving antiepileptic drugs. Neurology 41:961–964, 1991.

205. Perkin JE, and Hartje J: Diet and migraine: A review of the literature. J Am Diet Assoc 83(4): 459–463, 1983.

206. Pinnas JL, and Vanselow NA: Relationship of allergy to headache. Res Clin Stud Headache 4:85–95, 1978.

207. Portenoy RK, Abissi CJ, Lipton RB, et al: Headache in cerebrovascular disease. Stroke 15:1009–1012, 1984.

208. Poukkula E: The problem of post-spinal headache. Ann Chir Gynaecol 73(3):139–142, 1984.

209. Pradalier A, Clapin A, and Dry J: Treatment review: Nonsteroidal anti-inflammatory drugs in the treatment and long term prevention of migraine attacks. Headache 28:550–557, 1988.

210. Price R, and Posner JB: Chronic paroxysmal hemicrania: A disabling headache syndrome responding to indomethacin. Ann Neurol 3:183, 1978.

211. Pulec JL: Geniculate neuralgia: Diagnosis and surgical management. Laryngoscope 86(7):955–964, 1976.

212. Rappaport NB, McAnulty DP, Waggoner CD, et al: Cluster analysis of Minnesota Multiphasic Personality Inventory (MMPI) profiles in a chronic headache population. J Behav Med 10(1):49–60, 1987.

213. Raskin N: Migraine: Pathogenesis. In Raskin N (ed): Headache, ed 2. Churchill Livingstone, New York, 1988.

214. Raskin NH: Migraine: Clinical aspects. In Raskin N (ed): Headache, ed 2. Churchill Livingstone, New York, 1988, p 36.

215. Raskin NH: Repetitive intravenous dihydroergotamine as therapy for intractable migraine. Neurology 36:995–997, 1986.

216. Raskin NH: Migraine: Treatment. In Raskin N (ed): Headache ed 2. Churchill Livingstone, New York, 1988.

217. Raskin NH: Tension headache. In Raskin N (ed): Headache ed 2. Churchill Livingstone, New York, 1988, p 215.

218. Raskin NH: Headache: An overview. In Raskin N (ed): Headache ed 2. Churchill Livingstone, New York, 1988, p 20.

219. Raskin NH, and Knittle SC: Ice cream headache and orthostatic symptoms in patients with migraine. Headache 16:222–225, 1976.

220. Rasmussen BK, and Olesen J: Epidemiology of migraine and tension-type headache. Curr Opin Neurol 7(3):264–271, 1994.

221. Ratner EJ, Langer B, and Evins ML: Alveolar cavitational osteopathosis. J Periodont 57:593–603, 1986.

222. Ratner EJ, Person P, Kleinman DJ, et al: Jawbone cavities and trigeminal and atypical facial neuralgias. Oral Surg 48:3–20, 1979.

223. Rizzo PA, Pierelli F, Pozzessere G, et al: Subjective posttraumatic syndrome: A comparison of visual and brainstem auditory evoked responses. Neuropsychobiology 9(2–3):78–82, 1983.

224. Roberts CA, Tallents RH, Katzberg RW, et al: Comparison of arthrographic findings of temporomandibular joint with palpation of the muscles of mastication. Oral Surg Oral Med Oral Pathol 64: 275, 1987.

225. Rockcliff BW, and Davis EH: Controlled sequential trials of carbamazepine in trigeminal neuralgia. Arch Neurol 15:129, 1966.

226. Roll TW, and Schleifer LS: Drugs effective in the epilepsies. In Goodman AG, Gilman S, Rall TW, et al: (eds): The Pharmacological Basis of Therapeutics, ed 8. Pergamon Press, New York, 1990, p 448.

227. Roth AM, Milsow L, and Keltner JL: The ultimate diagnoses of patients undergoing temporal artery biopsies. Arch Ophthalmol 102(6):901–903, 1984.

228. Rothner AD: Headaches in adolescents: Diagnosis and management. Med Clin North Am 75(3): 653–660, 1991.

229. Rugh JD, and Solberg WK, cited by Sharav, Y: Orofacial pain. In Wall PD, and Melzack R (eds): Textbook of Pain. Churchill Livingstone, Edinburgh, 1984, p 343.

230. Rupa V, Saunders RL, and Weider DJ: Geniculate neuralgia: The surgical management of primary otalgia. J Neurosurg 75(4):505–511, 1991.

231. Rush JA: Pseudotumor cerebri. Clinical profile and visual outcome in 63 patients. Mayo Clin Proc 55:541–546, 1980.

232. Sahota RK, and Dexter JD: Sleep and headache syndromes: A clinical review. Headache 30(2):80–84, 1990.

233. Sands GH: A protocol for butalbital, aspirin, and caffeine (BAC) detoxification in headache patients. Headache 30:491–486, 1990.

234. Sansome MEG, and Ziegler DK: Lithium toxicity: A review of neurologic complications. Clin Neuropharmacol 8:242–248, 1985.

235. Saper JR: Long-term efficacy of microvascular decompression in trigeminal neuralgia. In Saper JR (ed): Topics in Pain Management. Current Concepts and Treatment Strategies. Williams & Wilkins, Baltimore, 1988, Vol 4(5).

236. Saper JR: Chronic headache syndromes. Neurol Clin 7(2):387–412, 1989.

237. Saper JR, and Jones JM: Ergotamine tartrate dependency: Features and possible mechanisms. Clin Neuropharmacol 9(3):244–256, 1986.

238. Schoenen J: Beta blockers and the central nervous system. Cephalalgia 6(5):47–54, 1986.

239. Schor DI: Headache and facial pain—the role of the paranasal sinuses: A literature review. Cranio 11(1):36–47, 1993.

240. Selby G, and Lance JW: Observations on 500 cases of migraine and allied vascular headache. J Neurol Neurosurg Psychiatry 23:23–32, 1960.

241. Seltzer S: Foods, and food and drug combinations, responsible for head and neck pain. Cephalalgia 2(2):111–124, 1982.

242. Sergott RC: Neuro-ophthalmology: Diagnosis and management of vision-threatening papilledema. Semin Neurol 6(2):176–184, June, 1986.

243. Sheftell FD: Chronic daily headache. Neurology 43(3 Suppl 2):32–36, 1992.

244. Sicuteri F, Nicolodi M, Fusco BM, et al: Idiopathic headache as a possible risk factor for phantom tooth pain. Headache 31:557–581, 1991.

245. Silberstein SD, and Young WB: Safety and efficacy of ergotamine tartrate and dihydroergotamine in the treatment of migraine and status migrainosus. Neurology 45:577–584, 1995.

246. Skyhoj Olsen T, Friberg L, and Lassen NA: Ischemia may be the primary cause of the neurologic deficits in classic migraine. Arch Neurol 44:156–161, 1987.

247. Smith I, Mullen PE, and Hanington E: Dietary migraine and tyramine metabolism. Nature 230:246–248, 1971.

248. Solomon GD: Pharmacology and use of headache medications. Cleve Clin J Med 57(7):627–635, Oct, 1990.

249. Solomon GD, and Spaccavento LJ: Verapamil prophylaxis of migraine: A double-blind, placebo-controlled trial. JAMA 250:2500–2502, 1983.

250. Solomon S, and Lipton RB: Atypical facial pain: A review. Semin Neurol 8:332, 1988.

251. Solomon SS, Lipton RB, and Newman LC: Prophylactic therapy of cluster headaches. Clin Neuropharmacol 14(2):116–130, 1991.

252. Spoor TC, and McHenry JG: Long-term effectiveness of optic sheath decompression for pseudotumor cerebri. Arch Ophthalmol 11(5):632–635, 1993.

253. Stewart WF, Schechter A, and Rasmussen BK: Migraine prevalence. A review of population-based studies. Neurology 44(Suppl 4) S17–S23, 1994.

254. Sumatriptan Auto-Injector Study Group. Self-treatment of acute migraine with subcutaneous sumatriptan using an auto-injector device. Eur Neurol 31(5):323–331, 1991.

255. Sweet WH: Percutaneous methods for the treatment of trigeminal neuralgia and other facio-cephalic pain; comparison with microvascular decompression. Semin Neurol 8(4):272–279, 1988.

256. Sweet WH: Surgical treatment of chronic cluster headache. Headache 29:669–670, 1988.

257. Sweet WH, Poletti CE, and Macon JB: Treatment of trigeminal neuralgia and other facial pains by retrogasserian injection of glycerol. Neurosurgery 9:647, 1981.

258. Sweet WH, and Wepsic JG: Controlled thermocoagulation of trigeminal ganglion and rootlets for differential destruction of pain fibers. I. Trigeminal neuralgia. J Neurosurg 40:143, 1974.

259. Tarsh MJ, and Royston C: A follow-up study of accident neurosis. Br J Psychiatry 146:18–25, 1985.

260. Tfelt-Hansen P: Efficacy of beta-blockers in migraine. A critical review. Cephalalgia 6(5):15–24, 1986, Suppl.

261. Tfelt-Hansen P, Lous I, and Olesen J: Prevalence and significant of muscle tenderness during common migraine attacks. Headache 21:49–54, 1981.

262. Tomsak RL: Ophthalmologic aspects of headache. Med Clin North Am 75(3):693–706, 1991.

263. Tunis MM, and Wolff HG: Long term observations of the reactivity of the cranial arteries in subjects with vascular headache of the migraine type. Archives of Neurology and Psychiatry 70:551–557, 1953.

264. Vander Ark GD, Kempe LG, and Smith DR: Pseudotumor cerebri treated with lumbar-peritoneal shunt. JAMA 217:1832–1834, 1971.

265. van Gijn J, and van Dongen KJ: Computerized tomography in subarachnoid hemorrhage: Difference between patients with and without an aneurysm on angiography. Neurology 30(5):538–539, 1980.

266. Wadsworth M, Butterfield W, and Blaney R: Health and Sickness: The Choice of Treatment. Tavistock, London, 1971.

267. Waters WE: Migraine: Intelligence, social class and familial prevalence. British Medical Journal 2:77–81, 1971.

268. Weingarten S, Kleinman M, Elperin L, et al: The effectiveness of cerebral imaging in the diagnosis of chronic headache. Arch Intern Med 152(12):2457–2462, 1992.

269. Welch KMA: Relationship of stroke and migraine. Neurology 44(Suppl 7): S33–S36, 1994.

270. Wilkinson M, and Blau JN: Are classical and common migraine different entities? Headache 25:211–212, 1985.

271. Wolff HG: Personality features and reactions of subjects with migraine. Arch Neurol Psychiatry 37:895–921, 1937.

272. Ziegler DK: Genetics of migraine. Headache 16: 330–331, 1977.
273. Ziegler DK, and Ellis DJ: Naproxen in prophylaxis of migraine. Arch Neurol 42:582–584, 1985.
274. Ziegler DK, Hassanein RS, and Couch JR: Characteristics of life headache histories in a non-clinic population. Neurology 27:265–269, 1977.
275. Ziegler DK, Hassanein RS, Harris D, et al: Headache in a non-clinic twin population. Headache 14:213–218, 1975.
276. Zimm S, Wampler GL, Stablein D, et al: Intracerebral metastases in solid-tumor patients: Natural history and results of treatment. Cancer 48:384–394, 1981.

APPENDIX I.

International Headache Society Classification of Headache Syndromes

I. Migraine
    1.1 Migraine without aura
    1.2 Migraine with aura
        1.2.1 Migraine with typical aura
        1.2.2 Migraine with prolonged aura
        1.2.3 Familial hemiplegic migraine
        1.2.4 Basilar migraine
        1.2.5 Migraine aura without headache
        1.2.6 Migraine with acute onset aura
    1.3 Ophthalmoplegic migraine
    1.4 Retinal migraine
    1.5 Childhood periodic syndromes that may be precursors to or associated with migraine
        1.5.1 Benign paroxysmal vertigo of childhood
        1.5.2 Alternating hemiplegia of childhood
    1.6 Complications of migraine
        1.6.1 Status migrainosus
        1.6.2 Migrainous infarction
    1.7 Migrainous disorder not fulfilling above criteria
2. Tension-type headache
    2.1 Episodic tension-type headache
        2.1.1 Episodic tension-type headache associated with disorder of pericranial muscles
        2.1.2 Chronic tension-type headache unassociated with disorder of pericranial muscles
    2.2 Chronic tension-type headache
        2.2.1 Chronic tension-type headache associated with disorder of pericranial muscles
        2.2.2 Chronic tension-type headache unassociated with disorder of pericranial muscles
    2.3 Headache of the tension-type not fulfilling above criteria
3. Cluster headache and chronic paroxysmal hemicrania
    3.1 Cluster headache
        3.1.1 Cluster headache periodicity undetermined
        3.1.2 Episodic cluster headache
        3.1.3 Chronic cluster headache
            3.1.3.1 Unremitting from onset
            3.1.3.2 Evolved from episodic
    3.2 Chronic paroxysmal hemicrania
    3.3 Cluster headache-like disorder not fulfilling above criteria
4. Miscellaneous headaches unassociated with structural lesion
    4.1 Idiopathic stabbing headache
    4.2 External compression headache
    4.3 Cold stimulus headache
        4.3.1 External application of a cold stimulus
        4.3.2 Ingestion of a cold stimulus
    4.4 Benign cough headache
    4.5 Benign exertional headache
    4.6 Headache associated with sexual activity
        4.6.1 Dull type
        4.6.2 Explosive type
        4.6.3 Postural type
5. Headache associated with head trauma
    5.1 Acute posttraumatic headache
        5.1.1 With significant head trauma and/or confirmatory signs
        5.1.2 With minor head trauma and no confirmatory signs

The general rules listed for classification are the following:

1. If the patient has more than one headache disorder, all should be diagnosed in the order of importance indicated by the patient.
2. To make a diagnosis, all letter headings of a set of diagnostic criteria must be fulfilled.
3. After each diagnosis add estimated number of headache days per year in brackets.
4. Diagnostic criteria given at the one- or two-digit level must generally be met by the subforms, but exceptions and/or more specific criteria are listed under the subforms.
5. Patients who, for the first time, develop a particular form of headache in close temporal relation to onset of one of the disorders listed in groups 5–11 are coded to these groups using the fourth digit to specify type of headache. A causal relationship is not necessarily indicated, however. Preexisting migraine, tension-type headache, or cluster headache aggravated in close temporal relation to one of the disorders listed in groups 5–11 is still coded as migraine, tension-type headache, or cluster headache (groups 1–3). If number of headache days increases by 100 percent or more, the aggravating factor may be mentioned in parentheses, but it is not coded for.
6. Code to the degree (number of digits) that suits your purpose.
7. If one headache type fits the diagnostic criteria for different categories of headache, code to the first headache category in the classification for which the criteria are fulfilled (1.7, 2.3, and 3.3). The headache type is not diagnostic if the headache also fulfills another diagnosis.
8. If a patient has a form of headache fulfilling one set of diagnostic criteria, similar episodes that do not quite satisfy the criteria also usually occur. This can be due to treatment, lack of ability to remember symptoms exactly, and other factors. Ask the patient to describe a typical untreated attack or an unsuccessfully treated attack and ascertain that there have been enough of these attacks to establish the diagnosis. Then estimate the days per year with this type of headache, adding also treated attacks and less typical attacks.
9. A major obstacle to an exact diagnosis is the reliance on patient's history to determine whether criteria are met. In less clear cases it is recommended to let the patient record attack characteristics, prospectively, using a headache diary before the diagnosis is made.
10. If a fourth digit is to be used in association with a diagnosis at the two-digit level, insert 0 as the third digit.

CHAPTER 5

NEUROPATHIC PAIN

Russell K. Portenoy, M.D.

NEUROPATHIC PAIN SUSTAINED BY
   CENTRAL MECHANISMS
Reflex Sympathetic Dystrophy/Causalgia
Deafferentation Pain
NEUROPATHIC PAIN DUE PRIMARILY TO
   PERIPHERAL CAUSES
Mechanisms
Specific Syndromes

The term *neuropathic pain* is applied to any acute or chronic pain syndrome in which the sustaining mechanism for the pain is inferred to involve aberrant somatosensory processing in the peripheral or central nervous system. Most previous classifications of the diverse syndromes constituting neuropathic pain have grouped them on the basis of diagnosis or syndrome[152] or the site of the inciting lesion (Fig. 5–1). Recently, a classification based on inferred pathophysiology[57,173] has offered clinical insights that could lead ultimately to the development of diagnostic approaches and management strategies based on mechanism. According to this taxonomy, some neuropathic pains are primarily sustained by processes in the central nervous system and others by processes in the peripheral nervous system (Fig. 5–2). Although this distinction has not been established in studies of human diseases, it is suggested by both clinical and experimental data (Table 5–1) and provides a heuristic structure for these disorders.

NEUROPATHIC PAIN SUSTAINED BY CENTRAL MECHANISMS

Neuropathic pains that are presumably sustained predominantly by aberrant central somatosensory processing can be broadly divided into two groups: (1) reflex sympathetic dystrophy (RSD)/causalgia and (2) deafferentation pains. Each of these groups, in turn, subsumes many specific syndromes.

Reflex Sympathetic Dystrophy/Causalgia

The nomenclature for the pain syndromes now commonly termed RSD/causalgia is confusing,[163] and many other diagnoses have been used in the past to describe similar entities (Table 5–2). A recent taxonomy developed by the International Association for the Study of Pain suggests that the term *complex regional pain syndrome* (type I for RSD and type II for causalgia) be used as a general descriptive label for all these syndromes.[152] A recent consensus statement retained the term RSD and offered the following operational definition:

> RSD is a descriptive term meaning a complex disorder or group of disorders that may develop as a consequence of trauma affecting the limbs, with or without an obvious nerve le-

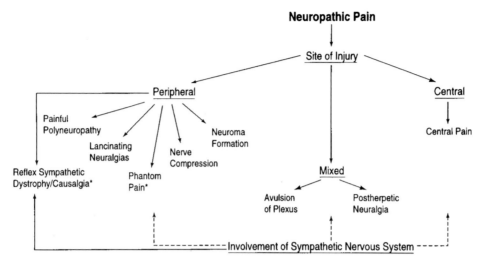

Figure 5–1. Classification of neuropathic pains by the site of the neural injury. The dependence of the pain on sympathetic efferent activity has been reported for lesions at all locations, although it is far more prevalent with peripheral lesions and predominates in reflex sympathetic dystrophy (RSD) and causalgia. *Usually a peripheral lesion. (From Portenoy RK: Issues in the management of neuropathic pains. In Basbaum A, and Besson J-M [eds]: Towards a New Pharmacotherapy of Pain. John Wiley & Sons, Chichester, 1991, p 394, with permission.)

sion. RSD may also develop after visceral diseases, and central nervous system lesions, or, rarely, without an obvious antecedent event. It consists of pain and related sensory abnormalities, abnormal blood flow and sweating, abnormalities in the motor system and changes in structure of both superficial and deep tissues ("trophic" changes). It is not necessary that all components are present. It is agreed that the name "reflex sympathetic dys-

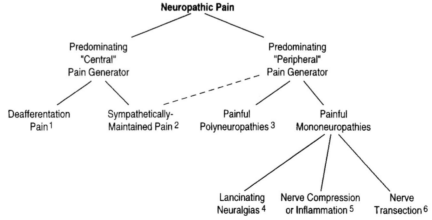

Figure 5–2. Classification of neuropathic pains by putative predominating mechanism. [1]Response to either peripheral or central nervous system injury. [2]Associated with focal autonomic dysregulation (e.g. edema, vasomotor disturbances), involuntary motor responses, or trophic changes that may improve with sympathetic nerve block. [3]Multiple mechanisms probably involved. [4]The patterns of peripheral activity, or peripheral and central interaction, that yield the lancinating quality of these pains are unknown. [5]Nociceptive nervi nervorum (small afferents that innervate larger nerves) may account for neuropathic pain accompanying nerve compression or inflammation. [6]Injury to axons may be followed by neuroma formation, a source of aberrant activity likely to be involved in pain. (Adapted from Portenoy RK: Issues in the management of neuropathic pain. In Basbaum A, and Besson J-M [eds]: Towards a New Pharmacotherapy of Pain. John Wiley & Sons, Chichester, 1991, p 386.)

Table 5–1. **PATHOPHYSIOLOGIC CLASSIFICATION OF NEUROPATHIC PAIN; EVIDENCE AND CAVEATS**[*]

Evidence	Caveat
Historical data regarding the efficacy of neurolysis suggest that some pains have a central mechanism that continues to cause pain after the painful part is isolated from the CNS.	Data are limited and published cases have selection bias; evidence is meager that pains believed to have a peripheral mechanism respond reliably to neurolysis.
Some correlations have been demonstrated in specific syndromes (e.g., abnormal electrical activity in CNS structures in deafferentation pains and similar activity on microneuronography of nerves proximal to neuroma).	Correlations between findings and pain do not prove causality; there have been no simultaneous recordings from peripheral and central structures in humans.
Extrapolation from animal models suggests that the most salient changes may be either central or peripheral (e.g., neuroma model demonstrates characteristics, such as mechanosensitivity, that correspond to findings in humans with similar pathology).	Relationship between animal models and chronic neuropathic pain in humans is highly inferential; studies show that peripheral injury produces substantial changes in the CNS and that CNS injury may cause changes in the periphery.

[*]Evidence supporting the hypothesized division of neuropathic pains into those with a predominating central "pain generator" and those with a predominating peripheral "pain generator," along with appropriate caveats that indicate the unproven nature of this conceptualization.

CNS = central nervous system.

Source: Portenoy RK: Issues in the management of neuropathic pain. In Basbaum A, and Besson J-M (eds): Towards a New Pharmacotherapy of Pain. John Wiley & Sons, Chichester, 1991, p 395, with permission.

trophy" is used in a descriptive sense and does not imply specific underlying mechanisms.[105]

Most of this definition can be applied equally well to causalgia, which is typically considered to be the same syndrome produced by injury to a nerve trunk. Thus, RSD/causalgia and complex regional pain syndrome are fundamentally descriptive labels and do not specifically indicate an underlying pathophysiology.

Notwithstanding, the clinical characteristics that establish a diagnosis of RSD/causalgia do suggest the possibility that the pathophysiology of the pain involves efferent activity in the sympathetic nervous system and could potentially be ameliorated by sympathetic nerve block. The term "sympathetically maintained pain" (SMP) has been applied to any pain that is sustained, at least in part, by sympathetic efferent activity. Patients with RSD/causalgia may or may not improve with sympathetic block; some improve transiently. Pain relief with sympathetic nerve block confirms that the pain syndrome is also an SMP.

Although this classification of SMP as a subtype of RSD/causalgia fits well with clinical observations, there are unresolved issues with both nomenclature and diagnosis. For example, reliance on sympathetic interruption as a confirmatory test for SMP is problematic. Sympathetic interruption can be accomplished with neural blockage, a brief systemic infusion of the α-adrenergic blocker phentolamine, or a regional intravenous infusion of a drug that depletes norepinephrine. These procedures are typically performed clinically without a placebo control. The placebo response to putative analgesic approaches, including phentolamine infusion,[64] can be profound and sustained,[227] and the outcome of sympathetic interruption is difficult to interpret without separately measuring this response. There have been no placebo-controlled studies of sympathetic nerve blocks, and placebo-controlled trials of the phentolamine infusion have yielded mixed results.[181,229,230] At minimum, the negative studies of the phentolamine infusion question the validity of this procedure as a diagnostic test for SMP. Some authors suggest that these negative findings actually question the SMP construct itself, contradicting the widely held view that some neuropathic pains are sustained by sympathetic efferent activity.[229,230]

Table 5–2. SOME TERMS PREVIOUSLY USED TO DESCRIBE REFLEX SYMPATHETIC DYSTROPHY OR CAUSALGIA

Major causalgia
Minor causalgia
Shoulder-hand syndrome
Sympathalgia
Sudeck's atrophy
Posttraumatic pain syndrome
Chronic traumatic edema
Posttraumatic sympathetic dystrophy
Traumatic angiospasm
Traumatic vasospasm
Posttraumatic osteoporosis
Algodystrophy
Thermalgia
Acute peripheral trophoneurosis
Neurovascular reflex dystrophy
Mimocausalgia
Neurovascular reflex sympathetic dystrophy
Neurovascular posttraumatic painful syndrome
Posttraumatic chronic edema
Spreading neuralgia

Source: Adapted from Portenoy RK: Issues in the management of neuropathic pain. In Basbaum A, and Besson J-M (eds): Towards a New Pharmacotherapy of Pain. John Wiley & Sons, Chichester, 1991, p 398, with permission.

Thus, the diagnosis of RSD/causalgia is suggested by the coexistence of pain and autonomic dysregulation or trophic changes (see following). The clinical findings should alert the clinician to the possibility of an SMP, which may or may not be confirmed by a procedure that blocks sympathetic efferent activity. An unequivocal response to sympathetic interruption establishes the diagnosis of SMP, but the empirical foundation for this procedure is limited and the use of a label that indicates a specific mechanism is problematic in the clinical setting, particularly when the response to sympathetic blockade may be transient, equivocal, or negative.

MECHANISMS

RSD/causalgia has been ascribed to both peripheral and central factors (Table 5–3).[132,136,157,160] Although it is now recognized that the syndrome may not respond to sympathetic nerve block (i.e., may not be SMP), the involvement of the sympathetic nervous system in the pathophysiology of RSD/causalgia has been assumed for many decades on the basis of several clinical observations. These include the therapeutic response to sympathetic interruption in some patients, the worsening of causalgia following stimulation of the ipsilateral sympathetic chain,[234] and the flare in pain that may be produced by subcutaneous injection of epinephrine in the affected area.[236] A recent alternative hypothesis, which rejects the importance of sympathetic efferent activity and posits a role for nociceptive visceral afferents traveling with the sympathetics, has no direct empirical support at this time.

Peripheral Processes. Presumably, some peripheral processes that underlie the pain of RSD/causalgia are unrelated to the sympathetic nervous system. RSD/causalgia following local trauma could be sustained, in part, by sensitization of primary afferent nociceptors, "backfiring" by injured polymodal C fibers (leading to peripheral release of substances, such as substance P, that activate primary nociceptors), and ectopic electrical activity originating in the damaged nociceptors.[50,52,235]

Other processes may explain the link between the sympathetic nervous system and the pain of RSD/causalgia. An early hypothesis suggested that sympathetic hyperactivity alters peripheral tissues in a manner that can activate nociceptors, thus creating a so-called vicious circle.[132] There is no evidence that RSD/causalgia is associated with sympathetic hyperactivity, however, and more recent hypotheses have focused on other links between sympathetic fibers and both nociceptive and nonnociceptive primary afferent nerves.[84,186,187,200]

After local trauma, sympathetic efferent activity could excite primary afferent neurons through several mechanisms. First, damaged nerves may have increased sensitivity to the catecholamines released by sympathetic terminals. The number of α-adrenergic receptors on regenerating nerve fibers (neuroma) increases, and ectopic activity produced by these fibers fluctuates with levels of circulating catecholamines.[55] A recent hypothesis suggests that α_1-adrenergic receptors on dam-

Table 5–3. **MECHANISMS THAT MAY BE INVOLVED IN REFLEX SYMPATHETIC DYSTROPHY/CAUSALGIA**

Peripheral Processes

Activity in nociceptive visceral afferents that travel with sympathetic efferent fibers.

Processes unrelated to sympathetic nervous system that increase activity in somatic nociceptors.

    Sensitization following injury.

    C-fiber "backfiring" with release of algogenic substances.

    Ectopic electrical activity from neuroma or areas of focal demyelination.

Processes involving sympathetic-somatic link.

    Sympathetic hyperactivity changes peripheral tissues in a way that activates nociceptors ("vicious circle").

    Damaged nociceptors have increased sensitivity to catecholamines released by sympathetic nerves.

    Prostaglandins released by sympathetic nerves may sensitize nociceptors.

    Sympathetic-nociceptor ephapses may form.

Central Processes

Any of the putative mechanisms of the deafferentation pains.

Sympathetically driven activity in nonnociceptive afferents may increase firing of sensitized wide–dynamic-range neurons in the spinal cord (Robert's hypothesis).

---

aged peripheral nerves specifically contributes to the development of SMP.[31] Second, prostaglandins are released from sympathetic nerve terminals in regions of local tissue injury.[131] These compounds could sensitize nociceptors. Third, the formation of *ephapses,* or abnormal connections, between efferent sympathetic nerves and primary afferent nociceptors could increase nociceptor input.[104]

Although one or more of the described phenomena may be involved in RSD/causalgia, none explains all observations. For example, these mechanisms do not address the pathogenesis of the autonomic and trophic changes that characterize RSD/causalgia. Equally puzzling, they provide no basis for the observation that RSD/causalgia can evolve without obvious peripheral injury or after injury to structures (such as pure sensory nerves or dorsal roots) that lack a sympathetic supply.

Central Processes. The most compelling evidence that central mechanisms are fundamental in RSD/causalgia is that complete isolation of the painful part from the central nervous system (by neurectomy or rhizotomy, for example) does not reliably eradicate the pain.[214] This characteristic is shared by the deafferentation pains (see following). Other relevant observations include the occurrence

of classic RSD/causalgia following damage to the central nervous system or viscera, the immediate appearance of the pain after injury in many patients (before neuroma can develop), and the development of spreading pain and bilateral signs in many patients.

A variety of central mechanisms may be involved in the pathogenesis of RSD/causalgia. Most could apply to any or all of the deafferentation pains as well (see following). A recent model that addresses SMP, but which may be more relevant to RSD/causalgia, suggests that the pathophysiology of the pain depends on an interaction between sensitized central neurons and sympathetically driven activity in nonnociceptive afferents.[185] Wide-dynamic-range neurons in the dorsal horn of the spinal cord receive input from both nociceptive and nonnociceptive primary afferents. Activation of nociceptors by peripheral injury can sensitize these neurons (see Chapter 2), which could then respond inappropriately to activity in nonnociceptive afferents, including activity driven by sympathetic efferent firing.

Although this hypothesis does not explain some observations, such as the occurrence of SMP without hypersensitivity of the skin, the concept of a sensitized central neuron is appealing and may be applicable to the pathogenesis of diverse neuropathic pains. A unifying model (Fig. 5–3) of the pathophysiologic changes that may underlie the pain induced by peripheral injury also posits this concept and highlights the dynamic interaction that may occur among peripheral nociceptive and nonnociceptive processes, sympathetic efferent activity, and central changes.[51]

CHARACTERISTICS

The diagnosis of RSD/causalgia is suggested by the history and physical findings, supported if necessary by ancillary tests. SMP is confirmed in a proportion of patients by a favorable response to sympathetic blockade.

Epidemiology. Relatively little is known about the epidemiology of RSD/causalgia. Surveys of veterans suggest that the incidence of causalgia following injury to a peripheral nerve is 1 to 5 percent.[214] The incidence of RSD following injury to other tissues is unknown but is presumed to be extremely small.

Many traumatic and nontraumatic processes cause RSD/causalgia. The classic lesion that predisposes to the development of causalgia is a high-speed missile injury that stretches, but does not transect, a peripheral nerve. The injury is above the knee or elbow 90 percent of the time; most often involved are the sciatic nerve (40 percent), median nerve (35 percent), medial cord of the brachial plexus (12 percent), and other nerves (13 percent).[214] The cause of this selective vulnerability is unknown but has been speculated to be related to the relatively high proportion of postganglionic sympathetic fibers in these nerves.

Although injury to bone or soft tissue in an extremity appears to be the most common predisposing factor for RSD, there have been no systematic epidemiologic studies of this phenomenon. RSD can also occur in the head and trunk.[101]

Clinical Features. RSD/causalgia can develop immediately after an inciting event or be delayed for months or longer. As it develops, patients typically report a continuous fluctuating pain, which is usually burning in quality.[6,203,214,218] A throbbing, aching, or tingling component is also common. This continuous pain may flare with movement or touch, emotional upset, or environmental disturbances such as a change in temperature, weather patterns, or loud noises. Many patients additionally describe an intermittent, paroxysmal pain that may be spontaneous or precipitated by touch or movement.

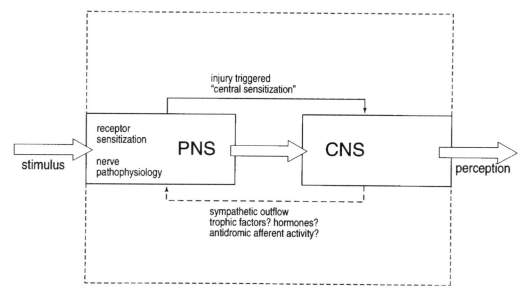

Figure 5–3. Proposed model of the pathophysiologic processes that may underlie the pain induced by peripheral injury. (From Devor M, Basbaum AI, Bennett GJ, et al: Group report: Mechanisms of neuropathic pain following peripheral injury. In Basbaum AI, and Besson J-M (eds): Towards a New Pharmacotherapy of Pain. John Wiley & Sons, Chichester, 1991, p 418, with permission.

Evidence of autonomic dysregulation, specifically some combination of local edema, vasomotor instability, or sudomotor disturbances, is generally the feature that first suggests the diagnosis of RSD/causalgia (Fig. 5–4). These findings have been used by some investigators to define diagnostic categories for RSD[123]: (1) "definite" RSD, indicated by pain in association with vasomotor instability and edema; (2) "probable" RSD, including patients with pain and either vasomotor instability or edema; and (3) "possible" RSD, describing patients with the typical pain alone. Although its simplicity is helpful in the clinical situation, there is no empirical evidence for this formulation.

Similar to other chronic pain states, RSD/causalgia is often associated with adverse psychologic and behavioral phenomena. The assessment of these patients must clarify the degree of disability and existence of psychiatric comorbidity. These factors may be important targets for therapy.

The neurologic examination of patients with RSD/causalgia yields variable findings. There may be raised thresholds for sensory stimuli (hypesthesia or hypalgesia), exaggerated responses to suprathreshold events (hyperesthesia, hyperalgesia, allodynia, or hyperpathia), or, paradoxically, a combination of these phenomena. These findings can occur independently of one another and do not correlate well with the degree or quality of spontaneous pain.[178]

Like the pain and autonomic features, the trophic changes that may occur in patients with RSD/causalgia are highly variable. Some patients demonstrate few or no such changes and others develop profound alterations within months of onset. The pattern of trophic changes within any individual is similarly variable.

Some authors have described the progression of RSD in three stages that may evolve at 3- to 6-month intervals (Table 5–4).[203] Many patients do not conform to this course, however, and long-term outcomes are variable. There are many reports of remission following early and intensive therapy, and some patients appear to remit spontaneously. Others remit and relapse or have a course characterized by persistent or worsening pain.

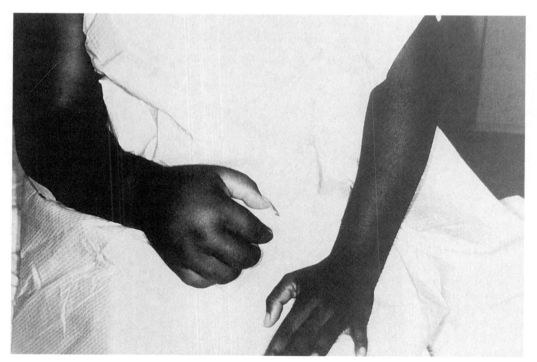

Figure 5–4. Chronic RSD affecting the right hand of a patient who sustained a soft tissue injury. Observable findings include edema, posturing of the hand, and abnormal nail growth.

Table 5–4. **PUTATIVE STAGES OF REFLEX SYMPATHETIC DYSTROPHY/CAUSALGIA***

Stage	Characteristics
Acute	Severe burning pain
	Local edema
	Skin that may be warm, dry, and erythematous, or cool, sweating, and cyanotic
	Increased hair growth
	Increased nail growth
	Decreased range of motion
	Early evidence of trophic changes
Dystrophic	Pain may be spreading
	Edema may be brawny or indurated
	Skin may be cool and cyanotic, erythematous, or characterized by livedo reticularis
	Increased sweating
	Decreased hair growth or hair loss
	Cracked, grooved, or ridged nails
	Decreased range of motion
	Muscle wasting and osteoporosis
Atrophic	Pain may lessen
	Skin cool, thin, shiny, and either cyanotic or pale
	Subcutaneous atrophy with thin, tapering digits
	Ankylosis of joints
	Muscle wasting and osteoporosis

*Although patients are very variable and seldom progress through well-defined stages, the characteristics indicate the spectrum of findings observed in this condition.

Given this variability, prognostication is difficult.

ANCILLARY TESTS

Supporting evidence of autonomic dysregulation or trophic changes may be diagnostically useful, particularly in equivocal cases. Radiography may demonstrate patchy demineralization,[91] and bone scintigraphy may reveal abnormal radionuclide uptake in the painful region.[123] A three-phase bone scintigram, preferred by some clinicians on the grounds that it may be a more sensitive indicator of RSD/causalgia, should be requested, if available. Thermography may depict subtle asymmetry of skin temperature and thereby provide evidence for local autonomic dysregulation. Other measures of local autonomic function, such as the sympathetic skin response and sweat testing, could potentially be applied in the same way as thermography, but are rarely used clinically. The sensitivity, specificity, and predictive value of these tests for the diagnosis of RSD/causalgia are unknown.

RESPONSE TO SYMPATHETIC INTERRUPTION

As noted previously, a therapeutic response to sympathetic interruption confirms that the patient with a clinical diagnosis of RSD or causalgia also has SMP.[105] This may be difficult to interpret, however. Clinical series that describe the response to sympathetic interruption do not apply placebo controls, identical techniques, or standardized criteria for a favorable outcome. Placebo-controlled studies of systemic phentolamine infusion have reported positive[181] and negative[229,230] outcomes. The responses to sympathetic interruption have not been described in terms of the acceptability of pain relief, effect on associated phenomena, improvement in functional capacity, or long-term outcomes. Although most clinicians view a positive response as one in which the patient experiences substantial relief for a period that exceeds the duration of the local anesthetic by many hours or days, the placebo reaction could still explain this outcome. These inconsistencies may account for a large variability in reported response rates to sympathetic blockade.[86,142,214,239]

In sum, the possibility of SMP should be considered in all patients who have findings consistent with RSD/causalgia, that is, all patients with persistent pain accompanied by evidence (clinical or on ancillary tests) of autonomic dysregulation or trophic changes. Patients should undergo diagnostic sympathetic nerve blocks with local anesthetic, if possible. The routine use of the phentolamine test as a substitute for sympathetic nerve block is controversial and cannot be recommended. A clear-cut response to sympathetic interruption is generally taken to confirm SMP and to suggest the value of sympathetic interruption as therapy (see following). Many patients respond with partial or transitory relief, so that often the diagnosis of RSD or causalgia is retained on clinical grounds, but the diagnosis of SMP remains equivocal.

MANAGEMENT

All patients with suspected RSD/causalgia require a comprehensive assessment of the organic and psychosocial contributions to the pain and the relationship of the pain to coexisting physical, psychologic, and behavioral impairments. Some patients with severe neuropathic pain have surprisingly little psychologic distress or functional impairment. These patients may be appropriate candidates for therapeutic trials of primary analgesic modalities alone. Other patients, whose pain is complicated by severe affective disturbances or disability, may benefit from the type of multidisciplinary approach employed by pain clinics. The assessment provides the information needed to target therapeutic approaches to the unique needs of the patient.

Anesthetic Approaches. Anesthetic approaches have traditionally been the mainstay of analgesic therapy for patients with RSD/causalgia (see Chapter 12). As discussed previously, sympathetic blockade is both a diagnostic tool and a major treatment modality for this disorder.

Sympathetic Blockade. Most patients undergo a trial period during which at least several sympathetic blocks are performed before the technique is considered a failure. The standard approach varies from clinician to clinician. Some recommend the procedure daily, whereas others perform it weekly or less often during this initial period. In some severe cases, continuous sympathetic blockade using local anesthetic infusion is attempted.

Responses to sympathetic blockade vary:
1. No analgesia or analgesia that persists only for several hours
2. Transitory relief that outlasts the duration of local anesthetic effect and lengthens with each block
3. Transitory relief that outlasts the duration of the local anesthetic effect but does not increment with subsequent blocks
4. Transitory relief that gradually diminishes with each block, until the block is entirely ineffective
5. A prolonged favorable response after one or a few blocks.

The size of each of these groups relative to the entire population is unknown, and although anecdotal reports suggest that early therapy and the presence of hyperpathia predict a favorable response,[142] there are no confirmed prognostic indicators.

The small minority of patients who develop a pattern of response to sympathetic blockade characterized by repeated short-lived periods of analgesia have traditionally been considered for permanent sympathetic interruption via chemical or surgical sympathectomy. Reported response rates for these procedures vary greatly.[214]

Intravenous Regional Sympathetic Blockade. Sympathetic interruption in a limb can also be performed via the intravenous injection of a drug that depletes adrenergic transmitters from sympathetic nerve endings.[87] In this approach, a sympatholytic agent is injected into a vein in the distal limb following inflation of a compression cuff proximally. The sympathetic block produced by this procedure can be prolonged and spares local sweating, a sympathetic function mediated by acetylcholine. Clinical experience has been greatest with the use of guanethidine as the sympatholytic agent[85,86]; however, the parenteral formulation of this drug is not approved in the United States, and trials have also been performed with reserpine and bretylium.[13,96] Although clinical experience has suggested that the regional intravenous technique is safe and can be effective, confirmatory controlled trials are lacking, and a recent meta-analysis of published data failed to demonstrate any benefit whatsoever.[100] Nonetheless, a regional intravenous infusion is still considered for those patients with suspected SMP who are unable or unwilling to undergo neural blockade.

Other Anesthetic Approaches. Myofascial trigger points may complicate RSD/causalgia, leading to increased pain and impairment of function. Local anesthetic injection of trigger points may also be useful. Trigger points may also be addressed with other techniques, most importantly the "spray and stretch" approach, in which application of a vapocoolant to the skin is followed by controlled stretching of the affected muscle.[224]

Physiatric Approaches. Although many experienced clinicians believe that physical therapy is essential to maintain the relief provided by sympathetic blocks, this idea has not been confirmed empirically. Nonetheless, it is prudent to attempt to normalize the function of the painful part, and formal physical therapy should be recommended for virtually all patients. Additionally, rehabilitative approaches can potentially prevent joint and muscle dysfunction produced by disuse and trophic changes, optimize function at any given level of impairment, and improve psychologic well-being (see Chapter 14). Unfortunately, the value of specific techniques has not been studied.

Pharmacologic Approaches. There are very few controlled studies of pharmacologic agents in the management of RSD/causalgia. A recent controlled evaluation of intranasal calcitonin yielded favorable results[76] and supports a trial of calcitonin in patients with RSD/causalgia who do not respond to sympathetic blockade. The mode of action of calcitonin in this condition is unknown.

Many other drugs, including anti-inflammatory drugs, opioids,[174,176] and adjuvant analgesics,[90] have been used empirically in the treatment of RSD/causalgia. A group of adjuvant analgesic drugs, including the oral sympatholytic agents, are administered specifically for SMP. Many others, including antidepressants, oral local anesthetics, and anticonvulsants, are used nonspecifically for RSD/causalgia and other types of neuropathic pain. All of these drugs are discussed in Chapters 10 and 11.

Neurostimulatory Approaches. The analgesic potential of afferent stimulation has been accepted for over two decades, and there is extensive clinical experience in the use of various stimulation modalities for neuropathic pain.[82,139] Although only a few patients attain long-term analgesia from transcutaneous electrical nerve stimulation (TENS), the safety of this approach supports a trial in patients with RSD/causalgia who fail to respond promptly to sympathetic blockade combined with adjunctive physiatric and pharmacologic approaches. Regardless of the pain syndrome, an optimal trial of TENS should involve a period of experimentation with electrode placement and stimulation timing, intensity, amplitude, and frequency.

Invasive neurostimulatory procedures include acupuncture, percutaneous electrical nerve stimulation, dorsal column stimulation, and deep brain stimulation. With the exception of a small survey of patients successfully treated for causalgia with dorsal column stimulation,[25] the utility of these approaches has not been assessed in RSD/causalgia. Invasive approaches should be reserved for patients who fail sympathetic blockade and conservative pharmacologic and nonpharmacologic measures. Practitioners who are experienced in the management of RSD/causalgia should be involved in the decision to implement invasive approaches.

Surgical Approaches. Procedures designed to isolate the painful part from the central nervous system have been disappointing in RSD/causalgia (see Chapter 13). These procedures, which include neurectomy, rhizotomy, cordotomy, mesencephalic tractotomy, and thalamotomy, are not recommended in the management of this condition. Clinical experience with amputation of the painful part has likewise been unfavorable, and this course should never be pursued for analgesic purposes. Little support exists for the dorsal root entry zone (DREZ) lesion and for those approaches designed to reduce the affective concomitants of pain, including cingulotomy and lobotomy. Although the latter procedures are occasionally considered for patients with severe and intractable pain, their use has been supplanted by newer analgesic techniques. Thus, excepting sympathectomy in selected cases, surgical approaches are usually ineffective, and their use must be discouraged.

Psychologic Approaches. Numerous psychologic approaches have been applied in the management of chronic nonmalignant pain, including neuropathic conditions such as RSD/causalgia. Formal psychotherapy and psychotropic drugs targeted to symptoms other than pain may be appropriate for some patients. Others benefit from the use of specific cognitive or behavioral approaches (see Chapter 15).[134,228]

All clinicians can help reduce maladaptive behaviors and increase satisfying ones. An activities diary may be useful to document the level of function and provide the information necessary for suggestions to discourage unwanted behavior and reinforce improvements.

Deafferentation Pain

The term *deafferentation pain* is applied to neuropathic pains that are inferred to have a sustaining central mechanism that is independent of activity in the sympathetic nervous system.[173] Phantom pain, avulsion of roots, postherpetic neuralgia, central pain, and a variety of miscellaneous disorders are commonly subsumed under this rubric.

MECHANISMS

"Deafferentation" is a descriptive label and does not refer to any specific set of known mechanisms. Studies of nerve injury in experimental animal models have demonstrated that denervation hypersensitivity of neurons and ectopic foci of spontaneous neuronal activity can develop in the dorsal horn of the spinal cord, thalamus, and perhaps cerebral cortex following an injury to afferent pathways.[1,140,144] Such activity has also been recorded at similar sites in humans with chronic pain due to nerve injury.[141,220] This "central sensitization" may be an important process common to the deafferentation syndromes. It may also be involved in the pathogenesis of RSD/causalgia and could be a necessary, but not sufficient, condition for some of the neuropathic pains that are believed to be sustained predominantly by peripheral factors.

The specific mechanisms that produce central sensitization are unknown, and presumably vary across syndromes (Table 5–5). Deafferentation states that follow peripheral injury (e.g., phantom limb pain) may involve the sensitization of central neurons by a barrage of activity in nociceptors,[51] a process that may be mediated by an interaction between excitatory amino acids (specifically glutamate) and the N-methyl-D-aspartate receptor.[57,249]

A variety of other processes could also contribute to the hyperexcitable state of central neurons.[220,248] Both changes in the receptive fields of central neurons[9,54,220] and functional alteration of thalamic neurons (e.g., pain response on stimulation of the intralaminar nuclei in patients with preexistent deafferentation pain)[220] have been described. Lesions in afferent pathways may also interfere with normal inhibitory pro-

Table 5–5. **CHANGES IN CENTRAL NEURONS THAT MAY BE INVOLVED IN A STATE OF "CENTRAL SENSITIZATION"**

Functional
Lowered threshold for activation
Exaggerated activation
Ectopic discharges
Enlarging receptive fields
Loss of normal inhibition

Structural
Transsynaptic and transganglionic degeneration
Collateral sprouting

cesses at any of the multiple levels of the central nervous system. Loss of inhibition, in turn, may result in hyperexcitability of neurons or enhanced stimulation of nociceptive neurons by incoming pathways.

Structural alterations in the central nervous system also occur following injury to afferent pathways. These alterations include degeneration, regeneration, and gliosis in regions that mediate processing of somatosensory input[118]; transsynaptic degeneration of cortical neurons following spinal cord section[62]; and both transganglionic degeneration of axons entering the central nervous system[245] and sprouting of collateral central nervous system axons following peripheral nerve damage.[9,145] Although the relationship of these findings to chronic pain in humans is conjectural, these phenomena affirm the plasticity of central connections and represent potential correlates of disturbances in central somatosensory processing.

The importance of peripheral input in deafferentation pain states is suggested by the phenomena of allodynia and hyperpathia and by the transitory relief of deafferentation pain that is commonly observed following interruption of proximal somatosensory pathways.[150] Rarely, prolonged relief occurs following proximal denervation, suggesting that peripheral activity can have a predominating effect in some patients who are believed to have a central pathogenesis for the pain.

SPECIFIC SYNDROMES

There is remarkable diversity among the various deafferentation pain syndromes (Table 5–6). Although the therapeutic implications of syndrome recognition are yet limited, proper diagnosis may provide direction for diagnostic evaluation and aid in prognostication.

Phantom Pain. Although the prototype phantom pain follows limb amputation, the term is now generally applied to pain following amputation of any body part. The term is also used to describe pain in regions of the body that are totally denervated but not amputated, such as that which occurs after spinal cord transection[150] or peripheral nerve injury. To avoid confusion, however, it is preferable to avoid this usage. Pains that may be ascribed to a lesion in the central nervous system should be labeled as *central pain* or one of its subtypes (see following). Pains that follow injury to nerve root or peripheral nerve and are inferred to have a predominating central mechanism should be labeled by either the nonspecific term, *deafferentation pain,* or the older term, *anesthesia dolorosa.*

Mechanisms. The specific mechanisms involved in the development or persistence of phantom pain are not known. The conceptualization of pain as a somatosensory "memory" has been advocated on the basis of an exhaustive review of clinical material.[114] This

Table 5–6. **CATEGORIES OF DEAFFERENTATION PAIN**

Syndrome	Subtypes
Phantom pain	Phantom limb pain
	Phantom pain following amputation of other structures (e.g., breast, tooth, anus)
	Phantom body pain*
Avulsion of roots	Avulsion of the brachial plexus
	Avulsion of the lumbosacral plexus
Postherpetic neuralgia	
Central pain	Pain due to a spinal cord lesion (trauma, focal demyelination, or other)
	Pain due to a brainstem lesion (vascular or other etiology)
	Pain due to a cerebral lesion

*Pain that is inferred to have a sustaining central mechanism and occurs in an insensate, but otherwise intact, part of the body. This usage may be confusing; see text for alternatives.

view suggests that the pathophysiologic processes that underlie phantom phenomena, including pain, involve complex interactions of neural networks in the brain and do not reside in a specific region of the central nervous system. The term "neuromatrix" has been applied to these proposed networks.[149] Presumably, the processes that induce or sustain such a neuromatrix could include the varied pathophysiologic mechanisms (e.g., sensitization of central neurons) described previously. Support for the potential relevance of neural networks as an underpinning for phantom phenomena can be adduced from the clinical observation that these phenomena are not reliably eliminated through neurolysis or surgical isolation of any central site.

Characteristics. The incidence, natural history, and characteristics of phantom pain have been most extensively described for phantom limb pain following traumatic amputation, typically during wartime. These data are generalized to related syndromes on the basis of clinical observation.

EPIDEMIOLOGY. Older surveys reported transitory or occasional discomfort in the phantoms of 25 to 98 percent of amputees, with severe pain in fewer than 10 percent. Among veterans with traumatic amputations, phantom pain has been reported in 78 to 85 percent.[206–208] A survey of patients undergoing medical amputation identified phantom limb pain in 72 percent of patients at 8 days, 65 percent at 6 months, and 59 percent at 2 years.[109]

Several studies have attempted to define predisposing factors for the development of phantom pain. Phantom limb pain is rare in congenital amputees or in children who lose a limb before the age of 6 years,[211] suggesting that a degree of maturity of the nervous system is required for this outcome. Pain in the amputated body part prior to amputation predisposes to phantom pain in some,[109] but not all,[92] surveys. A strong association between stump pain and phantom pain also has been reported.[109,208] Other surveys have suggested that older age, proximal amputations, upper limb lesions, sudden amputations, and preexisting psychologic disturbances may increase the likelihood of phantom pain, but these factors have not been confirmed in the more recent studies. Phantom pain is unrelated to the use of a prosthesis following amputation.[208]

NATURAL HISTORY. Phantom sensations and phantom pain may develop at any time after denervation; most patients develop symptoms immediately after the nerve injury. Over time, substantial improvement occurs in approximately one-half of patients.[109,208]

CLINICAL FEATURES. Phantom pain must be distinguished from stump pain, which is managed differently, and nonpainful phantom sensations, which usually require no treatment. Although these phenomena are best described following limb amputation, any or all can occur after amputation of other body parts. For example, surveys have characterized phantom phenomena following mastectomy,[103,125] tooth extraction,[172] and resection of the anus.[16,165]

Phantom limb sensation may be divided into several categories, as listed in Table 5–7. All these sensations are usually most vivid immediately after the amputation and gradually fade over time.

Phantom sensation may replicate the size and position of the body part or may be experienced as distortions of it.[33,92] The distal part of the limb is usually more prominent than proximal portions. The size of the phantom often shrinks over time, and in a curious phenomenon known as *telescoping,* this shrinkage usually takes the form of grad-

Table 5–7. **VARIOUS PERCEPTIONS OF PHANTOM SENSATION**

Kinesthetic Sensation
Unusual postures
Foreshortening of limb ("telescoping")
Distortions in the size of body parts—usually reduction in proximal regions and expansion of distal regions

Kinetic Sensation
Spontaneous movement
Willed movement

Exteroceptive Sensation
Pain
Touch
Temperature
Tingling
Pressure
Itch

ual diminution of the proximal part of the limb with relatively retained sensation of the distal part. This may culminate in the perception of a normal hand or finger attached to a stump seemingly too small to accommodate it.

The characteristics of phantom pain are extremely diverse and typically evolve over time. Some patients experience continuous burning, squeezing, or throbbing; others report stabbing or shooting pains. Many have pains of both types. Similarity between phantom pain and preamputation pain has been described[109] but is not universal. A recent study revealed that 57 percent of patients who experienced pain immediately before amputation developed phantom pain that resembled the preexisting pain in quality and location.[114] Once phantom pain is established, many factors may influence its intensity or the vividness of associated sensations. Stress, contact with the stump, and changes in climate may increase pain; rest, distraction, or elevation of the stump may reduce it.

In contrast to phantom pain, in which the inferred "generator" of the pain is in the central nervous system, stump pain is a prototypic peripheral neuropathic pain (see following). Patients usually report some combination of aching, squeezing, throbbing, stabbing, and electrical discomfort localized to the distal stump. Pains are usually precipitated or exacerbated by contact, and point tenderness can usually be discerned along the scar. The onset of the pain is usually delayed for months, and the incidence is lower than for phantom pain.[63,109] Local pathology, such as infection or bone spurs, appears to increase the likelihood of persistent stump pain, but it is not a necessary condition.

Management. Surveys of amputees have portrayed the therapy of phantom pain in discouraging terms.[208] Given the challenges encountered during the treatment of this condition, prevention would clearly be preferable. This possibility was suggested by a small randomized trial that demonstrated the efficacy of a 72-hour preoperative epidural infusion of local anesthetic and/or morphine in reducing phantom pain among patients with preamputation limb pain.[5] Such "preemptive analgesia" supports the hypothesis that an intense afferent barrage,

which occurs at the moment of amputation, may be critical in establishing the pathophysiology of phantom pain. Although the data are yet too limited to recommend regional anesthesia to block this afferent barrage prior to all planned amputations, a consensus appears to be in support of this approach in patients who have intense preexisting pain.

Patients with established phantom pain should be evaluated for a multimodality therapeutic program that targets the dual goals of pain reduction and functional improvement. All patients should also be evaluated for the existence of potentially treatable factors that may be exacerbating the pain, such as stump neuroma or depression.

PHARMACOLOGIC APPROACHES. On the basis of anecdotal reports and clinical experience, patients with phantom pain are usually offered trials of adjuvant analgesic drugs in the same manner as patients with other types of neuropathic pain (see Chapter 10).[90] The only controlled trial evaluated salmon calcitonin (200 IU via brief intravenous infusion) in patients with phantom pain of recent onset[102]; the favorable results of this study support a therapeutic trial of calcitonin in established cases as well. The long-term use of opioids, which can sometimes be effective in phantom pain, is discussed in Chapter 11.

ANESTHETIC APPROACHES. Although sympathetic nerve blocks may have immediate benefit in some patients with phantom pain, this effect is usually transitory.[111] Rare patients experience long-term benefit. Nonetheless, the potential for long-term favorable effects, albeit small, warrants a trial of sympathetic blockade in selected patients with refractory pain. The patients who obtain prolonged relief from sympathetic blockade presumably represent a subgroup with a unique mechanism in which the phantom pain is an SMP.

Prolonged relief from blockade of sensory nerves is rare. Sensory blockade paradoxically increases the pain in some patients,[204] an observation that supports both the existence of a central "generator" in this disorder and the importance of peripheral modulation of this site.[151]

Local injection into the stump usually has limited efficacy in the management of phantom pain but should be considered by patients with coexistent stump pain. A report of four patients who obtained prolonged relief following repeated instillation of local anesthetic into hyperalgesic points in the contralateral limb[81] suggests another option for intractable cases.

SURGICAL APPROACHES. Surgical interruption of proximal somatosensory pathways is no longer accepted for the treatment of patients with phantom pain, despite a long history of attempts to manage the pain in this way.[210] Although each reported series of cases note occasional patients with long-lasting relief of pain following an operation, the duration of follow-up in these reports is generally short, and most patients monitored for a prolonged period developed recurrence of pain.

The dorsal root entry zone lesion has had promising results in some types of deafferentation syndromes, such as plexus avulsion injuries (see following). Few cases have been reported in which the procedure was used to treat phantom pain, and the results have not been encouraging.

NEUROSTIMULATORY APPROACHES. The inherent safety of TENS warrants a trial of this modality in virtually all patients with phantom pain. Unfortunately, long-term results are poor.[65,207]

A large experience with invasive neurostimulatory procedures has yielded mixed results. In one survey of 64 patients treated with dorsal column stimulation,[124] 45 percent reported a 50 to 100 percent pain reduction and 11 percent noted 25 to 50 percent relief early on, but only 23 percent described the pain as more than half gone at a 5-year follow-up. Surveys of patients treated with deep brain stimulation[98,126,256] have included small numbers of patients with phantom pain and similarly suggest mixed results. Invasive neurostimulatory approaches should not be considered until conservative treatments have failed and the patient has undergone a comprehensive evaluation.

PHYSIATRIC APPROACHES. There is no compelling evidence that a prosthesis or physical therapy yields analgesic effects in patients with phantom pain. Nonetheless, rehabilitative therapies can have salutary effects on function and should be considered on this basis (see Chapter 14).

PSYCHOLOGIC APPROACHES. The dual goals of comfort and functional gains cannot be advanced without a comprehensive psychologic assessment and appropriate interventions (see Chapter 15). Change in body image and physical impairments may compound the distress related to phantom pain and augment the importance of psychologic treatments.

Avulsion of Nerve Plexus. Severe deafferentation pain can complicate avulsion of one or more nerve roots at any level of the nervous system. Plexus avulsion following massive trauma to a limb is the most common entity. Although injury to either the brachial plexus or the lumbosacral plexus is possible, the latter is rare, and virtually all published literature has evaluated lesions of the brachial plexus.

Mechanisms. The mechanisms that underlie the pain following root avulsion have not been elucidated. The effectiveness of the dorsal root entry zone lesion in this disorder (see following) suggests that the pathophysiology is situated in the dorsal horn of the spinal cord. Presumably, the mechanism or mechanisms at this level include those described previously (see Table 5–5).

Characteristics. Proper management of a proximal nerve injury requires accurate diagnosis of the neurologic lesion. The distinction between injury to the nerve root itself and avulsion of the root is critical, because the former lesion may be amenable to nerve grafting. The combination of clinical findings, electrodiagnostic studies, and imaging procedures is usually adequate to characterize the damage (Table 5–8).

EPIDEMIOLOGY. Avulsion injuries are uncommon, but, paradoxically, the incidence of pain following these injuries is much higher than with other types of nerve damage. Chronic pain is reported after brachial plexus avulsions in 26 to 91 percent of patients.[154,251–253] The severity of pain is associated with the number of roots avulsed and involvement of the lower plexus.[154,251]

NATURAL HISTORY. The onset of the pain after plexus avulsion can be immediate or delayed for months. In the largest series of painful avulsion injuries,[252] about two-thirds of the 122 patients experienced spontaneous improvement of pain within 2 years of the injury. In the remainder, severe pain persisted and, in many, pain seriously interfered with function years after the injury.

Table 5–8. **CLINICAL DIFFERENTIATION OF AVULSION OF ROOT VERSUS INJURY TO DISTAL ROOT**

	Avulsion	Injury to Root or Nerve
Proximal muscles spared	No	Possibly
Tinel's sign over plexus	No	Possibly
Electrodiagnostic studies	Consistent with proximal lesion	Findings possibly consistent with lesion distal to DRG*
Myelography/magnetic resonance imaging	Meningoceles may be present	No meningocele

*DRG = dorsal root ganglia.

CLINICAL FEATURES. Virtually all patients with brachial plexus avulsion describe continuous burning dysesthesias, usually in the hand. Many patients also experience severe paroxysms of pain. Stress, intercurrent illness, and changes in the weather may increase the pain; discomfort is sometimes reduced by distraction, relaxation, or stereotyped maneuvers, such as gripping or swinging the arm, or massaging the neck or shoulder.[252] The limb, or portions of it, can be entirely anesthetic, and most patients do not experience allodynia or hyperpathia. Spontaneous paresthesias are common, however, and other phantom phenomena may be experienced in the insensate regions.

Many patients with avulsion injury develop a swollen and discolored extremity with atrophy of the muscles and subcutaneous tissues. Although these phenomena presumably reflect denervation and/or disuse, they could represent a coexistent RSD/causalgia. The possibility of SMP is underscored in such patients, and diagnostic sympathetic blockade with local anesthetic is usually indicated to clarify the mechanisms involved and determine the viability of sympathetic interruption as therapy.[17]

Management. The physical and psychologic functioning of patients with avulsion injuries is often profoundly impaired as a result of the loss of strength and sensation in the painful limb, other injuries sustained at the time of the avulsion, and the effects of chronic pain. A multimodality approach to therapy should strive to improve both comfort and function.

SURGICAL APPROACHES. The dorsal root entry zone lesion has a high likelihood of success in the treatment of pain associated with root avulsion.[57,155,156,253] In one series, this lesion produced excellent pain relief in 16 of 24 patients who were followed for a period of 6 months to 4 years.[253] Although major morbidity can result from this procedure, the risk is justified in patients with refractory pain. Other procedures designed to denervate the painful part, including neurectomy and cordotomy, are generally ineffective.

PHARMACOLOGIC APPROACHES. There are no controlled trials of drug therapy in the treatment of pain associated with avulsion injuries. The drugs used to treat other types of neuropathic pain should be considered (see Chapters 10 and 11).

NEUROSTIMULATORY APPROACHES. TENS has been reported to benefit a substantial proportion of patients with chronic pain from brachial plexus avulsion[251,253] and a trial of this modality is warranted in all patients. A few anecdotal reports suggest that invasive neurostimulatory procedures may be useful.[256,258]

ANESTHETIC APPROACHES. As noted, an occasional patient with an avulsion injury responds to sympathetic nerve blocks, suggesting that the injury has been complicated by the development of SMP. Diagnostic blocks are indicated if this disorder is suspected. Other types of neural blockade are not useful in pain due to avulsion injuries. The use of trigger-point injections should be considered, however, for patients with coexisting myofascial pain.

PSYCHOLOGIC APPROACHES. Patients with avulsion injuries may develop severe psychologic and behavioral disturbances, which must be addressed to optimize pain relief and function. All patients should undergo a careful assessment and appropriate interventions (see Chapter 15).

PHYSIATRIC APPROACHES. Splinting of the paralyzed arm is an important intervention after severe brachial plexus lesions.[252] Splinting prevents the flail arm from interfering with activity, encourages function by facilitating the manipulation of objects, and potentially improves analgesia. Intensive physical therapy is also essential to retain residual strength and prevent contractures and joint ankylosis, either of which can become independent sources of pain. Other aspects of rehabilitation, including vocational retraining, may not have direct analgesic consequences, but can have favorable effects on function.

Postherpetic Neuralgia. An unfortunate minority of patients with acute herpes zoster develop a persistent neuropathic pain known as postherpetic neuralgia (PHN). The failure of peripheral interventions in most patients with this syndrome supports the inference of a predominating central pain "generator."

Mechanisms. Herpes zoster produces diffuse inflammation of peripheral nerve, dorsal root ganglia, and, in some cases, spinal cord.[49] Autopsy material from patients with PHN has confirmed the existence of chronic inflammation in the periphery, neuronal loss in dorsal root ganglia, and a reduction of both axons and myelin in affected nerve.[241,244] The central nervous system processes that result from this pathology and sustain the pain in PHN are unknown. Presumably, any of the mechanisms imputed to be involved in deafferentation pains (see Table 5–5) could play a role in this condition. The pathology also indicates that peripheral processes may be involved, and one study suggests that patients vary in the influence of these peripheral processes on the pain.[192] Selective loss of large peripheral nerve fibers in several cases[160,244] suggests that reduced peripheral inhibitory processes may contribute.

Characteristics. Inherent in the diagnosis of PHN is an arbitrary interval, the duration of pain required before acute herpetic neuralgia becomes PHN. This criterion for PHN has been variably defined as pain persisting beyond the crusting of lesions,[30] or beyond 1,[189] 1.5,[26] 8,[56] or 24[184] weeks following reso-

lution of the rash. For research, it is probably best to set a period of 4 months from lesion onset (1 month for lesion healing followed by 3 months of pain). This criterion is used to define an early period, during which therapies for acute herpes zoster are appropriate, and an open-ended period that follows, during which treatments appropriate for PHN should be implemented.[175]

EPIDEMIOLOGY. Herpes zoster has an incidence of 1.3 to 4.8 cases per 1000 person-years.[95,179] The incidence of the acute syndrome rises with age.[30,95] Immunosuppressed patients, including those with cancer and AIDS, are more likely to be afflicted than those who are immunocompetent. The incidence may be influenced by systemic insults, such as surgery, toxic exposures and infections, and focal pathologic processes affecting the spine or roots.[110]

Overall, approximately 10 percent of those who develop acute herpes zoster experience pain for more than one month.[179] Age strongly influences the likelihood of prolonged pain. In one large survey, the prevalence of pain one year after the eruption was 4.2 percent in patients younger than 20 years of age and 47 percent in those older than age 70 years.[47]

NATURAL HISTORY. As might be expected from the declining prevalence of pain over time, PHN gradually improves in most patients. Given this potential for spontaneous resolution, any intervention would appear to be useful if administered relatively early in the course, particularly in younger patients. This phenomenon has led to the introduction of many ineffective treatments on the basis of favorable effects observed during uncontrolled trials (Table 5–9).

The best predictor of improvement is the course during the recent past. Continued optimism is in order for patients whose pain has recently diminished, even modestly. Patients who develop a pattern of stable pain for a period of months are likely to experience pain indefinitely.

CLINICAL FEATURES. Herpes zoster, and hence PHN, affects the thoracic dermatomes in more than 50 percent of patients. Next most common are trigeminal eruptions, which most often affect the ophthalmic division. Lumbar and cervical zoster are least common, each occurring in 10 to 20 percent of patients.[30,244]

The pain of PHN is usually similar to that

Table 5–9. **SOME SUPERANNUATED TREATMENTS FOR POSTHERPETIC NEURALGIA**

Adrenocorticotropic hormone	Posterior pituitary extract
Applied galvanism	Protamide
Psychosurgery	Quinine
Cobra venom	Radiotherapy
Radiant heat	Rhizotomy
Cordotomy	Skin undermining
Cortisone	Skin excision
Dihydroergotamine mesylate	Smallpox vaccine
Diphtheria antitoxin	Histamine
Tetraethylammonium chloride	Immune globulin
Nicotinic acid	Ultraviolet light
	Vitamins B_1 and B_{12}

of herpes zoster neuralgia, with combinations of burning dysesthesias, aching or itching, and severe paroxysms of stabbing or burning pain. Some patients report allodynia or hyperpathia.[192] Like other neuropathic pains, PHN may or may not become associated with affective disturbances and maladaptive behaviors.

Management. The management of PHN can be considered from the perspective of preventive approaches and analgesic therapy.

PREVENTION. A varicella vaccine has recently been approved for the use in the United States. If the vaccine does not itself cause zoster, which is yet to be determined, a true reduction in the incidence of this disorder will be observed many years after its use becomes widespread. Primary prevention, therefore, continues to be a possibility for the distant future.

Antiviral drugs administered during the acute phase of herpes zoster, including interferon,[58] vidarabine,[246] and acyclovir,[170] produce short-term analgesia and improved healing of the eruption. There is no evidence that any of these drugs reduces the likelihood of PHN. Newer antivirals, including famciclovir and valacyclovir, may favorably influence the incidence of prolonged pain. Additional experience with these drugs is needed.

There is no good evidence that any other therapy for acute herpes zoster prevents PHN. Several trials that purported to demonstrate this effect for corticosteroids[56,115] were disconfirmed by a more recent, well-controlled

study.[60] Although corticosteroids can have valuable analgesic effects during acute zoster, they do not prevent the recurrence of pain. Suggestive data from controlled trials of amantadine[72] and levodopa[117] have not been replicated, and although the efficacy of sympathetic blockade was suggested in older surveys,[39] a recent series could not confirm that the early use of nerve blocks prevents PHN.[255]

TREATMENT. Acute herpetic neuralgia usually can be controlled with a combination of local measures, analgesic drugs (nonsteroidal anti-inflammatory drugs or opioids) and other treatments, including other drugs (most importantly, acyclovir and corticosteroids), sympathetic blockade, or both.[73] The more challenging problem is the management of PHN. Similar to other types of chronic pain, PHN is best treated with the aim of addressing both analgesia and function.

PHARMACOLOGIC APPROACHES. Topical agents usually have few systemic side effects and may be advantageous in patients with PHN, most of whom are predisposed to side effects by advanced age.[189] Anecdotal reports suggest that occasional patients benefit from a topical formulation of an anti-inflammatory drug, such as aspirin in chloroform.[121] These compounds are seldom used clinically.

Other reports suggest benefit from topical local anesthetics.[191,192] Dense cutaneous anesthesia can be produced by application of an eutectic mixture of lidocaine and prilocaine (EMLA), which is now available in the United States. Patients who are able to apply this compound effectively should be considered for a trial of topical application several times a day. Contact with the eye must be avoided, and PHN of the face may not be treatable for this reason. If cutaneous anesthesia is needed to produce pain relief, it can be obtained only by application of the cream to the skin for at least 1 hour under an occlusive dressing. This may not be feasible if the painful area is very large or situated over joints.

Another topical therapy, capsaicin cream, has been similarly advocated based on uncontrolled observations.[14,243] Capsaicin is a naturally occurring compound that selectively depletes peptide neurotransmitters (such as substance P) from small-diameter primary afferent neurons. Current experience suggests that an adequate trial of this drug, which requires 3 to 4 applications daily for approximately 4 weeks, will identify a small proportion of patients who report substantial pain relief. Perhaps one-quarter of patients develop local burning and are unable to proceed with a trial. Those who benefit should continue with the drug indefinitely. Although long-term safety has not been studied systematically, there has been no suggestion of any accruing risk with the formulations available commercially.

Systemic drug therapy for PHN follows the same general approach recommended for other types of neuropathic pain (see Chapter 10).[90] Among the adjuvant analgesics commonly used in all these disorders, several have been specifically evaluated in the PHN population. These include amitriptyline,[147,242] desipramine,[122] maprotiline,[240] clonidine,[148] and carbamazepine.[120] Sequential trials with these agents and other adjuvant analgesics comprise the major approach to the pharmacotherapy of PHN. Occasional patients benefit from a nonsteroidal anti-inflammatory drug or long-term opioid therapy (see Chapters 10 and 11).[174,176]

ANESTHETIC APPROACHES. Numerous anesthetic approaches have been advocated for PHN, including skin infiltration with local anesthetic[192] or local anesthetic and steroids,[59] intravenous local anesthetic,[205] temporary or permanent blocks of peripheral nerves or nerve roots,[94] sympathetic blocks,[39] epidural steroid administration,[169] and application of a cryoprobe to painful scars.[215] Although these reports are uncontrolled and lack long-term

follow-up in many cases, they suggest that a subgroup of patients responds favorably to peripheral manipulation.[192] Unfortunately, there is no reliable way to predict this response, and patients with severe refractory pain are usually offered empirical trials of temporary nerve blocks with local anesthetic (including sympathetic nerve blocks) and subcutaneous instillation of local anesthetic or local anesthetic plus a corticosteroid. Neurolysis is not considered except in the most extreme situations because of the uncertain nature of the results and concern about the possible adverse effects of increased denervation.

NEUROSTIMULATORY APPROACHES. Although a trial of TENS yielded disappointing results,[75] many anecdotal reports have suggested that some patients benefit from a noninvasive neurostimulatory approach, including TENS, counterirritation, application of vapocoolant spray, local vibration, or ultrasound.[158,167,221] Given their safety, an empirical trial of such an approach cannot be faulted. Occasional patients also appear to benefit from acupuncture, notwithstanding one negative trial.[133]

Patients with PHN have been included within case series describing the utility of invasive neurostimulatory techniques, specifically dorsal column stimulation and deep brain stimulation.[98,159,209] These cases suggest that some patients with severe pain refractory to conservative approaches could benefit. Given the empirical nature of these techniques, however, patient selection and treatment should be performed only by experienced practitioners.

SURGICAL APPROACHES. Patients with PHN have been reported to benefit from surgical procedures directed at every level from skin to cerebrum, including neurectomy, rhizotomy, sympathectomy, cordotomy, trigeminal tractotomy, mesencephalotomy, mesencephalothalamotomy, and thalamotomy.[82] The dorsal root entry zone lesion has also been reported to be effective.[68] In all these series, supporting documentation is meager and long-term follow-up is usually limited. Overall, the accumulated clinical experience with these techniques has been disappointing, and none is recommended routinely (see Chapter 13).

PHYSIATRIC APPROACHES. Although physiatric approaches have not been systematically evaluated in patients with PHN, some patients appear to benefit from physical or occupational therapy. These techniques should be particularly considered for those patients whose pain causes immobilization of a limb or general inactivity.

PSYCHOLOGIC APPROACHES. Patients with PHN can develop severe affective disturbances or maladaptive behaviors. Specific treatment should be directed at the psychologic and social impairments identified during a comprehensive assessment of these patients (see Chapter 15).

Central Pain Syndromes. The term "central pain" describes the many deafferentation pain syndromes that can occur following injury to the central nervous system.[166] Some of these syndromes have been named by the location of the lesion (e.g., thalamic pain) and some have been named by the inciting injury (e.g., poststroke pain). Some do not conform to a named syndrome (e.g., pain associated with syringobulbia) and are best described as central pain. Recognition of these central pain syndromes began with the original description of thalamic pain in 1906.[49]

Mechanisms. Although the existence of central pains provides incontrovertible evidence of the potential for a pain "generator" in the central nervous system, relatively little is known of the processes involved, the relationship between these processes and clinical phenomenology, or the similarities and differences among the types of central pain or other deafferentation syndromes. Any of the mechanisms described previously could contribute to central pain. Conceptually, there may be three critical determinants (Fig. 5–5): (1) dysfunction in specific thalamic neurons, (2) alterations in excitatory and inhibitory activity along nociceptive or modulatory pathways that are induced by a lesion at a particular site, and (3) delayed and persistent changes in receptor function that result from these alterations in activity.[35] Clinical observations suggest that damage to spinothalamocortical pathways is a fundamental element in the development of central pain following a lesion at any level of the neuraxis.[19,94,129,166] Possibly, deafferentation or disinhibition of central nociceptive neurons in the thalamus can follow such a lesion and result in the pathophysiologic changes that underlie the phenomenology of central pain.

Characteristics. The diagnosis of central pain syndromes is most clear when typical symptoms and signs can be combined with radiographic confirmation of an appropriate lesion in the central nervous system.[183] Most patients with central pain have overt neurologic dysfunction, evaluation of which demonstrates a lesion that can be imputed as the cause of the pain. Occasionally, the diagnosis can be difficult because associated neurologic symptoms or signs are lacking, and imaging studies are equivocal or normal.

Given the limited information available about the mechanisms that may underlie central pains, a simple classification based on topography is most useful at the present time (Table 5–10). From this perspective, central pains can be divided into those related to lesions of the spinal cord, brainstem, and cerebrum.

SPINAL CORD LESIONS. Central pain following damage to the spinal cord has been characterized best in patients with traumatic or demyelinating lesions. Other pathologic entities, however, may result in a similar outcome.

SPINAL CORD TRAUMA. Following acute spinal cord injury, 10 to 49 percent of patients de-

Table 5–10. TYPES OF CENTRAL PAIN

Pain From Spinal Cord Lesions
Trauma
Focal demyelination
Infection
Vascular lesions
Neoplasms
Syringomyelia
Others

Pain From Brainstem Lesions
Vascular lesions
Trauma (including surgical)
Infection
Neoplasms
Syrinx
Focal demyelination

Pain From Cerebral Lesions
Vascular lesions
Trauma (including surgical)
Neoplasm
Associated with seizures

velop chronic pain.[20,250] Pain may be related to any of a variety of processes,[61,250] a subgroup of which is neuropathic (Table 5–11). Radicular pain can follow injury to any level of the spine and presumably involves a peripheral pathogenesis from damage to nerve roots (see following). Deafferentation pain is inferred when dysesthesias occur in a nonsegmental distribution below the level of the injury. If the damage involves the spinal cord, the term "central pain" is appropriate. If the cauda equina is involved, the lesion can still be inferred to involve deafferentation, just as sectioning of peripheral nerve during amputation precipitates phantom pain. The inference that injury to the cauda equina can lead to either radicular pain (with a presumed peripheral pathophysiology) or deafferentation pain (with a presumed central pathophysiology) is based on clinical observation and should be viewed as a construct in need of empirical validation. It is likely that many patients have more than one process concurrently.

The clinical features of central pain following spinal cord injury are variable. Spontaneous and evoked dysesthesias may be associated with uncomfortable paresthesias described as tingling, numbness, or squeezing. These sensations can be experienced in any region below the injury. Some patients experience phantom sensations in the insensate regions.[43] Painful areas may be small or large, unilateral or bilateral, and stable or fluctuating in size and location. Pain may increase spontaneously or in response to changes in climate, stress, smoking, or other factors. Flexor or extensor spasms, which

may be spontaneous or precipitated by movement or by distention of the bladder or bowel, can contribute significantly to the pain. A few patients describe ill-defined visceral pains, which are usually experienced in the lower abdomen or pelvis; these pains are usually acute, often precipitated by blad-

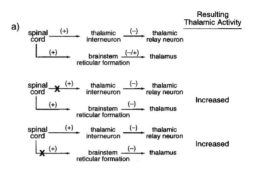

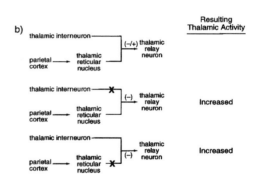

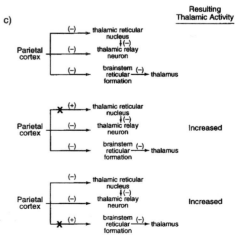

Figure 5–5. Conceptual framework for factors that may be important in the pathophysiology of central pain syndromes. "**X**" indicates a lesion; "(+)" indicates excitatory activity; and "(−)" indicates inhibitory activity. In this model, it is assumed that excessive or abnormal thalamic activity can lead to pain. This potentially may result from dysfunction of thalamocortical relay cells, inhibitory interneurons, or the thalamic reticular nucleus. A lesion anywhere along the neuraxis, including spinal cord (a), brainstem (a and c), thalamus (b), or cerebrum (c), can produce central pain through disinhibition of thalamic neurons. (Adapted from Casey, KL: Pain and central nervous system disease: A summary and overview. In Casey KL [ed]: Pain and Central Nervous System Disease: The Central Pain Syndromes. Raven Press, New York, 1991, pp 1–11.)

Table 5–11. TYPES OF CHRONIC PAIN THAT MAY FOLLOW SPINAL CORD INJURY

Type of Pain	Typical Description
Central (deafferentation)	Dysesthesia, often burning below the level of the injury; may follow injury to spinal cord or cauda equina
Radicular	Aching or dysesthetic (usually lancinating) pain in a segmental distribution; may follow injury to any level of the spine
Mechanical	Aching in the region of the injured spine
Visceral	Ill-defined, focal or diffuse pain in the abdomen (may be limited to epigastrium or lower abdomen; may be associated with increased pressure in bladder or bowel; in some circumstances, associated with headache).

der or rectal distention, and can be accompanied by nausea, headache, or autonomic disturbances (e.g., piloerection, hypertension, or diaphoresis).

FOCAL DEMYELINATION. Focal demyelination of the spinal cord can result in a central pain syndrome that usually affects the legs or lower trunk. This pain syndrome is most likely to occur in patients with established multiple sclerosis, and it is useful to describe it within a broader discussion of pain in this disorder.

Both acute pains and chronic pains are prevalent in multiple sclerosis. The most common acute syndromes comprise paroxysmal lancinating pains, which occur in 1 to 17 percent of patients.[193] The best-characterized pain is trigeminal neuralgia, which is identical to the idiopathic syndrome except for a younger age of onset and a greater likelihood of bilaterality. Other paroxysmal pains also occur, including a painful Lhermitte's sign, lancinating pains in a radicular distribution, stabbing pelvic pains, painful tonic seizures, and brief episodes of burning pain.[37,153]

The overall prevalence of chronic pain ranges from 23 to 80 percent and is higher in older patients, those with long-standing disease, and possibly women.[37,112,153] Central pain, the most prevalent type, usually occurs with disease of long duration, but, rarely, it can precede other signs by years.[177] The pain is usually described as continuous burning. It is sometimes associated with other types of dysesthesias or lancinating pains and may

fluctuate in intensity spontaneously or in response to activity, stress, or change in weather. The pain is most often in the distal legs and feet but occasionally occurs in a dermatomal distribution or asymmetric nondermatomal region of the trunk or extremity.

As with spinal cord injury, other types of chronic pain may complicate the course of established multiple sclerosis. Aching back pain, presumably musculoskeletal, relates to weakness or spasticity of paraspinal muscles. Pain from osteoporosis or degenerative arthropathy may be accelerated by immobility and abnormal postures. Some patients develop painful leg spasms, and occasional patients with severe spinal cord dysfunction experience a chronic visceral pain syndrome.[153]

OTHER SPINAL CORD PATHOLOGY. Other spinal cord lesions may be complicated by the development of neuropathic pain, the characteristics of which overlap those of the two syndromes described previously. Pain may occur in association with vascular lesions of the spinal cord, syringomyelia, intramedullary and extramedullary neoplasms, cervical spondylosis, inflammatory lesions (e.g., syphilitic myelitis), AIDS myelopathy, subacute combined degeneration, and toxic myelopathy.[166] Central pain can also be iatrogenic, occasionally complicating spinal surgery or cordotomy. For example, approximately 5 percent of patients who undergo cordotomy develop dysesthesias that are rarely severe and usually appear after weeks or months in an anesthetic area or in one regaining sensation.[41]

LESIONS IN THE BRAINSTEM. As noted, the deafferentation pain that follows a vascular lesion of the thalamus is the prototype for the central pain syndromes. Similar pains, however, have been described with other lesions in varying locations.

THALAMIC PAIN. Although thalamic pain has been best characterized following ischemic or hemorrhagic vascular lesions,[18,45,166] an identical syndrome is observed occasionally in association with nonsurgical or surgical trauma, or with structural lesions, including arteriovenous malformation, aneurysms, infection, or tumors.[78,166,223,238] The pain, which usually occurs months to years after the injury, can be experienced in the entire hemibody or be localized to a small region. Occasional patients have a pseudoradicular distribution or a so-called cheiro-oral distribution (perioral region and ipsilateral hand). The pain is usually dysesthetic (manifested by continuous burning, often with intermittent stabbing) and may be associated with uncomfortable paresthesias (e.g., squeezing, gnawing, crawling, or tingling). Allodynia is common, and some patients experience dramatic hyperpathia with diffuse radiation, duration far in excess of the stimulus, and extreme distress. Such exacerbations of pain may be unprovoked or induced by environmental changes (e.g., loud noises, bright lights, inclement weather) or emotional upset.

Like other severe neuropathic pains, the psychologic and social consequences of thalamic pain can be devastating. Patients often become withdrawn, inactive, and profoundly depressed. Pain may be increased by psychologic factors or the adverse effect of immobility, such as contractures, joint ankylosis, myofascial pains, and osteoporosis.

The neurologic deficits associated with thalamic pain are diverse. Most, but not all, patients have an obvious sensory disturbance in some part of the affected hemibody. A deficit in pain and temperature sensation appears to be a constant,[19,129] and disturbances in the perception of other sensory modalities may also occur. Patients may or may not have associated hemiparesis or choreoathetoid movements. Occasional patients demonstrate unilateral dysmetria or Horner's syndrome.

OTHER BRAINSTEM LESIONS. Central pain from a lesion in the brainstem caudal to the diencephalon may result from mass lesions such as intrinsic or extrinsic tumors, syringobul-bia or hematobulbia, focal demyelination, or surgical lesions.[166] Similar to central pain related to spinal cord or thalamic lesions, these syndromes have variable times of onset, topographies, and pain characteristics. One recent study[129] suggested that central pain due to brainstem lesions is more likely to have a burning quality and is less likely to be lancinating than is thalamic pain.

LESIONS IN THE CEREBRUM. The nature of the cortical processing of noxious stimuli has been in question since the influential work of Head and Holmes,[88] who hypothesized that pain perception occurs at a thalamic level. The occurrence of central pain following trauma, vascular lesions, or neoplasm in the cerebral hemisphere[19,129,166] suggests that the cerebral cortex is important in the experience of pain. Other evidence includes the development of disturbed pain perception from suprathalamic lesions,[15] the identification of nonnociceptive cortical neurons in primates,[188] and reports of pain following stimulation of parietal regions during cortical mapping experiments.[168]

The rare occurrence of central pain with seizures also suggests a cortical influence in pain processing. Pain may occur as an aura preceding a generalized seizure or as a manifestation of a focal epileptiform discharge without secondary generalization.[146,168,225] Pain varies greatly, ranging from diffuse abdominal discomfort with a visceral quality to focal pain in an extremity. The duration is typically minutes.

Management. The management of central pain is challenging,[77] and the goal of comfort is unattainable for many patients. In this population, therefore, it is particularly important to address physical and psychologic rehabilitation, in addition to analgesia, from the start of therapy.

PHARMACOLOGIC APPROACHES. A controlled trial in patients with central poststroke pain demonstrated a clear analgesic effect from amitriptyline and equivocal benefits from carbamazepine.[128] Favorable effects have been reported anecdotally from a variety of tricyclic antidepressants, anticonvulsants (including carbamazepine), naloxone (administered as a brief infusion), mexiletine and other local anesthetics, diphenhydramine, propranolol, anticholinesterase inhibitors, chlorpromazine, L-dopa, and 5-hydroxytryptophan.[128,166]

Currently, treatment should begin with a tricyclic antidepressant. Should an adequate trial with one or more of these drugs prove ineffective, further trials of other adjuvant analgesics can proceed. These sequential trials can include the drugs reported anecdotally for central pain and others commonly selected for the treatment of other types of neuropathic pain (see Chapter 10). Some patients respond favorably to opioid drugs, and selected patients may be considered for this therapy as well (see Chapter 11).

NEUROSTIMULATORY APPROACHES. Peripheral stimulation, specifically TENS, is usually attempted in those with focal or regional pain complaints due to a central lesion. Results are usually disappointing, but occasional patients benefit.

Invasive neurostimulatory techniques, particularly deep brain stimulation, have been used to manage central pain for more than a decade (see Chapter 13). Most experienced practitioners advocate stimulation of sites along the dorsal column–medial lemniscal system (including sensory thalamus).[219] Based on anecdotal reports and case series, it appears that as many as one-half of patients obtain relief. Although some of those who benefit initially experience a return of pain, durable effects have been reported. Unfortunately, there are currently no reliable predictors of long-term outcome. Invasive techniques should be implemented by experienced practitioners who can properly assess the nature of the pain and associated physical and psychosocial disability and can ensure that previous therapeutic trials have been administered appropriately.

ANESTHETIC APPROACHES. Temporary somatic nerve blocks with local anesthetic may provide short-lived relief of central pain, presumably reflecting the modulation of abnormally active central nociceptive pathways by peripheral input. Similar effects can be seen in some patients after sympathetic blockade.[143] Local anesthetic blockade is not predictive of long-term outcome with neurolysis, the results of which have been consistently disappointing.

SURGICAL APPROACHES. Surgical neurolytic techniques for central pain have been described in case reports and small series, which generally suggest that sustained benefit is rare.[219] At the present time, stimulation of central pathways is the preferred approach. The only possible exception to this is the use of the DREZ lesion for so-called "end zone" pain in patients with spinal cord injury.[67] It has been proposed that intermittent and evoked pain may also be more responsive to neurolysis than other types of central pain (see Chapter 13), but this remains to be confirmed.

PHYSIATRIC APPROACHES. Central pain is often associated with functional impairments, some of which may predispose to secondary painful complications. Physiatric interventions may forestall these complications and potentially improve function (see Chapter 14).

PSYCHOLOGIC APPROACHES. The benefits of psychologic approaches in patients with central pain have not been evaluated systematically, but the potential for favorable effects on pain, coping, and function are apparent. Skilled psychologic assessment is essential in the evaluation of these patients.

Miscellaneous Deafferentation Syndromes. Any peripheral nerve injury, including surgical sectioning of cutaneous sensory nerves at any site, can result in chronic neuropathic pain. In some cases, the mechanisms sustaining this pain are in the periphery, such as an active neuroma. When the clinical evidence supports this conclusion, the syndrome may be labeled a painful peripheral mononeuropathy (see following). In other cases, the sustaining mechanisms are in the central nervous system and are somehow related to other deafferentation pains, such as phantom pain. This inference cannot be proved, of course, but may be strongly suggested by its characteristics (such as pain that gradually "spreads") or its response to interventions (such as persistence of the pain despite proximal sensory block). As noted previously, the nonspecific term, *deafferentation pain,* and the older term, *anesthesia dolorosa,* may be appropriately applied to these syndromes. Other labels, either nonspecific (such as *postsurgical pain syndrome*) or specific (such as *postthoracotomy pain*) are merely descriptive and imply nothing about the mechanisms of the pain.

NEUROPATHIC PAIN DUE PRIMARILY TO PERIPHERAL CAUSES

Although profound central changes occur after peripheral injury, some types of neuropathic pain appear to have a sustaining peripheral pathogenesis. These chronic pains can be eradicated by peripherally directed interventions (e.g., resection of neuroma, decompression of a nerve, or isolation of the painful part from the central nervous system by rhizotomy or cordotomy). The label "peripheral neuropathic pain" should not be taken to imply that central mechanisms are absent or unimportant; rather, the sustaining mechanisms are in the periphery.

Mechanisms

Many processes can lead to peripheral neuropathic pains (Table 5–12). A broad division has been proposed in which these mechanisms are separated into those characterized by activation of normal nociceptors and those characterized by pathologic processes precipitated by axonal injury and attempts at regeneration.[3]

ACTIVATION OF NORMAL NOCICEPTORS

Some types of peripheral neuropathic pains may be caused by the persistent activation of otherwise normal nociceptors (see Table 5–12). Among the possible mechanisms are (1) sensitization of nociceptors (see Chapter 2), either directly or through the release of inflammatory mediators from local tissues or from the peripheral nerves themselves (including persistently "backfiring" C fibers, which may be the major pathophysiology in some disorders); (2) preferential loss of large fibers leading to diminished inhibitory processes and increased nociceptor input; and (3) activation of putative nociceptive nervi nervorum. Some nervi nervorum have the response characteristics of polymodal C nociceptors[7] and could presumably mediate pain produced by a nerve injury that does not sever axons (e.g., compression). The term "nerve sheath pain" has been proposed for these pains.[3]

AXONAL INJURY AND REGENERATION

As discussed previously, pathologic processes induced by axonal injury also result in chronic pain.[50] The term "dysesthetic pain" has been proposed for these pains.[3]

Neuroma formation is probably the most important process in the pathophysiology of

Table 5–12. **MECHANISMS THAT MAY BE INVOLVED IN NEUROPATHIC PAIN SUSTAINED BY PERIPHERAL PROCESSES**

Activation of "Normal" Nociceptors ("Nerve Sheath Pain"*)

Sensitization of C and A-delta nociceptors

Disinhibition due to large-fiber loss

Activation of nociceptive nervi nervorum

"Backfiring" C fibers, with peripheral release of algogenic substances

Aberrant Activity From Injured Nerves ("Dysesthetic Pain"*)

Neuroma formation (severed nerve or incontinuity)

Focal demyelination

Ephapse formation

*The distinction between "nerve sheath pain" and "dysesthetic pain" was proposed originally by Asbury AK, and Fields HL: Pain due to peripheral nerve damage: An hypothesis. Neurology 34:1587–1590, 1984.

pain following axonal injury. Neuromas, which may form at the end of a cut nerve or develop along the course of a successfully regenerated nerve (so-called neuroma-in-continuity), generate spontaneous discharges both locally and at the level of the dorsal root ganglia.[50,235] Once these regions of aberrant activity are established, ectopic discharges can be evoked by mechanical stimulation and changes in the local environment, including increased concentration of catecholamines, ischemia, and electrolyte disturbances. As illustrated by Tinel's sign and microneuronographic studies of neuroma,[161] these evoked discharges can be associated with pain.

Other processes may also mediate the peripheral "generator" responsible for some types of neuropathic pain. Ectopic impulse generation can result from focal demyelination along an otherwise intact peripheral nerve or from the formation of ephapses, abnormal synapses between peripheral nerve fibers, which develop at the site of nerve injury.[53]

Specific Syndromes

Currently, the most relevant taxonomy divides the peripheral neuropathic pains into the painful polyneuropathies and painful mononeuropathies (see Fig. 5–2).

PAINFUL POLYNEUROPATHY

Pain can occur in many types of neuropathy, but it is a prevalent symptom in relatively few. Although some painful neuropathies can be treated, with analgesic consequences, the pain itself becomes an independent problem for many patients and must be addressed directly.

Mechanisms. Many studies have related pain to selective fiber-type dysfunction. Small-diameter nerve fibers mediate pain,[217,222] and ectopic activity originating from these small fibers, either from direct injury or from regeneration, could cause pain in some polyneuropathies. Pathologic material from diabetics with painful neuropathy appears to support this hypothesis.[28]

A disorder of small primary afferent nerve fibers cannot explain all observations, however. Some painless neuropathies have selective small-fiber loss, and some painful neuropathies have either no selective damage or damage limited to large fibers. The painful polyneuropathy associated with the dysproteinemias, for example, is associated with injury to both large and small fibers,[237] and preferential loss of large fibers has been demonstrated in patients with painful neuropathy due to isoniazid ingestion[162] or hypothyroidism.[171]

The occurrence of pain in several neuropathies with selective large-fiber loss suggests an alternative hypothesis, namely that pain may relate to the loss of peripheral inhibition. This explanation fails to account for painless neuropathies with selective large-fiber loss, as in Friedreich's ataxia.

These observations suggest that the pain associated with polyneuropathy cannot be ascribed solely to selective small- or large-fiber disease. Although these processes could be involved, at least in some types of painful polyneuropathy, other mechanisms are certainly involved as well.

Characteristics. Despite the variability of the painful polyneuropathies, the pain complaints are remarkably uniform, at least among disorders characterized by a generalized axonopathy. Patients usually report burning or other dysesthesias of the feet and distal legs (and the hands, when the lesion is advanced), paroxysmal lancinating pains that may be spontaneous or provoked, deep aching in the feet and legs, and muscle cramping. Some have severe allodynia, or even hyperpathia, and accompanying paresthesias that can become aversive. These paresthesias include the perception of swelling of the feet, squeezing as if shoes were too tight, paradoxical cold (despite skin that may be red and warm), and the sense of walking on sandpaper or ground glass.

Pain associated with myelinopathy, specifically the acute inflammatory polyneuropathy of Guillain-Barré syndrome, is generally aching in quality and experienced in both the back and limbs. The distal-to-proximal distribution of pain and other symptoms that characterize the axonopathies may not be observed. Muscle cramps occur as well.

Rare patients pose difficulties in the localization of the disorder. Lesions of the spinal cord or cauda equina can produce dysesthesias that begin in the feet and slowly ascend, mimicking painful polyneuropathy. Coexistence of lesions is common in patients with disorders such as cancer or AIDS, and patients whose diagnosis remains uncertain despite electrodiagnostic testing should undergo imaging of the spinal epidural space. Myopathies may produce generalized muscle cramps that can suggest acute inflammatory polyneuropathy or one of the axonopathies. Severe cramping occasionally can accompany motor neuron disease as well. Lancinating pains can be observed in tabes dorsalis or subacute combined degeneration. In all these cases, clinical assessment and electrodiagnostic studies usually resolve the differential diagnosis.

Causes. Elucidation of factors that precipitate or sustain the neuropathy has obvious implications for treatment and prognosis. It is essential that the clinician evaluate the patient for the systemic disorders that may cause the syndrome (Table 5–13).

Metabolic Disorders. Painful polyneuropathy can occur with many metabolic diseases, including diabetes, nutritional deficiencies, hypothyroidism, uremia, amyloidosis, and Fabry's disease. Of these, diabetes is the best characterized.

DIABETES. Polyneuropathy is a common manifestation of diabetes mellitus. The neuropathies in this disorder are divided into dis-

Table 5–13. **PAINFUL POLYNEUROPATHIES**

Painful Polyneuropathy Due to Metabolic Disorders
Diabetic neuropathy
Neuropathy associated with insulinoma
Nutritional deficiency
   Alcohol–nutritional neuropathy
   Thiamine deficiency
   Niacin deficiency
   Pyridoxine deficiency
   Strachan's syndrome
Hypothyroid neuropathy
Uremic neuropathy
Amyloid neuropathy
Neuropathy associated with Fabry's disease

Painful Neuropathy Due to Drugs or Toxins
Isoniazid
Gold
Misonidazole
Nitrofurantoin
Vincristine
Cisplatin
Arsenic
Cyanide
Thallium

Painful Polyneuropathy Due to Neoplasm
Subacute sensory neuronopathy
Sensorimotor neuropathy associated with carcinoma
Sensorimotor neuropathy associated with dysproteinemias

Hereditary Painful Polyneuropathy

Painful Polyneuropathies Associated with Guillain-Barré Syndrome

tal symmetric polyneuropathies, symmetric proximal motor neuropathy, and focal and multifocal neuropathies.[27] The distal symmetric neuropathies can be divided into groups, each characterized by a predominant disorder of motor, sensory, or autonomic fibers, and a mixed group in which all fiber types are affected. The sensory neuropathy can, in turn, be divided into a large-fiber type, a small-fiber type, and a mixed type.

The pathogenesis of diabetic polyneuropathy is unknown, and the specific pathophysiology of the pain is conjectural. A study of sural nerve biopsies from 32 patients with diabetic neuropathy provided support for the concept that fiber loss is primary in the diabetic neuropathies and that ischemia plays a central role in this occurrence.[55] The spectrum of fiber loss ranged from relative depletion of small fibers to relative depletion of large fibers, and it was speculated that the extremes of this spectrum define the clinical syndromes of large- and small-fiber polyneuropathies, respectively. Although these results do not clarify the interactions among symptoms, sensory abnormalities, and morphology, earlier work adduced a relationship between pain and small-fiber disease.[28,197]

Quantitative sensory testing has been used to assess sensory thresholds for vibratory and thermal stimuli in patients with diabetic neuropathy. Thresholds for vibratory stimuli have been inferred to reflect large-fiber function, and those for thermal stimuli, to reflect small-fiber function. Threshold elevations occur in both painful and nonpainful sensory neuropathies, with relatively greater abnormalities in thermal sensation among those with pain.[257]

Although a vascular etiology for diabetic polyneuropathy is likely, given the available pathologic data, metabolic processes also may be involved.[40] Reports of patients with painful neuropathy suggest that symptomatic relief may follow normalization of serum glucose.[2,22]

INSULINOMA. Painful polyneuropathy has been observed rarely with hypoglycemia due to insulinoma.[108] Dysesthesias and weakness affect the upper extremities more than the lower. Removal of the tumor can benefit the neuropathy.

NUTRITIONAL DEFICIENCY. Painful polyneuropathy complicates many nutritional deficiencies. The major syndromes include the following:

ALCOHOL-NUTRITIONAL DEFICIENCY. Pain and paresthesias in the feet and distal legs occur in approximately one-quarter of alcoholics with neuropathy.[231] Although well-nourished alcoholics can present with this disorder, the pathogenesis in most patients probably involves multiple vitamin deficiencies. With abstinence and vitamin supplementation, symptoms and signs may improve. The onset of symptoms is usually insidious, and acute worsening occurs occasionally. A subgroup develops the so-called "burning feet" syndrome, which can occur with or without clinical evidence of polyneuropathy and is identical to a syndrome of the same name that can develop in association with nutritional deficiencies unrelated to alcoholism.[212]

THIAMINE DEFICIENCY. The clinical features of the neuropathy accompanying specific thiamine deficiency (so-called "dry" beriberi) are indistinguishable from those associated with the alcohol-nutritional neuropathy. Many other neuropsychologic (Wernicke-Korsakoff syndrome) and cardiac ("wet" beriberi) manifestations may occur with this deficiency. In an animal model, thiamine repletion reversed the pathologic changes of this axonopathy.[216]

NIACIN DEFICIENCY. Pellagra is associated with a polyneuropathy characterized by painful dysesthesias and severe aching legs. Inadequate niacin intake is also one of the causes of the "burning feet" syndrome.

PYRIDOXINE DEFICIENCY. Painful polyneuropathy may complicate pyridoxine deficiency. Naturally occurring pyridoxine (vitamin B_6) deficiency is rare, owing to the ubiquity of the vitamin. Symptomatic deficiencies are almost always due to ingestion of pyridoxine antagonists. Virtually all cases are attributable to the use of the antituberculous agent isoniazid.[74]

STRACHAN'S SYNDROME. The triad of painful polyneuropathy, amblyopia, and orogenital dermititis, which may occur in beriberi or pellagra, has been considered to be a separate entity known as Strachan's syndrome or Jamaican neuropathy. No single nutritional deficiency has been associated with these findings, and the precise nature of the entity is controversial.

HYPOTHYROIDISM. Hypothyroidism may be accompanied by a predominantly sensory polyneuropathy, with associated pain and paresthesias in the legs.[10] Muscle cramping occurs frequently and may be a manifestation of subclinical neuropathy. Signs of polyneuropathy, once evident, suggest relative impairment of large peripheral nerve fibers, an impression supported by morphologic studies of several patients.[171]

Hypothyroid patients are predisposed to painful mononeuropathies. Carpal tunnel syndrome is by far the most common, and like the symmetric polyneuropathy, may precede other evidence of hypothyroidism. Evaluation of thyroid function is indicated in all patients with unexplained painful polyneuropathy or entrapment syndromes.

UREMIA. A predominantly sensory polyneuropathy, uremic polyneuropathy, is extremely common among those with chronic renal failure. Quantitative analysis of nerve biopsy specimens suggests that any of a variety of nerve injuries can occur, including acute axonopathy, progressive axonopathy with segmental demyelination, and a predominantly demyelinating neuropathy.[195] A large proportion of patients experience dysesthesias, and occasional patients develop severe dysesthesias, which can mimic the "burning feet" syndrome. Muscle cramping and "restless legs" (often accompanied by uncomfortable paresthesias) are common in those with the polyneuropathy but can occur without evidence of this disorder. Although the pathogenesis of uremic polyneuropathy is unknown, a role for dialyzable toxins is suggested by improvement with renal transplantation and, at times, with dialysis.

AMYLOIDOSIS. A progressive sensory polyneuropathy may occur in both primary and secondary amyloidosis. Pain is common and usually accompanies evidence of impaired small-fiber function, including loss of pain and thermal sensibility and signs of autonomic neuropathy such as postural hypotension, impaired sweating, and gastrointestinal dysmotility. Electrophysiologic and pathologic studies reveal decreased lightly myelinated and unmyelinated axons. Amyloid deposits around capillaries are evident throughout nerve and perineural structures.

FABRY'S DISEASE. Fabry's disease (angiokeratoma corpus diffusum) is a rare lipid storage disorder with sex-linked genetics that results from a deficiency of the enzyme ceramide trihexosidase. A severe, painful polyneuropathy often is the presenting feature.[24] Pathologic studies demonstrate selective loss of small myelinated and unmyelinated fibers.[164] Patients report episodes of severe pain, which may be spontaneous or precipitated by activity or other factors. Some also experience continuous burning dysesthesias of the distal extremities. Another early sign is a rash, the so-called angiokeratoma corpuscum, which is most prominent in the lower abdomen, inguinal region, perineum, and buttocks. In time, multisystem dysfunction develops as lipid accumulates in the kidneys, heart, and other organs. Most patients live only to the fourth or fifth decade.

Toxins or Drugs. Although scores of drugs and toxins have been associated with symptomatic polyneuropathy,[130] few are characterized by severe dysesthesias. The pathogenesis of pain in most of these syndromes is not known. Removal of the drug or toxin leads to gradual improvement in most cases.

Painful polyneuropathy is common following long-term isoniazid therapy. This disorder is due to drug-induced interference with pyridoxine metabolism and can be prevented by coadministration of this vitamin. Other drugs associated with a painful polyneuropathy include gold, misonidazole, nitrofurantoin, and the chemotherapeutic agents vincristine, cisplatin, and paclitaxel. Although pain can accompany other drug-induced neuropathies, its prevalence is unknown. Most surveys do not specifically assess pain, and patients may not volunteer the complaint if the intensity is mild.

Toxic neuropathies also can be painful. Dysesthesias or uncomfortable paresthesias can accompany the neuropathies associated with acute and chronic exposure to arsenic, sublethal cyanide poisoning, and acute and subacute ingestion of thallium salts.

Neoplasms. Nerve injury may result from direct effects of cancer, antineoplastic therapy, comorbid metabolic disturbances, or poorly understood remote (paraneoplastic) effects. All these etiologies are prevalent, including remote effects. A recent study that used quantitative sensory testing to evaluate 29 patients with cancer who were carefully screened to exclude other causes of neuropathy revealed large-fiber sensory dysfunction in 31 percent of patients and small-fiber sensory dysfunction in 43 percent.[135]

SUBACUTE SENSORY NEURONOPATHY. Subacute sensory neuronopathy is a well-described subtype of paraneoplastic neuropathy that usually begins with aching pain, dysesthesias, and paresthesias in the distal extremities. Symptoms progress during weeks to months and ultimately become associated with severe impairment of sensory functions, particularly those mediated by large fibers. Some patients have concurrent dysfunction of other parts of the nervous system (e.g., limbic or brainstem

encephalitis). Small cell carcinoma is the most common associated tumor, but other carcinomas and lymphomas have been reported. The neurologic syndrome usually precedes the clinical appearance of the neoplasm by many months and, rarely, years, and the course of the neuropathy is usually independent of the neoplasm. Degeneration of sensory neurons in the dorsal root ganglia is the major pathologic finding,[97] and strong evidence links a humoral immunologic insult to this lesion.[79] The factors that induce the production of the offending antibody remain speculative.

CARCINOMA. A relatively nonspecific paraneoplastic sensorimotor neuropathy can complicate any tumor type.[42] The clinical features, including the onset and course are variable. Pain may or may not occur, and the incidence, characteristics, and course of this symptom have not been defined.

DYSPROTEINEMIA. Sensorimotor polyneuropathy is a well-recognized complication of the dysproteinemias, including multiple myeloma,[44] Waldenström's macroglobulinemia,[99] solitary plasmacytoma,[182] and osteosclerotic plasmacytoma.[233] A cryoglobulinemia can result in a pain syndrome described as acral pain on exposure to cold. In all cases, symptoms and signs often precede the diagnosis of the underlying neoplasm by many months.

The pathogenesis of these neuropathies and the pain that may accompany them is not known. Although amyloid deposition may occur, it is not the cause of the neuropathy in most cases.[232] Pathologically, there is a loss of nerve fibers of all diameters.[237] Deposition of immunoglobulin along the course of the nerve suggests a likely immunologic mechanism for at least a component of the lesion.

Heredity. Hereditary sensory neuropathy type I is a rare, dominantly inherited neuropathy that predominantly affects small myelinated and unmyelinated fibers.[48] Patients can develop aching or lancinating pain in denervated regions. The loss of pain and temperature sensibility may be accompanied by penetrating foot ulcers and gradual destruction of denervated joints.

Miscellaneous. As noted previously, pain can be prominent in Guillain-Barré syndrome. Pain occurs early in 55 percent of patients, and 72 percent experience pain during the course.[190] Most patients describe a deep aching in large muscles, which is typically moderate in intensity and worsens at night. Some patients also report a superficial burning pain, which can be proximal. Pain does not correlate with weakness or electrophysiologic findings, but an association with elevated creatine kinase levels has been observed.[190]

Pain severe enough to impair function occasionally characterizes other neuropathies. Patients with chronic inflammatory demyelinating polyneuropathy or porphyric neuropathy, for example, may report pain as a prominent symptom, and occasional patients with polyneuropathy associated with an autoimmune disease note significant dysesthesias. Rarely, idiopathic neuropathy is accompanied by disabling pain.

Management. The management of painful polyneuropathy requires a comprehensive assessment and skillful integration of analgesic treatments and therapies to improve function. Assessment must include an assiduous search for the etiology of the neuropathy. Primary treatment may provide symptomatic relief and should be implemented whenever appropriate. Other approaches are directed at pain or associated physical, psychologic, or social disturbances.

Pharmacologic Approaches. The neuropathy associated with a deficiency state should be treated with repletion of the missing compound. Primary therapy with insulin or another hypoglycemic agent should similarly be considered an analgesic approach in painful diabetic neuropathy. Therapies designed to reverse the metabolic consequences of hyperglycemia may be useful; for example, a single-blind, incompletely controlled trial suggested that an aldose reductase inhibitor could be analgesic in these patients.[107]

Adjuvant analgesics have been evaluated in patients with painful neuropathy. Controlled trials of selected tricyclic antidepressants[147] and oral local anesthetics[46] justify trials with these drugs, and anecdotal reports provide the rationale for the use of numerous others (see Chapter 10). Topical capsaicin is commonly tried on the basis of a favorable trial in painful diabetic neuropathy.[32] Occasional patients obtain relief from the use of a nonsteroidal anti-inflammatory drug, an observation consistent with a favorable controlled trial of ibuprofen and sulindac in diabetic neuropathy.[38] Clinical experience also supports the long-term use of opioid drugs in some patients with refractory pain (see Chapter 11).

Neurostimulatory Approaches. There have been no surveys of any of the neurostimulatory modalities in the treatment of painful polyneuropathy. Patients can rarely use TENS effectively because of the location of the pain, and invasive techniques such as dorsal column stimulation are considered only in extreme cases.

Anesthetic Approaches. Injection of trigger points is occasionally helpful in patients with secondary myofascial pains, which may develop in limbs weakened by neuropathy. Other anesthetic approaches are seldom useful. Sympathetic blocks have been reported to benefit rare patients transiently.

Surgical Approaches. There is no evidence that surgical interruption of afferent neural pathways is effective in painful neuropathies.

Physiatric Approaches. The use of a lift to elevate the bedsheets at night and shoe orthotics to provide support for the weakened foot may enhance the patient's comfort. Physical therapy and occupational therapy may forestall or alleviate the development of secondary painful complications such as myofascial trigger points, muscle contractures, or ankylosis of relatively immobile joints.

Psychologic Approaches. There have been no studies of specific psychologic interventions for the management of painful polyneuropathy. Nonetheless, a potential role for these approaches should be clarified as part of a comprehensive assessment.

LANCINATING NEURALGIAS

As typically applied, the term "neuralgia" refers to pain that is caused by damage to a peripheral nerve and is experienced in the distribution of the nerve. This label can be confusing, however, given the great diversity of the chronic pains that follow nerve injury and the commonplace use of this descriptor to refer to pains that mimic trigeminal neuralgia. Consequently, it is useful to clarify the nomenclature by distinguishing a group of disorders, which can be labeled the "lancinating neuralgias" (see Fig. 5–2), that are related to nerve injury and are characterized by brief paroxysmal pains (similar to trigeminal neuralgia). These disorders may be considered a subtype of painful mononeuropathy.

Mechanism. In one current hypothesis, both a peripheral process and a central process are necessary elements in the pathogenesis of trigeminal neuralgia.[69,71] A peripheral lesion, such as an arterial loop, chronically injures the trigeminal nerve, leading to both ectopic impulses from a focal region of demyelination and diminution of segmental inhibition. These processes predispose to paroxysmal discharges of interneurons in the trigeminal nucleus, which may be incited by peripheral stimulation of trigger zones. The subsequent paroxysmal firing of trigeminothalamic projection neurons may account for lancinating facial pain. The details of this model remain to be elucidated and confirmed.

From the standpoint of classification and management, the putative peripheral element in the pathogenesis of the lancinating neuralgias is most relevant. A structural lesion that distorts or compresses the trigeminal nerve adjacent to the brainstem is identified in a large majority of surgically managed patients with trigeminal neuralgia. This is most often an aberrant arterial loop, but other lesions have been observed, including vascular malformations, ectatic basilar artery, neoplasms, and fibrous bands.[71,106] Patients with glossopharyn-geal neuralgia have been found to have injury to cranial nerves IX and X by a tortuous blood vessel, tumor, abscess, carotid aneurysm, or ossified stylohyoid ligament.[29,127]

Characteristics. The lancinating neuralgias are characterized by brief, usually shocklike pains. These may occur in isolation or in runs of variable duration. The severity of each attack varies within and across patients. Many patients also report a mild aching or burning pain in the same region, which may occur for a brief period after a severe attack of the lancinating pain, or continuously during periods of frequent attacks.

Types

THE HEAD. The best-characterized neuralgias involve peripheral nerves of the face and head. Trigeminal neuralgia is most common (see Chapter 4). Other well-described, but rare, cranial neuralgias include glossopharyngeal neuralgia, occipital neuralgia, geniculate (or nervus intermedius) neuralgia, and superior laryngeal (or vagal) neuralgia (Table 5–14).[138]

OTHER SITES. Focal nerve injuries at other sites occasionally result in chronic neuropathic pain characterized by predominant lancinating dysesthesias. These disorders can be named according to the nerve affected. For example, *intercostal neuralgia* refers to lancinating chest pains that may follow injury to the intercostal nerves, and *ilioinguinal neuralgia*

Table 5–14. **UNCOMMON CRANIAL NEURALGIAS**

	Location of the Pain	Associated Features	Precipitating Factors	Involved Nerve*
Glossopharyngeal neuralgia	Tonsillar fossa; pharynx	Syncope; cardiac arrhythmias	Swallowing; talking; coughing; yawning	C.N. IX
Occipital neuralgia	Suboccipital; occipital (unilateral)	Local tenderness	Head movement	Greater or lesser occipital
Geniculate neuralgia	Deep in ear	Vertigo; tinnitus; herpes zoster (Ramsay-Hunt syndrome)	Contact with ear canal; talking; swallowing	Nervus intermedius (C.N.VII)
Superior laryngeal neuralgia	Larnyx; throat; angle of the jaw	Hiccups; cough	Coughing; swallowing; talking; yawning	Superior laryngeal nerve (branch of vagus)

*Inference based on location of the pain and potential efficacy of nerve blocks.

describes intense inguinal stabbing pain that can complicate injury to the ilioinguinal or genitofemoral nerve. In each of these cases, the same clinical injury can also produce a neuropathic pain syndrome in which continuous dysesthesias predominate and lancinating pains are a minor component or are altogether absent. Although the latter syndromes are also sometimes termed "neuralgia," it is more appropriate to label them *painful mononeuropathies*. This distinction is not based on known pathophysiologic differences but, rather, derives from the observation that the therapeutic approach may vary with the specific characteristics of the pain.

Management. The treatment of trigeminal neuralgia is the model for all the lancinating neuralgias (see Chapter 4). In most cases, trials of anticonvulsant drugs and other agents, such as baclofen[70] and the oral local anesthetics, should be administered first. Patients who fail to respond to these drugs are offered other adjuvant analgesics (see Chapter 10) or invasive treatments that restore normal anatomy at the site of injury or destroy the offending nerve (see Chapter 13).

PAINFUL MONONEUROPATHIES

The painful mononeuropathies refer to a diverse group of pain syndromes, all of which are inferred to have a sustaining peripheral pathogenesis. The pain is typically associated with a known peripheral nerve injury and is experienced, at least partly, in the distribution of the damaged nerve. The injury to the nerve may be traumatic, vascular, neoplastic, or inflammatory. The timing of the injury (acute, subacute, or chronic) may or may not correlate with the temporal characteristics of the pain, which may follow the injury immediately and then persist, or occur days, weeks, months, or, rarely, years after the nerve damage appears.

Mechanisms. The mechanisms responsible for a painful mononeuropathy are largely unknown.[51] Although some extensively investigated processes, such as neuroma formation or nerve compression, have been linked to pain, none of the known mechanisms adequately explain the clinical phenomena, including the critical observation that most patients who develop the structural consequences of nerve injury never experience chronic pain. Recent studies in an animal model of nerve injury suggest that genetic factors may be important,[53] but there is yet no confirmation of this finding in any human disorder. Presumably, complex interactions among predisposing factors and elements specific to nerve injury lead to the peripheral and central changes associated with chronic pain.

Characteristics. Patients with painful nerve injury may use descriptors that are usually applied to nociceptive pains—such as aching, throbbing, or sharp—or terms that are consistent with dysesthesia—such as burning, electrical, or stabbing. The painful area may include a region of sensory loss (i.e., a raised threshold to response), with or without accompanying areas of hyperesthesia, hyperalgesia, allodynia, or, sometimes, hyperpathia. Focal tenderness is common, and some patients have a highly localized area of exquisite sensitivity along the course of a nerve, which suggests the site of neuroma formation or entrapment.

Complete temporary eradication of pain following local anesthetic infiltration of a trigger zone or tender area suggests the predominance of local factors but should not be taken as confirmatory. A prominent placebo reaction may result in a similar outcome, and many patients with central pain appear to gain transient relief from reduced afferent input. In contrast, the lack of pain relief following a complete sensory block that effectively denervates the painful area is usually accepted as evidence that a peripheral mechanism is insufficient to explain the pain.

Nerve Trauma. Acute or chronic trauma to any nerve, including relatively small cutaneous nerves, may be followed by persistent pain. The lesion may involve transection, stretch, inflammation, or compression of the nerve. The specific processes that lead to pain are unknown but presumably involve any or all of the peripheral processes described previously.

Pains associated with neuroma and those due to compression are probably the most common traumatic painful mononeuropathies. The prototype pain syndrome related to neuroma is stump pain, discussed previously. The characteristics of other chronic pains related to nerve transection, such as those following surgical incision, are similar.

Nerve root compression due to spine disease (see Chapter 6) and nerve compression at sites of entrapment are some of the most frequent disorders in neurologic practice.[213] The incidence of pain relative to the electrophysiologic or pathologic evidence of compression is not well-defined, and may actually be low; for example, one study identified pain as a complaint in only 17 of 116 cases of peroneal mononeuropathy.[113] The factors that cause pain to complicate some traumatic mononeuropathies and not others are unknown.

Inflammation of Nerve. Acute herpetic neuropathy is the prototype for pain from nerve inflammation (see previously). The peripheral contribution to the pain may relate to a number of processes, including activation of nociceptors and axonal damage with resultant ectopic activity or ephapse formation (see Table 5–12).

An inflammatory lesion is assumed to underlie the conditions of acute brachial plexus neuropathy (also known as brachial plexitis) and a similar condition that affects the lumbosacral plexus.[199,226] Acute brachial plexopathy begins with severe arm and shoulder pain, which typically persists for hours to weeks. Progressive weakness in the shoulder girdle begins after the pain. Sensory symptoms and signs are uncommon. The neurologic deficits gradually improve and chronic pain develops rarely. The pathogenesis is unknown, but the diversity of antecedent events, including viral infections and immunizations, and the similarity between this condition and brachial plexopathy associated with serum sickness suggest an immunologic disorder.

In idiopathic lumbosacral plexopathy, unilateral pain occurs in the buttock, thigh, and leg, and is followed by weakness of the limb. Most patients worsen for weeks, then gradually improve. Some patients have elevated erythrocyte sedimentation rates and appear to improve with immunosuppressive therapy.[23]

A rare inflammatory neuropathy, sensory perineuritis, is characterized by pain and paresthesias that usually involve the feet.[4] Nerve biopsy from several patients revealed chronic inflammation affecting regions of cutaneous nerves. The etiology is unknown.

Vascular Nerve Lesions. The most common vascular insult to nerve is infarction from small vessel disease. As discussed previously, diabetes mellitus is the most common underlying disorder. Diabetic mononeuropathies include a discrete femoral neuropathy, classic diabetic amyotrophy, and a more extensive lumbar radiculoplexopathy.[11,36] These disorders typically present with a relatively brief progressive phase, which usually lasts days to weeks and is characterized by severe aching pain in the thigh and knee associated with weakness in the proximal musculature. The pain usually improves gradually, and strength slowly returns over months. The pain associated with other diabetic focal neuropathies has a similar course. These syndromes include cranial neuropathies, the most common of which is oculomotor neuropathy, and thoracoabdominal neuropathies, which may mimic the pain of cardiac ischemia or acute cholecystitis.[119]

Pain may also accompany a mononeuritis or mononeuritis multiplex due to vasculitis. Polyarteritis nodosa is the prototype disorder in this group, but a large number of other diseases also produce this lesion, including rheumatoid arthritis, Sjögren's syndrome, Churg-Strauss syndrome, and others.[21] An isolated vasculitis of the peripheral nervous system has been described.[196] The incidence, characteristics, and natural history of pain associated with these disorders are poorly defined.

Large vessel occlusion is a rare cause of painful focal neuropathy.[247] The pain in this condition may be due to ischemia of muscle and other soft tissue, as well as injury to the nerve.

Neoplastic Nerve Lesions. Peripheral nerve tumors produce focal pain or pain that radiates in the distribution of the nerve. The pain from benign tumors, such as neurofibroma, is modest and precipitated by local pressure, whereas pain from malignant lesions is usually severe and spontaneous. Malignant tumors typically produce an obvious mass and focal neurologic signs.[66]

Management. The diagnosis of a painful peripheral mononeuropathy suggests the potential utility of interventions directed at the site of the lesion. Invasive interventions can be dramatically effective, but the risks must be recognized. In one survey, for example, 48 of 103 patients with pain due to nerve injury underwent surgery; 21 were made worse, 10 were unchanged, and 17 were improved.[254] Neither the type of surgery, which included transposition of nerves, resection of neuromas, and nerve grafting, nor the specific type of painful injury predicted the response to surgery. Invasive therapies must be implemented cautiously in patients with painful mononeuropathy.

Pharmacologic Approaches. With the exception of acute herpes zoster (see previously), the pharmacotherapy of the painful peripheral mononeuropathies is nonspecific, involving empirical trials of nonopioid analgesics, adjuvant analgesics, and opioids (see Chapters 10 and 11).[90,174,201] Trials of nonsteroidal anti-inflammatory drugs have been recommended on theoretical grounds,[34] but there is no evidence of specific benefit from these agents. Systemic and epidural corticosteroid therapy has been advocated for painful radiculopathy,[12,80,116] but controlled trials do not support the use of systemic steroids[83,89] and the use of epidural steroids remains controversial. Most experienced clinicians will consider the use of epidural steroid injection in selected cases of patients with painful radiculopathy that has not responded to conservative management.

Neurostimulatory Approaches. The focal nature of the painful peripheral mononeuropathies is well-suited to trials of noninvasive neurostimulatory approaches, such as counterirritation and TENS. Invasive neurostimulatory procedures are used rarely.

Anesthetic Approaches. Randomized trials of anesthetic approaches for painful mononeuropathies have not been performed, and treatment is guided by anecdotal experience. Some patients obtain long-term pain relief following repeated temporary nerve blocks or a prolonged block using a local anesthetic infusion technique.[180] Although neurolysis is sometimes considered for patients who report transitory relief after each of many nerve blocks, this approach should be undertaken cautiously. Pain commonly recurs after neurolysis, and some patients develop new pains induced by the procedure.

Cryoblock yields a longer-lasting interruption of nerve function than local anesthetic instillation.[8,137] The risks of this procedure are less than for chemical neurolysis. Although limited data are available, cryoblock may be considered an alternative to chemical or surgical neurolysis in selected patients with painful mononeuropathy.

Surgical Approaches. The prospect of cure impels repeated consideration of surgical therapy for patients with painful peripheral mononeuropathies. Unfortunately, the potential for dramatic success must be balanced by the risk of deterioration.[254] Surgery should be considered only after reasonable conservative measures have failed and a comprehensive assessment, which may include a trial of local anesthetic blocks, suggests that the pain could potentially improve if the peripheral focus were eliminated.

Many surgical approaches have been attempted to manage painful mononeuropathies (see Chapter 13). Some procedures address etiologic factors. Release of entrapment may relieve the pain produced by compression of a nerve root or peripheral nerve, and surgical resection is often considered for symptomatic neuromas that are unresponsive to medical management. Comparative trials of different techniques have not been performed and, currently, the selection of patients and operative approaches is empirical.

Surgical procedures to denervate the painful part should be considered only rarely. Occasional patients benefit from procedures such as neurectomy, rhizotomy, or cordotomy,[93] but the potential for serious morbidity limits these approaches. Similarly, the dorsal root entry zone lesion has been helpful in several patients with peripheral lesions,[198] but the data are so limited that no conclusions are possible.

Physiatric Approaches. The potential for favorable analgesic and functional effects from physiatric interventions has been emphasized previously (see Chapter 14). These approaches should be considered in all patients with painful peripheral mononeuropathies.

Psychologic Approaches. There have been no trials of psychologic interventions in patients with peripheral neuropathic pain. The selection of patients and specific approaches is, therefore, the same as for other types of chronic pain.

SUMMARY

The term "neuropathic pain" characterizes a diverse group of syndromes that share a spectrum of putative mechanisms but vary in presentation, natural history, and response to therapy. The sustaining mechanisms for these syndromes presumably involve aberrant somatosensory processing in the peripheral or central nervous system. A simple topographic classification based on the location of the inciting lesion can be usefully complemented by a proposed pathophysiologic classification, in which syndromes are divided by the location of the inferred sustaining "generator." Syndromes inferred to have predominating central mechanisms comprise RSD/causalgia and the so-called deafferentation pains. Syndromes inferred to have a predominating peripheral mechanism can be divided into the painful polyneuropathies, painful mononeuropathies, and the lancinating neuralgias.

All patients with neuropathic pain should undergo a comprehensive assessment designed to characterize the pain, associated neurologic lesions, concurrent medical disorders, and other pain-related phenomena, including psychosocial and functional comorbidity. Although some patients with neuropathic pain syndromes may be amenable to specific therapy targeted to the underlying etiology, many must be treated with nonspecific therapeutic approaches intended to improve comfort, if possible, and address the needs for physical and psychosocial rehabilitation. The nonspecific analgesic therapies include sequential trials of systemic and topical analgesic drugs, stimulation techniques (such as transcutaneous electrical nerve stimulation), physiatric and psychologic interventions, and, in carefully selected patients, invasive approaches that are classified as anesthetic (such as intraspinal opioid or local anesthetic), neurostimulatory (such as dorsal column stimulation), or neurosurgical.

RSD/causalgia and complex regional pain syndrome are descriptive terms that refer to a complex syndrome of persistent pain, autonomic dysregulation, motor findings, and trophic changes. The underlying pathophysiology of these disorders is not known, but the assumption has been that efferent activity in the sympathetic nervous system can precipitate or sustain the pain, at least in some patients. A favorable response to sympathetic blockade confirms that the

pain is also sympathetically maintained. The nature of this response has not been evaluated systematically, however, and many patients with RSD/causalgia do not have SMP. If the diagnosis of RSD/causalgia is suspected, sympathetic blockade is needed to clarify the diagnosis and determine the potential value of sympathetic interruption as therapy. If sympathetic nerve block and mobilization of the painful part fail to resolve the syndrome, therapeutic modalities are offered in a manner that parallels the nonspecific treatment of other neuropathic pains.

The deafferentation pains include phantom pain, pain due to avulsion of nerve roots, postherpetic neuralgia, and central pains. These pains are believed to be sustained by central mechanisms such as central neuronal sensitization.

Phantom pain can occur after amputation of any body part. One study suggested that the likelihood of phantom pain could be reduced by treatments, such as intraspinal infusion of opioid or local anesthetic, that interrupt the afferent barrage that presumably accompanies acute denervation (such as at the time of amputation). Once established, the presentation of phantom sensation and phantom pain is extremely variable and often changes over time. A controlled trial of calcitonin demonstrated efficacy in relatively short-lived phantom limb pain, but experience with this drug is limited. Other therapies are used on the basis of anecdotal reports; neurolytic approaches should be eschewed.

Avulsion of nerve roots can produce a neuropathic pain that appears to be unique in its response to a specific neurolytic procedure, the dorsal root entry zone lesion. The favorable response to this technique suggests that the sustaining mechanism for this disorder is localized in the dorsal horn of the spinal cord. Given the potential efficacy of a specific therapy, accurate diagnosis is important. The demonstration of lateral meningoceles in the damaged region and evidence of proximal neural damage clinically or on electrodiagnostic studies should suggest the diagnosis. Patients who fail a surgical approach, or are not candidates for surgery, should be managed by use of the same nonspecific spectrum of analgesic approaches applied in other neuropathic pains.

Postherpetic neuralgia is prolonged pain following resolution of acute herpes zoster. The duration of pain required for the diagnosis is arbitrary, but a period of 4 months from the onset of the infection is recommended as the definition. Antiviral therapy during the acute attack can reduce pain and hasten resolution of the disorder; the potential for this treatment to prevent postherpetic neuralgia is undergoing investigation. Other treatments for the acute zoster, such as systemic corticosteroids, can reduce pain but do not reduce the risk of postherpetic neuralgia. The treatment of established postherpetic neuralgia is challenging and typically involves empirical use of the nonspecific therapies used in any refractory neuropathic pain syndrome.

A lesion of any type at any level of the central nervous system can eventuate in central pain. These pain syndromes are often very difficult to treat and are typically approached with the same nonspecific therapies for neuropathic pain.

Neuropathic pains sustained by peripheral mechanisms may relate to any of a spectrum of specific pathophysiologies. Some may involve the activation of normal nociceptive nervi nervorum, which may underlie the pain produced by nerve compression or inflammation; others may involve pathologic processes induced by axonotmesis, such as neuroma formation. When pain is focal, the inference of a peripheral mechanism may suggest the potential utility of peripherally focused treatment approaches.

Painful polyneuropathies are diverse. Although the hypothesis that pain relates to selective fiber damage has been suggested repeatedly, the observation that pain may accompany small-fiber, large-fiber, and mixed-fiber polyneuropathies indicates that this explanation is insufficient. Some progress has been made in understanding the pathophysiology of several specific disorders; for example, painful diabetic polyneuropathy appears likely to involve both ischemic injury to small fibers and metabolic dysfunction related to hyperglycemia.

Some patients with painful polyneuropathy respond to primary therapy directed against the identified etiology, such as vitamin repletion for nutritional neuropathies. Many patients do not respond adequately, however, or lack an identifiable or treatable etiology. In such cases, treatment usually requires sequential trials of topical and systemic analgesic drugs.

Painful mononeuropathies, most often associated with nerve trauma, may be amenable to invasive peripheral approaches, such as injection or resection of neuroma. If not effective, other analgesic therapies are applied empirically. A distinct type of painful mononeuropathy, which may be labeled lancinating neuralgia, is characterized by paroxysmal, stabbing pains. Trigeminal neuralgia is the prototypic disorder. These syndromes may be particularly amenable to treatment with a specific group of adjuvant analgesic drugs, including the anticonvulsants, baclofen, and the oral local anesthetics.

REFERENCES

1. Albe-Fessard D, and Lombard MC: Use of an animal model to evaluate the origin of and protection against deafferentation pain. In Bonica JJ, Lindblom U, and Iggo A (eds): Advances in Pain Research and Therapy, Vol 5. Raven Press, New York, 1983, pp 691–700.
2. Archer AG, Watkins PJ, Thomas PK, et al: The natural history of acute painful neuropathy in diabetes mellitus.. J Neurol Neurosurg Psychiatry 46:491–499, 1983.
3. Asbury AK, and Fields HL: Pain due to peripheral nerve damage: An hypothesis. Neurology 34:1587–1590, 1984.
4. Asbury AK, Picard EH, and Baringer JR: Sensory perineuritis. Arch Neurol 26:302–312, 1972.
5. Bach S, Noreng MF, and Tjellden NU: Phantom limb pain in amputees during the first 12 months following limb amputation, after preoperative lumbar epidural blockade. Pain 33:297–301, 1988.
6. Backonja M: Reflex sympathetic dystrophy/sympathetically-maintained pain/causalgia: The syndrome of neuropathic pain with dysautonomia. Semin Neurol 14:263–271, 1994.
7. Bahns E, Ernsberger U, Janig W, et al: Discharge properties of mechanosensitive afferents supplying the retroperitoneal space. Pflugers Arch 407:519–525, 1986.
8. Barnard D, Lloyd J, and Evans J: Cryoanalgesia in the management of chronic facial pain. Journal of Maxillofacial Surgery 9:101–102, 1981.
9. Basbaum AI, and Wall PD: Chronic changes in the response of cells in adult cat dorsal horn following partial deafferentation. The appearance of responding cells in a previously nonresponsive region. Brain Res 116:181–204, 1976.
10. Bastron JA: Neuropathy in diseases of the thyroid and pituitary glands. In Dyck PJ, Thomas PK, Lambert EH, et al (eds): Peripheral Neuropathy, Vol II. WB Saunders, Philadelphia, 1984, pp 1833–1846.

11. Bastron JA, and Thomas JE: Diabetic polyradiculopathy: Clinical and electromyographic findings in 105 patients. Mayo Clin Proc 56:725–732, 1981.
12. Benzon HT: Epidural steroid injections for low back pain and lumbosacral radiculopathy. Pain 24:277–295, 1986.
13. Benzon HT, Chomka CM, and Brunner EA: Treatment of reflex sympathetic dystrophy with regional intravenous reserpine. Anesth Analg 59:500–502, 1980.
14. Bernstein JE, Bickers DR, Dahl MV, et al: Treatment of chronic postherpetic neuralgia with topical capsaicin. J Am Acad Dermatol 17:93–96, 1987.
15. Berthier M, Starkstein S, and Leiguarda R: Asymbolia for pain: A Sensory-limbic disconnection syndrome. Ann Neurol 24:41–49, 1988.
16. Boas RA: Phantom anus pain syndrome. In Bonica JJ, Lindblom U, and Iggo A (eds): Advances in Pain Research and Therapy, Vol 5. Raven Press, New York, 1983, pp 947–951.
17. Boas RA, and Cousins MJ: Diagnostic neural blockade. In Cousins MJ, and Bridenbaugh PO (eds): Neural Blockade in Clinical Anesthesia and Management of Pain, Ed 2. Philadelphia, JB Lippincott, 1988, pp 885–898.
18. Bogousslavsky J, Regli F, and Uske A: Thalamic infarcts: Clinical syndromes, etiology and prognosis. Neurology 38:837–848, 1988.
19. Boivie J, Leijon G, and Johansson I: Central poststroke pain—a study of the mechanisms through analyses of the sensory abnormalities. Pain 37:173–185, 1989.
20. Botterell EH, Callaghan JC, and Jousse AT: Pain in paraplegia: Clinical management and surgical treatment. Proceedings of the Royal Society of Medicine 47:281–288, 1954.
21. Bouche P, Leger JM, Travers MA, et al: Peripheral neuropathy in systemic vasculitis: Clinical and electrophysiologic study of 22 patients. Neurology 36:1598–1602, 1986.
22. Boulton AJM, Drury J, Clarke B, et al: Continuous subcutaneous insulin infusion in the management of painful diabetic neuropathy. Diabetes Care 5:386–390, 1982.
23. Bradley WG, Chad D, Verghese JP, et al: Painful lumbosacral plexopathy with elevated erythrocyte sedimentation rate: A treatable inflammatory syndrome. Ann Neurol 15:457–464, 1984.
24. Brady RO: Fabry disease. In Dyck PJ, Thomas PK, Lambert EH, et al (eds): Peripheral Neuropathy, Vol II. WB Saunders, Philadelphia, 1984, pp 1717–1727.
25. Broesta J, Roldan P, Gonzalez-Darder J, et al: Chronic epidural dorsal column stimulation in the treatment of causalgic pain. Applied Neurophysiology 45:190–194, 1982.
26. Brown GR: Herpes zoster: Correlation of age, sex, distribution, neuralgia and associated disorders. South Med J 69:576–578, 1976.
27. Brown MJ, and Asbury AK: Diabetic neuropathy. Ann Neurol 15:2–12, 1984.
28. Brown MJ, Martin JR, and Asbury AK: Painful diabetic neuropathy: A morphometric study. Arch Neurol 33:164–171, 1976.
29. Bruyn GW: Glossopharyngeal neuralgia. In Vinken PJ, Bruyn GW, Klawans HL, et al (eds): Handbook of Clinical Neurology, Vol 48. Elsevier, Amsterdam, 1986, pp 459–473.
30. Burgoon CF, Burgoon JS, and Baldridge GD: The natural history of herpes zoster. JAMA 164:265–269, 1957.
31. Campbell JN, Meyer RA, and Raja SN: Is nociceptor activation by alpha-1 adrenoreceptors the culprit in sympathetically maintained pain? American Pain Society Journal 1:3–11, 1992.
32. Capsaicin Study Group: Effect of treatment with capsaicin on daily activities of patients with painful diabetic neuropathy. Diabetes Care 15:159–165, 1992.
33. Carlen P, Wall P, Nadvorna H, et al: Phantom limbs and related phenomena. Neurology 28:211–217, 1978.
34. Casey KL: Toward a rationale for the treatment of painful neuropathies. In Dubner R, Gebhart GF, and Bond MR (eds): Proceedings of the Vth World Congress on Pain. Elsevier, Amsterdam, 1988, pp 165–174.
35. Casey KL: Pain and central nervous system disease: A summary and overview. In Casey KL (ed): Pain and Central Nervous System Disease: The Central Pain Syndromes. Raven Press, New York, 1991, pp 1–11.
36. Chokroverty S, Reyes MG, Rubino FA, et al: The syndrome of diabetic amyotrophy. Ann Neurol 2:181–194, 1977.
37. Clifford DB, and Trotter JL: Pain in multiple sclerosis. Arch Neurol 41:1270–1272, 1984.
38. Cohen KL, and Harries S: Efficacy and safety of nonsteroidal anti-inflammatory drugs in the therapy of diabetic neuropathy. Arch Intern Med 147:1442–1444, 1987.
39. Colding A: The effect of sympathetic blocks on herpes zoster. Acta Anaesthesiol Scand 13:133–141, 1969.
40. Committee on Health Care Issues, American Neurological Association: Does improved control of glycemia prevent or ameliorate diabetic polyneuropathy? Ann Neurol 19:288–290, 1986.
41. Cowie RA, and Hitchcock ER: The late results of antero-lateral cordotomy for pain relief. Acta Neurochir 64:39–50, 1982.
42. Croft PB, Henson RA, and Wilkinson M: Peripheral neuropathy of sensorimotor type associated with malignant disease. Brain 90:31–66, 1967.
43. Davis L, and Martin J: Studies upon spinal cord injuries. II. The nature and treatment of pain. J Neurosurg 4:483–491, 1947.
44. Davis LE, and Drachman DB: Myeloma neuropathy: Successful treatment of two patients and a review of cases. Arch Neurol 27:507–511, 1972.
45. Dejerine J, and Roussy G: La syndrome thalamique. Rev Neurol (Paris) 12:521–532, 1906.
46. Dejgard A, Petersen P, and Kastrup J: Mexiletine for treatment of chronic painful diabetic neuropathy. Lancet 1:9–11, 1988.
47. Demorgas JM, and Kierland RR: The outcome of patients with herpes zoster. Arch Dermatol 75:193–196, 1957.
48. Denny-Brown D: Hereditary sensory radicular neuropathy. J Neurol Neurosurg Psychiatry 14:237–242, 1951.
49. Denny-Brown D, Adams RD, and Fitzgerald PJ: Pathologic features of herpes zoster: A note on

"geniculate" herpes. Arch Neurol Psychiatry 51:216–231, 1944.

50. Devor M: The pathophysiology of damaged nerve. In Wall PD, and Melzack R (eds): Textbook of Pain, ed 3. Churchill Livingston, New York, 1994, pp 79–100.

51. Devor M, Basbaum AI, Bennett GJ, et al: Group report: Mechanisms of neuropathic pain following peripheral injury. In Basbaum AI, and Besson J–M (eds): Towards a New Pharmacotherapy of Pain. John Wiley & Sons, Chichester, 1991, pp 417–440.

52. Devor M, Govrin-Lippman R, and Raber PL: Corticosteroids suppress ectopic neuronal discharge originating in experimental neuromas. Pain 22:127–137, 1985.

53. Devor M, and Raber P. Heritability of symptoms in an experimental animal model of neuropathic pain. Pain 42:51–68, 1990.

54. Devor M, and Wall PD: The effect of peripheral nerve injury on receptive fields of cells in the cat spinal cord. J Comp Neurol 199:277–291, 1981.

55. Dyck PJ, Karnes JL, O'Brien P, et al: The spatial distribution of fiber loss in diabetic polyneuropathy suggests ischemia. Ann Neurol 19:440–449, 1986.

56. Eaglestein WH, Katz R, and Brown JA: The effects of early corticosteroid therapy on the skin eruption and pain of herpes zoster. JAMA 211:1681–1683, 1970.

57. Elliott KJ: Taxonomy and mechanisms of neuropathic pain. Semin Neurol 14:195–205, 1994.

58. Emodi G, Rufli T, Just M, and Hernandez R: Human interferon therapy for herpes zoster in adults. Scand J Infect Dis 7:1–5, 1975.

59. Epstein E: Treatment of zoster and postzoster neuralgia by the intralesional injection of triamcinolone: A computer analysis of 199 cases. Int J Dermatol 15:762–769, 1976.

60. Esmann V, Kroon S, Peterslund NA, et al: Prednisolone does not prevent post-herpetic neuralgia. Lancet 2:126–129, 1987.

61. Farkash AE, and Portenoy RK: The pharmacological management of chronic pain in the paraplegic patient. J Am Paraplegia Soc 9:41–50, 1986.

62. Feringa ER, Gilberltie WJ, and Vahlsing HL: Histologic evidence for death of cortical neurons after spinal cord transection. Neurology 34:1002–1006, 1984.

63. Finch DRA, MacDougal M, Tibbs DJ, et al: Amputation for vascular disease: The experience of a peripheral vascular unit. Br J Surg 67: 233–237, 1980.

64. Fine PG, Roberts WJ, Gillette RG, et al: Slowly developing placebo responses confound tests of intravenous phentolamine to determine mechanisms underlying idiopathic chronic low back pain. Pain 56:235–242, 1994.

65. Finsen V, Persen L, Lovlien M, et al: Transcutaneous electrical nerve stimulation after major amputation. J Bone Joint Surg Br 70:109–112, 1988.

66. Foley KM, Woodruff JM, Ellis FT, et al: Radiation-induced malignant and atypical peripheral nerve sheath tumors. Ann Neurol 7:311–318, 1980.

67. Friedman AH, and Bullitt E: Dorsal root entry zone lesions in the treatment of pain following brachial plexus avulsion, spinal cord injury and herpes zoster. Applied Neurophysiology 51:164–169, 1988.

68. Friedman AH, and Nashold BS: DREZ lesions for postherpetic neuralgia. Neurosurgery 15:969–970, 1984.

69. Fromm GH: Etiology and pathogenesis of trigeminal neuralgia. In Fromm GH (ed): The Medical and Surgical Management of Trigeminal Neuralgia. Futura Publishing, Mt Kisco, NY, 1987, pp 31–41.

70. Fromm GH, Terence CF, and Chatta AS: Baclofen in the treatment of trigeminal neuralgia. Ann Neurol 15:240–247, 1984.

71. Fromm GH, Terrence CF, and Maroon JC: Trigeminal neuralgia: Current concepts regarding etiology and pathogenesis. Arch Neurol 11:309–312, 1984.

72. Galbraith AW: Prevention of postherpetic neuralgia by amantadine hydrochloride. Br J Clin Pract 37: 304–306, 1983.

73. Galer BS, and Portenoy RK: Acute herpetic and postherpetic neuralgia: Clinical features and management. Mt Sinai J Med 58:257–266, 1991.

74. Gammon GD, Burge FW, and King G: Neural toxicity in tuberculous patients treated with isoniazid (isonicotinic acid hydrazide). Arch Neurol Psychiatry 70:64–69, 1953.

75. Gerson GR, Jones RB, and Luscombe DK: Studies on the concomitant use of carbamazepine and clomipramine for the relief of post-herpetic neuralgia. Postgrad Med J 54:104–109, 1977.

76. Gobelet C, Waldburger M, and Meier GAL: The effect of adding calcitonin to physical treatment of reflex sympathetic dystrophy. Pain 48:171–175, 1992.

77. Gonzales GR: Central pain. Semin Neurol 14:255–263, 1994.

78. Gonzales GR, Herskovitz S, Rosenblum M, et al: Central pain from cerebral abscess: Thalamic syndrome in AIDS patients with toxoplasmosis. Neurology 42:1107–1109, 1992.

79. Graus F, Elkon KB, Cordon-Cardo C, et al: Sensory neuronopathy and small cell lung cancer: Antineuronal antibody that also reacts with the tumor. Am J Med 80:45–52, 1986.

80. Green LN: Dexamethasone in the management of symptoms due to herniated lumbar disc. J Neurol Neurosurg Psychiatry 38:1211–1217, 1975.

81. Gross D: Contralateral local anaesthesia in the treatment of phantom limb and stump pain. Pain 13: 313–320, 1982.

82. Gybels JM, and Sweet WH: Neurosurgical Treatment of Persistent Pain. New York: Karger, 1989, pp 283–317.

83. Haimovic IC, and Beresford HR: Dexamethasone is not superior to placebo for treating lumbosacral radicular pain. Neurology 36:1593–1594, 1986.

84. Hallin RG, and Wiesenfeld-Hallin A: Does sympathetic activity modify afferent inflow at the receptor level in man? J Auton Nerv Syst 7:391–397, 1983.

85. Hannington-Kiff JG: Intravenous regional sympathetic block with guanethidine. Lancet 1:1019–1020, 1974.

86. Hannington-Kiff JG: Relief of causalgia in limbs by regional intravenous guanethidine. British Medical Journal 2:367–368, 1979.

87. Hannington-Kiff JG: Antisympathetic drugs in limbs. In Wall PD, and Melzack R (eds): Textbook of Pain. Churchill Livingstone, New York, 1984, pp 566–576.

88. Head H, and Holmes G: Sensory disturbances from cerebral lesions. Brain 34:102–254, 1911.

89. Hedeboe J, Buhl M, and Ramsing P: Effects of using dexamethasone and placebo in the treatment of prolapsed lumbar disc. Acta Neurol Scand 65:6–10, 1982.

90. Hegarty A, and Portenoy RK: Pharmacotherapy of neuropathic pain. Semin Neurol 14:213–224, 1994.

91. Helms CA, O'Brien ET, and Katzberg RW: Segmental reflex sympathetic dystrophy syndrome. Radiology 135:67–68, 1980.

92. Henderson WR, and Smyth GE: Phantom limbs. J Neurol Neurosurg Psychiatry 11:88–112, 1948.

93. Hitchcock E: A comparison of analgesic ablative and stimulation techniques. Zentralbl Neurochir 42:189–199, 1981.

94. Holmgren H, Leijon G, Boivie J, et al: Central post-stroke pain—somatosensory evoked potentials in relation to location of the lesion and sensory signs. Pain 40:43–52, 1990.

95. Hope-Simpson RE: The nature of herpes zoster: A long-term study and a new hypothesis. Proc R Soc Lond (Biol) 58:9–20, 1965.

96. Hord AH, Rooks MD, Stephens BO, et al: Intravenous regional bretylium and lidocaine for treatment of reflex sympathetic dystrophy: A randomized, double-blind study. Anesth Analg 74:818–821, 1992.

97. Horwich MS, Cho L, Porro RS, et al: Subacute sensory neuropathy: A remote effect of carcinoma. Ann Neurol 2:7–19, 1977.

98. Hosobuchi Y: Subcortical electrical stimulation for control of intractable pain in humans. J Neurosurg 64:543–553, 1986.

99. Iwashita H, Argyrakis A, Lowitzsch K, and Spaar FW: Polyneuropathy in Waldenstrom's macroglobulinaemia. J Neurol Sci 21:341–354, 1974.

100. Jadad AR, Carroll D, Glynn CJ, and McQuay HJ: Intravenous regional sympathetic blockade for pain relief in reflex sympathetic dystrophy: A systematic review and a randomized, double-blind crossover study. Journal of Pain Symptom Management 10:13–20, 1995.

101. Jaeger B, Singer E, and Droening R: Reflex sympathetic dystrophy of the face. Arch Neurol 43:693–695, 1986.

102. Jaeger H, and Maier C: Calcitonin in phantom limb pain: A double-blind study. Pain 48:21–27, 1992.

103. Jamison K, Wellisch DK, Katz R, et al: Phantom breast syndrome. Arch Surg 114:93–95, 1979.

104. Janig W: Causalgia and reflex sympathetic dystrophy: In which way is the sympathetic nervous system involved? Trends Neurosci 8:471–477, 1985.

105. Janig W, Blumberg H, Boas RA, et al: The reflex sympathetic dystrophy syndrome: Consensus statement and general recommendations for diagnosis and clinical research. In Bond MR, Charlton JE, and Woolf CJ (eds): Proceedings of the VIth World Congress on Pain. Elsevier, Amsterdam, 1991, pp 373–376.

106. Jannetta PJ: Structural mechanisms of trigeminal neuralgia: Arterial compression of the trigeminal nerve at the pons in patients with trigeminal neuralgia. J Neurosurg 26:159–162, 1967.

107. Jaspan JB, Maselli R, Herold K, and Bartkus C: Treatment of severely painful diabetic neuropathy with an aldose reductase inhibitor: Relief of pain and improved somatic and autonomic nerve function. Lancet 1:758–762, 1983.

108. Jaspan JB, Wollran RZ, Bernstein L, et al: Hypoglycaemic peripheral neuropathy in association with insulinoma: Implications of glucopenia rather than hyperinsulinism. Medicine (Baltimore) 61:33–44, 1982.

109. Jensen TS, Krebs B, Nielsen J, et al: Immediate and long-term phantom limb pain in amputees: Incidence, clinical characteristics and relationship to pre-amputation limb pain. Pain 21:267–278, 1985.

110. Juel-Jensen BE, and MacCallum PO: Herpes Simplex, Varicella and Zoster. JB Lippincott, Philadelphia, 1972, pp 127–132.

111. Kallio KE: Permanency of results obtained by sympathetic surgery in the treatment of phantom pain. Acta Orthop Scand 19:391–397, 1950.

112. Kassirer MR, and Osterberg DH: Pain in chronic multiple sclerosis. Journal of Pain Symptom Management 2:95–97, 1987.

113. Katirji MB, and Wilbourn AJ: Common peroneal mononeuropathy: A clinical and electrophysiologic study of 116 lesions. Neurology 38:1723–1728, 1988.

114. Katz J, and Melzack R: Pain "memories" in phantom limbs: Review and clinical observations. Pain 43:319–336, 1990.

115. Keczkes K, and Basheer AM: Do corticosteroids prevent post-herpetic neuralgia? Br J Dermatol 102:551–555, 1980.

116. Kepes ER, and Duncalf D: Treatment of backache with spinal injections of local anesthetics, spinal and systemic steroids: A review. Pain 22:33–47, 1985.

117. Kernbaum S, and Hauchecorne J: Administration of levodopa for relief of herpes zoster pain. JAMA 246:132–134, 1981.

118. Kerr FWL: Central nervous system changes and deafferentation pain. In Bonica JJ, Lindblom U, and Iggo A (eds): Advances in Pain Research and Therapy, Vol 5, Raven Press, New York, 1983, pp 663–676.

119. Kikta DG, Breuer AC, and Wilbourn AJ: Thoracic root pain in diabetes: The spectrum of clinical and electromyographic findings. Ann Neurol 11:80–85, 1982.

120. Killian JM, and Fromm GH: Carbamazepine with treatment of neuralgia. Arch Neurol 19:129–136, 1968.

121. King RB: Concerning the management of pain associated with herpes zoster and of postherpetic neuralgia. Pain 33:73–78, 1988.

122. Kishore-Kumar R, Max MB, Schafer SC, et al: Desipramine relieves postherpetic neuralgia. Clin Pharmacol Ther 47:305–312, 1990.

123. Kozin F, Ryan LM, Carerra GF, et al: The reflex sympathetic dystrophy syndrome III: Scintigraphic studies, further evidence for the therapeutic efficacy of systemic corticosteroids, and proposed diagnostic criteria. Am J Med 70:23–30, 1981.

124. Krainick JU, Thoden U, and Riechert T: Pain reduction in amputees by long-term spinal cord stimulation. J Neurosurg 52:346–350, 1980.

125. Kroner K, Krebs B, Skoy J, et al: Immediate and long-term phantom breast syndrome after mastectomy: Incidence, clinical characteristics and rela-

tionship to pre-mastectomy breast pain. Pain 36:327–335, 1989.

126. Kumar K, Wyant GM, and Nath R: Deep brain stimulation for control of intractable pain in humans, present and future: A ten-year follow-up. Neurosurgery 26:774–782, 1990.

127. Laha RK, and Janetta PJ: Glossopharyngeal neuralgia. J Neurosurg 47:316–320, 1977.

128. Leijon G, and Boivie J: Central post-stroke pain—a controlled trial of amitriptyline and carbamazepine. Pain 36:27–36, 1989.

129. Leijon G, Boivie J, and Johansson I: Central post-stroke pain—neurological symptoms and pain characteristics. Pain 36:13–25, 1989.

130. Le Quesne PM: Neuropathy due to drugs. In Dyck PJ, Thomas PK, Lambert EH, et al (eds): Peripheral Neuropathy, Vol II. WB Saunders, Philadelphia, 1984, pp 2162–2179.

131. Levine JD, Dardick SJ, Basbaum AI, et al: Reflex neurogenic inflammation. 1. Contribution of the peripheral nervous system to spatially remote inflammatory responses that follow injury. J Neurosci 5:1380–1386, 1985.

132. Lewis T: Pain. Macmillan, New York, 1942.

133. Lewith GT, Gield J, and Machin D: Acupuncture compared with placebo in post-herpetic pain. Pain 17:361–368, 1983.

134. Linton SJ: Behavioral remediation of chronic pain: A status report. Pain 24:125–142, 1986.

135. Lipton RB, Galer BS, Dutcher JP, et al: Large and small fibre type sensory dysfunction in patients with cancer. J Neurol Neurosurg Psychiatry 54:706–709, 1991.

136. Livingston WK: Pain Mechanism: A Physiological Interpretation of Causalgia and Its Related States. Macmillan, New York, 1944, pp 83–113.

137. Lloyd JW, Barnard JDW, and Glynn CJ: Cryoanalgesia: A new approach to pain relief. Lancet 2:932–934, 1976.

138. Loeser JD: Cranial neuralgias. In Bonica JJ (ed): The Management of Pain, ed 2. Lea & Febiger, Philadelphia, 1990, 676–686.

139. Loeser JD, Black RG, and Christman A: Relief of pain by transcutaneous stimulation. J Neurosurg 42:308–314, 1975.

140. Loeser JD, and Ward AA: Some effects of deafferentation on neurons of the cat spinal cord. Arch Neurol 17:629–636, 1967.

141. Loeser JD, Ward AA, and White LE: Chronic defferentation of human spinal cord neurons. J Neurosurg 29:48–50, 1968.

142. Loh L, and Nathan PW: Painful peripheral states and sympathetic blocks. J Neurol Neurosurg Psychiatry 41:664–671, 1978.

143. Loh L, Nathan PW, and Schott G: Pain due to lesions of the central nervous system removed by sympathetic block. British Medical Journal 282:1026, 1981.

144. Lombard MC, and Larabi Y: Electrophysiological study of cervical dorsal horn cells in partially deafferented rats. In Bonica JJ, Lindblom U, and Iggo A (eds): Advances in Pain Research and Therapy, Vol 5. Raven Press, New York, 1983, pp 147–154.

145. Lynch G, Deadwyler S, and Cotman CW: Post lesional axonal growth produces permanent functional connections. Science 180:1364–1366, 1973.

146. Mauguire F, and Courjon J: Somatosensory epilepsy: A review of 127 cases. Brain 101:307–332, 1978.

147. Max MB, Culnane M, Schafer SC, et al: Amitriptyline relieves diabetic neuropathy pain in patients with normal or depressed mood. Neurology 37:589–594, 1987.

148. Max MB, Schafer SC, Culnane M, et al: Association of pain relief with drug side effects in postherpetic neuralgia: A single-dose study of clonidine, codeine, ibuprofen, and placebo. Clin Pharmacol Ther 43:363–371, 1988.

149. Melzack R: Phantoms and the concept of a neuromatrix. Trends Neurosci 13:88–92, 1990.

150. Melzack R, and Loeser JD: Phantom body pain in paraplegics: Evidence for a central "pattern generating mechanism" for pain. Pain 4:195–210, 1978.

151. Melzack R, and Wall PD: Pain mechanisms: A new theory. Science 150:971–978, 1965.

152. Merskey H, and Bogduk N (eds): Classification of Chronic Pain. Descriptions of Chronic Pain Syndromes and Definitions of Pain Terms, ed. 2. IASP Press, Seattle, 1994, pp 40–43.

153. Moulin DE, Foley KM, and Ebers GC: Pain syndromes in multiple sclerosis, Neurology 38:1830–1834, 1988.

154. Narakas A: The effects on pain of reconstructive neurosurgery in 160 patients with traction and/or crush injury to the brachial plexus. In Siegfried J, and Zimmermann M (eds): Phantom and Stump Pain. Springer Verlag, Berlin, 1981, pp 126–147.

155. Nashold BS: Current status of the dorsal root entry zone lesion: 1984. Neurosurgery 15:942–944, 1984.

156. Nashold BS, and Ostdahl RH: Dorsal root entry zone lesions for pain relief. J Neurosurg 51:59–69, 1979.

157. Nathan PW: Involvement of the sympathetic nervous system in pain. In Kosterlitz HW, and Terenius LY (eds): Pain and Society. Verlag Chemie, Deerfield Beach, FL, 1980, pp 311–324.

158. Nathan PW, and Wall PD: Treatment of post-herpetic neuralgia by prolonged electrical stimulation. British Medical Journal 3:645–647, 1974.

159. Nielson KD, Adams JE, and Hosobuchi Y: Experience with dorsal column stimulation for relief of chronic intractable pain: 1968–1973. Surg Neurol 4:148–152, 1975.

160. Noordenbos W: Pain. Elsevier, Amsterdam, 1959.

161. Nystrom B, and Hagbarth KE: Microelectrode recordings from transected nerves in amputees with phantom limb pain. Neurosci Lett 27:211–216, 1981.

162. Ochoa J: Isoniazid neuropathy in man. Brain 93:831–850, 1970.

163. Ochoa JL: Essence, investigation and management of "neuropathic" pains: Hopes from acknowledgement of chaos [Editorial]. Muscle Nerve 16:997–1008, 1993.

164. Ohnishi A, and Dyck PJ: Loss of small peripheral sensory neurons in Fabry's disease. Arch Neurol 31:120–127, 1974.

165. Ovensen P, Kroner K, Ornsholt J, et al: Phantom-related phenomena after rectal amputation: Prevalence and characteristics. Pain 44:289–291, 1991.

166. Pagni CA: Pain due to central nervous system lesions: Physiopathological considerations and therapeutical implications. In Bonica JJ (ed): Advances in Neurology, Vol 4. Raven Press, New York, pp 339–348, 1989.
167. Payne C: Ultrasound for post-herpetic neuralgia. Physiotherapy 70:96–97, 1984.
168. Penfield W, and Gage L: Cerebral localization of epileptic manifestations. Arch Neurol Psychiatry 30:709–727, 1933.
169. Perkins HM, and Hanlon PR: Epidural injection of local anesthetic and steroids for relief of pain secondary to herpes zoster. Arch Surg 113:253–254, 1978.
170. Peterslund NA, Seyer-Hansen K, Ipsen J, et al: Acyclovir in herpes zoster. Lancet 2:827–830, 1981.
171. Pollard JD, McLeod JG, Honnibal TGA, et al: Hypothyroid polyneuropathy: Clinical, electrophysiological and nerve biopsy findings in two cases. J Neurol Sci 53:461–471, 1982.
172. Pollmann L: Studies on phantom toothache. In Sicuteri F, Terenius L, Vecchiet L, and Maggi CA (eds): Advances in Pain Research and Therapy, Vol 20: Pain Versus Man. Raven Press. New York, 1991, pp 281–283.
173. Portenoy RK: Issues in the management of neuropathic pain. In Basbaum A, and Besson J–M (eds): Towards a New Pharmacotherapy of Pain. John Wiley & Sons, Chichester, 1991, pp 393–416.
174. Portenoy RK: Opioid therapy for chronic nonmalignant pain: Current status. In Fields HL, and Liebeskind JC (eds): Pharmacologic Approaches to the Treatment of Chronic Pain: New Concepts and Critical Issues. Progress in Pain Research and Management, Vol 1. IASP Press, Seattle, 1994, pp 247–287.
175. Portenoy RK, Duma C, and Foley KM: Acute herpetic and postherpetic neuralgia: Clinical review and current management. Ann Neurol 20:651–664, 1986.
176. Portenoy RK, and Foley KM: Chronic use of opioid analgesics in non-malignant pain: Report of 38 cases. Pain 25:171–186, 1986.
177. Portenoy RK, Yang K, and Thorton D: Chronic intractable pain. An atypical presentation of multiple sclerosis. J Neurol 235:226–228, 1988.
178. Price DD, Long S, and Huitt C: Sensory testing of pathophysiological mechanisms of pain in patients with sympathetic dystrophy. Pain 49:163–173, 1992.
179. Ragozzino MW, Melton LJ, Kurland LT, et al: Population-based study of herpes zoster and its sequelae. Medicine (Baltimore) 61:310–316, 1982.
180. Raj PP: Prognostic and therapeutic local anesthetic blockade. In Cousins MJ, and Bridenbaugh PO (eds): Neural Blockade in Clinical Anesthesia and Management of Pain. JB Lippincott, Philadelphia, 1988, pp 899–933.
181. Raja SN, Treede RD, Davis KD, et al: Systemic alpha-adrenergic blockade with phentolamine: A diagnostic test for sympathetically maintained pain. Anesthesiology 74:691–698, 1991.
182. Read D, and Warlow C: Peripheral neuropathy and solitary plasmacytoma. J Neurol Neurosurg Psychiatry 41:177–184, 1978.
183. Riddoch G: The clinical features of central pain. Lancet 234:1093–1098, 1150–1156, 1205–1209, 1938.
184. Riopelle JM, Naraghi M, and Grush KP: Chronic neuralgia incidence following local anesthetic therapy for herpes zoster. Arch Dermatol 120:747–750, 1984.
185. Roberts WJ: An hypothesis on the physiological basis for causalgia and related pains. Pain 24:297–311, 1986.
186. Roberts WJ, and Elardo SM: Sympathetic activation of A-delta nociceptors. Somatosens Mot Res 3:33–44, 1985.
187. Roberts WJ, and Elardo SM: Sympathetic activation of unmyelinated mechanoreceptors in cat skin. Brain Res 339:123–125, 1985.
188. Robinson CJ, and Burton H: Somatic submodality distribution within the second somatosensory (SII), 7b, retroinsular, postauditory and granular insular cortical areas of M. fascicularis. J Comp Neurol 192:93–108, 1980.
189. Rogers RS, and Tindall JP: Geriatric herpes zoster. J Am Geriatr Soc 19:495–503, 1971.
190. Ropper AH, and Shahani BT: Pain in Guillain-Barré syndrome. Arch Neurol 41:511–514, 1984.
191. Rowbotham MC: Topical analgesic agents. In Fields HL, and Liebeskind JC (eds): Pharmacologic Approaches to the Treatment of Chronic Pain: New Concepts and Critical Issues. Progress in Pain Research and Management, Vol 1. IASP Press, Seattle, 1994, pp 211–227.
192. Rowbotham MC, and Fields HL: Postherpetic neuralgia: The relation of pain complaint, sensory disturbance and skin temperature. Pain 39:129–144, 1989.
193. Rushton JG, and Olafson RA: Trigeminal neuralgia associated with multiple sclerosis: Report of 35 cases. Arch Neurol 13:383–386, 1965.
194. Russell WR, Espir MLE, and Morganstern FS: Treatment of post-herpetic neuralgia. Lancet 1:242–245, 1957.
195. Said G, Boudier L, Selva J, et al: Different patterns of uremic polyneuropathy: Clinicopathologic study. Neurology 33:567–574, 1983.
196. Said G, Lacroix-Coaid C, Fujimura H, et al: The peripheral neuropathy of necrotizing arteritis: A clinicopathological study. Ann Neurol 23:461–465, 1988.
197. Said G, Slama G, and Salva J: Progressive centripetal degeneration of axons in small fiber diabetic polyneuropathy. Brain 106:791–807, 1983.
198. Samii M, and Moringlane JR: Thermocoagulation of the dorsal root entry zone for the treatment of intractable pain. Neurosurgery 15:953–955, 1984.
199. Sander JE, and Sharp FR: Lumbosacral plexus neuritis. Neurology 31:470–473, 1981.
200. Sato J, and Perl ER: Adrenergic excitation of cutaneous pain receptors induced by peripheral nerve injury. Science 251:1608–1610, 1991.
201. Scadding W, Wall PD, Parry CBW, et al: Clinical trial of propranolol in post-traumatic neuralgia. Pain 14:283–292, 1982.
202. Schott GD: Visceral afferents: Their contribution to "sympathetic dependent" pain. Brain 117:397, 1994.
203. Schwartzman RJ, and McLellan TL: Reflex sympathetic dystrophy: A review. Arch Neurol 44:555–561, 1987.
204. Sellick BC: Phantom limb pain and spinal anesthesia. Anesthesiology 62:801–802, 1985.

205. Shanbrom E: Treatment of herpetic pain and posttherpetic neuralgia with intravenous procaine. JAMA 12:1041–1043, 1961.
206. Sherman R, and Sherman C: Prevalence and characteristics of chronic phantom limb pain among American veterans: Results of a trial survey. Am J Phys Med 62:227–238, 1983.
207. Sherman R, Sherman C, and Gall N: A survey of current phantom limb pain treatment in the United States. Pain 8:85–99, 1980.
208. Sherman RA, Sherman CJ, and Parker L: Chronic phantom and stump pain among veterans: Results of a survey. Pain 18:83–95, 1984.
209. Siegfried J: Monopolar electrical stimulation of ventroposteriomedialis thalami for postherpetic facial pain. Applied Neurophysiology 45:179–184, 1982.
210. Siegfried J, and Cetinalp E: Neurosurgical treatment of phantom limb pain: a survey of methods. In Siegfried J, and Zimmermann M (eds): Phantom and Stump Pain. Springer Verlag, Berlin, 1981, pp 148–155.
211. Simmel ML: Phantom experiences following amputation in childhood. J Neurol Neurosurg Psychiatry 25:69–78, 1962.
212. Simpson J: "Burning feet" in British prisoners of war in the Far East. Lancet 1:959–961, 1946.
213. Stewart JD: Focal Peripheral Neuropathies. Elsevier, New York, 1987.
214. Sunderland S: Nerves and Nerve Injuries, ed 2. Churchill Livingston, New York, 1978, pp 377–420.
215. Suzuki H, Ogawa S, Nakagawa H, et al: Cryocautery of sensitized skin areas for the relief of pain due to postherpetic neuralgia. Pain 9:355–362, 1980.
216. Swank RL, and Prados M: Avian thiamine deficiency. II. Pathologic changes in the brain and cranial nerves (especially vestibular) and their relation to the clinical behaviour. Arch Neurol Psychiatry 47:97–131, 1942.
217. Swanson AG, Buchan GC, and Alvord EC: Anatomic changes in congenital insensitivity to pain. Arch Neurol 12:12–18, 1965.
218. Tahmoush AJ: Causalgia: Redefinition as a clinical pain syndrome. Pain 10:187–197, 1981.
219. Tasker RR, de Carvalho G, and Dostrovsky JO: The history of central pain syndromes, with observations concerning pathophysiology and treatment. In Casey KL (ed): Pain and Central Nervous System Disease: The Central Pain Syndromes. Raven Press, New York, 1991, pp 31–58.
220. Tasker RR, and Dostrovsky JO: Deafferentation and central pain. In Wall PD, and Melzack R (eds): Textbook of Pain, ed 2. Churchilll Livingstone, Edinburgh, 1989, pp 154–180.
221. Taverner D: Alleviation of post-herpetic neuralgia. Lancet 2:671–673, 1960.
222. Torebjork HE, and Hallin RG: Perceptual changes accompanying controlled preferential blocking of A and C fibre responses in intact human skin nerves. Exp Brain Res 16:321–332, 1973.
223. Tovi D, Schisano G, and Liljeqvist B: Primary tumours of the region of the thalamus. J Neurosurg 18:730–740, 1961.
224. Travell JG, and Simons DG: Myofascial Pain and Dysfunction. Williams & Wilkins, Baltimore, 1983.
225. Trevathan E, and Cascino GD: Partial epilepsy presenting as focal paroxysmal pain. Neurology 38:329–330, 1988.
226. Tsairis P, Dyck PJ, and Mulder DW: Natural history of brachial plexus neuropathy: Report on 99 patients. Arch Neurol 27:109–117, 1972.
227. Turner JA, Deyo RA, Loeser JD, et al: The importance of placebo effects in pain treatment and research. JAMA 271:1609, 1994.
228. Turner JA, and Romano JM: Evaluating psychologic interventions for chronic pain: issues and recent developments. In Benedetti C, Chapman CR, and Moricca G (eds): Advances in Pain Research and Therapy, Vol 7. Raven Press, New York, 1984, pp 257–296.
229. Verdugo RJ, Campero M, and Ochoa JL: Phentolamine sympathetic block in painful polyneuropathy. II. Further questioning of the concept of sympathetically-maintained pain. Neurology 44:1010–1014, 1994.
230. Verdugo RJ, and Ochoa JL: Sympathetically-maintained pain. I. Phentolamine block questions the concept. Neurology 44:1003–1010, 1994.
231. Victor M: Polyneuropathy due to nutritional deficiency and alcoholism. In Dyck PJ, Thomas PK, Lambert EH, et al (eds): Peripheral Neuropathy, Vol II. WB Saunders, Philadelphia, 1984, pp 1899–1941.
232. Vital C, Vallat JM, Deminiere C, et al: Peripheral nerve damage during multiple myeloma and Waldenstrom's macroglobulinemia: An ultrastructural and immunopathologic study. Cancer 50:1491–1497, 1982.
233. Waldenstrom JG, Adner A, Gydell K, et al: Osteosclerotic "plasmacytoma" with polyneuropathy, hypertrichosis and diabetes. Acta Medica Scandinavica 203:297–303, 1978.
234. Walker AE, and Nulson F: Electrical stimulation of the upper thoracic portion of the sympathetic chain in man. Arch Neurol Psychiatry 5:559–560, 1948.
235. Wall PD, and Devor M: Sensory afferent impulses originate from dorsal root ganglia as well as from the periphery in normal and nerve injured rats. Pain 17:321–339, 1983.
236. Wallin BG, Torebjork E, and Hallin R: Preliminary observations on the pathophysiology of hyperalgesia in the causalgic pain syndrome. In Zotterman Y (ed): Sensory Functions of the Skin in Primates With Special Reference to Man. Pergamon Press, Oxford, 1976, pp 15–35.
237. Walsh JC: The neuropathy of multiple myeloma. Arch Neurol 25:404–414, 1971.
238. Waltz TA, and Ehni G: The thalamic syndrome and its mechanisms: Report of two cases, one due to arteriovenous malformation in the thalamus. J Neurosurg 24:735–742, 1966.
239. Wang JK, Hohnson KA, and Ilstrup DM: Sympathetic blocks for reflex sympathetic dystrophy. Pain 23:13–17, 1985.
240. Watson CPN, Chipman M, Reed K, et al: Amitriptyline versus maprotiline in postherpetic neuralgia: A randomized, double-blind, crossover trial. Pain 48:29–36, 1992.
241. Watson CPN, Deck JH, Morshead C, et al: Post-herpetic neuralgia: Further post-mortem studies of cases with and without pain. Pain 44:105–117, 1991.

242. Watson CPN, Evans RJ, Reed K, et al: Amitriptyline versus placebo in postherpetic neuralgia. Neurology 32:671–673, 1982.

243. Watson CPN, Evans RJ, and Watt VR: Post-herpetic neuralgia and topical capsaicin. Pain 33:333–340, 1988.

244. Watson CPN, Morshead C, Van der Kooys D, et al: Postherpetic neuralgia: Postmortem analysis of a case. Pain 34:129–138, 1988.

245. Westrum LE, and Canfield RE: Light and electron microscopy of degeneration in the brainstem spinal trigeminal nucleus following tooth pulp removal in adult cats. In Anderson DJ, and Matthews B (eds): Pain in the Trigeminal Region, Elsevier, Amsterdam, 1977, pp 171–180.

246. Whitley RJ, Soong SJ, Dolin R, et al: Early vidarabine therapy to control the complications of herpes zoster in immune suppressed patients. N Engl J Med 307:971–975, 1982.

247. Wilbourn A, and Hulley W: Monomelic ischemic neuropathies. Neurology 27:363–370, 1977.

248. Willis WD: Central neurogenic pain: Possible mechanisms. In Nashold BS, and Ovelmen-Levitt J (eds): Deafferentation Pain Syndromes: Pathophysiology and Treatment. Raven Press, New York, 1991, pp 81–102.

249. Woolf CJ, and Ghompson SWN: The induction and maintenance of central sensitization is dependent on N-methyl-D-aspartic acid receptor activation: Implications for the treatment of post-injury pain hypersensitivity states. Pain 44:293–299, 1991.

250. Woolsey RM: Chronic pain following spinal cord injury. J Am Paraplegia Soc 9:39–41, 1986.

251. Wynn Parry CB: Pain in avulsion lesions of the brachial plexus. Pain 99:41–53, 1980.

252. Wynn Parry CB: Management of pain in avulsion lesions of the brachial plexus. In Bonica JJ, Lindblom U, and Iggo A (eds): Advances in Pain Research and Therapy, Vol 5. Raven Press, New York, 1983, pp 751–761.

253. Wynn Parry CB: Pain in avulsion of the brachial plexus. Neurosurgery 15:960–965, 1984.

254. Wynn Parry CB, and Withrington R: The management of painful peripheral nerve disorders. In Wall PD, and Melzack R (eds): Textbook of Pain. Edingurgh, Churchill Livingstone, 1984, pp 395–401.

255. Yanagida H, Suwa K, and Corssen G: No prophylactic effect of early sympathetic blockade on postherpetic neuralgia. Anesthesiology 66:73–76, 1987.

256. Young RF, Kroening R, Fulton W, et al: Electrical stimulation of the brain in the treatment of chronic pain: Experience over 5 years. J Neurosurg 62:389–396, 1985.

257. Ziegler D, Mayer P, Wiefels K, et al: Assessment of small and large fiber function in long-term type 1 (insulin-dependent) diabetic patients with and without painful neuropathy. Pain 34:1–10, 1988.

258. Zorub DS, Nashold BS, and Cook WA: Avulsion of the brachial plexus: A review with implications on the therapy of intractable pain. Surg Neurol 2:347–353, 1974.

CHAPTER 6

LOW BACK PAIN

Ronald M. Kanner, M.D.

"The majority of adults in the United States will have back pain at some point in their lives."[56] Although only a small percentage of these individuals seek medical attention, chronic low back pain is the single largest cause of lost work days (see Chapter 3).[34] Because the age group affected is often in the prime working years, the financial impact is enormous.[85]

The human spine is ideally constructed to cause pain. Pain-sensitive structures are constantly exposed to minor trauma, and normal movements stress pain-sensitive articulations. Understanding the structure of the spine can improve diagnosis of acute back pain or persistent back pain due to nociceptive or neuropathic mechanisms. This chapter addresses the mechanisms of back pain, the diagnostic approach to patients with back pain, available treatment modalities, evaluation of outcome data, and treatment of the failed low back.

MECHANISMS OF BACK PAIN

The pain-sensitive structures of the back include supporting bones (vertebrae and laminae), articulations (facet joints), meninges, nerves, muscles, and aponeuroses.[25] One or more of these structures may be the origin of acute or chronic back pain.

The vertebral body is composed of cancellous bone with hard end plates of cortical bone. Innervation is supplied directly from the dorsal roots. The most common causes of pain originating in the vertebral bodies are osteoporotic collapse, tumor, and infection. Pain tends to be localized and aching, unless roots are involved. Occasionally, the L-1 vertebral body refers pain to the hips, and L-5 may refer to the posterior thighs.[62]

The facet joints, through which the vertebrae articulate, are true diarthrodial joints with a joint capsule. Both the joints and the capsules are innervated by small posterior rami off the dorsal roots (facet nerves). Pain originating in the facets is exacerbated by dorsiflexion of the spine, and there is marked limitation of movement.

The intervertebral disks that form a cushion between vertebral bodies are made up of a spongy nucleus pulposus, surrounded by a dense annulus fibrosus. The nucleus pulposus does not contain nociceptive fibers, but the annulus is innervated. Distention of the annulus produces the initial pain in disk herniation, even before the nucleus extrudes. Pain is characteristically exacerbated by Valsalva maneuvers.

Although the meninges are highly vascular and richly innervated, they are rarely a primary cause of pain. Rather, they are affected by pathologic processes in the surrounding structures. The meninges follow the nerve root out into the intervertebral foramen. This "root sleeve" is a pain-sensitive structure that may be the focus of pain in nerve root compression. Pain from dural encroachment may be referred in a radicular distribution, even without nerve root involvement.[94]

Nerve roots are not pain-sensitive unless they are inflamed. Compression of a normal peripheral nerve or nerve root may cause numbness but usually does not cause pain. Experimental investigations on human nerves have shown that numbness results from ischemia and demyelination rather than from mechanical compression.[78] If the nerve root or peripheral nerve is inflamed, however, even minor mechanical deformation may cause radiating pain. This has been demonstrated by placing sutures or inflatable catheters around nerve roots at the time of surgery for herniated disks, and postoperatively inducing stretching or compression of the nerve root.[84] When nerve roots compressed by herniated intervertebral disks are exposed surgically, they are sometimes described as flattened and, at other times, as inflamed or edematous.[80] Inflammation may explain the pain felt on nerve stretching in straight leg-raising. Intraneural edema and demyelination seem to be critical factors in radicular pain.

Four sets of muscle groups surround the lumbar spine: the psoas major, quadratus lumborum, transversospinalis, and the erector spinae. The innervation of the paraspinal muscle groups is segmental. The primary role of muscle injury in the production of low back pain remains uncertain, even though sprains and strains of the lower back are the most common diagnoses in back pain.

Pain-sensitive structures are not isolated or static. It may be the interaction of these structures that gives rise to pain. From this perspective, the spine can be considered in three different functional segments: the motion

segment, the superficial tissues, and the nerve trunks. This "geographic" approach is particularly useful in acute back pain. For patients with chronic pain, a more pathophysiologic approach, which attempts to infer the predominating mechanism for the pain (nociceptive, neuropathic, or psychogenic pain), may be more illuminating (see Chapter 2).

CLINICAL APPROACH TO PATIENTS WITH BACK PAIN

Accurate diagnosis of low back pain requires a guided history and physical examination, as well as the judicious selection of ancillary procedures. The first step in a diagnostic algorithm[21] determines whether the back pain is acute or chronic. If acute, the next step is to determine whether emergency attention is required.

Acute Back Pain

More than 80 percent of the general population suffers acute back pain at some time, but more than 90 percent of these resolve spontaneously, typically within 2 weeks.[20] In these cases, an etiologic diagnosis is not made, and most are considered "low back sprain."

To make an etiologic diagnosis in the remaining cases, the history should elicit the precipitating event, the location and character of the pain, and any exacerbating or relieving factors. Associated illnesses with fever or weight loss should raise the suspicion of metastatic disease or infection, which may require immediate attention. Psychosocial history should stress any life events that may perpetuate pain (stress, secondary gain, job-related problems, or history of substance abuse). Physical examination should be focused on any obvious deformities or areas of tenderness, range of motion, and neurologic function.[21]

Radiologic procedures are not needed in most patients with acute low back pain. It may be difficult to convince patients and many physicians of this fact, but plain radiographic findings of degenerative disease are as common in patients who have had no symptoms of back pain as they are in patients with back pain.[19,35] MRI scanning is even more sensitive and less specific; 52 percent of asymptomatic subjects showed a disk bulge at one lumbar level or more, and 27 percent had a protrusion.[48] Nonetheless, imaging should be considered if there is severe point tenderness over the spine or if other historical data raise the suspicion of tumor involvement or infection.[5] Practice guidelines and clinical algorithms are being developed to provide more specific indications.[54] Discussion of procedure selection follows the clinical presentations.

PHYSICAL EXAMINATION OF THE LUMBOSACRAL SPINE

The spine should be examined with the patient at rest and in motion. With the patient standing, back to the examiner, the vertical axis is checked for curvature. Normally, a gentle lordosis should be in both the cervical and lumbar regions. Areas of hyperlordosis or of flattening of the normal curvatures are often compensatory postures and indicate underlying pathology. Lateral tilt of the spine produces narrowing of the ipsilateral intervertebral foramen, with compromise of the corresponding root. In lateral disk herniations, patients tend to list away from the side of the herniation. In this condition, pain usually increases with tilt toward the side of the herniation.

The normal range of motion for forward flexion of the lumbar spine is 40 to 60 degrees from the vertical. Extension should be from 20 to 35 degrees. Extension of the spine increases pain in patients with facet joint involvement. Pain on flexion of the spine or on straight leg-raising is more indicative of nerve root pathology.

Hip disease can sometimes mimic radicular disease on straight leg-raising. To differentiate the two, the leg is raised with the knee bent and the thigh rotated laterally (Patrick's maneuver); this produces pain in hip disease but not in radicular disease.

The paraspinal areas should be palpated carefully, from the cervical to the lumbar levels, and areas of spasm or trigger points sought. Localized muscle spasm is usually the result of some other pain-related pathology, rather than the cause of the pain. For a trigger point to be considered as a cause of pain, local pressure on the point must reproduce the clinical pain syndrome.

Pain on percussion of the spine itself should raise the suspicion of collapse, metastatic disease, or infection. It is uncommon for disk disease or degenerative osteoarthritis to produce local spine tenderness.

CLINICAL SYNDROMES

Acute Pain Originating in the Bony Elements. Structural bone disease may produce pain syndromes that are commonly considered to have somatic nociceptive mechanisms (see Chapter 2). Treatment of the underlying cause is of primary importance.

Vertebral metastases. Back pain is the presenting complaint in more than 95 percent of patients with epidural spinal cord compression from tumor.[37] Patients with a history of cancer and back pain should be assumed to have vertebral metastases until proved otherwise. Pain is deep, localized, and aching. Compromise of the neural canal can result in radicular radiation and associated neurologic symptoms or signs. Characteristically, pain increases in intensity over days to weeks, without any clear precipitating cause. It is exacerbated by weight bearing and Valsalva maneuvers and is often unrelieved or even exacerbated by recumbency. In patients without a history of cancer, these characteristics and associated constitutional symptoms, including weight loss, fatigue, and anorexia, should impel an evaluation for malignancy.

Physical examination usually reveals tenderness to percussion at the level of the metastasis. Neurologic dysfunction depends on the site and extent of the lesion. If the epidural or foraminal spaces are not compromised, the neurologic examination is normal. Even in patients with epidural compression, one-quarter may have no complaints of weakness.[37]

In patients without neurologic compromise, plain radiographs should be obtained. Most tumors produce lytic lesions, but breast and prostate metastases may appear sclerotic. When there are multiple vertebral collapses from tumor, the disk spaces are usually spared (Fig. 6–1).

Even without abnormal neurologic findings, patients with cancer who have pain and

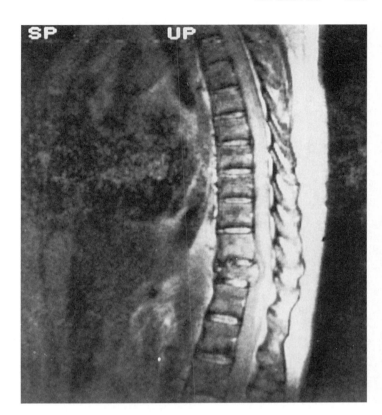

Figure 6–1. Metastatic involvement of two adjacent vertebral bodies by carcinoma of the breast, with epidural extension, shown on magnetic resonance imaging (MRI). Note the normal signal from the intervening disk. (Film courtesy of Dr. M. Patel, Long Island Jewish Medical Center.)

positive radiographs have more than a 50 percent chance of having epidural tumor.[72] A systematic evaluation for this condition is described in Chapter 9.

Metastatic involvement of the vertebral bodies is the quintessential somatic nociceptive pain syndrome. Nociceptors are activated by destruction of bone trabeculae, expansion of the periosteum, and stretching of the dura. Pain often responds to a combination of a nonsteroidal anti-inflammatory drug and an opioid. In severe pain or in patients with epidural extension, systemic administration of a corticosteroid almost invariably provides temporary relief. As with metastatic lesions of other bony structures, radiation therapy provides pain relief in approximately 70 percent.

Osteoporosis. Demineralization of bone is painless unless weight-bearing bones are fractured. In the case of vertebral bodies, microfractures of the trabeculae can produce intermittent pain. Pain is localized, deep, and aching in quality. With involvement of the lumbar spine, pain may radiate to the hips. Pain is exacerbated by weight bearing and by Valsalva maneuvers, and there is often tenderness to percussion. In contrast to tumor-related pain, osteoporotic pain is almost invariably relieved by recumbency. Patients usually avoid weight bearing, leading to further demineralization and collapse.[59] The neurologic examination is usually normal, even with compression of thoracic vertebrae. This normality is probably due to the manner in which the vertebral body "accordions" on itself, rather than extruding a mass as happens in metastatic collapse.

Postmenopausal women and patients treated with corticosteroids are most at risk for osteoporotic collapse. Even in this group, however, it should not be assumed that the osteoporosis is idiopathic. Initial evaluation should include a complete blood count, as well as serum calcium, phosphorus, alkaline phosphatase, blood urea nitrogen, creatinine, sedimentation rate, and serum protein electrophoresis. Plain radiography should be performed, both to document the collapse and to seek findings that may suggest an alternative diagnosis, such as metastatic disease.

Pain usually subsides over a few weeks. During the period of acute pain, ice packs and analgesics are usually helpful. As noted earlier, prolonged bed rest should be avoided because of the risk of increased bone loss.

Chronic pain in osteoporosis is probably more accurately defined as recurring acute pain. Minor trabecular fractures may go unnoticed radiographically but produce pain. Progressive loss of vertebral height may be too gradual to notice on repeated visits.

The treatment of pain due to osteoporosis usually should include primary therapy of the underlying condition. The goal is prevention of further mineral loss. Therapeutic regimens include estrogen replacement; calcium and vitamin D supplements; and treatment with sodium fluoride, bisphosphonates, or calcitonin.[1] Any therapeutic regimen should also include rehabilitation exercises tailored to increased weight bearing. One effective analgesic regimen provides an oral opioid (such

as one of the oxycodone combinations) 15 to 30 minutes before an exercise period, which is followed by slow walking and relaxation (a cool-down period). Specific goals should be set for each exercise period, as well as for total "up time" during a day or week.

Vertebral Osteomyelitis. Vertebral osteomyelitis presents as subacute back pain, increasing over a period of days to weeks. In the general population, it most commonly affects men over age 50 years, and the lumbar spine is affected more often than the thoracic and cervical spines. In the AIDS population, the affected patient is generally younger and the cervical spine is affected more frequently.

Physical examination of patients with vertebral osteomyelitis reveals local tenderness and limitation of range of motion. Plain radiographs may show involvement of the vertebral body end plates and the intervening disk space (as opposed to tumor involvement, which usually spares the disk space). Figure 6–2 illustrates the complete destruction of vertebral bodies and the intervening

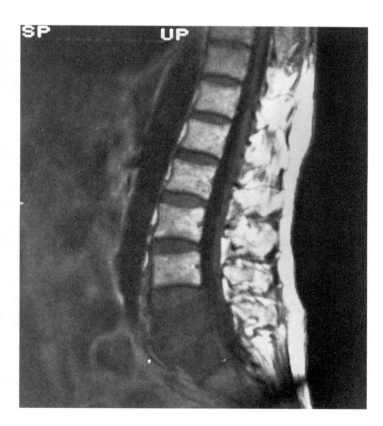

Figure 6–2. Infectious involvement of the L-5 and S-1 vertebral bodies shown on MRI. Note the involvement of the intervening disk space. (Film courtesy of Dr. M. Patel, Long Island Jewish Medical Center.)

disk space that can be caused by *Staphylococcus aureus* infection.

The posterior elements of the spine are usually spared in osteomyelitis, unless the infection is caused by actinomycosis or coccidioidomycosis.[79]

As with other somatic nociceptive pain syndromes, the most specific therapy is identification and treatment of the underlying cause—specifically, antibiotic therapy of the organism. While antimicrobial therapy is being instituted, initial pain relief can be obtained with bed rest and opioid analgesics.

Acute Pain Originating in Muscles, Aponeuroses, and Nerves.

Low Back Strain. Many patients report pain following exertion or prolonged sitting.[28] This is the most common type of back pain and is presumed to be nociceptive in origin. It responds to analgesics, physical medicine approaches (e.g., local application of heat or cold), and brief bed rest; recovery occurs rapidly in the vast majority of patients. On evaluation, there is tenderness in the paraspinal muscles but no clear focal abnormality. Flexion of the spine and rapid movements of any type are limited and increase pain. Neurologic examination is negative, and imaging procedures are not helpful.

Locked Back Syndrome. Locked back syndrome is an acute pain syndrome that is often misdiagnosed as a herniated disk or missed completely. Patients typically complain of acute pain after a twisting movement or of awakening with pain. There is no history of trauma or strain that is necessary to herniate a disk. On examination, there is an abnormal posture, associated with an area of severe paraspinal muscle spasm at the level of the pain. Radiologic and electromyographic studies are unrevealing.

The cause of the acute locked back syndrome is slippage of an articular facet, with encroachment on the pain-sensitive joint capsule.[81] The severe, localized pain sets off muscle spasm that is painful in its own right and maintains the abnormal posture.

The pain of an acute locked back can be relieved by a distraction-rotation technique. The patient lies in a lateral decubitus position, with the painful side up. The leg on the affected side is allowed to dangle forward, off the examining table. The shoulders and hips are then rotated in opposite directions (hip rotated forward), while downward pressure is applied on the hips. There may be an audible "pop" as the facets realign.

Pain Originating in Neural Structures. Acute pain of neural origin has stereotyped symptomatology. Pain is typically lancinating (described as shooting or stabbing) and is in the distribution of specific roots or nerves. Occasionally, the pain may have a dysesthetic quality (burning or tingling), but that usually occurs later. Neurologic dysfunction depends on the nerves or roots affected (Table 6–1).

The term "sciatica" is loosely applied to pain radiating down the leg; pain of this type may be due to radiculopathy, plexopathy, or true sciatic nerve dysfunction.

Radicular Pain Without Spinal Pathology. The acute onset of lumbar or sacral pain in a radicular distribution prompts a search for a causative spinal lesion. Acute pain of this type without structural pathology is unusual but is occasionally caused by inflammatory or demyelinating lesions of the dorsal root entry zone of the spinal cord, lumbar roots, or lumbosacral plexus. Pain can be accompanied by weakness, reflex changes, and, after a few weeks, atrophy.

The sciatic nerve itself may be compromised as it passes through the piriformis muscle. The "piriformis syndrome"[26] is characterized by pain that radiates in a sciatic distribution and is exacerbated by straight leg-raising and by prolonged sitting. Direct palpation of the piriformis muscle through rectal or vaginal examination may reproduce the pain.

Herniated Lumbar Intervertebral Disks. Three questions must be answered in patients suspected of having a herniated lumbar disk:

1. Is there a herniated disk?
2. Is the herniated disk the cause of the current pain problem?
3. When should surgery be considered?

Disk herniation rarely occurs without significant antecedent trauma, usually in the form of heavy lifting. Patients experience an initial jolt of pain in the back, probably corresponding to pressure on or through the annulus fibrosus. Pain is markedly exacerbated by Valsalva maneuver and, in lateral extrusions, by tilting toward the side of the herniation. As the acute back pain subsides,

Table 6–1. **ROOT COMPRESSION SYNDROMES**

Root Level	Pain	Reflex	Motor	Sensory Distribution
L-1	Iliac crest Inguinal canal	None	Psoas	Inguinal
L-2	Inguinal canal	None	Psoas ± Quads*	Anterolateral thigh
L-3	Anterior thigh	Patellar Adductor	Quads* Adductor	Medial thigh and knee
L-4	Anterior thigh Medial calf	Patellar Adductor	Quads* Adductor Dorsiflexors	Medial calf
L-5	Buttocks Lateral leg	Post tib*	Dorsiflexors Invertors ± Evertors EHL*	Lateral shin Medial dorsal foot
S-1	Buttocks Posterior thigh	Achilles	Plantar flexors Evertors ± Invertors	Lateral dorsal foot Plantar foot

*Quads = quadriceps femoris; Post tib = posterior tibial; EHL = extensor hallucis longus.

it may be followed by radicular pain, as the nucleus or fragment impinges on the nerve root. As noted earlier, some of the early radicular pain may actually be from compromise of the dural nerve root sleeve rather than the nerve itself. Partial relief is obtained by recumbency.

The vast majority of lumbosacral disk herniations occur at the L4-5 or L5-S1 interspaces (Fig. 6–3).[21] In these conditions, pain radiates either down the lateral aspect of the shin and across the dorsum of the foot (L-5) or down the posterior aspect of the leg (S-1).

A number of syndromes with pain radiating from the back can simulate a herniated disk. Nephrolithiasis commonly presents with paraspinal pain that radiates into the groin, simulating L-1 pathology. The character of renal colic pain is more intense and is not affected by leg movement. Hip pathology may simulate radicular pain in the leg, but it does not go below the knee. Pain intensity alone is not a good indicator because patients with myofascial pain may complain of more intense pain and dysfunction than patients with documented disk disease.[7]

Straight leg-raising is positive on the affected side in over 90 percent of herniated disks, but it is nonspecific. Pain on raising the contralateral leg is less sensitive but more specific. If straight leg-raising is negative, either there is no herniated disk, or it is at a higher level. "Reverse" straight leg-raising, in which the patient lies prone and the leg is extended at the hip, may be positive in higher lumbar herniations.

Reflex changes are not noted with L-5 radiculopathies, because the tibialis posterior reflex, the only one subserved by L-5, is difficult to elicit and usually not tested. Both the dorsiflexors of the foot and the extensor hallucis longus (EHL) are supplied by L-5 and can be affected by compression of the L-5 root. The EHL, however, is more sensitive because of the smaller muscle size. Sensory loss can be found over the lateral leg and dorsal or medial foot.

The Achilles reflex is the first affected in S-1 radiculopathies. The hamstring reflex is less sensitive. Weakness of plantar flexion may be missed on manual motor testing and is elicited more readily by having the patient try to stand on the toes on the affected side. Sensory defects, if present, are most pronounced on the lateral aspect on the foot.

Almost all patients with acute back pain have plain radiographs of the lumbosacral spine, despite the poor diagnostic yield of

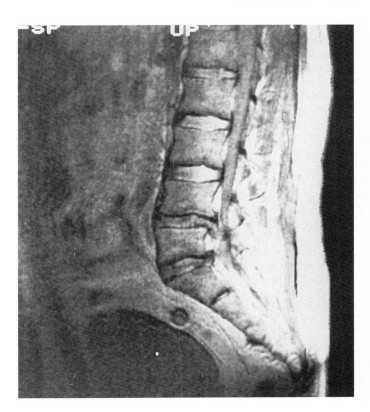

Figure 6–3. Herniated intervertebral disk at the L4-5 level, shown on MRI. Note the abnormal signal from the disk and the impingement on the spinal canal. (Film courtesy of Dr. M. Patel, Long Island Jewish Medical Center.)

the test. Plain films are unnecessary in most patients with acute low back pain. After age 50, degenerative changes of the spine are common and may not be more prevalent in patients with pain than in those who are asymptomatic.[2,19,35] Narrowing of a disk space or the presence of osteophytes does not correlate well with pain complaints. Plain radiographs are helpful and mandatory when tumor or infection is suspected of causing the radiculopathy. Otherwise, radiographs should be used only for persistent pain.

Computed tomography (CT) and magnetic resonance imaging (MRI) are both widely used for the initial evaluation of patients with low back pain, and there is no clear consensus as to which is more efficacious. Selection of a given imaging procedure may depend more upon the physician making the selection than on the symptoms or signs presented by the patient.[12] MRI offers the advantages of better soft tissue definition, information on the composition of the disk, and clearer visualization of the area

of the conus medullaris.[63] MRI can also identify nerve roots within the foramina and demonstrate sequestered disk fragments. Given its sensitivity, MRI may demonstrate false positive findings: Up to one-third of asymptomatic patients have abnormalities, and as many as 20 percent of normal young patients may show a herniated disk.[2] Although MRI yields information about disk composition, no particular pattern (white, dark, or speckled) is uniformly diagnostic.[44] In patients with pain, disk abnormalities at multiple levels, and no clear neurologic deficit, it is difficult to determine which, if any, disk is responsible for the symptoms.

CT is less expensive than MRI, is more readily available, and provides good bone visualization. Like MRI, it can identify lateral disk herniations, lateral recess stenosis, and foraminal stenosis.[42] Soft tissues are not well defined, and disk morphology is not as clear as with MRI.

Myelography should not be used as the only imaging procedure. When used in conjunction with CT, however, it can provide very detailed images of intradural pathology and clear definition of small lesions. Myelography also has the advantage of yielding cerebrospinal fluid (CSF) for analysis when the cause of the radiculopathy is in doubt.

Diskography is sometimes used to determine which herniated disk is the cause of pain in patients with multiple herniations. Reproduction of the pain when contrast material is injected into a disk is presumed to be diagnostic of a symptomatic disk. A high false-positive rate has been reported, however, and its use remains controversial.[64,67,83]

Studies that clarify the role of thermography in the diagnosis of low back pain are scant and difficult to interpret.[43] Reports have shown that limbs affected by radiculopathy can be warmer than, cooler than, or the same temperature as unaffected limbs and that the pattern of temperature change does not necessarily follow radicular patterns.[52] Thermography is rarely used in the diagnosis of acute radiculopathies, but in chronic pain it may be useful in focal autonomic changes and in documenting the efficacy of sympathetic blockade.

Electrophysiologic studies are most useful in defining the site and extent of the neurologic lesion. In acute radiculopathy, electromyography is normal for up to 3 weeks, but the H reflex is affected early. When performed adequately, electrophysiologic studies can differentiate root lesions from plexus involvement and can help to define the number of roots involved.

TREATMENT OF HERNIATED LUMBAR DISKS. Pain from a herniated disk resolves spontaneously in most cases.[15] Bed rest is commonly recommended, based on the theory that reduced intradiskal pressure accelerates healing. Sitting produces the highest intradiskal pressure and should be avoided during the early phases of recovery. The lateral decubitus position actually raises intradiskal pressure to the same level as standing.[20]

The most appropriate duration of enforced bed rest is disputed. More than 2 days is probably excessive, and more than a week can lead to deconditioning. Patients kept at bed rest for more than a week have a lower rate of return to work than those who are mobilized early.[17] Mobilization and some exercise should start even before the pain resolves entirely.[32] No data suggest that any particular type of exercise is more beneficial than another, and programs should be tailored to the individual.

If recumbency does not fully relieve the back pain, nonsteroidal anti-inflammatory drugs are the first line of pharmacologic therapy. If pain is severe, a brief course of opioid analgesics can be added. The role of "muscle relaxants," such as a benzodiazepine or cyclobenzaprine, is poorly documented, and some authors believe that the relief reported by some patients may be due to the sedative effect of these drugs. It is probably best to give patients a specific timetable for rest, exercise, and medications to reduce the chance of excessive medication use or deconditioning.

Lumbar traction, long a standard of therapy for back pain, is useless, regardless of the weight applied or the duration of treatment. There is no evidence that traction even as strong as inversion of the body produces any significant change in disk morphology. There is no advantage for traction over bed rest in patients with herniated disks, sciatica, or uncomplicated low back pain.[74] In 1988, hospitalizations for "medical back problems" constituted the seventh most common diagnosis related group. About half of these admissions were for pain control and half for further diagnostic workup, and it is not clear that these hospitalizations were therapeutically beneficial.[11]

The efficacy of heat or cold is purely anecdotal, but some patients with severe pain respond to the local application of ice packs for short periods of time. The pack should be separated from the skin by a thin towel and applied for no more than 20 minutes at a time.

Epidural steroid injections do not alter the long-term outcome of disk herniations.[73] Some studies have shown a more rapid resolution of pain than seen with bed rest alone, but other studies have been contradictory.[14,23] Relative benefit may depend on more accurate diagnosis, patient selection, and technical expertise.[86]

Numerous reports have evaluated invasive therapies for radiculopathy due to herniated lumbar disks. The data are difficult to evaluate. Chymopapain injection appears to be more effective than placebo but may not offer significant advantages over open procedures.[29,47]

Similar to many surgical procedures, appropriate patient selection is the most important influence on the outcome of lumbar laminectomy.[3,31,41] In selected patients, lumbar laminectomy with diskectomy is very effective in relieving acute radicular pain and slightly less effective in relieving back pain. Unfortunately, selection criteria are not uniformly accepted. Although most surgeons require an imaging procedure that shows disk pathology at the appropriate level to explain the symptoms and signs, radiographic findings may not be the most important factor, and some studies have shown that even postoperative imaging may not correlate exactly with success or failure.[39] If muscle weakness, sensory loss, reflex asymmetry and pain on straight leg-raising are present, there is a 98 percent chance that a herniated disk will be confirmed at surgery.[45] The degree of relief provided by surgery declines progressively as the surgical findings change from complete herniation to bulging disk to no herniation.[56]

Although most authors agree that surgery in the appropriately selected patient will bring about more rapid resolution of symptoms than will conservative therapy, the long-term results are less clear. Surgical results are difficult to evaluate because of the obvious problems with blinding and randomization. One prospective study[91] demonstrated that patients randomized to undergo surgery had a better outcome at 1 year than those randomized to physiotherapy, but the difference was less pronounced at 4 years and not statistically significant at 10 years. Another 10-year study[53] showed somewhat better results for surgery, presumably because of more stringent radiographic evidence of disk herniation as a requirement for inclusion in the study. Despite the difficulty in interpreting surgical results, the proportion of surgical admissions for back pain was still rising in 1988.[89]

Laminectomy with diskectomy is most clearly indicated for patients who have: (1) failed 4 to 6 weeks of conservative therapy, (2) symptoms and signs that are attributable to a herniated disk, and (3) limited contributing psychosocial factors. Surgery is usually essential for severe or progressive neurologic deficit, and it is indicated emergently for cauda equina dysfunction.

Other surgical approaches, such as percutaneous techniques and microsurgical diskectomy, have been advocated for the management of selected patients with herniated disks.[61,93] Comparative data are limited, and the controversies that continue to prevent a consensus on the relative efficacy of laminectomy and conservative therapy extend as well to these procedures.

The influence of psychologic factors on the outcome of laminectomy in acutely herniated lumbar disks is complex. A number of screening techniques have been used to identify psychologic characteristics to predict success or failure, but most of these were done on chronic pain patients.[6,40,41] Issues of pending litigation, workmen's compensation, and other forms of secondary gain have not been clearly elucidated.[27,46]

Chronic Low Back Pain

Patients with chronic low back pain rarely have an easily identifiable cause that can be corrected quickly, and management should be centered around a comprehensive program of rehabilitation.[55,76] Within the framework of a multidisciplinary approach, amelioration of symptoms is aided by a pathophysiologic diagnosis, with specific treatments tailored to the dominant pathophysiology.

SOMATIC NOCICEPTIVE PAIN

The hallmark of somatic nociceptive pain is an aching quality that is exacerbated by movement or weight bearing. This pathophysiologic diagnosis reflects the clinician's inference that the pain is due to ongoing activity of nociceptors due to persistent pathology affecting pain-sensitive structures.

"Degenerative Disease of the Spine." The term *degenerative joint disease* (DJD) is one of the most commonly used diagnoses but provides little insight. Pain-free patients are commonly encountered with pronounced degenerative changes and large osteophytes. Marked disk-space narrowing at multiple levels correlates better with pain.

In the absence of neurologic signs, emphasis should be on restoration of function. In the acute phase, supportive orthoses may provide transient relief, but there is no evidence that they alter outcome, and they may lead to deconditioning. Along with analgesics, they should probably be used only for acute exacerbations. Back schools and techniques aimed at long-term strengthening of the supportive muscles may be effective. This also holds true for chronic pain related to osteoporosis, in which progressive weight bearing is of even greater importance.

Facet Disease. Hypertrophy of the articular facets has been cited as a cause of chronic back pain, but the evidence is not overwhelming that facet disease can be the isolated cause. Facet pathology is inferred when pain is exacerbated by dorsiflexion of the spine and plain radiographs show facet hypertrophy, occasionally with encroachment on the intervertebral foramina. A small subgroup of patients may respond to injections of the facet joints with anesthetics or steroids. If facet hypertrophy is severe, it may encroach on the neural foramen or cause a lateral recess syndrome, with more prominent neuropathic symptoms.

Spondylolisthesis. A small degree of anterior slippage of a vertebral body may be seen in as many as 10 to 15 percent of elderly patients. Most cases are caused by spondylolysis, the incidence of which increases with age and with repeated trauma. This abnormality may contribute to pain and produce instability, although the radiographic appearance of anteroposterior vertebral malalignment does not necessarily indicate spinal instability. When pain is prominently exacerbated on movement and plain radiographs reveal spondylolisthesis, flexion/extension films should be performed to evaluate instability. Initial treatment of spondylolisthesis is the same as for other types of degenerative disease of the spine, but short-term bracing may provide dramatic relief in the early stages. In cases of severe slippage and/or neurologic compromise, spinal fusion may provide relief.

Fibromyalgia/Myofascial Pain Syndrome. Numerous terms have been used to describe patients who have stiff, aching muscles.[95,96] The term *fibromyalgia* is now applied to a syndrome of widespread pain associated with multiple tender points.[97] Some patients with this condition have back pain as the predominant complaint. Patients may also have sleep and mood disturbance, as well as functional disability. The management of fibromyalgia is challenging and must address both pain and functional impairments (see Chapter 7).

The term *myofascial pain syndrome* is usually used to describe a more localized pain syndrome in which pain is associated with trigger points.[33,88] Major and minor diagnostic criteria have been proposed.[97] The syndrome commonly occurs after "muscular overload," such as may occur with acute injury (e.g., following a near fall or intense exertion). Patients complain of a deep, aching pain that does not have a radicular distribution. They may have disturbed sleep patterns and morning stiffness. Examination reveals mild limitation of range of motion in all directions and palpable tender points or "taut bands" in muscles. Injection of local anesthetics or "spray and stretch" techniques may provide relief.

VISCERAL NOCICEPTIVE PAIN

Pain from pelvic organs, the retroperitoneal space, the gallbladder, and the pancreas can be referred to the back. The pattern of referral is devoid of neurologic patterns and is not exacerbated by movement. It is characteristically crescendo/decrescendo in nature. In this instance, determining the underlying cause is more urgent than pain control.

NEUROPATHIC PAIN

Lateral Recess Syndrome. The lateral recess is a triangular space bordered by the pedicle, the vertebral body, and the superior articular facet. The lumbar nerve root exiting at the next lower level can be affected when facet hypertrophy or an extruded lateral disk encroaches on the lateral recess, producing a space of less than 5 mm.[13] The space can become sharply angulated, compromising the nerve root (Fig. 6–4).

When a disk herniates into the lateral recess (Fig. 6–5), symptoms may be similar to spinal claudication, except that they are limited to fewer roots. Paresthesia may dominate over lancinating pain, and straight leg-raising is often negative. The space may be poorly visualized on routine studies, but CT myelography can define the dimensions well.[24] In well-defined cases that do not respond to conservative measures, surgical decompression of the space can be accomplished by laminectomy or

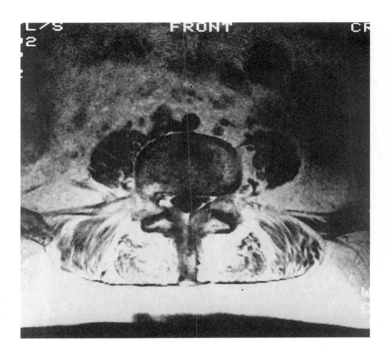

Figure 6–4. Lateral recess syndrome, shown on MRI. Note the very acute angle formed by the lateral recess on the right side of the film. (Film courtesy of Dr. M. Patel, Long Island Jewish Medical Center.)

laminotomy—removal of part of the ligamentum flavum and hypertrophied facet.

Spinal Stenosis. Spinal stenosis can develop with aging, as a result of facet hypertrophy, ligamentous hardening, and spondylolisthe-

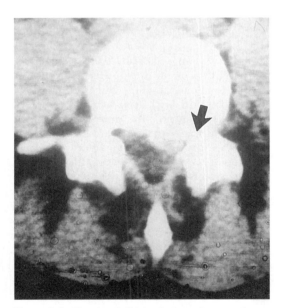

Figure 6–5. Herniated disk in the lateral recess, shown on MRI. (Film courtesy of Dr. M. Patel, Long Island Jewish Medical Center.)

sis (Fig. 6–6). Congenital spinal stenosis is unusual. When stenosis leads to pain, the hallmark is "neurogenic claudication."[30] After the patient walks a short distance, pain develops in both legs and is relieved by anteroflexion of the spine. The presumed mechanism is compromise of the radicular arteries, with relief brought on by the anatomic opening of the foramina with anteroflexion. Transient relief may be afforded by epidural steroid injections,[23] but these should be coupled with an intensive rehabilitation program aimed at progressive exercise. The number of epidural steroid injections should be limited to three or fewer in any 6-month period because of the risk of ligamentous deterioration. In intractable cases, wide lumbar laminectomy may be indicated, but it carries the added risk of spinal instability.

Lumbar Arachnoiditis. Arachnoiditis is most commonly an iatrogenic illness caused by either repeated lumbar myelography or multiple surgeries. Pain is polyradicular in distribution and is not exacerbated by straight legraising. Neurologic findings depend on the degree of radicular compromise but are usually less severe than the complaints.[16] Three common patterns are found on MRI: a central conglomeration of roots, a peripheral conglomeration of roots (leading to the appear-

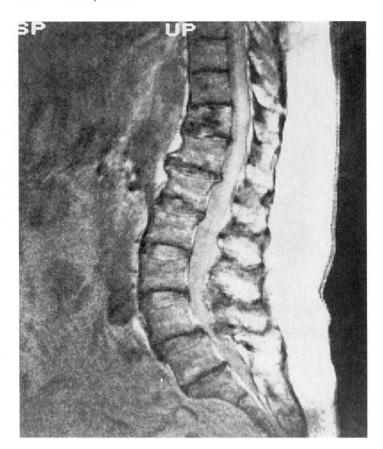

Figure 6–6. Spinal stenosis at multiple levels of the lumbar spine, shown on MRI. (Film courtesy of Dr. M. Patel, Long Island Jewish Medical Center.)

ance of an empty dural sac), and soft tissue mass replacing the subarachnoid space. Neither subarachnoid steroid injections nor lysis of adhesions has been shown to be effective.

Adjuvant medications are most often used to manage the neuropathic component of the foregoing syndromes (see Chapter 10). A small subset of patients may respond to chronic opioid therapy, but this should be undertaken only by physicians with experience in managing the treatment (see Chapter 11).[49,71] Chronic spinal electrical stimulation is also used, with results that are extremely dependent on patient selection and the experience of the team performing the stimulation (see Chapter 13).[69]

Neoplasm. Tumors of the cauda equina, filum terminale, or lumbar dura can occasionally present with chronic neuropathic pain. Examination ultimately shows significant neurologic compromise, with bowel or bladder involvement.

PSYCHOGENIC PAIN

Purely psychogenic pain, with no underlying pathology, is unusual and is represented by delusional pain, malingering, Munchausen syndrome, and hysterical conversion reactions. It is important to differentiate among these syndromes and to separate them from the clinical presentations of patients with underlying structural disease and psychologic factors complicating medical illness.

Malingering. Malingering is not entirely appropriate for inclusion in psychogenic pain, because it represents a conscious effort to deceive rather than psychiatric dysfunction leading to symptoms. Secondary gain is clearly apparent, and symptoms tend to be exaggerated. Verbal descriptors of pain are inconsistent and less emotionally loaded than in patients with hysteria.

"Hysterical Features." Hysterical features are often mentioned in the description of patients with back pain and are supported by scores on the Minnesota Multiphasic Personality Inventory (MMPI).[66,75] True hysterical conversion reactions, which show strong evidence that the symptom serves the purposes of primary and secondary gain in the absence of physical pathology, are uncommon. More commonly, patients have or develop styles that embellish existing symptoms.[51] In either case, it is not a conscious effort to deceive; rather, it is a psychologic style of dealing with perceived illness. Cognitive and behavioral treatment methods should be tailored to the individual patient.

Delusional Pain. In delusional pain, the patient has a fixed belief about the origin, severity, and meaning of the pain, despite clear medical demonstration of health. Such pains are seen only in conjunction with severe psychiatric disturbances and in some patients with nondominant hemispheric disease.

Depression. Depression is three to four times as prevalent in patients with chronic back pain than in the general population but not significantly higher than in patients with other chronic symptomatic diseases.[10,26,92] The expression of depression in back pain may depend more on the chronicity of the problem than on the severity. In the treatment of clinical depression in back pain patients, the doses and duration of antidepressant therapy should be the same as in primary depression.[87]

Secondary Gain. The role of monetary compensation in chronic pain is open to controversy.[27,38] Conventional wisdom has been that patients with compensation are less motivated to return to work and to heal, but studies exist that dispute this.[27] The issue becomes even more complicated when the secondary gain is emotional or interpersonal rather than monetary.

Unfortunately, physicians are often put in the position of judging "disability." Disability is a societal issue rather than a medical one per se. Physicians can evaluate subjective complaints and note objective signs of disease, but it is the interaction of these findings with the environment that produces or sustains disability. Whether or not that disability should be monetarily compensable is a legal decision.

Somatization. The process of somatization, in which patients express emotional issues in somatic terms, appears to be extremely common. Some patients who somatize demonstrate hysterical features on medical evaluation and some have a diagnosable psychiatric disorder, such as major depression. Other patients have only a suggestive medical history, which characteristically contains numerous medical complaints without evidence of disease. These patients may not be helped by medical therapy and are often resistant to psychologic interventions. They are best treated in a multidisciplinary setting. Unfortunately, even the MMPI, which is the most commonly employed psychologic tool in pain clinics, cannot predict outcome in multidisciplinary treatment of back pain.[9]

Failed Low Back Syndrome

The term *failed low back* is used to define a heterogeneous and difficult group of patients with persistent low back pain, despite usually efficacious therapy. In its most limited meaning, it refers to patients who still have pain after surgery to correct the presumed cause. The most important causes of the phenomenon are as follows:

INCORRECT PATIENT SELECTION

"[T]he single most striking factor influencing the outcome of surgery is poor patient selection prior to the initial operative procedure."[57,58] Inattention to psychosocial factors influencing pain is a sure road to disaster.[55] Indeed, the radiologic diagnostic procedures may not be as important as an accurate history. The presence of a herniated disk does not necessarily mean that the disk causes the pain syndrome or that its removal will relieve pain.

INCORRECT SURGERY

Surgical procedures fail less commonly for technical reasons than for reasons of selection.[68] In patients who have had relief from surgery for months or years and then have a recurrence of pain, a structural cause for that recurrence should be sought. Unfortunately, imaging procedures performed in postoperative patients may be similar in cured and symptomatic cases.[4,8,77] When pain persists from the time of surgery, investigation should be aimed at persistent pathology or incorrect indication for surgery. As noted earlier, the clearer the disk herniation at the site of pain, the higher the likelihood of surgical success.

COMPLICATIONS OF SURGERY

Arachnoiditis can be a complication of surgery and can result in chronic neuropathic pain. The removal of posterior elements can lead to spinal instability and mechanical, nociceptive pain. Given the risk of these complications, reoperation is rarely indicated in patients with failed low back syndrome. Surgery should be considered only with clear structural pathology and no significant psychosocial dysfunction. Most patients should be treated in a multidisciplinary setting with the emphasis on rehabilitation.

Chronic Nonmalignant Pain Syndrome

The chronic nonmalignant pain syndrome is conceptualized as pain and disability disproportionate to any recognizable organic cause (see Chapter 1). Patients may become regressed and develop abnormal interpersonal relationships that tend to perpetuate the pain syndrome. The specific site of pain may be less relevant than the pain-related behaviors that surround it. Some patients with chronic back pain are usefully categorized in this manner.[55]

REVIEW OF COMMONLY USED THERAPEUTIC MODALITIES

Chronic low back pain results from a heterogeneous group of disorders with varying contributions from nociceptive, neuropathic, and psychosocial sources. Judging the validity of any therapeutic measure aimed at the disorder requires clear outcome measures, and these are not yet available. A number of multifactorial measures have been suggested, including patient ratings, return to work, and increased function.[50] The Back Pain Outcome Assessment Team (BOAT) is currently addressing this issue,[18] but, given the dearth of verifiable treatment outcomes, the best that can be offered is an outline of techniques that have achieved wide clinical use.

Pharmacological Therapies

ANALGESIC MEDICATIONS

Nonsteroidal anti-inflammatory drugs are widely used for acute exacerbations of back pain. Although their use in chronic noninflammatory pain may be difficult to support, some patients do respond for prolonged periods. There are, however, no studies to document the efficacy of prolonged use. Long-term complications of renal impairment and gastrointestinal side effects further limit their usefulness in chronic low back pain. A detailed discussion of nonopioid analgesics is provided in Chapter 10.

Early in the development of the field of pain management, one of the main goals was to eliminate analgesic medications, particularly opioids, from patients' treatment regimens. Recently, it has become clear that some select patients can be managed well, with acceptable risks of complications, on long-term opioid therapy. In properly selected and managed patients, the risk of addiction is low and side effects are few. This type of therapy should be limited to patients without a prior history of addiction, who can understand the limitations and risks, and who will be carefully followed by a physician knowledgeable about these drugs in an environment capable of dealing with the difficult issues that arise (see Chapter 11).

ADJUVANT ANALGESICS

Tricyclic antidepressants may be efficacious in chronic low back pain, regardless of an effect on depressive symptomatology.[90] Other adjuvant analgesics are used empirically, depending on the nature of the pain (see Chapter 10).

Physical Medicine Approaches

Physical therapy can provide general conditioning, strengthen weakened muscles, and minimize mechanical stress on the spine (see Chapter 14). Extended walks or exercise on a stationary bike can be performed with intermittent resting in a supine position. Swimming may also be beneficial. The duration of exercise should be increased gradually, with specific goals set for each patient and with progress verified through family members or other observers. Prolonged sitting produces maximal stress on the lumbosacral spine,[65] and behaviors should be modified to keep sitting to a minimum. Although bracing reduces mechanical stress on the spine, long-term use may lead to deconditioning. It can be useful on a PRN basis, such as when prolonged standing is required. Chiropractic manipulations may provide transient relief in some cases, but long-term efficacy has not been established.[82]

Hot packs, cold packs, and massage may provide symptomatic relief, but efficacy of these modalities varies greatly (and possibly idiosyncratically) from patient to patient.

NEURAL STIMULATION

Transcutaneous electrical nerve stimulation (TENS) was initially met with great enthusiasm because of early reports of efficacy and low morbidity. The mechanism was explained by the gate control theory of pain and was believed to be enkephalin-mediated. Under closer scrutiny, sustained efficacy has not been demonstrated conclusively in controlled studies.[22,60]

In experienced hands (with as much experience in patient selection), spinal stimulation has been shown to be effective in a small group of carefully selected patients (see Chapter 13). Patient selection requires psychologic screening and a successful trial of percutaneous stimulation before implantation of electrodes.

Despite anecdotal reports of success and patient testimonials, there are no rigorous scientific studies of acupuncture in low back pain. It remains in use probably because of low morbidity, patient requests, and physician frustration.[17]

Psychologic Management

A recent study reported that 77 percent of patients presenting to a functional restoration program for back pain met lifetime diagnostic criteria for at least one psychiatric diagnosis and 59 percent demonstrated current psychiatric symptoms, even with the exclusion of the somatoform disorder.[70] The most common diagnoses were anxiety, depression, and substance abuse. Although patients tend to deny the influence of psychologic issues on their pain syndrome and attribute any psychologic disturbance to the pain, target symptoms of anxiety and depression may need to be treated independently. As discussed in Chapter 15, pain that leads to suffering and abnormal pain behaviors may need to be addressed in a behavioral fashion while rehabilitation issues are being pursued.

Multidisciplinary Pain Centers

Most workers in the field believe that a subset of patients with chronic low back pain are best managed in a multidisciplinary pain center. In this setting, pharmacologic, psychologic, and physical modalities can be used in an integrated manner by clinicians experienced in their use. The goals are directed more toward physical rehabilitation than toward pure symptom control.[50,76]

The lack of reliable and generally applicable outcome measures has impeded evaluation of these treatments. Return to work is one of the commonly used end-points, but it has clear limitations. Patients who were not part of the workforce before the back pain cannot use this criterion for outcome. If it is broadened to include housework or other tasks, the measure becomes less quantifiable. Reduction of analgesic intake is also a false end-point. In some patients, the use of analgesics may allow for a return to work and a more normal lifestyle.

The Back Pain Outcome Assessment Team (BOAT) is putting together criteria for judging success in the treatment of back pain.[18] Until adequate outcome data are available and agreed upon by experts in the field, most recommendations for treatment will be influenced by personal bias and belief, rather than rooted in solid clinical studies.

SUMMARY

Back pain affects the majority of adults and is the single greatest cause of lost work days. Acute low back pain usually resolves spontaneously, without specific treatment or clear etiologic diagnosis. A few days of rest and minor analgesics suffice. Imaging procedures are generally not helpful and even can be misleading. The exception to this is when weight loss, fever, or local tenderness suggests the diagnosis of tumor or infection.

Chronic low back pain is probably best addressed from a pathophysiologic point of view, in which the clinician infers a specific mechanism or mechanisms based on the character of the pain and the physical examination. Pain resulting from facet degeneration, spondylolisthesis, and musculoskeletal syndromes may be categorized as somatic nociceptive pain syndromes. Pain induced by nerve root injury, which may occur in the lateral recess syndrome, spinal stenosis, and arachnoiditis, may be categorized as neuropathic pain. All patients should be carefully evaluated for the impact of psychologic factors on pain and disability.

There is a lack of consensus on the best treatment for chronic low back pain. Acute pain usually responds to conservative approaches. Pain that persists and is inferred to be predominantly somatic nociceptive may respond well to analgesics and physical medicine approaches. Chronic neuropathic pains are often more difficult to treat and may require a combination of analgesics and other therapeutic modalities. When the history implies a significant psychogenic component, the specific psychologic syndrome should receive the appropriate pharmacologic or psychotherapeutic intervention. Comfort and function are usually both considered to be important goals, and rehabilitative approaches must be considered in every case. Some patients, particularly those who are highly disabled, may benefit from a formal multidisciplinary pain program. The use of surgery in the management of chronic pain should be limited to carefully selected patients.

REFERENCES

1. Ambrus JL, Hoffman M, Abrus CM, et al: Prevention and treatment of osteoporosis. One of the most frequent disorders in American women: a review. J Med 23(6):369–388, 1992.
2. Boden SD, David DO, and Dina MD: Abnormal magnetic-resonance scans of the lumbar spine in asymptomatic subjects. J Bone Joint Surg Am 72:3:403–406, 1990.
3. Brodsky AE, Kovalsky ES, and Khalil MA: Correlation of radiologic assessment of lumbar spine fusions with surgical exploration. Spine 16(6 Suppl) S261–265, 1991.
4. Bundschuh CV, Stein L, Slusser JH, et al: Distinguishing between scar and recurrent herniated disk in postoperative patients: Value of contrast-enhanced CT and MR imaging. American Journal of Neuroradiology 11(5):949–958, 1990.
5. Butt WP: Radiology for back pain. Clin Radiol 40:6–10, 1989.
6. Campbell J, Levin S, and Long D: A comparison between the MMPI and the Mensana Clinic Back Pain Test for validating the complaint of chronic back pain in women. Pain 23:243–251, 1985.
7. Cassisi JE, Sypert GW, Lagana L, et al: Pain, disability, and psychological functioning in chronic low back pain subgroups: Myofascial versus herniated disc syndrome. Neurosurgery 33(3):379–385, 1993.
8. Cerevellini P, Curri D, Volpin L, et al: Computed tomography of epidural fibrosis after discectomy: A comparison between symptomatic and asymptomatic patients. Neurosurgery 23(6):710–713, 1988.
9. Chapman SL, and Pemberton JS: Prediction of treatment outcome from clinically derived MMPI clusters in rehabilitation for chronic low back pain. Clin J Pain 10:267–276, 1994.
10. Cheatle MD, Brady JP, and Ruland T: Chronic low back pain, depression, and attributional style. Clin J Pain 6(2):114–117, 1990.
11. Cherkin DC, and Deyo RA: Nonsurgical hospitalization for low-back pain. Is it necessary? Spine 18(13):1728–1735, 1993.
12. Cherkin DC, Deyo RA, Wheeler K, et al: Physician variation in diagnostic testing for low back pain. Who you see is what you get. Arthritis Rheum 37(1):15–22, 1994.
13. Ciric I, and Mikhael MA: Lumbar spinal–lateral recess stenosis. Neurol Clin 3(2):417–423, 1985.
14. Cuckler JM, Bernini PA, Wiesel SW, et al: The use of epidural steroids in the treatment of lumbar radicular pain: A prospective, randomized, double-blind study. J Bone Joint Surg Am 67:63–66, 1985.
15. Curd JG, and Throne RP: Diagnosis and management of lumbar disk disease. Hosp Pract 24:9:135–148, 1989.
16. Delamarter RB, Ross JS, Masaryk TJ, et al: Diagnosis of lumbar arachnoiditis by magnetic resonance imaging. Spine 15(4):304–310, 1990.
17. Deyo RA: Conservative therapy for low back pain: Distinguishing useful from useless therapy. JAMA 250:1057–1063, 1983.
18. Deyo RA, Cherkin D, and Conrad D: The back pain outcome assessment team. Health Serv Res 25(5):733–777, 1990.
19. Deyo RA, Diehl AK, and Rosenthal M: Reducing roentgenography use. Can patient expectations be altered? Arch Intern Med 147:141–145, 1987.
20. Deyo RA, Loeser JD, and Bigos SJ: Herniated lumbar intervertebral disc. Ann Intern Med 112:598–603, 1990.
21. Deyo RA, Rainville J, and Kent DL: What can the history and physical examination tell us about low back pain? JAMA 268:760–765, 1992.
22. Deyo RA, Walsh N, and Martin D: A controlled trial of transcutaneous electrical nerve stimulation and

exercise for low back pain. N Engl J Med 322:1627–1634, 1990.

23. Dilke TFW, Burry HC, and Grahame R: Extradural corticosteroid injection in management of lumbar nerve root compression. British Medical Journal 2: 635–637, 1973.

24. Donmez T, Caner H, Cila A, et al: Diagnostic value of computed tomography in spinal and lateral recess stenosis, preoperatively and for long-term follow-up: A prospective study in 50 cases. Radiat Med 8(4):111–115, 1990.

25. Dowart RH, and Genant HK: Anatomy of the lumbosacral spine. Radiol Clin North Am 21(2):201–220, 1983.

26. Durrani Z, and Winnie AP: Piriformis muscle syndrome: An underdiagnosed cause of sciatica. Journal of Pain Symptom Management 6(6):374–379, 1991.

27. Dworkin RH: Compensation in chronic pain patients: Cause or consequence? (Letter) Pain 43(3): 387–388, 1990.

28. Dwyer AP: Backache and its prevention. Clin Orthop 222:35–43, 1987.

29. Ejeskar A, Machemson A, Herberts P, et al: Surgery versus chemonucleolysis for herniated lumbar disks. A prospective study with random assignment. Clin Orthop 174:236–242, 1983.

30. Epstein JA, Epstein BS, and Lavine LS: Nerve root compression associated with narrowing of the lumbar spinal canal. J Neurol Neursurg Psychiatry 25: 165–176, 1982.

31. Finneson BE: A lumbar disc surgery predictive score card. Spine 3:186, 1978.

32. Fordyce WE, Brockway JA, Bergman JA, et al: Acute back pain: A control-group comparison of behavioral vs traditional management methods. J Behav Med 9:127–140, 1986.

33. Fricton JR: Myofascial pain syndrome. In Portenoy RK (ed): Pain: Mechanisms and Syndromes, Vol 7: Neurologic Clinics. WB Saunders, Philadelphia, 1989, pp 413–427.

34. Friedlieb OP: The impact of managed care on the diagnosis and treatment of low back pain: A preliminary report. Am J Med Qual 9(1):24–29, 1994.

35. Frymoyer JW: Back pain and sciatica. N Engl J Med 318(5):291–300, 1988.

36. Garron DC, and Leavitt F: Chronic low back pain and depression. J Clin Psychol 39(4):486–493, 1983.

37. Gilbert TW, Kim JH, and Posner JB: Epidural spinal cord compression from metastatic tumor: Diagnosis and treatment. Ann Neurol 3:40–51, 1978.

38. Guest GH, and Drummond PD: Effect of compensation on emotional state and disability in chronic back pain. Comment in: Pain 48(2):121–123, 1992.

39. Heilbronner R, Fankhauser H, Schnyder P, et al: Computed tomography of the postoperative intervertebral disc and lumbar spinal canal: Serial long-term investigation in 19 patients after successful operation for lumbar disc herniation. Neurosurgery 29(1):1–7, 1991.

40. Hendler N, Mollett A, Talo S, et al: A comparison between the Minnesota Multiphasic Personality Inventory and the Mensana Clinic Back Pain Test for validating the complaint of chronic back pain. J Occup Med 30(2):98–102, 1988.

41. Hendler N, Viernstein M, Gucer P, et al: A preoperative screening test for chronic back pain patients. Psychosomatics 20(12):801–808, 1979.

42. Herzog RJ: CT: Clinical efficacy and outcome in the diagnosis and treatment of low back pain. In Weinstein JN (ed): Raven Press, New York, 1992, pp 67–89.

43. Hoffman RM, Kent DL, and Deyo RA: Diagnostic accuracy and clinical utility of thermography for lumbar radiculopathy. A meta-analysis. Spine 16(6):623–628, 1991.

44. Horton WC, and Daftari TK: Which disc as visualized by magnetic resonance is actually a source of pain? Spine 17(6):S164–171 (Suppl), 1992.

45. Hudgins RW: Computer aided diagnosis of lumbar disc herniations. Spine 8:604–615, 1983.

46. Jamison RN, Matt DA, and Parris WC: Treatment outcome in low back pain patients: Do compensation benefits make a difference? Orthop Rev 17(12): 1210–1215, 1988.

47. Javid MJ, Nordb EJ, Ford LT, et al: Safety and efficacy of chymopapain (Chymodiactin) in herniated nucleus pulposus with sciatica. Results of a randomized, double-blind study. JAMA 249:2489–2494, 1983.

48. Jensen MC, Brant-Zawadzki MN, Obuchowski N, et al: Magnetic resonance imaging of the lumbar spine in people without back pain. N Engl J Med 331:69–73, 1994.

49. Kanner RM: Rehabilitation of patients with back pain. Journal of Neurologic Rehabilitation 5:153–160, 1991.

50. Klapow JC, Slater MA, Patterson TL, et al: An empirical evaluation of multidimensional clinical outcome in chronic low back pain patients. Pain 55(1): 107–118, 1993.

51. Leavitt F: Pain and deception: Use of verbal pain measurement as a diagnostic aid in differentiating between clinical and simulated low-back pain. J Psychosom Res 29(5):495–505, 1985.

52. LeRoy PL, Christian CR, and Filasky R: Diagnostic thermography in low back syndromes. Clin J Pain 1:4, 1985.

53. Lewis PJ, Weir BKA, and Broad RW: Long-term prospective study of lumbosacral discectomy. J Neurosurg 67:49–53, 1987.

54. Linden CN, and Alfonso M: An algorithm for imaging and treatment of patients with back pain. American Journal of Neuroradiology 15(6):1193, 1994.

55. Loeser JD, Bigos SJ, Fordyce WE, et al: Low back pain. In Bonica JJ (ed): The Management of Pain, ed 2. Lea & Febiger, Philadelphia, 1990, pp 1448–1483.

56. Loeser JD, and Volinn E: Epidemiology of low back pain. Neurosurg Clin North Am 2(4):713–718, 1991.

57. Long DM: Failed low back syndrome. Neurosurg Clin North Am 2(4):899–912, 1991.

58. Long DM, Filtzer DL, BenDebba M, et al: Clinical features of the failed-back syndrome. J Neurosurg 69(1):61–71, 1988.

59. Lukert BP: Osteoporosis—a review and update. Arch Phys Med Rehabil 63:480–487, 1982.

60. Marchand S, Charest J, Li J, et al: Is TENS purely a placebo effect? A controlled study on chronic low back pain. Pain 54(1):99–106, 1993.

61. Maroon JC, and Abla A: Microlumbar discectomy. Clin Neurosurg 33:407–417, 1986.

62. McCall IW, Park WM, and O'Brien JP: Induced pain referral from posterior lumbar elements in normal subjects. Spine 4(5):441–446, 1979.

63. Modic MT, and Ross JS: Clinical efficacy and outcome in the diagnosis and treatment of low back pain. In Weinstein JN (ed): Raven Press, New York, 1992, pp 57–66.

64. Nachemson A: Lumbar discography—where are we today? (Editorial) Spine 14:555–557, 1989.

65. Nachemson AL, Schultz AB, and Berkson MH: Mechanical properties of human lumbar spine motion segments. Influences of age, sex, disc level, and degeneration. Spine 4:1, 1979.

66. Nehemkis AM, Carver DW, and Evanski PM: The predictive utility of the orthopedic examination in identifying the low back pain patients with hysterical personality features. Clin Orthop 145:158–162, 1979.

67. North American Spine Society: Position statement on discography (Editorial). Spine 13:1343, 1989.

68. North RB, Campbell JN, James CS, et al: Failed back surgery syndrome: 5-year follow-up in 102 patients undergoing repeated operation. Neurosurgery 28(5): 685–691, 1991.

69. North RB, Ewend MG, Lawton MT, et al: Failed back surgery syndrome: 5-year follow-up after spinal cord stimulator implantation. Neurosurgery 28(5):692–699, 1991.

70. Polantin PB, Kinney RK, Gatchel RJ, et al: Psychiatric illness and chronic low-back pain. The mind and the spine—which goes first? Spine 18(1):66–71, 1993.

71. Portenoy RK, and Foley KM: Chronic use of opioid analgesics in non-malignant pain: Report of 38 cases. Pain 25:171–186, 1986.

72. Portenoy R, Lipton R, and Foley K: Back pain in the cancer patient: An algorithm for evaluation and management. Neurology 37(1):134–138, 1987.

73. Power RA, Taylor GJ, and Fyfe IS: Lumbar epidural injection of steroid in acute prolapsed discs. Spine 17(4):453–455, 1992.

74. Quebec Task Force on Spinal Disorders: Scientific approach to the assessment and management of activity-related spinal disorders: A monograph for clinicians. Report of the Quebec Task Force on Spinal Disorders. Spine 12:S1–S59, 1987.

75. Rosomoff HL, Fishbain DA, Goldberg M, et al: Physical findings in patients with chronic intractable benign pain of the neck and/or back. Pain 37:279–287, 1989.

76. Rosomoff HL, and Rosomoff RS: Comprehensive multidisciplinary pain center approach to the treatment of low back pain. In Loeser JD (ed): Neurosurgery Clinics of North America: Low Back Pain, Vol 2. WB Saunders, Philadelphia, 1991, pp 877–897.

77. Ross JS, Masaryk TJ, Schrader M, et al: MR imaging of the postoperative lumbar spine: Assessment with gadopentetate dimeglumine. American Journal of Roentgenology 155(4):867–872, 1990.

78. Rydevik B, Brown MD, and Lundborg G: Pathoanatomy and pathophysiology of nerve root compression. Spine 9(1):7–15, 1984.

79. Sapico FL, and Montogomerie JZ: Vertebral osteomyelitis. Infect Dis Clin North Am 4(3):539–551, 1990.

80. Schaumburg HH, and Spencer PS: Pathology of spinal root compression. Research Status of Spinal Manipulative Therapy, NINCDS Monograph No. 15. US Department of Health, Education and Welfare, Washington, DC, 1975, pp 141–148.

81. Seimon L: The acute locked back. In Seimon L (ed): Low Back Pain: Clinical Diagnosis and Management. Appleton, Century, Crofts, New York, 1983, pp 69–77.

82. Shekelle PG, Adams AH, Chassin MR, et al: Spinal manipulation for low-back pain. Ann Intern Med 117(7):590–598, 1992

83. Simmons JW, April CN, Dwyer AP, et al: A reassessment of Holt's data on "The question of lumbar discography." Clin Orthop 237:120–124, 1988.

84. Smyth MJ, and Wright V: Sciatica and the intervertebral disc. An experimental study. J Bone Joint Surg Am 40:1401–1418, 1958.

85. Social Security Bulletin Annual Statistical Supplement, 1986, Table 51, p 119.

86. Stolker RJ, Vervest ACM, and Groen GJ: The management of chronic spinal pain by blockades: A review. Pain 58:1–20, 1994.

87. Sullivan MJ, Reesor K, Mikail S, et al: The treatment of depression in chronic low back pain: Review and recommendations. Pain 50(1):5–13, 1992.

88. Travell J, and Simons DG: Myofascial Pain and Dysfunction: The Trigger Point Manual. Baltimore, Williams & Wilkins, 1983, pp 63–158.

89. Volinn E, Turczyn KM, and Loeser JD: Patterns in low back pain hospitalizations: Implications for the treatment of low back pain in an era of health care reform. Clin J Pain 10(1):64–70, 1994.

90. Ward NG: Tricyclic antidepressants for chronic low-back pain. Mechanisms of action and predictors of response. Spine 11(7):661–665, 1986.

91. Weber H: Lumbar disc herniation. Spine 8:131–140, 1983.

92. Wesley AL, Gatchel RJ, Polatin PB, et al: Differentiation between somatic and cognitive/affective components in commonly used measurements of depression in patients with chronic low-back pain. Let's not mix apples and oranges. Spine 16(6 Suppl): S213–S215, 1991.

93. Williams RW: Microlumbar discectomy. Spine 3:175–182, 1978.

94. Wirth FP, and Van Buren JM: Referral of pain from dural stimulation in man. J Neurosurg 34:630–642, 1971.

95. Wolfe F: Methodological and statistical problems in the epidemiology of fibromyalgia. In Fricton JR, and Award E (eds): Advances in Pain Research and Therapy, Vol 17. Raven Press, New York, 1990, pp 147–163.

96. Wolfe F, Smythe HA, Yunus MB, et al: The American College of Rheumatology 1990 Criteria for the Classification of Fibromyalgia. Report of the Multicenter Criteria Committee. Arthritis Rheum 33(2): 160–172, 1990.

97. Yunus MB: Primary fibromyalgia syndrome: A critical evaluation of recent criteria developments. Rheumatology 48(5):217–222, 1989.

CHAPTER 7

FIBROMYALGIA AND MYOFASCIAL PAIN SYNDROME

Frederick Wolfe, M.D.

FIBROMYALGIA

Definition and Criteria

Under various names and guises, the syndrome of fibromyalgia has been known to physicians for most of the twentieth century.[124] Although its current meaning is that of a widespread pain disorder associated with musculoskeletal tenderness, past definitions included both local and regional musculoskeletal problems and psychologically mediated musculoskeletal pain. The term "fibrositis" was applied to all of these disorders, and no accepted criteria existed to differentiate the constructs. For many, fibrositis was a wastebasket diagnosis used to categorize unexplainable musculoskeletal problems. With no clear definition, no criteria, and no general agreement as to meaning, the idea of fibrositis was in disrepute for many years.

In 1977, Hench first suggested the use of the term fibromyalgia instead of fibrositis.[62] This suggestion was taken up by Yunus et al,[167] who emphasized the noninflammatory nature of the syndrome. A similar name, generalized tendomyopathy (*Die generalisierte tendomyopathie*), was adopted in Europe.[96,97] The physical medicine literature, led by Simons,[134] also abandoned the term fibrositis and adopted "myofascial pain syndrome" to identify regional and local musculoskeletal syndromes.[120]

Anticipating these changes in nomenclature, a series of key papers proposed and later tested criteria for the fibromyalgia syndrome. In 1977, Smythe and Moldofsky promulgated testable criteria that included a physical sign: musculoskeletal tenderness (tender points).[125] For the first time, it became possible to apply criteria for a specific diagnosis. The work of these authors had a profound influence and began a spiral of investigations and papers that has not leveled off to this day. Only 16 papers dealing with fibromyalgia or fibrositis were listed in *Index*

From the Arthritis Research Center and the University of Kansas School of Medicine–Wichita.

Supported in part by grants from the Kansas and Southern California chapters of the Arthritis Foundation and the National Institute of Arthritis, Diabetes, Digestive, and Kidney Diseases (AM21393).

145

Medicus during 1977; more than 100 new papers per year were added between 1989 and 1994.

During the 1980s, more than half a dozen criteria for fibromyalgia continued to be in use.[145] The criteria developed by Yunus et al from the results of the first controlled study of this condition were most widely accepted,[167] but a sense of imprecision crept back into the fibromyalgia concept. Occam's razor, used by Smythe and Moldofsky in 1977,[125] had grown dull.

In 1990, the American College of Rheumatology (ACR) published Criteria for the Classification of Fibromyalgia based on a multicenter, blinded, controlled study of 558 patients and controls.[160] The 1990 ACR criteria met with wide acceptance (Fig. 7–1 and Table 7–1) and broke new ground by finding that fibromyalgia could be (and should be) diagnosed in the presence of other musculoskeletal and medical disorders.

Fibromyalgia currently has reliable and widely accepted criteria, which distinguish it from other musculoskeletal disorders. The syndrome is still often confused with other disorders, however, and its definition, criteria, and nomenclature must be underscored. The need to stress nomenclature is highlighted by modern publications that continue to misuse the term fibromyalgia when referring to regional musculoskeletal problems.[137]

Prevalence

Fibromyalgia is highly prevalent (Fig. 7–2). The disorder has been identified in 12 to 20 percent of patients in rheumatic disease clinics,[152,167] 5.6 percent of patients in a

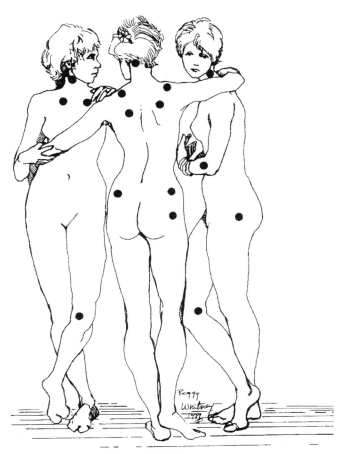

Figure 7–1. The 18 tender point sites of the 1990 American College of Rheumatology Criteria for the Classification of Fibromyalgia (*3 Graces*, after Baron Jean-Baptiste Regnault, 1793). See Table 7–1 for details of site locations.[160]

Table 7–1. **THE 1990 AMERICAN COLLEGE OF RHEUMATOLOGY CRITERIA FOR THE CLASSIFICATION OF FIBROMYALGIA**[*]

1. *History of widespread pain*[†]

Definition: Pain is considered widespread when all of the following are present: pain in the left side of the body, pain in the right side of the body, pain above the waist, and pain below the waist. In addition, axial skeletal pain (cervical spine or anterior chest or thoracic spine or low back) must be present. In this definition shoulder and buttock pain is considered as pain for each involved side. "Low back" pain is considered lower segment pain.

2. *Pain in 11 of 18 tender point sites on digital palpation*[†]

Definition: Pain, on digital palpation, must be present in at least 11 of the following 18 tender point sites:

Occiput: bilateral, at the suboccipital muscle insertions.

Low cervical: bilateral, at the anterior aspects of the inter-transverse spaces at C5 to C7.

Trapezius: bilateral, at the midpoint of the upper border.

Supraspinatus: bilateral, at origins, above the scapular spine near the medial border.

Second rib: bilateral, at the second costochondral junctions, just lateral to the junctions on upper surfaces.

Lateral epicondyle: bilateral, 2 cm distal to the epicondyles.

Gluteal: bilateral, in upper outer quandrants of buttocks in anterior fold of muscle.

Greater trochanter: bilateral, posterior to the trochanteric prominence.

Knees: bilateral, at the medial fat pad proximal to the joint line.

Digital palpation should be performed with an approximate force of 4 kg.

---

[*]For classification purposes, patients are said to have fibromyalgia if both criteria are satisfied. Widespread pain must have been present for at least 3 months. The presence of a second clinical disorder does not exclude the diagnosis of fibromyalgia.

[†]For a tender point to be considered "positive" the subject must state that the palpation is painful. "Tender" is not to be considered painful.

Source: Wolfe F, Smythe HA, Yunus MB, et al: The American College of Rheumatology 1990 Criteria for the Classification of Fibromyalgia: Report of the Multicenter Criteria Committee. Arthritis Rheum 33:160–172, 1990, with permission.

---

general medical clinic,[24] and 2.1 percent of patients in a family practice clinic.[56] A study of hospitalized patients in Switzerland diagnosed fibromyalgia in 7.5 percent.[95]

Prevalence rates in community-based surveys vary with the survey methodology and criteria used for identification of fibromyalgia. Earlier studies included patients identified in various community health surveys and used definitions of "widespread pain" that were modifications of the ACR criteria. More recent studies used the ACR definition. Jacobsson et al's community population survey of 900 subjects in Malmo, Sweden, yielded a prevalence estimate of 1 percent,[70] and Forseth and Gran estimated a 10 percent prevalence among women in Norway.[45] Wolfe and colleagues applied ACR criteria in a US population survey of

3000 subjects and noted an age- and sex-adjusted total prevalence of 2 percent (0.5 percent for men and 3.7 percent for women); the prevalence was 1 percent for those at or below age 50.[158] In a German study of 541 residents, the prevalence of fibromyalgia was 1.9 percent using non-ACR diagnostic criteria (excluding patients with a number of tender points at nondiagnostic sites [see following]) and 2.8 percent using the ACR criteria.[103] A lower prevalence rate for fibromyalgia (0.66 percent) was noted in one survey, but reanalysis of the data using the ACR criterion for the definition of tender points yielded a prevalence rate of approximately 1.8 percent.[154]

Yunus et al[165] and others[22] have called attention to the importance of fibromyalgia in children. In a carefully prepared report,

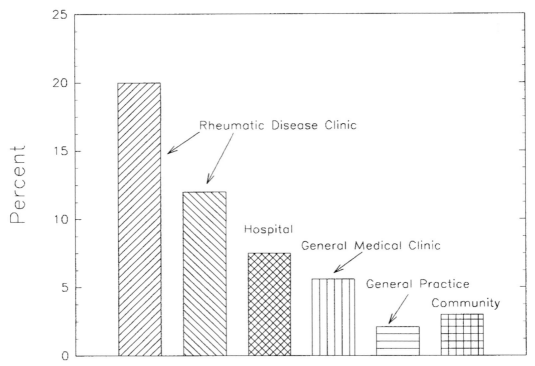

Figure 7–2. Prevalence of fibromyalgia in the clinic and the community. See text for details.

Buskila and colleagues reported an overall prevalence of 6.2 percent.[22] Approximately one-third of the 60 adolescents referred to a rheumatology clinic had this diagnosis.[32]

DEMOGRAPHIC FEATURES

Almost 90 percent of those with fibromyalgia are women.[160] Although originally thought of as a disorder of young women, this characterization was based on studies that excluded patients with concomitant conditions.[149] The mean age of patients with primary fibromyalgia (fibromyalgia without other musculoskeletal conditions) in the ACR criteria study was 44.7 years (SD 10.4) and the mean age of those with concomitant or secondary fibromyalgia (fibromyalgia associated with other disorders) was 51.9 years (SD 12.5).[160] Using a definition of fibromyalgia that incorporates primary and secondary fibromyalgia, the overall mean age in the ACR study was 49.1 years (SD 12.8). Similar age distributions have been reported in other clinical studies, and the ages reported in community-based studies have been slightly higher.[151]

The distribution of fibromyalgia appears to be worldwide. Studies of the syndrome have been conducted in Japan[99] and South Africa.[83] Although well-educated white patients predominate in studies of fibromyalgia, this skew probably reflects the referral bias of the clinics from which most research originates rather than the true demographics of the disease. Fibromyalgia has been noted in less–well-educated Hispanics in the United States,[31] and population data indicate that decreased income and lower education are associated with the syndrome.[158] Fibromyalgia patients have a higher divorce rate than others with rheumatic conditions.[60]

CLINICAL COURSE

Despite its prevalence, little is known of the natural history of the fibromyalgia syndrome. Most patients are evaluated well into the course of their illness, and few have been followed longitudinally. Studies that have assessed natural history have been performed in specialty clinics and reflect the experience of a selected population; patients with transitory or remittent fibromyalgia are under-represented at these clinics. Improvement can occur in a wide spectrum of chronic pain patients,[37,144] and it is possible that such improvement is the case for a subgroup of fibromyalgia patients.

In the selected populations studied, the symptoms of fibromyalgia have usually been constant over time, and remissions have been uncommon.[29,42,59,85] Hawley et al[59] assessed 75 patients monthly for 12 months using self-report measures of pain, global severity, functional disability, stiffness, and sleep; although patients varied widely, there were no significant within-patient changes. Felson and Goldenberg[42] observed that more than 60 percent of patients continued to report moderate to severe symptoms during a 2-year period, despite treatment for the disorder. Among 81 patients studied by Cathey et al,[146] only 23 percent reported remissions in the past; the median duration of remission was 12 months, or 21 percent of the time with the illness. In a recent detailed study, 97 percent of fibromyalgia patients had symptoms, and 85 percent fulfilled diagnostic criteria 4 years after initial examination; scores on the Health Assessment Questionnaire (HAQ) indicated clinically important self-reported functional disability at this time.[80]

DISABILITY

Work disability has also been investigated in the population with fibromyalgia.[10,29,30,85] A preliminary report of 544 patients from a multicenter longitudinal study in the United States found that 12 percent of working-age patients were receiving disability benefits and 15.4 percent had received benefits at some point during their working lives[31]; among the most important correlates of work disability were scores on the Stanford Health Assessment Questionnaire, a functional assessment instrument.[47] In one study,[27] the mean work loss per year among the 37 percent of patients with fibromyalgia who were employed was 9.8 days, compared with 8.0, 7.4, and 5.2 days in a national sample of patients with low back pain, rheumatoid arthritis (RA), and osteoarthritis (OA), respectively.[76] Only 6 percent of the patients with fibromyalgia in the latter study received disability payments, compared with 6 percent of patients with low back pain, 24 percent of patients with RA, and 29 percent of pa-

tients with OA in the national sample. A follow-up study of 176 fibromyalgia patients found that 5 days (SD 16.5) were lost from work during a 6-month period; 5.7 percent received disability payments, 9.3 percent considered themselves disabled, 30.4 percent stated that they changed jobs because of the fibromyalgia, and 17 percent reported that they stopped working because of the syndrome (Table 7–2).[30] In a comparative study,[85] 33 percent of fibromyalgia patients (N = 74) and 26 percent of RA patients (N = 186) reported job changes because of their disorder. A Swedish study[10] observed that 55 percent of 55 fibromyalgia patients were unable to manage household work alone, and 24 percent were receiving pensions.

Etiologic Considerations

In 1953, Graham suggested that fibromyalgia (fibrositis) was a final common pathway, rather than a distinct disorder.[52] Since then, three distinct views have emerged (Table 7–3). One places most stress on the psychologic aspects of the syndrome and the others ascribe the clinical features to organic processes.

PSYCHOLOGIC FACTORS

Although there have been few direct assertions that fibromyalgia is a primary psychologic disorder, psychologic factors have been associated with the disease* and with the tender points that are a fundamental element of the syndrome (see below).[138,157] Certainly, psychologic disturbances are common among fibromyalgia patients who are treated in specialty clinics. Using cutoff scores on a standardized depression inventory, Hawley and Wolfe[58] found that 48.6 percent of unselected clinic patients with fibromyalgia had possible clinical depression, and 29.3 percent had probable depression. Of all other clinic patients (N = 5610), 34.5 and 19.1 percent met these criteria. These data suggest that depression, variously defined, is 10 to 15 percent more common in those with fibromyalgia. Population data also indicate an association between fibromyalgia and both anxiety and depression.[158]

Notwithstanding these associations, a psychologic causation for fibromyalgia has been rejected by some investigators,[1,33,49,50] in-

---

*References 2,25,44,58–60,95,100,110,150,153,157.

Table 7–2. WORK STATUS OF FIBROMYALGIA PATIENTS (N=176) FROM AN OUTPATIENT RHEUMATIC DISEASE CLINIC

	Percent	Mean	SD
EMPLOYMENT STATUS			
Ever employed	94.7		
Current Employment Status			
Employed	54.0		
Homemaker	28.4		
Retired	14.2		
Seeking employment, student, or sick leave	2.3		
Employment Change			
Stopped working because of fibromyalgia	17.0		
Changed job because of fibromyalgia	30.4		
DISABILITY STATUS			
Reporting	9.3		
Receiving benefits	5.7		
WORK AND WORK LOSS[*]			
Hours worked		36.8	(11.95)
Days Unable to Work			
All		9.2	(23.47)
Employed		5.0	(16.55)
Not employed		14.3	(29.20)
Work Loss >7 Days			
All	18.8		
Employed	8.4		
Not employed	30.9		

[*]Days unable to work are days missed from work per 6-month period by employed patients and days unable to perform usual activities per 6-month period for those not working.

Source: Modified from Cathey MA, Wolfe F, Kleinheksel SM, et al: Functional ability and work status in patients with fibromyalgia. Arthritis Care and Research 1:85–98, 1988. Reprinted with permission from Arthritis Care and Research. © American College of Rheumatology.

cluding the author, who conclude from the available evidence that psychologic abnormalities are not necessary or sufficient for the diagnosis. Although psychologic factors influence the presentation of the syndrome, they are probably not its primary etiology.

MUSCLE ABNORMALITIES

The second view links the clinical signs and symptoms of the fibromyalgia syndrome with abnormalities in the muscle. This theory is based on the work of groups working in Denmark,[4,38,39,67–69] Sweden,[*] and the United States.[13–16,21,75] For these investigators, the muscle is the "'end organ': responsible for the pain . . ." of the syndrome.[13] Bengstsson et al[12] found decreases in ADP, ATP, and phosphoryl creatine in the tender points of fibromyalgia muscles and hypothesized that hypoxia or a metabolic defect may cause these changes. The latter investigators also noted decreased

[*]References 5,8,9,11,12,63,64,82,168.

Table 7–3. **SUGGESTED ETIOLOGIES FOR FIBROMYALGIA**

Etiology	Evidence	Objection
Psychologic	Psychologic abnormalities by testing and interview reported in most studies	Selection bias Criterion contamination May be due to chronic pain
Muscular	Decreased oxygen tension and blood flow in muscle Abnormal muscle biopsies Weakness	Does not explain pain distribution Biopsy abnormalities minimal Nonspecific; some abnormalities may be related to myofascial pain syndrome
Neurogenic	Generalized pain Increase in CSF substance P Decrease in serum and CSF serotonin Sympathetic blockade effective Similar to "radiation" patterns of axial skeletal disorders Similarity to disorders such as sympathetic dystrophy	May be a secondary phenomenon — Does not explain muscle abnormality

oxygen tension in "trigger points" of trapezius muscles (and in subcutaneous tissue), but not in brachioradialis muscles.[82] Brückle et al[19] noted hypoxia in taut areas of muscle (known as "myogelose") and higher oxygen tension in all other muscle areas, compared with normals. Bennett et al[16] provided physiologic evidence for the hypoxic hypothesis by demonstrating decreased muscle blood flow in exercising patients with fibromyalgia compared with sedentary controls. Capillary density, however, is normal in fibromyalgia patients.[11]

Other observations that may support the muscle hypothesis include an increased frequency of "ragged red" fibers, indicating mitochondrial abnormality, in trapezius biopsies[9]; evidence of decreased muscle strength[15,67,68,75]; and the finding of muscle antibodies.[69] A recent magnetic resonance study found an increased incidence of a phosphodiester peak in skeletal muscle of fibromyalgia patients, although the significance of this finding is unclear,[73] and recent studies have failed to confirm specific abnormalities of muscle.

The most important problem with the muscle hypothesis is that its main construct, hypoxia leading to pain and dysfunction, does not adequately explain the clinical picture. These muscle abnormalities are not convincing to many observers[164] and may be nonspecific.[78] The pain of fibromyalgia is located not only in muscle but also is noted in joints, periarticular regions, dermatomes,

and multiple organ regions including, for example, the gastrointestinal tract and bladder. In addition, the muscle abnormalities found in fibromyalgia patients may also characterize patients with myofascial pain syndromes and normals. Trapezial trigger points are frequent,[126] and the failure to find consistent abnormalities in areas removed from the trapezius is difficult to explain.

THE NEUROGENIC HYPOTHESIS

The third etiologic construct for fibromyalgia is the central or neurogenic hypothesis. This hypothesis was most succinctly stated by Littlejohn and Reilly,[104] and later by Yunus.[162] Supporting evidence includes the demonstration of decreased pain thresholds not only over tender point regions but also generally[109–111,160]; as well as the widespread pain in muscle, muscle-joint interface, joint, and nonarticular structures; and the association of the syndrome with other disorders, including headache, irritable bowel syndrome, and irritable bladder syndrome.[141,160] Some of the features of fibromyalgia, including regional pain, paresthesias, swelling, and sympathetic hyperactivity[5,7,61,81,140] are consistent with both central nervous system changes and regional pain syndromes such as reflex sympathetic dystrophy (see Chapter 5). Interestingly, sympathetic nerve blocks can abolish the tender points of fibromyalgia.[5,7]

A central pathogenesis is also suggested by

neurochemical and hormonal abnormalities. Vaeroy and Russell[127,139] reported elevated levels of substance P in the cerebrospinal fluid (CSF) of fibromyalgia patients but not in normals or patients with other painful diagnoses, and recent studies found decreased serotonin in CSF and plasma.[65,108,163] Hypothalamic-pituitary–adrenal axis dysfunction has been observed.[36,53,54,98]

The etiology of fibromyalgia remains unknown. Nonetheless, important discoveries during the past decade have advanced knowledge of the psychologic, neuroendocrine, and muscular abnormalities present in the syndrome.

Clinical Features

Fibromyalgia is a syndrome characterized by widespread pain, musculoskeletal tenderness, and associated symptoms (Figure 7–3).[148,150] According to the 1990 ACR criteria,[160] the core features are widespread pain and widespread tenderness. These features, which are necessary and sufficient for the diagnosis, indicate that fibromyalgia can be defined as a musculoskeletal pain disorder with widespread local tenderness.

Within the symptom complex of fibromyalgia, there are three characteristic features: fatigue, nonrefreshed or disturbed sleep, and morning stiffness (Table 7–4). These are present in more than 75 percent of patients but are not required for the diagnosis.[148]

Other features are common and occur in most patients with fibromyalgia (Table 7–4). These features are not necessary for the diagnosis but help identify the syndrome. They include irritable bowel and bladder syndromes, Raynaud's phenomenon, headache, subjective swelling, paresthesias, psychologic abnormality and functional disability, and modulation of symptoms by sleep, stress, and weather. There may also be symptoms and physical findings of coexistent rheumatic conditions, such as arthritis, low back and cervical disorders, and tendinitis. The symptoms of these disorders intertwine and overlap with those of fibromyalgia. It is the relative predominance and severity of the common features and the variable presence of coexisting rheumatic conditions that influence the clinical presentation of the patient.

PAIN

Widespread pain is the central dominating feature of the fibromyalgia syndrome (Fig.

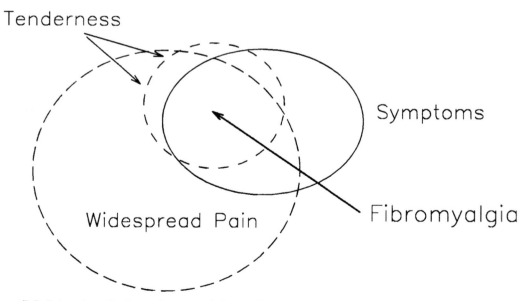

Figure 7–3. Interaction of pain, tenderness, and characteristic and common symptoms of fibromyalgia. A model of fibromyalgia in the clinic. This model reflects the prevalence of fibromyalgia in the clinic and the relative relationship among tenderness, pain, and symptoms found in the clinic. (From Wolfe F: Fibromyalgia: On diagnosis and certainty. Journal of Musculoskeletal Pain 1:17–36, 1993, Haworth Press, Inc., with permission.)

Table 7–4. **PREVALENCE OF PAIN AND SYMPTOMS IN THE 1990 ACR STUDY OF CRITERIA FOR THE CLASSIFICATION OF FIBROMYALGIA**

Criterion	Fibromyalgia Syndrome % Positive
Pain Symptoms	
Pain posterior thorax	72.3
15+ painful sites	55.6
Neck pain	85.3
Low back pain	78.8
Widespread pain	97.6
Symptoms	
Sleep disturbance	74.6
"Pain all over"	67.0
Fatigue	81.4
Morning stiffness >15 minutes	67.2
Anxiety	47.8
Headache	52.8
Prior depression	31.5
Irritable bowel syndrome	29.6
Sicca symptoms	35.8
Urinary urgency	26.3
Dysmenorrhea history	40.6
Raynaud's phenomenon	16.7
Modulating Factors	
Noise	24.0
Cold	79.3
Poor sleep	76.0
Anxiety	69.0
Humidity	59.6
Stress	63.0
Fatigue	76.7
Weather change	66.1
Warmth	78.0

Source: Modified from Wolfe, Smythe HA, Yunus MB, et al: The American College of Rheumatology 1990 Criteria for the Classification of Fibromyalgia: Report of the Multicenter Criteria Committee. Arthritis Rheum 33:160–172, 1990, with permission.

7–4 and 7–5).[148] In the ACR 1990 criteria report, 97 percent of patients with fibromyalgia had widespread pain, which was defined as pain above and below the waist, pain on the left and right sides of the body, and pain involving the axial skeleton. More than 75 percent of patients had pain in the cervical region, posterior thorax, and low back. When the body was divided into 30 regions, 56 percent had pain in at least 15 of these zones.

Similar data are available from other studies. Leavitt et al[79] described 24 regions in which at least 25 percent of patients complained of pain. These areas spanned all body areas, including the genitals and face. Similar to the ACR findings, the investigators noted pain in 15 of 25 body areas in more than 50 percent of patients.

Although patients may describe widespread pain when queried, they may concen-

VAS PAIN SCORES

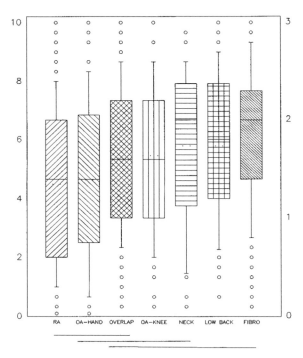

Figure 7–4. Visual Analog Pain Scores obtained in an outpatient rheumatic disease clinic for rheumatoid arthritis (RA) (N=624), osteoarthritis of the hand (OA-HAND) (N=100), patients with more than one disorder excluding RA and fibromyalgia (OVERLAP) (N=183), osteoarthritis of the knee (OA-KNEE) (N=165), cervical pain syndrome (NECK) (N=59), low back pain syndrome (LOW BACK) (N=143), and fibromyalgia (FIBRO) (N=248), respectively. Scale on the left represents 0–10 scaling. Scale on the right represents original 0–3 pain scale. Dotted lines represent means; solid lines represent medians. Boxes represent scores from the 25th to 75th percentiles. The cross bars at the end of the lines extending from the boxes are the 10th and 90th percentiles. Points beyond the 10th and 90th percentiles are individual patient scores. Solid lines below the disease categories indicate groups that do not differ ($p > 0.05$) in post hoc analyses. Pain scores are greatest in patients with fibromyalgia. (From Hawley DJ, and Wolfe F: Pain, disability, and pain/disability relationships in seven rheumatic disorders: Study of 1522 patients. J Rheumatol 18:1552–1557, 1991, with permission.)

trate on the areas that are currently most bothersome and not mention all painful areas unless specifically asked. The author has seen hundreds of patients whose complaints of neck and arm pain, or buttock and leg pain, led to extensive and expensive investigations (and sometimes surgical interventions) for what was really fibromyalgia. The diagnosis of fibromyalgia requires specific inquiries about other body regions. For example, the clinician should ask the patient with buttock and leg pain, "Do you have problems in your hands, . . . in your arms, . . . chest, . . ." and so on. The answers to such questions allow the interviewer to place the chief complaint into perspective. Is the pain fibromyalgia or is it related to a focal and potentially more serious etiology, which requires additional investigation?

The pain due to fibromyalgia is often severe. It is more severe than the pain reported by patients with rheumatoid arthritis and osteoarthritis, and it is similar to the pain reported by patients with low back pain and cervical pain syndromes.[57] Pain is the most important contributor to patients' ratings of

global disease severity, accounting for 58 percent of disease severity variance.[59]

Leavitt et al[79] noted that more than 60 percent of fibromyalgia patients described their pain as aching, exhausting, nagging, or hurting. The words that best differentiated fibromyalgia patients from those with RA were radiating, steady, spreading, and spasms. Together, these verbal descriptors suggest that the pain of fibromyalgia is characterized by chronicity, emotional content, severity, and radiation. In Figure 7–5, pain drawings from four fibromyalgia patients show the characteristics of widespread fibromyalgia pain. Although not all fibromyalgia patients have severe pain, and not all pain involves as many areas as noted in Figure 7–5, all patients satisfy the "widespread" pain definition.

TENDERNESS

The second core feature of fibromyalgia is the presence of widespread tenderness.[148] When palpated, specific regions in tendons, muscles, and other structures are painful in individuals with fibromyalgia. These consti-

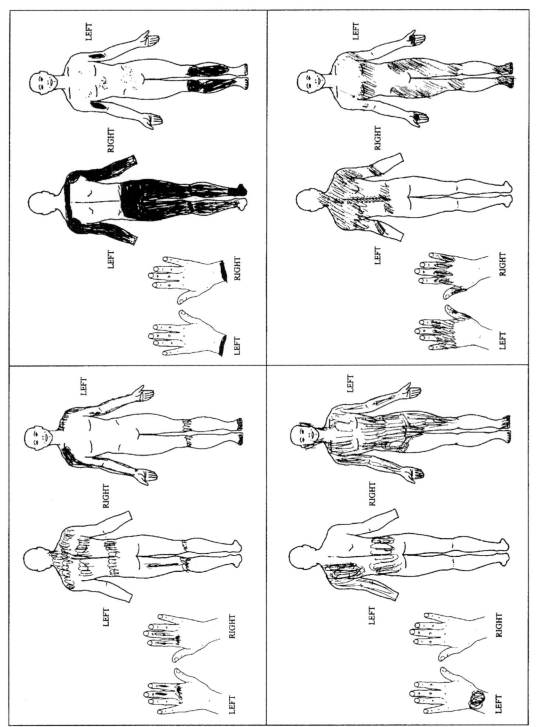

Figure 7–5. Pain diagrams from four patients with fibromyalgia. Note the widespread and contiguous nature of the pain complaint. (From Wolfe F: Fibromyalgia: On diagnosis and certainty. Journal of Musculoskeletal Pain 1:17–36, 1993, Haworth Press, Inc., with permission.)

tute "tender points." Although it was originally thought that fibromyalgia patients were tender only at specific tender point sites, it is now known that tenderness is generalized but that the tender point sites are areas with greater sensitivity. In a systematic search for widespread tenderness, these sites are more often positive. *Dolorimetry*, a technique of quantitating pain threshold, has demonstrated that fibromyalgia patients differ from both normal and other rheumatic disease controls at "fibrositic" tender point sites (those sites usually positive in individuals with fibromyalgia) and at "control" sites (tender point locations that are usually negative or nontender).[24] In addition, statistically significant differences can be clearly discerned between the two types of sites within both patients and controls.

Scudds et al compared three kinds of painful stimuli in fibromyalgia patients and normal controls.[110] Fibromyalgia patients did not have a significantly lower threshold to electrical stimuli or to constant pressure, but changing pressure (dolorimetry) differentiated the fibromyalgia patients from the other groups.

Although dolorimetry is a useful research tool, it is impractical in the clinic. Digital palpation is a reliable and simple method for establishing fibromyalgia tenderness (Table 7–5).[160] An early debate about the location and number of tender points has been resolved with the adoption of the ACR 1990 criteria,[160] which operationalized the observation of Smythe[123] that "multiple tender points, widely and symmetrically distributed" are the characteristic feature of fibromyalgia. According to the ACR criteria, an examination should be labeled "positive" if it demonstrates that at least 11 of 18 specified tender point sites are positive (see Fig. 7–1 and Table 7–1). It is impossible to satisfy this requirement without having tender points present in all four body quadrants. Focal tenderness also occurs in regional musculoskeletal disorders,[112–115] but these syndromes will not be mistaken for fibromyalgia if this criterion, which confirms the existence of "widely and symmetrically distributed tenderness," is fulfilled.

Palpation technique involves contact with the tender point site using 1 to 3 fingers (including the thumb) at a force of about 4 kilograms. The appropriate amount of pressure is the maximum that can be tolerated without pain in individuals without fibromyalgia. This technique can generally be learned quickly in the clinic. According to the ACR criteria, a site is rated positive when the patient states that the examination is "painful"

Table 7–5. DOLORIMETRY AND TENDER POINT SCORES FOR FIBROMYALGIA PATIENTS AND CLINIC CONTROLS

	Range	Fibromyalgia		Controls			
		Mean*	SE	Mean*	SE	t	p-Value
*Dolorimetry Scores**							
Active sites	(0–6.5)	3.4	0.07	4.9	0.08	13.2	<.001
Control sites	(0–6.5)	5.1	0.79	5.7	0.74	6.1	<.001
Tender Pont Palpation Scores and Counts†							
Average Tenderness	(0–4)	1.5	0.04	0.5	0.04	−19.1	<.001
Mild or >	(0–24)	19.7	0.25	8.0	0.44	−23.0	<.001
Moderate or >	(0–24)	12.5	0.41	3.6	0.36	−16.6	<.001
Severe	(0–24)	5.0	0.33	1.3	0.17	−9.8	<.001

*Dolorimetry scores represent the mean of 6 "active" dolorimetry sites and 3 "control" sites. The maximum score at any site cannot exceed 6.5 because of study instrument limitations (see text).

†Tender point palpation scores and counts refer to the 24 active sites. Average tenderness is the total tender point score for the 24 sites divided by 24, or the mean score for tenderness per site. Other tender point variables are counts of the number of sites that are tender at "mild" or >, "moderate" or >, or "severe," respectively.

Source: Modified from Wolfe F, Smythe HA, Yunus MB, et al: The American College of Rheumatology 1990 Criteria for the Classification of Fibromyalgia: Report of the Multicenter Criteria Committee. Arthritis Rheum 33:160–172, 1990, with permission.

or "hurts."[160] If the patient complains that the area is tender, the examiner acknowledges the tenderness but then asks again if it is "painful." Only a statement of "pain" or "hurt" should be accepted as positive.

CHARACTERISTIC AND COMMON FEATURES

More than 75 percent of those with fibromyalgia report sleep disturbance, fatigue, or morning stiffness. All three of the features were found simultaneously in 56 percent of patients, emphasizing the prominent, but not universal, role they play in fibromyalgia. As originally defined by Moldofsky,[93] fibromyalgia sleep abnormality is an alpha delta sleep anomaly. In the clinic, "sleep disturbance" means to awaken "frequently or often" feeling "unrefreshed" or "tired."[155]

According to the ACR criteria study, more than 60 percent of patients report paresthesias and 50 percent note headaches. Psychologic symptoms (past depression in 31 percent and anxiety in 48 percent) are similarly frequent. Symptoms suggestive of connective tissue disease, such as fatigue (81 percent), morning stiffness (77 percent), joint and muscle pain, Raynaud's phenomenon (16.7 percent), and sicca symptoms (36 percent), are also common. These observations explain the frequent misdiagnosis of fibromyalgia.

Among these common symptoms, gastrointestinal (GI) and psychologic disturbances have attracted the most attention. Gastrointestinal complaints, which were first noted by Yunus and colleagues,[167] were described as irritable bowel syndrome and were recorded in 29.6 percent of patients in the ACR study.[160] Triadafilopoulos, Simms, and Goldenberg[136] studied these symptoms in 123 patients with fibromyalgia, 54 patients with degenerative joint disease (DJD), and 46 normal controls. Of patients with fibromyalgia, 73 percent reported altered bowel function, compared with 37 percent of those with DJD and none of the normals. Patients with fibromyalgia were significantly more likely than controls to report "alternating diarrhea and constipation," "irregular bowel function," "bowels worse when joints worse," "consulted physician for bowel symptoms," and "laxative use." In all, 60 percent met the criteria for irritable bowel syndrome used in a population survey.[40,41] Although the high proportion of GI symptoms in this study may reflect the true prevalence, other explanations must also be considered, including bias introduced by "suggestion" or "overreporting"[28] or a referral bias.[41,143,149]

As discussed previously, the psychologic status of patients with fibromyalgia is the subject of controversy. Psychologic distress, which is highly prevalent in this population, may be the cause or the effect of the pain. Psychologic screening instruments that have been used to assess these patients are biased by the observation that fibromyalgia symptoms, in and of themselves, constitute some criteria for psychologic abnormality.[102] For example, fatigue or malaise and frequent headaches are common in fibromyalgia and may also be criterion items in some psychologic tests, most notably the Minnesota Multiphasic Personality Index.[102] A profound selection bias directs patients with more severe fibromyalgia and more severe psychologic disturbance to specialty clinics, which have provided the populations that have been studied in psychologic research.[149]

The possibility of bias in the findings reported by specialty clinics was underscored in the study of Clark et al,[33] which found no differences in the responses on a psychologic instrument (the Symptom Checklist-90) between fibromyalgia patients who were attending a general medical clinic and controls in the same clinic. Interestingly, this finding duplicates studies of patients with irritable bowel syndrome, which have determined that a high prevalence of psychologic abnormalities is not found when patients are evaluated in the community rather than in the clinic.[41,143]

In the rheumatic disease specialty clinic, fibromyalgia patients almost always score more abnormally on standard psychometric measures than either control subjects or those with other rheumatic disorders. Studies that used the Basic Personality Index (BPI), various depression scales, and the Arthritis Impact Measurement Scales (AIMS) have shown that fibromyalgia patients have abnormal scores, although the differences between fibromyalgia and other patients are often small.[110,153]

The use of the MMPI to evaluate fibromyalgia patients has engendered controversy. The MMPI is an invalid test in fibromyalgia and other rheumatic conditions because many of the common symptoms in these disorders represent "abnormal" answers on this test.[102] Nonetheless, the findings of studies that have used the MMPI should not be automatically discounted, especially since recent changes in the scoring of this instrument, which reflect the influence of contemporary norms (as opposed to the mores of the 1930s, when the test was designed), place more fibromyalgia patients in the normal category.[1] Most MMPI studies indicate that fibromyalgia patients have more abnormal scores than do rheumatic and non–rheumatic disease controls.[1,2,79,100,153] These findings are similar to the results obtained from other psychologic instruments that do not have the same "criteria contamination" as the MMPI.[110,153] Although some evidence from community studies suggests that the psychologic abnormalities encountered in the clinic may be found in the community as well, investigations of the criteria developed for the *Disease and Statistical Manual* (DSM-III-R) of the American Psychiatric Association[3] found disparate results: One study indicated that fibromyalgia patients have little major psychiatric disease,[66] whereas another found evidence of major depression in many patients.[74]

Although a high prevalence of psychologic abnormality among those with fibromyalgia is generally accepted, it is essential to note that not all patients have psychopathology. The author and colleagues recently studied psychologic status in more than 6000 rheumatic disease patients.[58] Abnormalities consistent with "clinical depression" were noted in 29.3 percent with fibromyalgia, as opposed to 17.9 percent from other groups. Thus, although the prevalence of depression is relatively high among those with fibromyalgia, this diagnosis still occurs in only a minority of patients.

Diagnosis and Assessment

DIAGNOSIS

Fibromyalgia should be diagnosed in individuals with widespread pain, widespread tenderness, and characteristic symptoms of fibromyalgia, regardless of the presence of other musculoskeletal disorders. Fibromyalgia is not a diagnosis of exclusion, and a patient who has another disorder should also be diagnosed as having fibromyalgia if the syndrome is, in fact, present.

Although the 1990 ACR criteria[160] (Table 7–1 and Fig. 7–1) are useful, some patients who seem to have fibromyalgia clinically may not meet the rigorous classification criteria. The author has suggested that fibromyalgia may be diagnosed for clinical purposes if 50 percent of the tender point sites are positive and characteristic and common features are present.[148] It is an error, however, to diagnose fibromyalgia solely on the basis of symptomatology (without signs of tenderness).[151] No laboratory test, electrodiagnostic study, or imaging technique aids in the diagnosis of fibromyalgia.

DIFFERENTIAL DIAGNOSIS

Fibromyalgia may be confused with many other syndromes. Symptoms of muscle pain, fatigue, low-grade fever, and arthritis may suggest the diagnosis of *systemic lupus erythematosus (SLE)*, particularly when the antinuclear antibody (ANA) is positive. The latter finding is nonspecific (SLE is present in only 1 to 2 percent of ANA-positive individuals), and SLE should not be diagnosed unless the criteria of the American College of Rheumatology are met.[129]

Similarly, *rheumatoid arthritis* is sometimes diagnosed in those with fibromyalgia, based on the findings of joint swelling, joint tenderness, morning stiffness, and fatigue. Two factors lead to misdiagnosis. First, the tenderness in fibromyalgia is not just joint tenderness but is part of generalized tenderness. Second, the swelling reported by patients with fibromyalgia is subjective and not observable. Patients confuse the mild generalized soft tissue swelling that occurs diffusely in fibromyalgia with the synovial swelling associated with arthritis.

Various compressive and noncompressive *syndromes of the cervical and lumbar spine* may present diagnostic difficulties. Patients with fibromyalgia have high rates of hospitalization and surgery for such complaints,[29] although it is doubtful the actual prevalence and severity of the syndromes are increased. Because all painful conditions tend to be more severe in fibromyalgia, it may well be that the intensity of the complaint drives the physician to more testing, hospitalization, and surgery.

Many patients with fibromyalgia have undergone *carpal tunnel* surgery. Nerve conduction tests are performed frequently, because paresthesias are present in almost two-thirds of those with fibromyalgia. No studies have examined the prevalence of abnormal conduction times at the wrist in fibromyalgia, but true carpal tunnel syndrome is uncommon.

Polymyositis and *polymyalgia rheumatica (PMR)* are sometimes incorrectly diagnosed in patients with fibromyalgia. Tender points are not characteristic of these disorders, and neither clinical signs of myopathy nor muscle enzyme elevations occur in fibromyalgia. PMR may be confused with fibromyalgia when the sedimentation rate is elevated and pain and stiffness are generalized. Clues to fibromyalgia lie in the widespread tenderness, the duration of the pain (often years), and the location of pain beyond the shoulder girdle, pelvic girdle, and neck. Corticosteroid treatment, usually a good diagnostic test for PMR, is not as useful in fibromyalgia. In the author's experience, fibromyalgia patients often experience an immediate response to steroids, but pain tends to recur after a while, a pattern that is rare in PMR. Regardless of diagnosis, it may be difficult to discontinue steroids because dose reduction often leads to increased pain.

ASSESSMENT

There are no laboratory tests for fibromyalgia. Although it seems reasonable to assess improvement (or worsening) by measuring tenderness by either dolorimetry or the tender point count, it is not clear that such measures are sensitive to change. In a pain disorder such as fibromyalgia, visual analog pain scales, scales that measure global severity, and scales that record functional ability have great value. Simms and colleagues[112] have proposed methods to assess improvement, but these methods apply primarily to clinical trials. Burckhardt et al[20] have developed a Fibromyalgia Impact Questionnaire (FIQ), which integrates measures of pain, stiffness, sleep disturbance, func-

tional and work ability, and psychologic distress into a single short questionnaire.

Central to the issue of outcomes assessment is the question of which features are most important in fibromyalgia. The validity of creating a single score by adding items (the method used in the FIQ) has not been adequately investigated. Alternative methodology favors the use of standard health status instruments,[156] such as the Health Assessment Questionnaire (HAQ),[30,47] the Modified Health Assessment Questionnaire (MHAQ),[23] and the Arthritis Impact Measurement Scales (AIMS).[18,89] All of these instruments are useful in evaluating fibromyalgia and other rheumatic disorders. At a minimum, a pain severity scale and one of the health status instruments should be used in the long-term assessment of this disorder.

Treatment Considerations

Although primary treatment of fibromyalgia is generally unsatisfactory, much can be done and some patients improve considerably (Table 7–6). Making a diagnosis and explaining the nature of the syndrome constitute key steps in treatment. The use of medical resources, including expensive studies such as magnetic resonance imaging and computed tomography, is high prior to diagnosis,[29] and accurate diagnosis can lead to a decrease in service utilization.[31] Explanations to the patient also help to control anxiety and reduce psychologic distress (of both patients and physicians!). Some patients can do quite well with their fibromyalgia when they understand its nature, course, symptoms, and treatments.

PHARMACOLOGIC TREATMENT

The tricyclic antidepressants are "specific" therapy for fibromyalgia. The original rationale for this intervention was based on the observation of sleep disturbance in this disorder[91–93] and the ability of these drugs to improve stage I sleep.[123] Recently, however, Reynolds et al[106] reported no change in sleep physiology in 12 fibromyalgia patients during treatment with cyclobenzaprine, a tricyclic compound marketed as a muscle relaxant. This finding suggests that there may be alternative mechanisms for the improvement produced by tricyclic drugs.

Table 7–6. **THERAPEUTIC MEASURES IN FIBROMYALGIA**

Intervention	Effectiveness
Amitriptyline	Effective
Cyclobenzaprine	Effective
Alprazolam	Effective
Exercise	Effective
Analgesics	Effective
Education	Effective
Biofeedback	Possibly effective
Hypnotherapy	Possibly effective
Antidepressants	Possibly effective
Anxiolytics	Possibly effective
Corticosteroids	Not effective
NSAIDs	Not effective
Physical therapy	Not tested
Tender point injections	Not tested
Psychotherapy	Not tested

Goldenberg et al[51] compared amitriptyline (25 mg), amitriptyline (25 mg) plus naproxen (1000 mg), naproxen (1000 mg), and placebo during a 6-week trial. Statistically significant improvement in all studied outcomes was recorded in the amitriptyline group and the amitriptyline plus naproxen group; these groups benefited equally. Carette et al[26] found somewhat less improvement in a 9-week placebo-controlled trial of amitriptyline (50 mg). Cyclobenzaprine was better than placebo in another trial,[17] and the benefits of both amitriptyline and cyclobenzaprine were confirmed in a large (N = 208), placebo-controlled, 6-month trial.[25] Several other studies examined the effect of tricyclics on fibromyalgia, but methodologic flaws limit their interpretation.[35,161]

Although these studies indicate that tricyclic compounds can be useful in the treatment of fibromyalgia, others suggest that only a small proportion of patients gain sustained benefit. In an open-label trial of amitriptyline, approximately one-third of patients improved. Each of these patients was then studied in an N-of-1 trial, and only 65 percent subsequently benefited;[72] in all, then, less than 25 percent of the study group improved. In the trial conducted by Golden-

berg et al,[51] 69 percent of patients remained on therapy 1 year later, and in the Carette trial,[26] 47 percent of patients were receiving the study drug 9 months after the trial. The controlled comparison of amitriptyline and cyclobenzaprine could find no benefit for either drug beyond the first month of therapy.[25] A survey conducted by Cathey et al[29] found that 31 percent of fibromyalgia patients were taking amitriptyline at some point during a 1-year period, but only 18.5 percent were receiving the drug at the end of the year. Similar findings were reported from a multicenter survey of 544 patients.[31]

The failure of many patients to continue treatment with these drugs may reflect the modest benefit they provide or the side effects they produce. In the study[51] of amitriptyline that yielded the most improvement, for example, average pain scores declined from about 7.5 to about 5.5 on a 0 to 10 scale. Furthermore, none of the placebo-controlled trials found improvement in the tender point score. These data suggest that only some patients with fibromyalgia improve on tricyclic therapy, and that the degree of improvement is limited.

Other drugs have also been investigated in fibromyalgia patients. A placebo-controlled trial of alprazolam found that the drug was minimally effective overall, but that a subgroup of patients improved significantly.[107] A trend toward normalization of serotonin levels, as measured by a platelet binding essay, was associated with improvement.

Although nonsteroidal anti-inflammatory drugs (NSAIDs) are widely used by fibromyalgia patients, trials of naproxen[94] and ibuprofen[166] have not found them to be more effective than placebo. These observations are curious, because surveys report the use of these agents by approximately one-third of fibromyalgia patients. On the basis of this clinical experience, a subgroup of patients probably does benefit from NSAIDs. It is possible that this subgroup comprises those with concomitant nonfibromyalgic musculoskeletal disease—for example, osteoarthritis of varying degrees of severity.

Clark and coworkers[34] studied prednisone therapy in a double blind, placebo-controlled experiment. No benefit or trend toward benefit was found among those receiving this drug. This is an important study because an older study in the rheumatologic literature[6] suggested that corticosteroids have value in fibromyalgia.

NONPHARMACOLOGIC TREATMENT

A variety of nonpharmacologic treatments have been investigated in patients with fibromyalgia. Compared with control patients, hypnotherapy improved pain, fatigue, sleep, and global assessment but not tender point scores.[55] Baseline pain and psychologic distress were very abnormal in these patients, suggesting that the population was biased by selection for psychologic factors. Another study demonstrated benefit from biofeedback[44]; the methodology in this study has been criticized[147] and defended.[43]

Although many patients with fibromyalgia receive physical therapy in hospital and outpatient clinics, this approach has not been investigated. Anecdotally, the author is aware of no reports of substantial benefit from physical therapy. In the United States, manipulative therapy administered by chiropractors has been reported to benefit some patients.[29]

Acupuncture has generally been used in the more localized myofascial pain syndromes.[48,77,90,142] There have been no trials of this approach in fibromyalgia.

The most important therapy to emerge recently for the treatment of fibromyalgia has been aerobic exercise.[86] McCain and associates[87] randomized 42 fibromyalgia patients to receive either stretching exercise or aerobic exercises (stationary bicycle). The aerobic group improved in pain threshold measurements and in both patient and physician global assessments, but not in pain intensity, percent of the body involved in pain, disturbed sleep, or psychologic profile. This study was carried out very well and demonstrates the usefulness of aerobic exercise. It also suggests that ordinary physical therapy and limited exercise are not useful in fibromyalgia. Although McCain[86] has pointed out that the benefit from aerobic exercise is limited and that not all patients benefit, there are few other effective treatments for fibromyalgia, and exercise should be prescribed to almost all patients. The extent to which this difficult and potentially expensive therapy can and will be carried out in the community has not yet been determined.

The issue of psychologic therapy for fibromyalgia is complicated. Psychotherapy can be used for primary psychiatric disease, for psychologic abnormalities associated with chronic pain, or for the combination of the two. Some fibromyalgia treatment programs incorporate various forms of psychologic therapy and have claimed efficacy (for the program as a whole).[128] A trial[101] that evaluated amitriptyline and psychotherapy in patients with "chronic, intractable, 'psychogenic' pain" may have included patients with fibromyalgia and confirmed benefit only from amitriptyline; the effect of psychotherapy was complex and not clearly beneficial. Nonetheless, it is possible that the efficacy of antidepressant drugs in some patients[25,26,51,130] could be due to their effects on mood.

Because fibromyalgia may improve to a limited extent with the use of amitriptyline, psychologic therapy, exercise therapy, and some other treatments, centers that can integrate all of these therapies may offer the best therapeutic opportunities. Such combined therapeutic endeavors are expensive, however. For the cost of these centers to be justified, they must be able to demonstrate screening and follow-up, show sustained patient improvement and decreased utilization of services as outcomes, and confirm that the program as a whole is better than the individual parts alone. In general, the results of centers that use combined therapeutic approaches have been variable. The effective "agent" in such programs is unclear, but several preliminary reports suggest it may be the "program" itself, rather than specific components of the program, including exercise.

MYOFASCIAL PAIN SYNDROME

Fibromyalgia and the myofascial pain syndrome have shared terminologies but differ in important ways (Table 7–7). Whereas fibromyalgia represents a diffuse musculoskeletal pain syndrome, the myofascial pain syndrome is a local or regional disorder.[134,135] Recognition of the syndrome, particularly in deeper and less commonly involved muscles, is difficult and requires precise anatomic understanding.

The myofascial pain syndrome refers to patterns of local and referred pain and associated phenomena caused by a focal lesion in muscle or surrounding fascia known as a *trigger point.* Trigger points can be identified by palpation and reproduce the pain when pressure is applied. One muscle or a group of muscles may be involved. The differences in presentation suggest that trigger points and the pain they cause are variable and may develop acutely from sudden muscular overload or slowly (or, perhaps, repeatedly over time) from chronic overload of the affected muscles.[134]

Although myofascial pain has been recognized since the nineteenth century,[105] the need to improve its clinical recognition has been advocated only recently. The pioneering efforts of Travell and Simons have produced specific diagnostic terminologies, maps and descriptions of trigger points, specific suggestions regarding therapy, and speculations about etiology.[115–121,131–133] Based on this work, "myofascial trigger points" have been found in virtually every body location, from head to toe.[48,84]

Despite growing acceptance, the construct of myofascial pain remains problematic for some experienced clinicians. McCain and Scudds, for example, have noted "few controlled studies [of prevalence]," a "scarcity of randomized controlled trials [of treatment]," and an "absence of firm data [regarding diagnostic criteria]."[88] Little is known about the epidemiology because the literature describing the condition consists primarily of case reports and uncontrolled observations. In one prospective survey, Skootsky et al[122] studied the prevalence of trigger points and the myofascial pain syndrome within a general medical clinic and observed that 54 of 172 consecutive patients complained of pain and 30 percent of this group had myofascial trigger points.

Diagnosis and Assessment

According to Simons,[120] "myofascial pain syndromes are essentially single muscle syndromes that may combine to form complex patterns involving many muscles in several regions in the body." Through various mech-

Table 7–7. OVERLAPPING NOMENCLATURE OF FIBROMYALGIA AND MYOFASCIAL PAIN SYNDROMES

Preferred Name	Other Names	Preferred Names for Physical Descriptors	Other Names for Physical Descriptors
Fibromyalgia	Fibrositis	Tender points Myofibrositis Fibromyositis	Trigger points
Myofascial pain syndrome	Fibrositis Myofibrositis Fibromyositis	Trigger points Taut band	

anisms that begin with an "active trigger point," pain and/or sensations of "autonomic phenomena" can be referred to a distant region that coincides with the patient's pain problem.

One classification system distinguishes four types of trigger points[134]:

1. An *active trigger point* is an area of exquisite tenderness that is usually located in a taut band in the belly of a skeletal muscle, where it is associated with a local twitch response and a zone of reference (region at a distance from the trigger point). The zone of reference is the site of pain, sensation, or autonomic referral. Palpation of the active trigger point reproduces the patient's pain problem.

2. A *latent trigger point* is clinically quiescent. It is not associated with clinical pain but on palpation may have all the other features of an active trigger point.

3. A *secondary trigger point* is active because of the effects produced by another trigger point. This type of trigger point has been defined as a hyperirritable spot in muscle that becomes active because of overload in areas that are compensating for the effect of a muscle with an active trigger point.

4. A *satellite myofascial trigger point* has been defined as a focus of hyperirritability in a muscle or its fascia that becomes active because the muscle is located within the zone of reference of another trigger point. Satellite myofascial trigger points can be distinguished from "referred tenderness" by their palpable bands, local twitch responses, and induction of referred pain.

This classification of trigger points is complicated and hypothetical. It has not been well tested and is not universally accepted. A definition that is applied more often is operational: *A trigger point is identified in muscle by the presence of pain on palpation and the presence of referred pain that reproduces the patient's pain.*[46,159] Although simpler, this definition has also not been subjected to reliability and validity testing.

Although myofascial pain syndrome is conceptually an acute, single muscle disorder, chronicity may occur when perpetuat-

ing factors exist. For example, a leg length discrepancy, a severe scoliosis, or prolonged maintenance of abnormal postures can lead to persistent muscle overload. Additionally, other factors such as depression, fatigue, and behavioral disturbances may become associated when pain becomes chronic.[46]

Therapy

Active trigger points are treated with a variety of approaches, including "stretch and spray" and local injection.[134] In "stretch and spray," the muscle with the trigger point is identified and sprayed along its length several times with a coolant spray such as fluorimethane. This is followed by passively stretching the muscle and often spraying again to relieve pain that may have been caused by the stretch.

In the injection method, a small amount (perhaps 0.5 to 1.0 mL) of a local anesthetic is instilled into the trigger point using a very small (25-gauge) needle. Although there is no rationale for the use of corticosteroids, they are frequently coadministered in clinical practice.

Jaeger et al[71] have shown that passive stretch reduces trigger point sensitivity. In general, it is believed that the stretch rather than the injection or the spray is the effective treatment. The spray or the injection is merely a "distraction" from the pain. Unfortunately, trigger point therapy has not been subjected to appropriate scientific scrutiny using clinical trial methodologies. Long-term follow-up assessments have not been accomplished. Although it appears certain that some patients who receive these therapies improve strikingly, it is not clear how often such responses occur, how long they last, and whether they occurred because of, or in spite of, the treatment administered.

Although the literature on myofascial pain syndrome relates the failure to respond to "stretch and spray" or trigger point injection to a variety of "perpetuating factors," no studies are available to support or refute this hypothesis. Perpetuating factors identified anecdotally include mechanical stresses (e.g., leg length discrepancies), vitamin deficiencies (e.g., low levels of vitamin C, and "low normal" levels of B_1, B_6, and B_{12}), hypothyroidism, hyperuricemia, hypoglycemia, psychologic disturbances, chronic infection, allergy, and poor sleep.[134]

In practice, the identification and treatment of trigger points are sometimes clinically useful. Yet there are substantial problems with the concept of a myofascial pain syndrome, all of which continue because of a lack of scientifically valid studies. The definition of the syndrome and the various types of trigger points does not have general agreement, and trigger points identified by one definition may not be similarly identified by the next.[159] The reliability and validity of the myofascial pain examination have not been established. The techniques of trigger point identification in most muscles may be difficult to learn and may not be generally applicable.[159] No studies have investigated putative perpetuating factors. No valid clinical trials have tested treatments for myofascial pain syndrome, and little is known of the outcome of the treatments used anecdotally. No cost-benefit analyses exist.

Thus, the physician who administers a "stretch and spray" treatment may wonder if the approach makes sense or whether the intervention is merely "doing something" to assuage the patient or the physician. Clinical experience indicates that trigger points exist and may contribute to clinically important pain syndromes. Clinical science must be introduced to this intriguing and common disorder.

SUMMARY

The development of reliable criteria for fibromyalgia has led to an expansion of interest in the syndrome. Fibromyalgia is common in the clinic (5 to 20 percent) and exists in the community at a prevalence of about 2 percent. The fibromyalgia syndrome consists of widespread pain, decreased pain threshold, sleep disturbance, fatigue, stiffness, and often psychologic distress, among other symptoms. Fibromyalgia is diagnosed when widespread pain and tenderness at 11 of 18 specific sites are identified. The etiology of fibromyalgia is not known, but the pathogenesis has been linked to central pain dysfunction, psychologic factors, and muscle abnormalities.

The treatment of fibromyalgia is challenging. Pharmacologic therapy generally consists of a tricyclic antidepressant, which is usually administered in low doses. Drugs in this class can improve pain and sleep, but surveys indicate that a relatively small proportion of patients respond and that the duration of response among those who initially benefit is often limited. One study suggests that alprazolam can benefit some patients with fibromyalgia, but there is no evidence that nonsteroidal anti-inflammatory drugs and corticosteroids are effective. A controlled study of aerobic exercise indicates that this approach is an effective nonpharmacologic treatment for some patients. The data in support of psychologic therapies is equivocal, but many patients benefit from counseling about the disease.

In contrast to the generalized disorder of fibromyalgia, myofascial pain syndrome is a local or regional disorder characterized by focal and referred pain related to one or more trigger points in muscle. Various classifications of trigger points have been developed, but an understanding of these phenomena is limited by a lack of scientific investigation. Treatments for trigger points, which are applied on the basis of anecdotal observations, include a "stretch and spray" therapy and injection techniques. Some patients benefit from these interventions, but no information exists about the relative efficacy of different treatments and no therapeutic approach has been evaluated in a controlled clinical trial. Although myofascial pain due to trigger points appears to be a clinically important disorder, scientific investigations are needed to establish diagnostic criteria, determine etiologies and sustaining mechanisms, and identify the most effective treatments.

REFERENCES

1. Ahles TA, Yunus MB, Gaulier B, et al: The use of contemporary MMPI norms in the study of chronic pain patients. Pain 24:159–163, 1986.
2. Ahles TA, Yunus MB, Riley SD, et al: Psychological factors associated with primary fibromyalgia syndrome. Arthritis Rheum 27:1101–1106, 1984.
3. American Psychiatric Association: Diagnostic and statistical manual of mental disorders (DSM–III–R), ed 3. American Psychiatric Association, Washington, DC, 1987, pp 1–567.
4. Bartels EM, and Danneskiold-Samsoe B: Histological abnormalities in muscle from patients with certain types of fibrositis. Lancet 1:755–757, 1986.

5. Bäckman E, Bengtsson A, Bengtsson M, et al: Skeletal muscle function in primary fibromyalgia. Effect of regional sympathetic blockade with guanethidine. Acta Neurol Scand 77:187–191, 1988.
6. Beetham WPJ: Diagnosis and management of fibrositis syndrome and psychogenic rheumatism. Med Clin North Am 63:433–439, 1979.
7. Bengtsson A, and Bengtsson M: Regional sympathetic blockade in primary fibromyalgia. Pain 33:161–167, 1988.
8. Bengtsson A, Cederblad G, and Larsson J: Carnitine levels in painful muscles of patients with fibromyalgia. [Letter] Clin Exp Rheumatol 8:197–198, 1990.
9. Bengtsson A, and Henriksson KG: The muscle in fibromyalgia—a review of Swedish studies. J Rheumatol Suppl 19:144–149, 1989.
10. Bengtsson A, Henriksson KG, Jorfeldt L, et al: Primary fibromyalgia. A clinical and laboratory study of 55 patients. Scand J Rheumatol 15:340–347, 1986.
11. Bengtsson A, Henriksson KG, and Larsson J: Muscle biopsy in primary fibromyalgia. Light-microscopical and histochemical findings. Scand J Rheumatol 15:1–6, 1986.
12. Bengtsson A, Henriksson KG, and Larsson J: Reduced high-energy phosphate levels in the painful muscles of patients with primary fibromyalgia. Arthritis Rheum 29:817–821, 1986.
13. Bennett RM: Beyond fibromyalgia: Ideas on etiology and treatment. J Rheumatol Suppl 19:185–191, 1989.
14. Bennett RM: Muscle physiology and cold reactivity in the fibromyalgia syndrome. Rheum Dis Clin North Am 15:135–147, 1989.
15. Bennett RM: Physical fitness and muscle metabolism in the fibromyalgia syndrome: An overview. J Rheumatol Suppl 19:28–29, 1989.
16. Bennett RM, Clark SR, Goldberg L, et al: Aerobic fitness in patients with fibrositis: A controlled study of respiratory gas exchange and [133]xenon clearance from exercising muscle. Arthritis Rheum 32:454–460, 1989.
17. Bennett RM, Gatter RA, Campbell SM, et al: A comparison of cyclobenzaprine and placebo in the management of fibrositis: A double-blind controlled study. Arthritis Rheum 31:1535–1542, 1988.
18. Brown JH, Kazis LE, Spitz PW, et al: The dimensions of health outcomes: A cross-validated examination of health status measurement. Am J Public Health 74:159–161, 1984.
19. Brückle W, Suckfull M, Fleckenstein W, et al: [Tissue pO_2 measurement in taut back musculature (m. erector spinae)]. Z Rheumatol 49:208–216, 1990.
20. Burckhardt CS, Clark SR, and Bennett RM: The fibromyalgia impact questionnaire—development and validation. J Rheumatol 18:728–733, 1991.
21. Burckhardt CS, Clark S, and Nelson DL: Assessing physical fitness of women with rheumatic disease. Arthritis Care Research 1:38–44, 1988.
22. Buskila D, Press J, Gedalia A, et al: Assessment of nonarticular tenderness and prevalence of fibromyalgia in children. J Rheumatol 20:368–370, 1993.
23. Callahan LF, Smith WJ, and Pincus T: Self report questionnaires in five rheumatic diseases: Comparisons of health status constructs and associations with formal education level. Arthritis Care and Research 2:122–131, 1989.
24. Campbell SM, Clark S, Tindall EA, et al: Clinical characteristics of fibrositis. I. A "blinded," controlled study of symptoms and tender points. Arthritis Rheum 26:817–824, 1983.
25. Carette S, Bell MJ, Reynolds WJ, et al: Comparison of amitriptyline, cyclobenzaprine, and placebo in the treatment of fibromyalgia—a randomized, double-blind clinical trial. Arthritis Rheum 37:32–40, 1994.
26. Carette S, McCain GA, Bell DA, et al: Evaluation of amitriptyline in primary fibrositis. A double-blind, placebo-controlled study. Arthritis Rheum 29:655–659, 1986.
27. Caro XJ: Immunofluorescent studies of skin in primary fibrositis syndrome. Am J Med 81:43–49, 1986.
28. Caro XJ, Kinsted NA, Russell IJ, et al: Increased sensitivity of health related questions with primary fibrositis syndrome. {Abstract] Arthritis Rheum 30:S63, 1987.
29. Cathey MA, Wolfe F, Kleinheksel SM, et al: Socioeconomic impact of fibrositis. A study of 81 patients with primary fibrositis. Am J Med 81:78–84, 1986.
30. Cathey MA, Wolfe F, Kleinheksel SM, et al: Functional ability and work status in patients with fibromyalgia. Arthritis Care and Research 1:85–98, 1988.
31. Cathey MA, Wolfe F, Roberts FK, et al: Demographic, work disability, service utilization and treatment characteristics of 620 fibromyalgia patients in rheumatologic practice. [Abstract] Arthritis Rheum 33:S10, 1990.
32. Cicuttini F, and Littlejohn GO: Female adolescent rheumatological presentations: The importance of chronic pain syndromes. Aust Paediatr J25:21–24, 1989.
33. Clark S, Campbell SM, Forehand ME, et al: Clinical characteristics of fibrositis. II. A "blinded," controlled study using standard psychological tests. Arthritis Rheum 28:132–137, 1985.
34. Clark S, Tindall E, and Bennett RM: A double blind crossover trial of prednisone versus placebo in the treatment of fibrositis. J Rheumatol 12:980–983, 1985.
35. Connolly RG: Treatment of fibromyositis with fluphenazine and amitriptyline: A preliminary report. Del Med J 53:189–191, 1981.
36. Crofford LJ, Pillemer SR, Kalogeras KT, et al: Hypothalamic-pituitary-adrenal axis perturbations in patients with fibromyalgia. Arthritis Rheum 37:1583–1592, 1994.
37. Crook J, Weir R, and Tunks E: An epidemiological follow-up survey of persistent pain sufferers in a group family practice and specialty pain clinic. Pain 36:49–61, 1989.
38. Danneskiold-Samsoe B, Christiansen E, and Bach Andersen R: Myofascial pain and the role of myoglobin. Scand J Rheumatol 15:174–178, 1986.
39. Danneskiold-Samsoe B, Christiansen E, Lund B, et al: Regional muscle tension and pain (fibrositis): Effect of massage on myoglobin in plasma. Scand J Rehabil Med 15:17–20, 1982.
40. Drossman DA: A questionnaire for functional bowel disorders. Ann Intern Med 111:627–629, 1989.
41. Drossman DA, McKee DC, Sandler RS, et al: Psychosocial factors in the irritable bowel syndrome. Gastroenterology 95:701–708, 1988.

42. Felson DT, and Goldenberg DL: The natural history of fibromyalgia. Arthritis Rheum 29:1522–1526, 1986.

43. Ferraccioli GF, Fontana S, Scita F, et al: EMG-biofeedback in fibromyalgia syndrome. [Letter; comment] J Rheumatol 16:1013–1014, 1989.

44. Ferraccioli GF, Ghirelli L, Scita F, et al: EMG-biofeedback training in fibromyalgia syndrome. J Rheumatol 14:820–825, 1987.

45. Forseth KO, and Gran JT: The prevalence of fibromyalgia among women aged 20–49 years in Arendal, Norway. Scand J Rheumatol 21:74–78, 1992.

46. Fricton JR, Kroening R, Haley D, et al: Myofascial pain syndrome of the head and neck: A review of clinical characteristics of 164 patients. Oral Surg 60:615–623, 1985.

47. Fries JF, Spitz PW, and Kraines RG: Measurement of patient outcome in arthritis. Arthritis Rheum 23:137–145, 1980.

48. Garvey TA, Marks MR, and Wiesel SW: A prospective, randomized, double-blind evaluation of trigger-point injection therapy for low-back pain. Spine 14:962–964, 1989.

49. Goldenberg DL: Psychiatric and psychologic aspects of fibromyalgia syndrome. Rheum Dis Clin North Am 15:105–114, 1989.

50. Goldenberg DL: Psychological symptoms and psychiatric diagnosis in patients with fibromyalgia. J Rheumatol (Suppl 16) 19:127–130, 1989.

51. Goldenberg DL, Felson DT, and Dinerman H: A randomized, controlled trial of amitriptyline and naproxen in the treatment of patients with fibromyalgia. Arthritis Rheum 29:1371–1377, 1986.

52. Graham W: The fibrositis syndrome. Bull Rheum Dis 3:33–34, 1953.

53. Griep EN, Boersma JW, and Dekloet ER: Altered reactivity of the hypothalamic-pituitary-adrenal axis in the primary fibromyalgia syndrome. J Rheumatol 20:469–474, 1993.

54. Griep EN, Boersma JW, and Dekloet ER: Pituitary release of growth hormone and prolactin in the primary fibromyalgia syndrome. J Rheumatol 21:2125–2130, 1994.

55. Haanen HCM, Hoenderdos HTW, Van Romunde LKJ, et al: Controlled trial of hypnotherapy in the treatment of refractory fibromyalgia. J Rheumatol 18:72–75, 1991.

56. Hartz A, and Kirchdoerfer E: Undetected fibrositis in primary care practice. J Fam Pract 25:365–369, 1987.

57. Hawley DJ, and Wolfe F: Pain, disability, and pain/disability relationships in seven rheumatic disorders: Study of 1522 patients. J Rheumatol 18:1552–1557, 1991.

58. Hawley DJ, and Wolfe F: Depression is not more common in rheumatoid arthritis: A 10 year longitudinal study of 6,608 rheumatic disease patients. J Rheumatol 20:2025–2031, 1993.

59. Hawley DJ, Wolfe F, and Cathey MA: Pain, functional disability, and psychological status: A 12-month study of severity in fibromyalgia. J Rheumatol 15:1551–1556, 1988.

60. Hawley DJ, Wolfe F, Cathey MA, et al: Marital status in rheumatoid arthritis and other rheumatic disorders: A study of 7,293 patients. J Rheumatol 18:654–660, 1991.

61. Helme RD, Littlejohn GO, and Weinstein C: Neurogenic flare responses in chronic rheumatic pain syndromes. Clin Exp Neurol 23:91–94, 1987.

62. Hench PK: Nonarticular rheumatism (22nd Rheumatism review of 1973–1976 literature). Arthritis Rheum 19:1088, 1976.

63. Henriksson KG: Muscle pain in neuromuscular disorders and primary fibromyalgia. Eur J Appl Physiol 57:348–352, 1988.

64. Henriksson KG, Bengtsson A, Larsson J, et al: Muscle biopsy findings of possible diagnostic importance in primary fibromyalgia (fibrositis, myofascial syndrome). [Letter] Lancet 2:1395, 1982.

65. Houvenagel E, Forzy G, Cortet B, et al: 5-Hydroxy indol acetic acid in cerebrospinal fluid in fibromyalgia. Arthritis Rheum 33:S55, 1990.

66. Hudson JI, Hudson MS, Pliner LF, et al: Fibromyalgia and major affective disorder: A controlled phenomenology and family history study. Am J Psychiatry 142:441–446, 1985.

67. Jacobsen S, and Danneskiold-Samsoe B: Isometric and isokinetic muscle strength in patients with fibrositis syndrome. New characteristics for a difficult definable category of patients. Scand J Rheumatol 16:61–65, 1987.

68. Jacobsen S, and Danneskiold-Samsoe B: Inter-relations between clinical parameters and muscle function in patients with primary fibromyalgia. Clin Exp Rheumatol 7:493–498, 1989.

69. Jacobsen S, Höyer-Madsen M, Danneskiold-Samsoe B, et al: Screening for autoantibodies in patients with primary fibromyalgia syndrome and a matched control group. APMIS 98:655–658, 1990.

70. Jacobsson L, Lindgärde F, and Manthorpe R: The commonest rheumatic complaints of over six weeks' duration in a twelve-month period in a defined Swedish population. Prevalences and relationships. Scand J Rheumatol 18:353–360, 1989.

71. Jaeger B, and Reeves JL: Quantification of changes in myofascial trigger point sensitivity with the pressure algometer following passive stretch. Pain 27:203–210, 1986.

72. Jaeschke R, Adachi JD, Guyatt G, et al: Clinical usefulness of amitriptyline in fibromyalgia: The results of 23 N-of-1 randomized controlled trials. J Rheumatol 18:447–451, 1991.

73. Jubrias SA, Bennett RM, and Klug GA: Increased incidence of a resonance in the phosphodiester region of P-31 nuclear magnetic resonance spectra in the skeletal muscle of fibromyalgia patients. Arthritis Rheum 37:801–807, 1994.

74. Kirmayer LJ, Robbins JM, and Kapusta MA: Somatization and depression in fibromyalgia syndrome. Am J Psychiatry 145:950–954, 1988.

75. Klug GA, McAuley E, and Clark S: Factors influencing the development and maintenance of aerobic fitness: Lessons applicable to the fibrositis syndrome. J Rheumatol (Suppl) 19:30–39, 1989.

76. Kramer JS, Yelin EH, and Epstein WV: Social and economic impacts of four musculoskeletal conditions. Arthritis Rheum 26:901–907, 1983.

77. Langley GB, Sheppeard H, Johnson M, et al: The analgesic effects of transcutaneous electrical nerve stimulation and placebo in chronic pain patients. A double-blind non-crossover comparison. Rheumatol Int 4:119–123, 1984.

78. Larsson B, Libelius R, and Ohlsson K: Trapezius muscle changes unrelated to static work load—chemical and morphologic controlled studies of 22 women with and without neck pain. Acta Orthop Scand 63:203–206, 1992.

79. Leavitt F, Katz RS, Golden HE, et al: Comparison of pain properties in fibromyalgia patients and rheumatoid arthritis patients. Arthritis Rheum 29:775–781, 1986.

80. Ledingham J, Doherty S, and Doherty M: Primary fibromyalgia syndrome—an outcome study. Br J Rheumatol 32:139–142, 1993.

81. Littlejohn GO, Weinstein C, and Helme RD: Increased neurogenic inflammation in fibrositis syndrome. J Rheumatol 14:1022–1025, 1987.

82. Lund N, Bengtsson A, and Thorborg P: Muscle tissue oxygen pressure in primary fibromyalgia. Scand J Rheumatol 15:165–173, 1986.

83. Lyddell C: The prevalence of fibromyalgia in a South African community. [Abstract] Scand J Rheumatol (Suppl) 94:S143, 1992.

84. Mance D, McConnell B, Ryan PA, et al: Myofascial pain syndrome. J Am Podiatr Med Assoc 76:328–331, 1986.

85. Mason JH, Simms RW, Goldenberg DL, et al: The impact of fibromyalgia on work: a comparison with RA. [Abstract] Arthritis Rheum 32:S197, 1989.

86. McCain GA: Nonmedicinal treatments in primary fibromyalgia. Rheum Dis Clin North Am 15:73–90, 1989.

87. McCain GA, Bell DA, Mai FM, et al: A controlled study of the effects of a supervised cardiovascular fitness training program on the manifestations of fibromyalgia. Arthritis Rheum 31:1135–1141, 1988.

88. McCain GA, and Scudds RA: The concept of primary fibromyalgia (fibrositis): Clinical value, relation and significance to other chronic musculoskeletal pain syndromes. Pain 33:273–287, 1988.

89. Meenan RF, Gertman PM, and Mason JH: Measuring health status in arthritis: The arthritis impact measurement scales. Arthritis Rheum 23:146–152, 1980.

90. Melzack R: Myofascial trigger points: Relation to acupuncture and mechanisms of pain. Arch Phys Med Rehabil 62:114–117, 1981.

91. Moldofsky H: Rheumatic pain modulation syndrome: The interrelationships between sleep, central nervous system serotonin, and pain. Adv Neurol 33:51–57, 1982.

92. Moldofsky H, and Lue FA: The relationship of alpha and delta EEG frequencies to pain and mood in 'fibrositis' patients treated with chlorpromazine and L-tryptophan. Electroencephalogr Clin Neurophysiol 50:71–80, 1980.

93. Moldofsky H, Scarisbrick P, England R, et al: Musculoskeletal symptoms and non-REM sleep disturbance in patients with "fibrositis syndrome" and healthy subjects. Psychosom Med 37:341–351, 1975.

94. Moore SE, and Smiley JD: Neurogenic arthritis. Compr Ther 8:28–33, 1982.

95. Müller W: The fibrositis syndrome: Diagnosis, differential diagnosis and pathogenesis. Scand J Rheumatol (Suppl) 65:40–53, 1987.

96. Müller W, and Lautenschläger J: [Generalized tendomyopathy. I: Clinical aspects, follow-up and differential diagnosis]. Z Rheumatol 49:11–21, 1990.

97. Müller W, and Lautenschläger J: [Generalized tendomyopathy. II: Pathogenesis and therapy]. Z Rheumatol 49:22–29, 1990.

98. Neeck G, and Riedel W: Neuromediator and hormonal perturbations in fibromyalgia syndrome: Results of chronic stress? Baillieres Clin Rheumatol 8:763–775, 1994.

99. Nishikai M: Fibromyalgia in Japanese. J Rheumatol 19:110–114, 1992.

100. Payne TC, Leavitt DC, Garron DC, et al: Fibrositis and psychologic disturbance. Arthritis Rheum 25:213–217, 1982.

101. Pilowsky I, and Barrow CG: A controlled study of psychotherapy and amitriptyline used individually and in combination in the treatment of chronic intractable, "psychogenic" pain. Pain 40:3–19, 1990.

102. Pincus T, Callahan LF, Bradley LA, et al: Elevated MMPI scores for hypochondriasis, depression and hysteria in patients with rheumatoid arthritis reflect disease rather than psychological status. Arthritis Rheum 29:1456–1466, 1986.

103. Raspe HH, Baumgartner C, and Wolfe F: The prevalence of fibromyalgia in a rural German community: How much difference do different criteria make? Arthritis Rheum (Suppl 9) 36:S48, 1993.

104. Reilly PA, and Littlejohn GO: Fibrositis/fibromyalgia syndrome: the key to the puzzle of chronic pain. [Editorial] Med J Aust 152:226–227, 1990.

105. Reynolds MD: The development of the concept of fibrositis. J Hist Med Allied Sci 38:5–35, 1983.

106. Reynolds WJ, Moldofsky H, Saskin P, et al: The effects of cyclobenzaprine on sleep physiology and symptoms in patients with fibromyalgia. J Rheumatol 18:452–454, 1991.

107. Russell IJ, Fletcher EM, Michalek JE, et al: Treatment of primary fibrositis/fibromyalgia syndrome with ibuprofen and alprazolam—a double-blind, placebo-controlled study. Arthritis Rheum 34:552–560, 1991.

108. Russell IJ, Vaeroy H, Javors M, et al: Cerebrospinal fluid (CSF) biogenic amines in fibrositis/fibromyalgia syndrome (FS). Arthritis Rheum 33:S55, 1990.

109. Scudds RA: The relationship between pain responsiveness and disease activity in fibrositis and rheumatoid arthritis. Ph.D. thesis. The University of Western Ontario, London, Ontario, 1989, pp 1–275.

110. Scudds RA, Rollman GB, Harth M, et al: Pain perception and personality measures as discriminators in the classification of fibrositis. J Rheumatol 14:563–569, 1987.

111. Scudds RA, Trachsel LC, Luckhurst BJ, et al: A comparative study of pain, sleep quality and pain responsiveness in fibrositis and myofascial pain syndrome. J Rheumatol (Suppl) 19:120–126, 1989.

112. Simms RW, Felson DT, and Goldenberg DL: Development of preliminary criteria for response to treatment in fibromyalgia syndrome. J Rheumatol 18:1558–1563, 1991.

113. Simons DG: Muscle pain syndromes—Part I. Am J Phys Med Rehabil 54:289–311, 1975.

114. Simons DG: Muscle pain syndromes—Part II. Am J Phys Med Rehabil 55:15–42, 1976.

115. Simons DG: Myofascial trigger points: A need for understanding. Arch Phys Med Rehabil 62:97–99, 1981.

116. Simons DG: Myofascial pain syndromes. [Letter] Arch Phys Med Rehabil 65:561, 1984.

117. Simons DG: Myofascial Pain Syndrome Due to Trigger Points. CV Mosby, St Louis, 1987, pp 4–39.

118. Simons DG: Myofascial pain syndrome due to trigger points. In Goodgold J (ed): Rehabilitation Medicine. CV Mosby, Philadelphia, 1988.

119. Simons DG: Myofascial pain syndromes of head, neck and low back. In Dubner R, Gebhart GF, and Bond MR (eds): Pain Research and Clinical Management, Vol 3. Elsevier, Amsterdam, 1988.

120. Simons DG: Myofascial pain syndromes: Where are we? Where are we going. Arch Phys Med Rehabil 69:207–212, 1988.

121. Simons DG, and Travell JG: Myofascial origins of low back pain. Postgrad Med 73:66–108, 1983.

122. Skootsky SA, Jaeger B, and Oye RK: Prevalence of myofascial pain in general internal medicine practice. West J Med 151:157–160, 1989.

123. Smythe HA: "Fibrositis" and other diffuse musculoskeletal syndromes. In Kelley WN, Harris ED, Jr, Ruddy S, et al: (eds): Textbook of Rheumatology. WB Saunders, Philadelphia, 1985, pp 481–489.

124. Smythe HA: Fibrositis syndrome: A historical perspective. J Rheumatol (Suppl 19) 16:2–6, 1989.

125. Smythe HA, and Moldofsky H: Two contributions to understanding of the "fibrositis" syndrome. Bull Rheum Dis 28:928–931, 1977.

126. Sola AE, and Kuitert JH: Myofascial trigger point pain in the neck and shoulder girdle. Northwest Medicine Sep: 980–984, 1955.

127. Stokes MJ, Cooper RG, and Edwards RHT: Normal muscle strength and fatigability in patients with effort syndromes. British Medical Journal 297:1014–1017, 1988.

128. Strosberg JM, Thomas L, and Buchan AM: Fibromyalgia: Another viewpoint [letter]. J Rheumatol 16:247–248, 1989.

129. Tan EM, Cohen AS, Fries JF, et al: The 1982 revised criteria for the classification of systemic lupus erythematosus. Arthritis Rheum 25:1271, 1982.

130. Tavoni A, Vitali C, Bombardieri S, et al: Evaluation of S-adenosylmethionine in primary fibromyalgia. A double-blind crossover study. Am J Med 83:107–110, 1987.

131. Travell JG: Myofascial trigger points: Clinical review. In Bonica JJ, and Albe-Fessard D (eds): Advances in Pain Research and Therapy, Vol 1. Raven Press, New York, 1976, pp 919–926.

132. Travell JG: Identification of myofascial trigger point syndromes: A case of atypical facial neuralgia. Arch Phys Med Rehabil 62:100–106, 1981.

133. Travell JG, and Rinzler SH: The myofascial genesis of pain. Postgrad Med 11:425–434, 1952.

134. Travell JG, and Simons DG: Myofascial Pain and Dysfunction: The Trigger Point Manual. Williams & Wilkins, Baltimore, 1983.

135. Travell JG, and Simons DG: Myofascial Pain and Dysfunction: The Trigger Point Manual, Vol 2. Williams & Wilkins, Baltimore, 1992.

136. Triadafilopoulos G, Simms RW, and Goldenberg DL: Bowel dysfunction in fibromyalgia syndrome. Dig Dis Sci 36:59–64, 1991.

137. Truta MP, and Santucci ET: Head and neck fibromyalgia and temporomandibular arthralgia. Otolaryngol Clin North Am 22:1159–1171, 1989.

138. Urrows S, Affleck G, Tennen H, et al: Unique clinical and psychological correlates of fibromyalgia tender points and joint tenderness in rheumatoid arthritis. Arthritis Rheum 37:1513–1520, 1994.

139. Vaeroy H, Helle R, Frre O, et al: Elevated CSF levels of substance P and high incidence of Raynaud phenomenon in patients with fibromyalgia: New features for diagnosis. Pain 32:21–26, 1988.

140. Vaeroy H, Qiao ZG, Mökrid L, et al: Altered sympathetic nervous system response in patients with fibromyalgia (fibrositis syndrome). J Rheumatol 16:1460–1465, 1989.

141. Wallace DJ: Genitourinary manifestations of fibrositis: An increased association with the female urethral syndrome. J Rheumatol 17:238–239, 1990.

142. Waylonis GW, Wilke S, O'Toole D, et al: Chronic myofascial pain: Management by low-output helium-neon laser therapy. Arch Phys Med Rehabil 69:1017–1020, 1988.

143. Whitehead WE, Bosmajian L, Zonderman AB, et al: Symptoms of psychologic distress associated with irritable bowel syndrome. Gastroenterology 95:709–714, 1988.

144. Whitney CW, and Vonkorff M: Regression to the mean in treated versus untreated chronic pain. Pain 50:281–285, 1992.

145. Wolfe F: Development of criteria for the diagnosis of fibrositis. Am J Med 81:99–104, 1986.

146. Wolfe F: The clinical syndrome of fibrositis. Am J Med 81:7–14, 1986.

147. Wolfe F: EMG-biofeedback in fibromyalgia syndrome. [Reply] J Rheumatol 16:1014, 1989.

148. Wolfe F: Fibromyalgia: The clinical syndrome. Rheum Dis Clin North Am 15:1–18, 1989.

149. Wolfe F: Methodologic and statistical problems in the epidemiology of fibromyalgia. In Fricton JR, and Awad E: Myofascial Pain and Fibromyalgia. Raven Press, New York, 1990, pp 147–163.

150. Wolfe F: Fibromyalgia: On diagnosis and certainty. Haworth Press, Journal of Musculoskeletal Pain 1:17–36, 1993.

151. Wolfe F: The epidemiology of fibromyalgia. J Musc Med 1:137–148, 1993.

152. Wolfe F, and Cathey MA: Prevalence of primary and secondary fibrositis. J Rheumatol 10:965–968, 1983.

153. Wolfe F, Cathey MA, Kleinheksel SM, et al: Psychological status in primary fibrositis and fibrositis associated with rheumatoid arthritis. J Rheumatol 11:500–506, 1984.

154. Wolfe F, and Hawley DJ: Fibromyalgia in the adult Danish population. [Letter] Scand J Rheumatol 23:55, 1994.

155. Wolfe F, Hawley DJ, Cathey MA, et al: Fibrositis: Symptom frequency and criteria for diagnosis. An evaluation of 291 rheumatic disease patients and 58 normal individuals. J Rheumatol 12:1159–1163, 1985.

156. Wolfe F, and Pincus T: Standard self-report questionnaires in routine clinical and research practice—an opportunity for patients and rheumatologists. J Rheumatol 18:643–646, 1991.

157. Wolfe F, Ross K, Anderson J, et al: Aspects of fibromyalgia in the general population: Sex, pain threshold, and fibromyalgia symptoms. J Rheumatol 22:151–156, 1995.

158. Wolfe F, Ross K, Anderson J, et al: The prevalence and characteristics of fibromyalgia in the general population. Arthritis Rheum 38:19–28, 1995.

159. Wolfe F, Simons DG, Fricton JR, et al: The fibromyalgia and myofascial pain syndromes—a preliminary study of tender points and trigger points in persons with fibromyalgia, myofascial pain syndrome and no disease. J Rheumatol 19:944–951, 1992.

160. Wolfe F, Smythe HA, Yunus MB, et al: The American College of Rheumatology 1990 criteria for the classification of fibromyalgia: Report of the Multicenter Criteria Committee. Arthritis Rheum 33:160–172, 1990.

161. Wysenbeek AJ, Mor F, Lurie Y, et al: Imipramine for the treatment of fibrositis: A therapeutic trial. Ann Rheum Dis 44:752–753, 1985.

162. Yunus MB: Towards a model of pathophysiology of fibromyalgia—aberrant central pain mechanisms with peripheral modulation. J Rheumatol 19:846–850, 1992.

163. Yunus MB, Dailey PA, Masi AT, et al: Abnormal transport ratio of serum tryptophan in primary fibromyalgia. Arthritis Rheum 33:S55, 1990.

164. Yunus MB, and Kalyan-Raman UP: Muscle biopsy findings in primary fibromyalgia and other forms of nonarticular rheumatism. Rheum Dis Clin North Am 15:115–134, 1989.

165. Yunus MB, and Masi AT: Juvenile primary fibromyalgia syndrome. A clinical study of thirty-three patients and matched normal controls. Arthritis Rheum 28:138–145, 1985.

166. Yunus MB, Masi AT, and Aldag JC: Short term effects of ibuprofen in primary fibromyalgia syndrome: A double blind, placebo controlled trial [published Erratum appears in J Rheumatol 1989 Jun;16(6):855]. J Rheumatol 16:527–532, 1989.

167. Yunus MB, Masi AT, Calabro JJ, et al: Primary fibromyalgia (fibrositis): Clinical study of 50 patients with matched normal controls. Semin Arthritis Rheum 11:151–171, 1981.

168. Zidar J, Blackman E, Bengtsson A, et al: Quantitative EMG and muscle tension in painful muscles in fibromyalgia. Pain 40:249–254, 1990.

CHAPTER 8

CHRONIC ARTHRITIS AND PAINFUL DISEASES OF BONE

Milton L. Cohen, M.B., B.S., M.D., F.R.A.C.P.,
and Peter M. Brooks, M.B., B.S., M.D., F.R.A.C.P.,
F.A.C.R.M., F.A.F.P.H.M.

SCOPE OF THE PROBLEM OF MUSCULOSKELETAL PAIN

Epidemiology of Musculoskeletal Diseases and Pain

Musculoskeletal diseases are among the most common presentations to general practitioners in the United States, England, and Australia and are a major cause of disability.[82] There are over 150 different musculoskeletal pain syndromes, which include inflammatory forms of arthritis, such as rheumatoid arthritis or the seronegative arthropathies; degenerative arthritis (osteoarthritis); crystal arthritis (gout and calcium pyrophosphate disease); and the systemic connective tissue disorders, such as systemic lupus erythematosus and systemic sclerosis (Table 8–1). Soft tissue rheumatic complaints, including injury, enthesopathies, and diffuse ("fibromyalgia") and regional ("myofascial pain") syndromes, are probably the most common musculoskeletal problems, whereas metabolic bone disease, with subsequent vertebral and long bone fracture, is a major cause of musculoskeletal pain, particularly in the elderly.

The prevalence of the major rheumatic

Table 8–1. CAUSES OF MUSCULOSKELETAL PAIN

Inflammatory Arthropathies
Rheumatoid arthritis
Seronegative spondyloarthropathies
  Ankylosing spondylitis
  Reactive arthritis
  Psoriatic arthritis
  Gut-associated arthritis
Infectious
  Bacterial
  Viral (postviral)

Degenerative Arthropathies
Osteoarthritis

Crystal-Associated Arthropathies
Gout
Calcium pyrophosphate
Calcium hydroxyapatite

Soft Tissue Rheumatic Problems
Enthesopathies
Diffuse ("fibromyalgia") and regional ("myofascial pain") syndromes
Injury

Systemic Connective Tissue Diseases
Systemic lupus erythematosus
Vasculitides
Systemic sclerosis

Metabolic Bone Disease
Osteoporosis
Osteonecrosis
Osteomalacia
Paget's disease

diseases is relatively similar among countries (Table 8–2), although certain diseases (in particular, the HLA-B27–associated arthropathies) show marked differences in prevalence across populations. For example, the prevalence of ankylosing spondylitis in the Hiadas and Pimas is almost 20 percent, in contrast to less than 0.1 percent in whites. This difference is associated with the variation in prevalence of the genetic marker for ankylosing spondylitis (HLA-B27), which is found in almost 25 percent of the Native American population.

The etiology of a few rheumatic diseases, such as gout or viral arthropathies, is clear. The majority, however, have multifactorial etiologies, with risk factors that are now being studied. For example, risk factors in osteoarthritis of the knee include older age, obesity, knee injury, chondrocalcinosis, occupational knee bending, and physical labor.[39,164] Obesity is a predictor of knee osteoarthritis in population-based studies in the United States,[31] United Kingdom,[59] and Sweden.[5] The varying prevalence of osteoarthritis in different countries suggests that variation in posture and footwear might be relevant. Rheumatoid arthritis shows a fairly uniform prevalence throughout the world, although studies suggest that severity differs in tropical areas such as Africa and India.

The prevalence of both osteoporosis and bone fracture is high.[4] More than half of women 50 years of age will sustain an osteoporosis-related fracture during their lifetime.[25] Risk factors for osteoporosis include a thin body habitus, living in the city rather than in the country, dwelling in a nursing home, and drinking coffee.[1] These associations support the contention that environmental factors play some role in the genesis of osteoporosis, although genetic factors are important.[114]

Costs to the Community

In the United States, osteoarthritis accounts for 46 million physician visits and nearly 70 million lost working days each year.[30,83] The total cost of musculoskeletal disease in the United States is about 1 percent of the gross national product, or $21 billion in 1980.[172] This cost includes both the direct costs of treating patients with rheumatic diseases and the loss of productivity by those unable to work. Half the patients with rheumatoid arthritis who present to a hospital clinic will be unable to work 10 years after disease onset. Osteoarthritis and back pain are a major cause of lost productivity across all age groups. The direct costs of rheumatic diseases are likely to increase with an aging population. For example, the annual cost for knee arthroplasties is approximately $2 billion.[134] Rheumatoid

Table 8–2. **PREVALENCE OF MUSCULOSKELETAL DISEASES**

Disease	Prevalence* (%)	
Rheumatoid arthritis	1	
Osteoarthritis		
Hip (European, US)	7–25	>55 years
Hip (Chinese)	1	>55 years
Hand (Radiographic)	70	>65 years
Gout	0.5	
Ankylosing spondylitis	0.15	
Psoriatic arthritis	0.19	
Systemic lupus erythematosus	0.04	
Scleroderma	0.0004	
Polymyalgia rheumatica	0.02	
Fibromyalgia (Family Practice Clinic)	2	
Low back pain	40	

*Figures extracted from Hochberg M (ed): Epidemiology of rheumatic disease. Rheum Dis Clin North Am 3:499–789, 1990.

arthritis not only causes significant morbidity but also results in early death, with life span reduced up to 8 years. Risk factors for premature death in rheumatoid arthritis include age, male gender, single status, unemployment, and use of prednisone.[90] The burden of osteoporosis with subsequent hip fracture adds to the costs of rheumatic diseases.

Clinical Presentation Versus Pathoanatomic Change

In contrast to the standard biomedical model of disease, musculoskeletal disorders are characterized by discordance between clinical features and demonstrable pathoanatomic bases, especially in the soft tissue rheumatic disorders and osteoarthritis. Radiologic changes and symptoms correlate poorly in both degenerative and inflammatory arthropathies, where pain in a particular joint can vary dramatically from day to day while the radiologic picture remains unchanged. Radiologic changes of osteoarthritis and spondylosis increase with age; although the radiologic prevalence of knee osteoarthritis in the population 60 years and older is about 60 percent, only 25 to 30 percent complain of knee pain.[30,98] The factors responsible for symptoms are not clear, although one study of patients with radiographic evidence of knee osteoarthritis showed that symptoms were correlated with being white, female, smoking, suffering from hypertension, and having poor psychologic well-being.[89] By contrast, the investigation of a painful ankle in an otherwise well 25-year-old may reveal no structural abnormality, even with sophisticated imaging techniques. Anatomic normality in patients with musculoskeletal symptoms or radiologic pathology in the absence of symptoms implies that disturbances of function, rather than structure, may be the relevant pathogenesis.

Conceptual Frameworks

Perhaps nowhere else in the lay mind is the illness-disease link so strong as in the case of musculoskeletal problems. Musculoskeletal discomfort, especially when localized to a joint or joints, is all too readily labeled "rheumatism," which has no precise connotation, or "arthritis," which implies that the relevant pathophysiology is inflammation. This practice continues despite the discordance between radiologic signs and the clinical picture, and the small proportion of rheumatic complaints that can actually be explained by inflammatory diseases. The morbidity, disability, and socioeconomic costs of musculoskeletal disorders are attributable largely to the pain that characterizes them and not necessarily to an underlying disease process.

Other paradigms may prove more useful

for the problems of musculoskeletal pain than a biomedical model of disease that focuses on inflammation alone. A biopsychosocial theme embraces both the reductionist direction (from the person toward organs, tissues, cells, and molecules) and the cognitive-behavioral direction (reflecting the interaction of the person with family, friends, workplace, local community, national community, and the biosphere itself).[35,150] Three variations on this theme can be used interchangeably. First is the World Health Organization's classification of disability.[168] This classification includes the following:

1. *Impairment,* a disturbance in structure or function, physiologic or psychologic (at organ level)
2. *Disability,* the disturbance in functional activity or performance that is a consequence of impairment (at the level of the person)
3. *Handicap,* the disadvantage that results from impairment or disability and prevents fulfillment of a normal role (at the level of society)

Parallel frameworks of reference include, in ascending biopsychosocial hierarchic order, the levels of damage to tissue, to the nervous system, to the whole person (in terms of affect, cognition, and behavior), and to society (Table 8–3).[99,160] This discussion concentrates on the physical problem or impairment, specifically nociception.

ANATOMIC AND PHYSIOLOGIC BASES FOR JOINT AND BONE PAIN

Animal studies have been the predominant source of information about nociception from joints and bone. Extrapolation of this information to the human situation should be made with caution.

Neural Mechanisms in Joints

RECEPTORS AND PRIMARY AFFERENTS

Mammalian joints and surrounding structures have a rich array of receptors potentially able to signal nociception.[45,77,81,136,170]

Nociceptors homologous with C polymodal cutaneous nociceptors are found in a diffuse lattice throughout the joint capsule. Free nerve endings in internal and external joint ligaments correspond to the high-threshold A-delta nociceptors in the skin (see Chapter 2). Joint cartilage does not contain such receptors. The synovium itself has been considered largely insensitive, but neuropeptide-containing, small-diameter nerve fibers were recently identified immunohistochemically in healthy human synovium.[53,103,127] These fibers may be relevant in the process of neurogenic inflammation (see following), if not also in signaling nociception. The predominant populations of afferent fibers in the articular nerves of the cat knee are A-delta and C, which may imply that nociceptors dominate within the joint.[86] These receptors also may respond to nonnoxious mechanical and chemical stimuli.[54,144]

Mechanoreceptors potentially relevant to joint pain have also been described. These receptors are subserved by large-diameter, fast-conducting afferents.[46] Corpuscular structures within the outer (type I) or subsynovial (type II) layers of the fibrous capsule function as static or low-threshold dynamic mechanoreceptors, and others (type III), which function as dynamic mechanoreceptors, are situated on the surface of joint ligaments. These low-threshold receptors are considered to subserve proprioceptive functions, such as deep pressure and sense of movement. Although they do not appear to mediate nociception in the feline model of acute arthritis,[32] they may influence dorsal horn cell responses in the chronic situation.

Mechanically insensitive afferents (MIAs)[107] become responsive to mechanical stimuli only when the tissue becomes inflamed (see following). In the normal feline knee joint, about half of the C fibers in the posterior articular nerve are MIAs.[52]

SPINAL CONNECTIONS

At the spinal cord level, nociceptive-specific (NS) and wide-dynamic-range (WDR) neurons in the dorsal horn receive nociceptive inputs from articular tissues and may also respond to nonnoxious mechanical stimulation of limb joints. These dorsal horn neurons receive convergent inputs from

Table 8–3. **CONCEPTUAL FRAMEWORK FOR CHRONIC MUSCULOSKELETAL PAIN**

Biopsychosocial Hierarchy	WHO[168]	Loeser[99]	Waddell[160]	Example
Society	Handicap	—	Social interaction	Loss of job
Interpersonal	Handicap	Behavior	Illness behavior	Depression
Person	Disability	Suffering	Distress	Inability to use computer
Nervous system	Impairment	Pain	—	Pain
Tissue	Impairment	Nociception	Physical problem	Synovitis of fingers

cutaneous, muscle, and visceral afferents (see Chapter 2).[51,111,147] These sources provide an anatomic substrate for the poor localization and discrimination and the referral of pain and hyperalgesia that may accompany arthropathy.

SUPRASPINAL CONNECTIONS

Noxious joint inputs can reach a cortical level. In models of experimental arthritis, the populations of neurons and ascending pathways activated by inflamed joints appear to be different from those signaling noxious cutaneous inputs.[55] Spinal processing of afferent information from joints is subject to tonic descending inhibitory influences.[146]

OTHER SOURCES OF NOXIOUS INFORMATION

Activity in the central nervous system related to pain perception can be influenced by plasticity in the dorsal horn of the spinal cord and the class of mechanically insensitive or "sleeping" nociceptors. Plasticity at the spinal cord level is well established (see Chapter 2). In response to persistent nociceptive input, dorsal horn cells show increased activity, enhanced responsiveness to peripheral stimuli, and enlarged receptive field size. [33,34,65,117]

In the presence of an experimental arthritis, MIAs in joints, which do not normally respond even to noxious mechanical stimulation, acquire new response properties

characterized by spontaneous activity, discharge during nonnoxious movement, and enlarged receptive fields.[52,142,143] The central connections of MIAs remain uncertain.[117]

Neural Mechanisms in Bone

Little is known about bone nociception. Structurally the periosteum and bone marrow are richly innervated in normal but not in arthritic rats. Immunochemical studies have detected substance P (SP) and calcitonin gene-related peptide (CGRP) in these afferent fibers, which may establish their candidacy as nociceptors.[11,68]

Hyperalgesia of Joints

HYPERALGESIA AND SENSITIZATION

The characteristics of hyperalgesia, which is clinically recognized as *tenderness*, include decreased threshold to noxious stimuli and increased pain from suprathreshold stimuli. The neurophysiologic correlates at the receptor/afferent fiber level are decreased threshold to response and increased response to suprathreshold stimuli.

CUTANEOUS HYPERALGESIA

Two types of hyperalgesia have been described with cutaneous injury.[58,96] *Primary hy-*

peralgesia occurs in an area of injury, and *secondary hyperalgesia* occurs in the undamaged tissue surrounding the injury (see Chapter 2). The characteristics and mechanisms of these two types are distinct.[135,155] Regions of primary cutaneous hyperalgesia are characterized psychophysically by reduced pain threshold and pain tolerance to both thermal and mechanical stimuli; regions of secondary cutaneous hyperalgesia are identified by normal pain threshold to these stimuli and reduced pain tolerance to mechanical but not to thermal stimuli.

The main mechanism of primary cutaneous hyperalgesia to thermal stimuli is sensitization of A-delta and C-fiber afferents. Similar sensitization of nociceptors to mechanical stimuli has not been shown. Enlargement of the mechanical receptive field of the primary afferent nociceptor (spatial summation) may account for primary mechanical hyperalgesia, although sensitization of central nociceptive pathways may also be relevant. By contrast, the predominant mechanism subserving secondary (mechanical) hyperalgesia appears to be changes in dorsal horn neurons (plasticity), with both leftward shift in stimulus-response functions and increased size of receptive fields. As a result of these changes, input from low-threshold mechanoreceptors is processed as noxious.

SENSITIZATION OF JOINT RECEPTORS

Sensitization of joint nociceptors has been shown in two animal models of joint inflammation: acute feline arthritis of the knee induced by injection of kaolin and carrageenan[144] and polyarthritis in the rat induced by systemic administration of Freund's adjuvant.[54] As a result of inflammation, MIAs and afferents previously responding only to intense joint movement (high-threshold afferents) begin to respond to nonnoxious movements and develop increased resting activity. The response of some nonnociceptive (low-threshold) afferents is also enhanced. These changes manifest as reduction in threshold or enhancement of movement-induced responses, or both, and parallel the development and duration of hyperalgesia and pain behavior in the animals.

SPINAL AND SUPRASPINAL CHANGES

Acute or chronic arthritis can induce changes in central nociceptive pathways (dorsal horn, thalamus, and primary somatosensory cortex). These changes manifest as enhanced responsiveness to afferent activity from both the site of inflammation and other convergent inputs.[54,55,65,116,147] In the cat, projection neurons that normally show little response to knee flexion develop large responses soon after induction of acute inflammation,[148] and dorsal horn neurons with input from inflamed joints show enhanced responses to stimuli remote from the site of inflammation.[117] Adjuvant-induced arthritis in rats is associated with expansion of receptive fields and spontaneous activity of lamina I spinal cord dorsal horn neurons,[69] as well as enhanced response to mechanical stimuli.[21,110]

Chronic joint inflammation may influence cutaneous receptive fields of central somatosensory neurons. These neurons demonstrate the neurophysiologic correlates of hyperalgesia, including increased background activity and prolonged response to nonnoxious stimulation of skin.[110,147,148]

In the acute feline arthritis model, changes occur in tonic descending inhibition of spinal cord neurons that receive articular afferent input.[141,146] A tendency toward reduced inhibition during arthritis has been suggested.

In the rat model, studies of behavioral and thalamic responses suggest that central neurons increase activity following mechanical and heat stimuli from areas remote from the injury site.[54,57] The populations of central neurons that respond to intense stimulation may also differ in normal animals and in those with inflamed joints; this "sensitization" does not parallel that in the periphery.[55]

BIOCHEMISTRY AND PHARMACOLOGY OF JOINT NOCICEPTION

Prostaglandins are important in the activation and sensitization of joint afferents. Prostaglandin E (PGE) reverses the depressing effect of cyclooxygenase inhibitors on the spontaneous and movement-evoked activity of nociceptive afferents from inflamed joints.[56,62,63,145] Leukotrienes, products of arachidonic acid by the lipoxygenase pathway, sensitize nociceptors in animals and humans.[10,162] Bradykinin, serotonin, and histamine also activate these afferents, although the effects are short lived.[73] These inflammatory mediators may act synergistically: Bradykinin was shown to sensitize joint afferents to mechanical stimuli, an effect enhanced by PGE_2,[118] whereas serotonin also enhanced mechanical responsiveness.[9] Substance P (see following) may stimulate the release of prostaglandins from synovial cells.[100] At the spinal cord level, substance P and neurokinin A were released after innocuous mechanical stimulation of joints only after induction of experimental inflammation.[67,140]

NEUROGENIC INFLAMMATION

The involvement of the nervous system in inflammation has been recognized since the demonstration of the "axon reflex." This phenomenon of localized vasodilatation and exudation, which occurs in response to an irritant, requires intact sensory innervation[18,96] and can be induced by antidromic stimulation of peripheral sensory nerves.[37,72] C fibers are responsible for this phenomenon.[23,102]

This neurogenic inflammation is mediated through the local release of neuropeptides at the peripheral terminals of C fibers. These peptides are synthesized proximally in cell bodies in the dorsal root ganglia and are transported distally as well as centrally. They include SP, CGRP, somatostatin, vasoactive intestinal peptide (VIP), neurokinin A, and neurokinin B. As a group, they exert a variety of influences on inflammation, including changes in vascular tone and permeability, activation of neutrophils, proliferation and function of T and B lymphocytes, release of cytokines, production of oxygen free radicals and release of prostaglandins.[44,66,104]

Neurogenic inflammation contributes to acute and chronic arthritis. Intra-articular injection of SP in rats induces local inflammation,[85] and capsaicin, a compound that selectively depletes SP from primary afferent fibers, attenuates the development of adjuvant- and carrageenan-induced arthritis in the rat.[28,85] In animal models of chronic arthritis, injection of SP increases the local severity of inflammation, and the severity of

arthritis and the density of SP-containing nociceptive afferents are directly related.[92]

Sympathetic efferent fibers may also be involved in neurogenic inflammation in both experimental arthritis[27,93] and clinical human disease.[94] Neuropeptide Y, a powerful vasoconstrictor that co-localizes with catecholamine-synthesizing enzymes at sympathetic terminals, is reduced in rheumatoid synovium.[101,103] In human disease, clinical evidence indicates that the nervous system influences inflammatory joint disease.[80,95] Immunohistochemical techniques reveal that SP and CGRP are found in human synovium and have patterns of local release that suggest greater importance in inflammatory arthritis than in osteoarthrosis.[53,103,127] These observations establish the relevance of the efferent influence of primary nociceptive afferents on joint inflammation.

Thus, studies have demonstrated a convergence in the neurochemistry of nociception and inflammation. The implications of these findings are listed in Table 8–4.

PATHOPHYSIOLOGY OF JOINT AND BONE PAIN AND HYPERALGESIA

Nociception may be initiated by chemical or mechanical processes. These processes may occur together and influence each other. For example, chemical sensitization of nociceptors renders them susceptible to activation by mechanical stimuli, whereas the swelling that is the hallmark of inflammation may activate mechanoreceptors. Persistent nociception may induce large myelinated (A-beta) afferents, which normally respond to touch and proprioception, to signal mechanical allodynia.[22,133] Nociception that occurs in the muscles that control joints and bones may also be relevant.[174] Thus, mechanisms underlying both primary and secondary hyperalgesia must be considered.

Chemical Nociception: Inflammatory Model

Inflammation may be seen as the combination of (1) pain, which is attributable to activation of nociceptors; (2) primary hyperalgesia,

Table 8–4. **IMPLICATIONS OF KNOWLEDGE OF JOINT NOCICEPTION**

Findings	Implications
Prevalence and distribution of nociceptors in joints	Basis for chemical and mechanical pain and hyperalgesia
Response of sensitized receptors to nonnoxious movement	Spontaneous and movement-related pain in arthropathy
Convergent inputs from joint, muscle, cutaneous and visceral afferents	Projection of pain and hyperalgesia
Increased response of neurons remote from sites of inflammation	Poor localization and discrimination of joint pain
Thalamic and cortical connections	Changes in modulating influences (e.g., descending inhibition)

which is due to sensitization of nociceptors; and (3) swelling, which reflects the vascular effects of neuropeptide release. This conceptualization accounts for inflammation that occurs in response to either immunologic or neurogenic processes,[95,100] as well as the influence of ischemia.[12,71] The distribution of nociceptors in joint capsules and probably in synovial tissue, as described previously, provides an adequate anatomic substrate for such chemical nociception and primary hyperalgesia to develop within joints. This model conforms to the disease paradigm and readily accounts for most (but not all) of the pain and hyperalgesia of active (but not inactive) arthritides.

Mechanical Nociception: Mechanical Model

Changes in joint biomechanics per se may be responsible for pain and primary hyperalgesia without invoking inflammatory processes. It follows that mechanical nociception may be particularly relevant in joints that have been damaged by a pathologic process (e.g., osteoarthritis syndrome), especially if those nociceptors have been sensitized by prior influences.

Nociceptors in the capsules of joints and in bone, ligaments, entheses, and blood vessels may be activated by increased intra-articular pressure, abnormal posture, or changes in shape of joints or bone. Mechanoreceptors in joint capsules, but perhaps more importantly in periarticular tissues (especially musculotendinous junctions[120]), may also be activated

by the same processes. Although not usually considered to transduce nociception, these mechanoreceptors may become involved in the generation and maintenance of spinal cord plasticity such that mechanoreceptive information is processed as noxious.[33,137,171]

Allied to this mechanical model is the contribution to joint pain from surrounding musculoskeletal tissues, especially muscles, tendons, and entheses. Contraction of muscles by activation of spinal motor reflexes in response to a primary nociceptive stimulus may set up a vicious cycle of stimulation of muscle nociceptors, which in turn maintains reflex contraction. Such a nociceptive stimulus could come from a joint, tendon, entheses, or nerve.[46,112,169,174]

Role of Secondary Hyperalgesia: Neuropathic Model

Given the chronicity of the chronic arthropathies and the potential for sustained nociception over time, altered function of central nociceptive pathways may be involved in the pathogenesis of joint pain. Such a mechanism would correlate with regions of secondary hyperalgesia, which to date have not been characterized in this context.

Referred pain is recognized in chronic arthropathy. For example, pain from an osteoarthritic hip is commonly referred to the knee. Cutaneous hyperalgesia in regions of referred pain ("referred hyperalgesia") has the characteristics of secondary hyperalgesia and is considered to be due predominantly to central mechanisms.[148,155] Deep tissue hyperalgesia in regions of referred pain has been well documented and is probably also mainly centrally mediated.[58,97] The development of a regional pain syndrome, in which nociception in deep tissues such as joints is accompanied by a broader area of allodynia, deep hyperalgesia, and cutaneous hypesthesia, may also result from central processes. This type of pain has features similar to those that occur following nerve injury and has attracted the label "neuropathic pain," but it has not been investigated to any extent in human arthropathy.

CLINICAL ASSESSMENT OF JOINT AND BONE PAIN

Assessment of Impairment

JOINT PAIN

For the clinician, the challenge is to determine whether the symptom of arthralgia reflects an arthrosis and, if so, whether the underlying pathology is inflammatory and justifies the label "arthritis." A useful approach determines (1) the anatomic origin of pain, (2) the mechanisms of pain production, and (3) the associated disease process. This assessment derives from a background classification of arthropathy into inflammatory and noninflammatory entities.

The finding of hyperalgesia of a joint or joints in the region of pain confirms the probable anatomic origin, and swelling confirms the presence of arthrosis. Other signs such as crepitus and instability give clues to the degree of damage to joints and supportive structures. With inflammatory arthropathy, the pattern of joint involvement with associated extra-articular and systemic features may allow more precise syndrome or disease labels. Chronic inflammatory arthritides evolve slowly over time, and a provisional syndromic label may be all that is possible and appropriate.

This approach to evaluation is particularly relevant to the syndrome of osteoarthritis, or joint failure. Not all osteoarthritic joints are symptomatic, and the processes that make these joints painful, hyperalgesic, or swollen remain in question. Synovial fluid from symptomatic osteoarthritic joints, which is not always obtainable, is usually acellular or mildly cellular with a predominantly mononuclear count. Occasionally, known osteoarthritic joints present with typical signs of clinical inflammation, simplifying inferences about pathogenesis; sometimes, these joints are swollen but not hyperalgesic (Table 8–5).

In synovial inflammation, an example of primary hyperalgesia, nociceptors in the synovium are activated by chemical processes, possibly perpetuated by mechanical factors. In osteoarthritic joints, nociceptors and mechanoreceptors in joint capsule and presumably in periosteum could provide a sufficient anatomic substrate for mechanical nociception. Just as inflammation sensitizes nociceptors and MIAs, it is possible that damaged osteoarthritic joints sensitize primary afferent fibers and result in persistent sensitivity to movement.

The relevant clinical observation is that joints that do not move properly (usually hypomobile or, less commonly, hypermobile) may be painful, whether or not they are anatomically abnormal. Osteoarthritic joints may be symptomatic as a result of altered biomechanics, leading in turn to relevant nociceptor activation.

The role of secondary hyperalgesia in chronic arthritis has not been systematically evaluated. In laboratory animals, sensitization of both peripheral and central nociceptive neurons to nonnoxious movements has been demonstrated following joint inflammation. It seems reasonable that similar processes may contribute to chronic joint pain in humans.

Role of Laboratory Testing. In musculoskeletal medicine, the clinical assessment is of fundamental importance. The definitive laboratory test for inflammatory arthropathy is examination of synovial fluid for polymorphonuclear leukocytes. The presence of crystals, preferably within leukocytes, in the acute situation makes a diagnosis of the appropriate crystal arthritis highly probable. Other investigations are of limited use in diagnosis and in following the course of chronic arthritis. Radiographs may demonstrate anatomic changes in joints but cannot indicate whether such joints are symptomatic. Identification of typical synoviopathic or chondropathic changes[2] may

Table 8–5. **CLINICAL SPECTRUM OF CHRONIC INFLAMMATORY ARTHROPATHY**

Pattern of Joint Involvement	Extra-articular Features	Serologic Correlates	Nosology
POLYARTICULAR			
Erosive, symmetric, small joints	Systemic illness, vasculitis, sicca syndrome	Rheumatoid factor (RF)	Rheumatoid disease
Nonerosive, small joints	Sicca syndrome, renal disease	Antinuclear antibodies, anti-DNA*	SLE[†], Sjögren's syndrome
POLYARTICULAR OR MONOARTICULAR			
Small or large joints	Tophi	—	Gout
OLIGOARTICULAR			
Asymmetric, large joints, sacroiliac	Psoriasis, uveitis, conjunctivitis, urethritis, colitis	RF negative, HLA-B27[‡]	Psoriasis, reactive arthritis (including Reiter's syndrome); ankylosing spondylitis
Asymmetric, large joints	—	—	Pyrophosphate arthropathy

*Antibodies to double-stranded DNA.
[†]SLE = systemic lupus erythematosus.
[‡]Histocompatibility antigen B27.

help distinguish between inflammatory and noninflammatory processes once symptoms have been present for some months. In early disease, radiographs may not be helpful; in later disease, the radiographic features can largely be predicted from the clinical findings, so these studies need not be performed unless surgical management is contemplated.

The role of blood tests is also limited. The peripheral blood may not reflect what is happening within the synovial cavities. A nonspecific indicator of inflammation such as the erythrocyte sedimentation rate is commonly used, despite its inherent biologic and rheologic variability and the lack of information concerning its positive predictive value. C-reactive protein may be a superior indicator of inflammation because of its inherent biologic role in inflammation and its capacity for precise measurement and interpretation.[84,126] Chronic arthritis is often associated with a secondary anemia and thrombocytosis, each reflecting the degree of inflammation, although again the predictive value of anemia in this context has not been established.

Serologic tests do not assist in the important distinction between inflammatory and noninflammatory processes. The presence of rheumatoid factor (RF) by itself has little diagnostic utility: Assuming an 80 percent sensitivity and a 95 percent specificity for RF (as measured by the latex test at a cut-off titer of 80) in rheumatoid arthritis (RA)[165] and the population prevalence of RA of 1 percent, the predictive value of a positive test is 5 percent. In a population of patients with known inflammatory joint disease, however, use of the likelihood ratio of 16 (the quotient of 80 [the true positive rate] and 5 [the false positive rate] for the presence of RF in RA) is more appropriate to calculate posttest probability from pretest probability (prevalence) estimates.

Similarly, as the histocompatibility antigen HLA-B27 has a higher prevalence in the seronegative spondyloarthropathies,[78] its presence has been advocated as a diagnostic test. Assuming in ankylosing spondylitis the sensitivity and specificity for HLA-B27 each to be 90 percent, the likelihood ratio is 9. The rational use of this test in the context of back pain requires the same principle of calculating posttest probability, and it is rarely required.[79]

BONE PAIN

Pain in bones may be attributed to vascular, infective, neoplastic, or metabolic processes (Table 8–6). In destructive arthritis, the bone itself may become another source of nociception, a situation that can be readily determined clinically. In contrast to joint pain, bone pain is usually not influenced by posture or movement and is often noted to be worse at night. Discrete hyperalgesia over a painful bony site, especially vertebral, should suggest an underlying infective, neoplastic, or metabolic lesion. Again, clinical indicators are paramount and determine appropriate investigations.

Two situations of bone pain deserve further discussion. *Osteonecrosis* (aseptic necrosis), which commonly affects the femoral or humeral heads, may mimic arthropathy of those joints, with local and referred pain, hyperalgesia, and limited movement. Of the many associations with nontraumatic osteonecrosis,[152] corticosteroid therapy is the most common; the dose of steroid appears to be the major predictor of this risk.[40] Infection can be excluded from the differential diagnosis only by joint aspiration. Magnetic resonance imaging is the most sensitive technique for detecting osteonecrosis,[113] but the degree of bone or joint pathology in this study may be discordant with the clinical features. For example, bilateral changes may be seen when only one side is affected clinically. Once there is evidence of osteonecrosis on plain radiography or computed tomography, the opportunity to prevent joint damage has been lost, although the collapse of subchondral bone is not inevitable. Established osteonecrosis is essentially the clinical problem of joint damage (osteoarthritis), as described previously.

Osteoporosis, as defined by the clinical event of the fracture of an osteopenic bone, presents the problems of the acute fracture and its long-term mechanical consequences. In addition to identifying the factors that contribute to the osteopenia,[154] the clinical assessment of the pain associated with these processes is identical to that for pain arising

Table 8–6. **PAINFUL DISEASES OF BONE**

Vascular
Osteonecrosis

Infective
Osteomyelitis

Neoplastic
Secondary carcinoma

Metabolic
Paget's disease
Osteoporosis*
Hyperparathyroidism
Osteomalacia and rickets

*As defined by fracture in an osteopenic bone.

from joints. Osteopenia per se is not a cause of bone pain.

Assessment of Disability and Handicap

Identification of the tissue processes leading to joint or bone pain forms only part of the clinical picture. The consequences for function are of at least equal importance, especially with respect to the patient's ability to perform activities of daily living (see Chapter 1). Rheumatoid arthritis has been the focus for most of the work on outcome measures in musculoskeletal diseases. Quantitative measures, which assess disease activity and attempt to monitor and predict the course of a patient with rheumatoid arthritis, include process measures, such as the number of swollen and tender joints; radiographs and a variety of laboratory tests; and physical measures of functional status, such as grip strength and walking time.[130]

During the past decade, questionnaires developed to assess functional status have been shown to be valid, reliable, easy to administer in the clinical setting, and well correlated with traditional process measures.[131] These questionnaires, such as the Health Assessment Questionnaire (HAQ),[48] the Arthritis Impact Measurement Scales (AIMS),[108,109] and McMaster-Toronto Arthritis Questionnaire (MACTAR),[156] qualitatively assess dressing, rising, eating, walking, and outside activities, and take into account descriptive indices such as employment status, hours worked, and other demographic data. Similar measures, such as the Western Ontario McMaster Index,[8] have been developed for other rheumatic diseases.

The morbidity and mortality of rheumatoid arthritis are correlated with disease severity, as determined clinically and by radiographic and laboratory indices,[36,129] and disability is determined strongly by health status and socioeconomic variables, including educational status.* Psychologic morbidity in RA is a major contributor to disability, independent of disease activity indices. Anxiety and depression are common in cohorts of RA, and their development is related more to socioeconomic than to clinical indices.[60] Furthermore, disability is strongly correlated with attitude to illness.[106]

Pain is, of course, one of the three major determinants of health status in the arthritides, along with psychologic status and physical functioning.[74] Observed pain behaviors in RA correlate with self-report of pain and functional disability[105] as well as with disease activity.[3] Depression and anxiety are not significant predictors of pain behavior after demographic and socioeconomic variables are taken into account.[3] These findings underline the important contribution of ongoing nociception to pain behavior in inflammatory arthritis.

Cognitive factors, as assessed by pain coping strategies, also appear to modulate health status in both inflammatory and noninflammatory arthritis (see Chapter 15). In particular, the Coping Strategies Questionnaire reflects the tendency to use pain coping strategies and individual confidence in ability to manage pain problems. Changes in the latter scores correlate with changes in pain intensity and physical functioning and have been influenced by cognitive-behavioral therapy in both rheumatoid arthritis[123,124] and osteoarthritis.[75,76]

Outcome measures can be used in assessing the efficacy of a variety of interventions, including pharmacotherapy, and may also be used in determining prognosis. There is no simple single measure of disability and

*References 7, 48, 91, 130, 158, 159, 166.

handicap in rheumatic diseases, and impairment is not reliably reflected in disability. In rheumatoid disease, and possibly in other arthropathies, prognosis may be affected as much by cognitive, behavioral, and socioeconomic factors as by specific treatments. With chronic joint pain, however, the major determinant remains nociception. These two statements have profound implications for the comprehensive assessment and management of arthritis.

MANAGEMENT

A management plan based on an understanding of both physical and psychosocial pathology is optimal for the patient with chronic musculoskeletal pain. This approach may include treatments directed at nociceptive or neuropathic mechanisms, or at affective and evaluative components of the pain, aspects of the underlying disease, or disability and handicap.

Treatment of Pain

Pain can be managed with a range of drugs and adjunctive approaches. In inflammatory arthritis, nonsteroidal anti-inflammatory drugs (NSAIDs) tend to be used initially, followed after a period by the use of second-line agents (discussed under "Treatment of Underlying Disease," which follows).

NSAIDs are some of the most commonly prescribed drugs throughout the world (see Chapter 10).[87] Their use is rational when inflammation (causing pain and primary hyperalgesia) is the relevant pathophysiology, as these drugs influence a number of cellular and mediator aspects of the inflammatory process.[17] These include inhibition of cyclooxygenase, lipoxygenase, cell membrane processes, and a variety of other intracellular enzymes and lymphocyte functions. Responses to NSAIDs vary because of pharmacokinetic or pharmacodynamic differences or the common fluctuations in the intensity of inflammation. This fluctuation tends to confound many of the studies designed to address this problem. Although NSAIDs have variable plasma half-lives, the drug remains in the synovial fluid for much longer than in the plasma, which means that even drugs of short plasma half-life may be prescribed less frequently to provide 24-hour relief.

Adverse effects are a major problem with NSAIDs. These effects include gastrointestinal and renal dysfunction, skin rashes, and interactions with agents such as antihypertensive drugs, diuretics, and lithium (see Chapter 10).[153] The most common side effect is gastric erosion and ulcer formation; although the estimated absolute risk is relatively low (2 to 4 cases of NSAID-induced serious upper gastrointestinal adverse event per 10,000 person-months prescriptions[88]), this risk translates into a major public health problem when 20 percent or more of the population over the age of 65 is taking these drugs.[61] The physician must consider initially whether an NSAID is really required—that is, whether there is an inflammatory component—and then select an appropriate NSAID, taking into account the diagnosis and the previous experiences of physician and patient.[24]

In noninflammatory forms of arthritis (osteoarthritis), NSAIDs should be used judiciously and for the shortest possible time. Patients with osteoarthritis do just as well with acetaminophen as with NSAIDs.[163] Furthermore, higher ("anti-inflammatory") doses of NSAIDs are no better than low doses in this situation, whether or not there are signs of low-grade inflammation that are the usual rationale for their use.[14] In these clinical situations, the use of analgesics with a significantly lower incidence of side effects is more appropriate.

The use of acetaminophen should be considered for both inflammatory and noninflammatory arthropathy. In inflammatory arthritis, supplemental acetaminophen may provide as much analgesia as a higher dose of NSAID, thereby avoiding the adverse effects of the latter drug.[149] The mechanism of action of acetaminophen remains poorly understood, although there is evidence for direct effects on the central nervous system.[128] A major advantage is its lack of upper gastrointestinal toxicity, especially ulceration and bleeding. The well-known hazard of hepatotoxicity, seen virtually only with drug overdose, is increased with liver disease and alcoholism, and the daily dose should be carefully monitored in these situations. The risk for nephrotoxicity with chronic dosing remains uncertain, but it is probably very small.

Opioid analgesics have a place in the treatment of moderate and severe bone and joint pain. Although considered to work mainly through receptors in the central nervous system, either by inhibition of transmission of nociceptive messages to higher centers or by activation of descending antinociceptive pathways,[6] increasing evidence points to peripheral analgesic actions, especially in conditions characterized by inflammatory (primary) hyperalgesia (see Chapter 11).[151] The true place of these drugs in chronic musculoskeletal pain has not been determined, but in the context of a multidisciplinary approach to pain control, taken together with the low realistic risk of addiction,[43,132,173] an argument can be made for their more liberal, careful use (see Chapter 11).

Corticosteroids remain important in the rational pharmacology of inflammation, although their use as definitive or interim agents is controversial.[20] In the low doses (0.1 mg/kg per day) that appear to be required for control of joint inflammation, corticosteroids are safe, predictably effective, and unassociated with significant side effects (in particular, osteoporosis).[138]

Although the role of altered central nociception in the pain and secondary hyperalgesia associated with chronic musculoskeletal disorders awaits definition, the use of agents that may interfere with central mechanisms is justified when sensitization of dorsal horn neurons is highly likely. Candidates include the tricyclic antidepressants and anticonvulsants and the antagonists of excitatory amino acids that are under development (see Chapter 10).[33]

Antidepressant drugs may enhance the analgesia induced by other drugs. Their analgesic action is presumably mediated in the spinal cord, although their beneficial effect on sleep and on mood, where appropriate, suggests action elsewhere in the neuraxis. Debate continues over possible modes of action.[38,119,161] Definitive studies in chronic arthritis are awaited.

Nonpharmacologic approaches to pain therapy may be extremely useful in some cases. Chronic pain management programs, which emphasize cognitive-behavioral therapies, can address the disability (and hence prognosis) of patients with chronic arthritis.

Treatment of Underlying Disease

INFLAMMATORY ARTHRITIS

"Second-line," "remission-inducing," or "slow-acting" antirheumatic drugs (SAARDs) are useful mainly in rheumatoid disease (seropositive polyarticular pattern) and sometimes in the seronegative spondylarthropathies. These include gold, D-penicillamine, hydroxychloroquine, sulfasalazine, methotrexate, and immunosuppressive agents such as cyclophosphamide, chlorambucil, azathioprine, and cyclosporine. With the realization that rheumatoid arthritis is not a benign disease, that it may produce significant disability and some shortening of life, early use of second-line agents is being promoted.[16] This view derives from the observation that long-term disability is associated with the development of erosive joint disease and that 90 percent of RA patients who develop erosions do so within the first 2 years of disease.[15] Currently, however, few studies clearly demonstrate the efficacy of these agents in slowing the long-term progression of rheumatoid arthritis.

Evaluation of the effect of SAARDs in rheumatoid disease has been hampered by three factors. First, the natural history of the disease is one of relapse and remission. Second, the measures used to monitor disease process and functional outcome assess different aspects, among which there is poor correlation. Morbidity and mortality are predicted better by quantitative measures of functional status.[91,130] Third, studies of the SAARDs are often compromised by small numbers of patients.

Meta-analysis of published trials has been used to overcome the limits imposed by small numbers. Using disease process measures, a meta-analysis of injectable gold revealed modest improvement over a 6-month period.[26] Although only gold and cyclophosphamide were found by one meta-analysis to slow radiologic progression,[70] methotrexate and sulfasalazine have also been shown to reduce the rate of erosion. In a meta-analysis of 66 randomized, controlled trials of second-line agents, there was little difference in effi-

cacy among methotrexate, injectable gold, D-penicillamine, and sulfasalazine.[41] In the latter analysis, auranofin and hydroxychloroquine were significantly less effective than the other preparations. As the authors point out, however, few, if any, studies comparing SAARDs have had enough patients enrolled to differentiate more effective drugs from those that are less effective, and the duration of treatment required to demonstrate a favorable effect may be very prolonged. Most patients commencing a SAARD will take the drug for about 2 years (except for methotrexate, in which the mean continuation time is 4 years), until side effects arise or the disease flares up despite initial response.[167] Recent studies that have suggested a rank order of the SAARDs have favored methotrexate for efficacy and hydroxychloroquine for tolerability.[49,50]

The long-term morbidity of RA has led to early use of SAARDs and the principle that these drugs should be changed frequently if disability is not controlled: the so-called "sawtooth strategy."[47] In this approach, disability and other outcome variables are reviewed frequently so that disease progression can be serially plotted. A ceiling for disability is established a priori and is used as a decision point to trigger a treatment change. Combinations of SAARDs also have been used frequently, in a manner analogous to that of chemotherapy for malignant disease. There is no good evidence for additive or synergistic effects, however, and toxicity is greater with combination than with single therapy.[13,42,125]

Newer treatments include cyclosporin A[157] and a number of immunomodulating agents, such as anticytokine drugs and monoclonal antibodies.[121] These new approaches and drugs offer hope to patients with chronic rheumatoid arthritis, but they need to be tested in a properly controlled fashion.

Seronegative arthropathies (particularly those with a peripheral component) have also been shown to respond to SAARDs, especially sulfasalazine. Chronic gouty arthritis requires specific therapy with drugs such as allopurinol to lower the serum and total body urate, but NSAIDs, colchicine, or both also must be used to prevent recurrent painful attacks of the arthritis. Infectious forms of arthritis such as Lyme disease require specific antibiotic therapy; in most situations, these forms of disease can be easily controlled and cured.

THE ROLE OF SURGERY

Major advances in the surgical management of rheumatic diseases have occurred during the last two decades. Total joint replacements of hips and knees are rapidly becoming among the most frequently performed operations. Used judiciously, joint replacement can make an enormous difference to the ability of a patient with chronic rheumatic disease to perform daily tasks and live a more independent life.

BONE DISEASE

Specific management of early osteonecrosis (defined as positive findings on examination and MRI but negative findings on plain radiography or CT) remains undefined. Calcitonin stimulates osteoblast activity and is a rational therapy but has never been formally studied. Surgical management (core decompression of the femoral head), which is designed to limit ischemic damage, remains controversial.[29]

Established osteonecrosis (positive findings on plain radiography or CT) is essentially the clinical problem of joint damage. Management at this stage entails adequate pain control plus correction of mechanical factors, which may involve resolving leg-length discrepancy, providing isometric retraining of antigravity muscles, or training in the use of walking aids. Persistent pain, especially nocturnal, alone or with a significant mechanical disability, is an indication for joint replacement surgery. Surgery usually carries a good prognosis.

Amelioration of Disability and Handicap

As already discussed, the major determinants of disability and handicap in patients with chronic arthritis and diseases of bone are ongoing nociception, leading to persistent pain, and socioeconomic factors. Of these, pain and the functional impairments it causes are usually within the influence of

the health professions. Physical therapy is an important element in the multidisciplinary assessment and treatment of these patients.

The biomechanical consequences of joint disease include joint stiffness, instability, and muscle weakness. These impairments may be not only a result of but also a source of pain through altered movement and load bearing. The goals of physical therapy include increasing and maintaining muscle strength and endurance, increasing joint motion, decreasing joint instability, and improving capacity to perform activities of daily living (see Chapter 14). If attained, these goals improve the patient's overall well-being and capacity for social interaction.[64]

Despite its intuitive appeal, the role of physical modalities has only lately come under rigorous evaluation.[19,115,122] Nonetheless, these approaches are commonly used. As in the case of pharmacotherapy, prescriptions for physical therapy should be individualized and based on a biopsychosocial evaluation. In designing the therapy, the issues of comorbidity, pain control, and compliance should be considered.

SUMMARY

Chronic arthritis and painful bone diseases constitute a major category of chronic musculoskeletal pain that is associated with enormous human, social, and economic costs. These conditions should be approached through two conceptual frameworks: the pathophysiology of nociception at the level of impairment and a biopyschosocial approach to the consequences of impairment, including disability and handicap.

The neural basis of nociception from joints has been intensively investigated. Unmyelinated and lightly myelinated primary afferent fibers transmit information about noxious events, which can be mediated through local inflammation or mechanical disruption of the joint. Sensitization and the activation of afferents that become active only in areas of inflammation ("mechanically insensitive afferents") are involved in sustaining pain and hyperalgesia. Hyperalgesia may also be mediated by changes in central neurons in a manner analogous to the "central sensitization" produced by injury to other tissues. C-fiber nociceptors may also be involved in the development or perpetuation of inflammation through local release of neuropeptides, such as substance P. This neurogenic inflammation probably contributes to both acute and chronic arthritis.

In contrast to the growing knowledge about joint nociception, little is known about the specific mechanisms responsible for bone pain. Periosteum and bone marrow contain afferent fibers that may be nociceptive, but the function of these fibers has not been investigated.

The assessment of patients with chronic joint or bone pain is based, first, on clinical pathophysiologic explication rather than on disease labeling and second, on a multidisciplinary approach to disability. The activity of the disease, its associated symptoms, and the degree of disability expressed by the patient are poorly correlated. Hence, the standard biomedical model of disease is commonly inappropriate and should be replaced with a biopsychosocial model that encourages evaluation of overall health status, psychologic functioning, and socioeconomic variables, as well as assessment of the underlying disease.

The assessment of patients with chronic pain due to joint or bone disease should be comprehensive and provide a foundation for a management approach that offers treatments directed at the pathophysiology of the pain, the underlying disease, and the phenomena that contribute to associated disability or handicap. The traditional approach to the management of inflammation and primary hyperalgesia emphasizes the use of nonsteroidal anti-inflammatory drugs. These drugs have important adverse effects, such as gastrointestinal and renal dysfunction, and should be used cautiously. The administration or coadministration of acetaminophen should be considered to enhance analgesia in some patients.

The long-term administration of low-dose corticosteroid therapy may also be useful in the management of inflammatory pain. This approach is controversial, however, and risk versus benefits must be considered for each individual. Opioid analgesics and adjuvant analgesics, such as antidepressants or anticonvulsants, should be considered in selected cases of refractory pain. Nonpharmacologic approaches such as cognitive-behavioral therapies are particularly important in addressing high levels of disability.

The use of "slow-acting" antirheumatic drugs, including gold, D-penicillamine, hydroxychloroquine, sulfasalazine, methotrexate, and immunosuppressive agents such as cyclophosphamide, chlorambucil, azathioprine, and cyclosporine, is appropriate in rheumatoid disease and some cases of seronegative spondyloarthropathies. The long-term administration of these drugs is justified by the potential for substantial disability and shortening of life that may occur as a result of severe disease. Recent studies suggest that methotrexate is probably the most efficacious of these drugs and hydroxychloroquine is probably the best tolerated.

In some forms of arthritis, such as gout, treatment of the underlying disease is possible. Although these therapies may not obviate the need for pain management or other therapies, they should be pursued if possible. In some instances, such as in the use of calcitonin or surgical treatment to manage early osteonecrosis, primary therapy remains controversial.

Physical therapy may be helpful in reversing the disability and handicap associated with joint or bone diseases. This therapy must be individualized and must address comorbidity, unrelieved pain, and compliance. Surgical approaches must also be considered in selected cases. Joint replacement can dramatically improve quality of life for patients with refractory pain or functional impairment.

REFERENCES

1. Abyad A, and Boyer JT: Arthritis and aging. Curr Opin Rheumatol 4:153–159, 1992.
2. Alexander C: Use of a binary search pattern and discriminator analysis in the radiologic diagnosis of arthritis. Semin Arthritis Rheum 16:104–117, 1986.
3. Anderson LA, Keefe FJ, Bradley LA, et al: Prediction of pain behaviour and functional status in rheumatoid arthritis patients using medical status and psychological variables. Pain 33:25–32, 1988.
4. Avioli LJ: Significance of osteoporosis: A growing international health care problem. Calcif Tissue Int 49 (Suppl):55–57, 1991.
5. Bagge E, Bjelle A, Eden S, et al: Factors associated with radiographic osteoarthritis: Results from the population study: 70 year old people in Goteborg. J Rheumatol 18:1218–1222, 1991.

6. Basbaum AI, and Fields HL: Endogenous pain control systems: Brainstem spinal pathways and endorphin circuitry. Annu Rev Neurosci 7:309–338, 1984.
7. Bellamy N: Prognosis in rheumatoid arthritis. J Rheumatol 18:1277–1279, 1991.
8. Bellamy N, Buchanan W, and Goldsmith C: Validation study of WOMAC: A health status instrument for measuring clinically important outcomes to antirheumatic drug therapy of patients with osteoarthritis of the hip or knee. J Rheumatol 15:1833–1840, 1988.
9. Birrell GJ, McQueen DS, Iggo A, et al: The effects of 5-HT on articular sensory receptors in normal and arthritic rats. Br J Pharmacol 101:715–721, 1990.
10. Bisgaard H, and Kristensen JK: Leuokotriene B4 produces hyperalgesia in humans. Prostaglandins 30:791–797, 1985.
11. Bjurholm A, Kreibergs A, Brodin E, et al: Substance P and CGRP-immunoreactive nerves in bone. Peptides 9:165–171, 1988.
12. Blake DR, Merry P, Unsworth J, et al: Hypoxic reperfusion injury in the inflamed human joint. Lancet 1:289–293, 1989.
13. Boers M, and Ramsden M: Long acting drug combinations in rheumatoid arthritis—a formal review. J Rheumatol 18:316–324, 1991.
14. Bradley JD, Brandt KD, Katz BP, et al: Comparison of an antiinflammatory dose of ibuprofen, an analgesic dose of ibuprofen and acetaminophen in the treatment of patients with osteoarthritis of the knee. N Engl J Med 325:87–91, 1991.
15. Brook A, and Corbett M: Radiographic change in early rheumatoid disease. Ann Rheum Dis 36:71–73, 1973.
16. Brooks PM: Medical management of rheumatoid arthritis—slow acting drugs. Rheumatology Reviews 1:137–145, 1992.
17. Brooks PM, Day RO: Nonsteroidal antiinflammatory drugs—differences and similarities. N Engl J Med 324:1716–1725, 1991.
18. Bruce AN: Vasodilator axon reflexes. Quarterly Journal of Experimental Physiology 6:339–354, 1913.
19. Bunning RD, and Materson RS: A rational program of exercise for patients with osteoarthritis. Semin Arthritis Rheum 21 (Supp 2):33–43, 1991.
20. Caldwell JR, and Furst DE: The efficacy and safety of low-dose corticosteroids for rheumatoid arthritis. Semin Arthritis Rheum 21:1–11, 1991.
21. Calvino B, Villanueva L, and Lebars D: Dorsal horn convergent neurons in arthritic rats. I. Segmental excitatory influences. Pain 28:81–98, 1987.
22. Campbell JN, Raja SN, Meyer RA, et al: Myelinated afferents signal the hyperalgesia associated with nerve injury. Pain 32:89–94, 1988.
23. Celander O, Folkow B: The nature of the distribution of afferent fibres provided with the axon reflex arrangement. Acta Physiol Scand 29:359–370, 1953.
24. Champion GD: The therapeutic use of nonsteroidal anti-inflammatory drugs. Med J Aust 149 203–213, 1988.
25. Chrischilles EA, Butler CD, David CS, et al: A model of lifetime osteoporosis: Impact. Arch Intern Med 151:2026–2032, 1991.
26. Clark P, Tugwell P, Bennett K, et al: Meta-analysis of injectable gold in RA. J Rheumatol 16:442–447, 1989.
27. Coderre TJ, Basbaum AI, and Levine JD: Neural control of vascular permeability: Interactions between primary afferents, mast cells and sympathetic efferents. J Neurophysiol 62:48–58, 1989.
28. Colpaert FC, Donnerer J, and Lembeck F. Effects of capsaicin on inflammation and on the substance P content of nervous tissue in rats with adjuvant arthritis. Life Sci 32:1827–1834, 1983.
29. Colwell CW Jr: The controversy of core decompression of the femoral head for osteonecrosis. Arthritis Rheum 32:797–800, 1989.
30. Cunningham LS, and Kelsey JL: Epidemiology of musculoskeletal impairments and associated disability. Am J Public Health 74:574–579, 1984.
31. Davis MA, Ettinger WH, and Neuhams JM: Obesity and osteoarthritis of the knee: Evidence from the National Health and Nutrition Examination Survey (N HANES-1). Semin Arthritis Rheum 20 (Suppl 1):34–41, 1990.
32. Dorn T, Schaible H-G, and Schmidt RF: Response properties of thick myelinated group II afferents in the medical articular nerve of normal and inflamed knee joints of the cat. Somatosens Mot Res 8:127–136, 1991.
33. Dubner R: Neuronal plasticity and pain following peripheral tissue inflammation or nerve injury. In Bond MR, Charlton JE, and Woolf CJ (eds): Proc. VIth World Congress on Pain. Elsevier, Amsterdam, 1991, pp 263–276.
34. Dubner R: Neuronal plasticity in the spinal and medullary dorsal horns: A possible role in central pain mechanisms. In Casey KL (ed): Pain and Central Nervous System Disease: The Central Pain Syndromes. Raven Press, New York, 1991, pp 143–155.
35. Engel G: The clinical application of the biopsychosocial model. Am J Psychiatry 137:535–544, 1980.
36. Erhardt CC, Mumford PA, Venables PJW, et al: Factors predicting a poor life prognosis in rheumatoid arthritis: An eight-year prospective study. Ann Rheum Dis 48:7–13, 1989.
37. Fearn HJ, Kárády S, and West GB: The role of the nervous system in local inflammatory response. J Pharm Pharmacol 17:761–765, 1965.
38. Feinmann C: Pain relief by antidepressants: Possible modes of action. Pain 23:1–8, 1985.
39. Felson DT: The epidemiology of knee osteoarthritis: Results from the Framingham Osteoarthritis Study. Semin Arthritis Rheum 20 (Suppl 1):42–50, 1990.
40. Felson DT, and Anderson JJ: A cross-study evaluation of association between steroid dose and bolus steroids and avascular necrosis of bone. Lancet 1:902–905, 1987.
41. Felson D, Anderson J, and Meenan R: The comparative efficacy and toxicity of second-line drugs in rheumatoid arthritis. Arthritis Rheum 33:1449–1461, 1990.
42. Felson DT, Anderson JJ, and Meenan RF: The efficacy and toxicity of combination therapy in rheumatoid arthritis. Arthritis Rheum 37:1487–1491, 1994.
43. Fishbain DA, Rosomoff HL, Rosomoff RS: Drug abuse, dependence and addiction in chronic pain patients. Clin J Pain 8:77–85, 1992.
44. Foreman JC: Peptides and neurogenic inflammation. Br Med Bull 43:386–400, 1987.

45. Freeman MAR, and Wyke B: The innervation of the knee joint. An anatomical and histological study in the cat. J Anat 101:505–532, 1967.

46. Freeman MAR, and Wyke B: Articular reflexes at the ankle joint: An electromyographic study of normal and abnormal influences of ankle-joint mechanoreceptors upon reflex activity in the leg muscles. Br J Surg 54:990–1001, 1967.

47. Fries JF: Evaluating the therapeutic approach to rheumatoid arthritis—the sawtooth strategy. J Rheumatol Suppl 22:12–15, 1990.

48. Fries JF, Spitz PW, and Young DY: The dimensions of health outcomes: The Health Assessment Questionnaire, disability and pain scales. J Rheumatol 9:789–793, 1982.

49. Fries JF, Williams CA, Ramey D, et al: The relative toxicity of disease-modifying antirheumatic drugs. Arthritis Rheum 36:297–306, 1993.

50. Furst DE: Rheumatoid arthritis. Practical use of medications. Postgrad Med 87:79–92, 1990.

51. Gebhart GF, and Ness TJ: Central mechanisms of visceral pain. Can J Physiol Pharmacol 69:627–634, 1991.

52. Grigg P, Schaible H-G, and Schmidt RF: Mechanical sensitivity of group II and IV afferents from the posterior articular nerve in normal and inflamed cat knee. J Neurophysiol 55:635–643, 1986.

53. Grönblad M, Konttinen YT, Korkola O, et al: Neuropeptides in synovium of patients with rheumatoid arthritis and osteoarthritis. J Rheumatol 15:1807–1810, 1988.

54. Guilbaud G: Peripheral and central electrophysiological mechanisms of joint and muscle pain. In Dubner R, Gebhart GF, and Bond MR (eds): Proc. Vth World Congress on Pain. Elsevier, Amsterdam, 1988, pp 201–215.

55. Guilbaud G: Central neurophysiological processing of joint pain on the basis of studies performed in normal animals and in models of experimental arthritis. Can J Physiol Pharmacol 69:637–646, 1991.

56. Guilbaud G, Iggo A, and Teggner R: Sensory changes in joint-capsule receptors of arthritic rats: Effect of aspirin. In Fields HL, Dubner R, and Cervero F (eds): Advances in Pain Research and Therapy, Vol 9. New York, Raven Press, 1986, pp 81–90.

57. Guilbaud G, Kayser V, Benoist JM, et al: Modifications in the responsiveness of rat ventrobasal thalamic neurons at different stages of carrageenan-produced inflammation. Brain Res 385:86–98, 1986.

58. Hardy JD, Wolff HG, and Goodell H: Experimental evidence on the nature of cutaneous hyperalgesia. J Clin Invest 29:115–140, 1950.

59. Hart DJ, and Spector TD. The relationship of obesity, fat distribution and osteoarthritis in women in the general population: The Chingford Study. J Rheumatol 20:331–335, 1993.

60. Hawley DJ, and Wolfe F: Anxiety and depression in patients with rheumatoid arthritis: A prospective study of 400 patients. J Rheumatol 15:932–941, 1988.

61. Henry DA: Side-effects of non steroidal anti-inflammatory drugs. Bailliers Clin Rheumatol 2:425–454, 1988.

62. Heppelman B, Pfeiffer A, Schaible H-G, et al: Effects of acetylsalicylic acid and indomethacin on single group III and IV sensory units from acutely inflamed joints. Pain 26:337–351, 1985.

63. Heppelman B, Schaible H-G, and Schmidt RF: Effects of prostaglandins E1 and E2 on the mechanosensitivity of group III afferents from normal and inflamed cat knee joints. In Fields HL, Dubner R, and Cervero F (eds): Advances in Pain Research and Therapy, Vol 9. New York, Raven Press, 1986, pp 91–102.

64. Hicks JE: Exercise in patients with inflammatory arthritis and connective tissue disease. Rheum Dis Clin North Am 16:845–870, 1990.

64a. Hochberg M. (ed): Epidemiology of rheumatic disease. Rheum Dis Clin North Am 3:499–789, 1990.

65. Hoheisel U, and Mense S: Long-term changes in discharge behaviour of cat dorsal horn neurones following noxious stimulation of deep tissues. Pain 36:239–247, 1989.

66. Holzer P: Local effector functions of capsaicin-sensitive sensory nerve endings: Involvement of tachykinins, calcitonin gene-related peptide and other neuropeptides. Neuroscience 24:739–768, 1988.

67. Hope PJ, Jarrott B, Schaible H-G, et al: Release and spread of immunoreactive neurokinin A in the cat spinal cord in a model of acute arthritis. Brain Res 533:292–299, 1990.

68. Hukkanen M, Konttinen YT, Rees RG, et al: Innervation of bone from healthy and arthritic rates by substance P and calcitonin-gene-related-peptide-containing sensory fibres. J Rheumatol 19:1252–1259, 1992.

69. Hylden JK, Nahin RL, Traub RJ, et al: Expansion of receptive fields of spinal lamina I projection neurons in rats with unilateral adjuvant-induced inflammation: The contribution of dorsal horn mechanisms. Pain 37:229–243, 1989.

70. Iannuzzi I, Dawson N, Zein N: Does drug therapy slow radiological deterioration in rheumatoid arthritis? New Engl J Med 309:1023–1028, 1983.

71. James MT, Cleland LG, Rofe AM, et al: Intra-articular pressure and the relationship between synovial perfusion and metabolic demand. J Rheumatol 17:529–535, 1990.

72. Janscó N, Janscó-Gábor A, and Szolcsányi J: Direct evidence for neurogenic inflammation and its prevention by denervation and by pretreatment with capsaicin. Br J Pharmacol 31:138–151, 1967.

73. Kanaka R, Schaible H-G, and Schmidt RF: Activation of fine articular afferent units by bradykinin. Brain Res 327:81–90, 1985.

74. Kazis LE, Meenan RF, and Anderson JJ: Pain in the rheumatic diseases: Investigations of a key health status component. Arthritis Rheum 26:1017–1022, 1983.

75. Keefe FJ, Caldwell DS, Queen KT, et al: Pain coping strategies in osteoarthritis patients. J Consult Clin Psychol 55:208–212, 1987.

76. Keefe FJ, Caldwell DS, Williams DA, et al: Pain coping skills training in the management of osteoarthritic knee pain: A comparative study. Behavioural Therapy 21:49–62, 1990.

77. Kellgren JH, and Samuel EP: The sensitivity and innervation of the articular capsule. J Bone Joint Surg Br 32:84–92, 1950.

78. Khan MA, and Kellner H: Immunogenetics of spondyloarthropathies. Rheum Dis Clin North Am 18:837–864, 1992.

79. Khan DA, and Khan MK: Diagnostic value of HLA-B27 testing in ankylosing spondylitis and Reiter's syndrome. Ann Intern Med 96:70–76, 1982.

80. Kidd BL, Mapp PI, Blake DR, et al: Neurogenic influences in arthritis. Ann Rheum Dis 49:649–652, 1990.

81. Kniffki K-D, Mense S, and Schmidt RF: Responses of group IV afferent units from skeletal muscle to stretch, contraction and chemical stimulation. Exp Brain Res 31:511–522, 1978.

82. Koh KC: Epidemiology of the rheumatic diseases. Curr Opin Rheumatol 4:138–144, 1992.

83. Kramer JS, Yelin EH, and Epstein WV: Social and economic impacts of four musculoskeletal conditions: A study using national community-based data. Arthritis Rheum 26:901–907, 1983.

84. Kushner I: C-reactive protein in rheumatology. Arthritis Rheum 34:1065–1067, 1991.

85. Lam FY, and Ferrell WR: Inhibition of carrageenan-induced inflammation in the rat knee by substance P antagonist. Ann Rheum Dis 48:928–932, 1989.

86. Langford LA, and Schmidt RF: Afferent and efferent axons in the medial and posterior articular nerves in the cat. Anat Rec 206:71–78, 1983.

87. Langman MJS: Ulcer complications and non steroidal anti-inflammatory drugs. Am J Med 84 (Suppl 2A):15–19, 1988.

88. Langman MJS: Epidemiological evidence on the association between peptic ulceration and anti-inflammatory drug use. Gastroenterology 96(Suppl 2):640–646, 1989.

89. Lawrence RC, and Hochberg MC: Osteoarthritis of the knee—comparisons of signs, symptoms and comorbid conditions in those with and without current knee pain. Arthritis Rheum 29 (Suppl 4):S16, 1986.

90. Leigh JP, and Fries JF: Mortality predictors among 263 patients with rheumatoid arthritis. J Rheumatol 18:1307–1312, 1991.

91. Leigh JP, and Fries JF: Predictors of disability in a longitudinal sample of patients with rheumatoid arthritis. Ann Rheum Dis 51:581–587, 1992.

92. Levine JD, Clark R, Devor M, et al: Intraneuronal substance P contributes to the severity of experimental arthritis. Science 226:547–549, 1984.

93. Levine JD, Dardick SJ, Roizen MF, et al: Contribution of sensory afferents and sympathetic efferents to joint injury in experimental arthritis. J Neurosci 6:3243–3429, 1986.

94. Levine JD, Fye K, Heller PH, et al: Clinical response to regional guanethidine in patients with rheumatoid arthritis. J Rheumatol 13:1040–1043, 1986.

95. Levine JD, Goetzl EJ, and Basbaum AI: Contribution of the nervous system to the pathophysiology of rheumatoid arthritis and other polyarthritides. Rheum Dis Clin North Am 13:369–383, 1987.

96. Lewis T: Experiments relating to cutaneous hyperalgesia and its spread through somatic nerves. Clin Sci (Colch) 2:373–421, 1936.

97. Lewis T, and Kellgren JH: Observations relating to referred pain, viscero-motor reflexes and other associated phenomena. Clin Sci (Colch) 4:47–71, 1942.

98. Liang MH, and Fortin P: Management of osteoarthritis of the hip and knee. N Engl J Med 325:125–127, 1991.

99. Loeser JD: Concepts of pain. In Stanton-Hicks M, and Boas R (eds): Chronic Low Back Pain. Raven Press, Amsterdam, 1982.

100. Lotz M, Carson DA, and Vaughan JH: Substance P activation of rheumatoid synoviocytes: Neural pathways in the pathogenesis of arthritis. Science 235:893–895, 1987.

101. Lundberg JM, Terenius L, Hökfelt L, et al: Neuropeptide Y-like immunoreactivity in peripheral noradrenergic neurons and effects of neuropeptide Y on sympathetic function. Acta Physiol Scand 116:477–480, 1982.

102. Magerl W, Szolcsányi J, Westerman RA, et al: Laser Doppler measurement of skin vasodilatation elicited by percutaneous electrical stimulation of nociceptors in humans. Neurosci Lett 82:349–354, 1987.

103. Mapp PI, Kidd BL, Gibson SJ, et al: Substance P, CGRP and neuropeptide Y-immunoreactive nerve fibres are present in normal synovium but depleted in patients with rheumatoid arthritis. Neuroscience 37:43–153, 1990.

104. Matucci-Cerini M, and Partsch G: The contribution of the peripheral nervous system and the neuropeptide network to the development of synovial inflammation. Clin Exp Rheumatol 10:211–215, 1992.

105. McDaniel LK, Anderson LA, Bradley LA, et al: Development of an observation method for assessing pain behaviour in rheumatoid arthritis patients. Pain 24:165–184, 1986.

106. McFarlane AC, and Brooks PM: An analysis of the relationship between psychological morbidity and disease activity in rheumatoid arthritis. J Rheumatol 15:926–931, 1988.

107. McMahon S, and Koltzenburg, M: The changing role of primary afferent neurons in pain. Pain 43: 269–272, 1991.

108. Meenan RF, Gertman PM, and Mason JH: Measuring health status in arthritis: The Arthritis Impact Measurement Scales. Arthritis Rheum 23:277–284, 1980.

109. Meenan RF, Gertman PM, Mason JH, et al: The Arthritis Impact Measurement Scale. Further investigation of a health status measure. Arthritis Rheum 25:1048–1053, 1982.

110. Menétrey D, and Besson JM: Electrophysiological characteristics of dorsal horn cells in rats with cutaneous inflammation resulting from chronic arthritis. Pain 13:343–364, 1982.

111. Menétrey D, Chaouch A, and Besson JM: Location and properties of dorsal horn neurons at origin of spinoreticular tract in lumbar enlargement of the rat. J Neurophysiol 44:862–877, 1980.

112. Mense S: Considerations concerning the neurobiological basis of muscle pain. Can J Physiol Pharmacol 69:610–616, 1991.

113. Mitchell MD, Kundel HL, Steinberg ME, et al: Avascular necrosis of the hip: Comparison of MR, CT and scintigraphy. American Journal of Roentgenology 147:67–71, 1986.

114. Morrison NA, Qi JC, Tokito A, et al: Prediction of bone mineral density by vitamin D receptor alleles. Nature 367:284–287, 1994.

115. Namey TC (ed): Exercise and arthritis. Rheum Dis Clin North Am 16:1–1023, 1990.

116. Neugebauer V, and Schaible H-G: Peripheral and spinal components of the sensitization of spinal

neurones during an experimental acute arthritis. Agents Actions 25:234–237, 1988.

117. Neugebauer V, and Schaible H-G: Evidence for a central component in the sensitisation of spinal neurons with joint input during development of acute arthritis in the cat's knee. J Neurophysiol 64:299–311, 1990.

118. Neugebauer V, Schaible H-G, and Schmidt RF: Sensitization of articular afferents to joint stimuli by bradykinin. Pflugers Arch 415:330–335, 1989.

119. Onghena P, and Van Houdenhove B: Antidepressant-induced analgesia in chronic nonmalignant pain: A meta-analysis of 39 placebo-controlled studies. Pain 49:205–219, 1992.

120. Paintal AS: Functional analysis of group III afferent fibres of mammalian muscles. J Physiol (Lond) 152:250–270, 1960.

121. Panayi GS, Lanchbury JSS, and Kingsley G (eds): First International Symposium on the Immunotherapy of the Rheumatoid Diseases. Br J Rheumatol 30 (Suppl 2):3–9, 1991.

122. Panush RS: Does exercise cause arthritis? Longterm consequences of exercise on the musculoskeletal system. Rheum Dis Clin North Am 16:827–836, 1990.

123. Parker JC, Frank RG, Beck NC, et al: Pain management in rheumatoid arthritis patients: A cognitive-behavioural approach. Arthritis Rheum 31:593–601, 1988.

124. Parker JC, Smarr KL, Buescher KL, et al: Pain control and rational thinking; implications for rheumatoid arthritis. Arthritis Rheum 32:984–990, 1989.

125. Paulus H: The use of combinations of disease-modifying antirheumatic agents in rheumatoid arthritis. Arthritis Rheum 33:113–120, 1991.

126. Pepys MB: C-reactive protein and the acute phase response. Immunol Today 3:27–30, 1982.

127. Pereira da Silva JA, and Carmo-Fonseca M: Peptide-containing nerves in human synovium: Immunochemical evidence for decreased innervation in rheumatoid arthritis. J Rheumatol 17:1592–1599, 1990.

128. Piletta P, Porchet HC, and Dayer P: Distinct central nervous system involvement of paracetamol and salicylate. In Bond MR, Charlton JE, and Woolf CJ (eds): Proc. VIth World Congress on Pain. Elsevier, Amsterdam, 1991, pp 181–184.

129. Pincus T, and Callaghan LF: Taking mortality in rheumatoid arthritis seriously—predictive markers, socio-economic status and co-morbidity. J Rheumatol 13:841–845, 1986.

130. Pincus T, and Callaghan LF: Rheumatology function tests: Grip strength, walking time, button test and questionnaires document and predict longterm morbidity and mortality in rheumatoid arthritis. J Rheumatol 19:1051–1057, 1992.

131. Pincus T, Callaghan LF, Brooks RH, et al: Self report questionnaire scores in rheumatoid arthritis compared with traditional physical, radiographic and laboratory measures. Ann Intern Med 110:259–266, 1989.

132. Portenoy RK: Chronic opioid therapy in nonmalignant pain. Journal of Pain and Symptom Management 5(1S):S46–S62, 1990.

133. Price DD, Long S, and Huitt C: Sensory testing of pathophysiological mechanisms of pain in patients with reflex sympathetic dystrophy. Pain 49:163–173, 1992.

134. Quam JP, Michet CJ, Wilson MG, et al: Total knee arthroplasty: A population-based study. Mayo Clin Proc 66:589–595, 1991.

135. Raja SN, Meyer RA, and Campbell JN: Peripheral mechanisms of somatic pain. Anesthesiology 68:571–590, 1988.

136. Ralston HJ, Miller MR, and Kasahara M: Nerve endings in human fasciae, tendons, ligaments, periosteum and joint synovial membrane. Anat Rec 136:137–147, 1960.

137. Roberts WJ: A hypothesis on the physiological basis for causalgia and related pains. Pain 24:297–311, 1986.

138. Sambrook PN, Cohen ML, Eisman JA, et al: Effects of low dose corticosteroids on bone mass in rheumatoid arthritis: A longitudinal study. Ann Rheum Dis 48:535–538, 1989.

139. Samuel EP: The autonomic and somatic innervation of the articular capsule. Anat Rec 113:84–93, 1952.

140. Schaible H-G, Jarrott B, Hope PJ, et al: Release of immunoreactive substance P in the spinal cord during development of acute arthritis in the cat: A study with antibody microprobes. Brain Res 529:214–223, 1990.

141. Schaible H-G, Neugebauer V, Cervero F, et al: Changes in tonic descending inhibition of spinal neurons with articular input during the development of acute arthritis in the cat. J Neurophysiol 66:1021–1032, 1991.

142. Schaible H-G, and Schmidt RF: Effects of an experimental arthritis of the sensory properties of fine articular afferent units. J Neurophysiol 54:1109–1122, 1985.

143. Schaible H-G, and Schmidt RF: Direct observations of the sensitisation of articular afferents during an experimental arthritis. In Dubner R, Gebhart GF, and Bond MR (eds): Proc Vth World Congress on Pain. Elsevier, Amsterdam, 1988, pp 44–50.

144. Schaible H-G, and Schmidt RF: Time course of mechanosensitivity changes in articular afferents during a developing experimental arthritis. J Neurophysiol 60:2180–2195, 1988.

145. Schaible H-G, and Schmidt RF: Excitation and sensitisation of fine articular afferents from cat's knee joint by prostaglandin E2. J Physiol (Lond) 403P:91–104, 1988.

146. Schaible H-G, and Schmidt RF: Tonic descending inhibition of spinal cord neurones driven by joint afferents in normal cats and in cats with an inflamed knee joint. Exp Brain Res 83:675–678, 1991.

147. Schaible H-G, Schmidt RF, and Willis WD: Convergent inputs from articular, cutaneous and muscle receptors onto ascending tracts in the cat spinal cord. Exp Brain Res 66:479–488, 1987.

148. Schaible H-G, Schmidt RF, and Willis WD: Enhancement of the responses of ascending tract cells in the cat spinal cord by acute inflammation of the knee joint. Exp Brain Res 66:489–499, 1987.

149. Seideman P, and Melander A: Equianalgesic effects of paracetomal and indomethacin in rheumatoid arthritis. Br J Rheumatol 27:117–122, 1988.

150. Steig RL, and Williams RC: Chronic pain as a biosociocultural phenomenon: Implications for treatment. Semin Neurol 3:370–376, 1983.

151. Stein C: Peripheral analgesic effects of opioids. Journal of Pain and Symptom Management 6:119–124, 1991.

152. Steinberg ME, and Steinberg DR: Osteonecrosis. In Kelley WN, Harris ED, Ruddy S, et al (eds): Textbook of Rheumatology, ed 3. Philadelphia: WB Saunders, 1989, pp 1750–1754.

153. Tonkin AL, and Wing LMH: Interactions of non-steroidal anti-inflammatory drugs. Baillieres Clin Rheum 2:455–484, 1988.

154. Tosteson ANA, Rosenthal DI, Melton LJ, et al: Cost effectiveness of screening perimenopausal white women for osteoporosis: Bone densitometry and hormone replacement therapy. Ann Intern Med 113:594–603, 1990.

155. Treede R-D, Meyer RA, Raja SN, et al: Peripheral and central mechanisms of cutaneous hyperalgesia. Prog Neurobiol 38:397–421, 1992.

156. Tugwell P, Bombardier C, Buchanan WW, et al: The MACTAR Patient Preference Disability Questionnaire—an individualised functional priority approach for assessing improvement in physical disability in clinical trials in rheumatoid arthritis. J Rheumatol 14:446–451, 1987.

157. Van Rythoven AW, Dysmans B, and The HSG: Long term cyclosporine therapy in RA. J Rheumatol 18:19–23, 1991.

158. Verbrugge LM: From sneezes to adieux: Stages of health for American men and women. In: Ward RA, and Tobin SS (eds): Health in Ageing: Sociological Issues and Policy Directions. Berlin: Springer, 1987, pp 17–57.

159. Verbrugge LM, Lepkowski JM, and Konkol LL: Levels of disability among U.S. adults with arthritis. J Gerontol 46:871–873, 1991.

160. Waddell G: A new clinical model for the treatment of low-back pain. Spine 12:632–644, 1987.

161. Watson CPN: Antidepressant drugs as adjuvant analgesics. Journal of Pain and Symptom Management 9:392–405, 1994.

162. White DM, Basbaum AI, Goetzl EJ, et al: The 15-lipoxygenase product, 8R, 15S-diHETE stereospecifically sensitises C-fiber mechanoheat receptors in hair skin of rat. J Neurophysiol 63:966–970, 1990.

163. Williams HJ, Ward JR, Egger MK, et al: Comparison of naproxen and acetaminophen in a two-year study of treatment of osteoarthritis of the knee. Arthritis Rheum 36:1196–1206, 1993.

164. Wilson MG, Michet CJ, Ilstrum DM, et al: Idiopathic symptomatic osteoarthritis of the hip and knee: A population-based incidence study. Mayo Clin Proc 65:1214–1221, 1990.

165. Wolfe F, Cathey MA, and Roberts RK: The latex test revisited: Rheumatoid factor testing in 8,287 rheumatic disease patients. Arthritis Rheum 34:951–960, 1991.

166. Wolfe F, Hawley DJ, and Cathey MA: Clinical and health status measures over time: Prognosis and outcome assessment in rheumatoid arthritis. J Rheumatol 18:1290–1297, 1991.

167. Wolfe F, Hawley DJ, and Lathem MA: Termination of slow acting anti-rheumatic drug therapy in rheumatoid arthritis—a 14 year prospective evaluation of 1017 consecutive starts. J Rheumatol 17:994–1002, 1990.

168. Wood PHN: Appreciating the consequences of disease: The international classification of impairments, disabilities and handicaps. WHO Chronicle 34:76–380, 1980.

169. Woolf CJ, and Wall P: Relative effectiveness of C primary fibres of different origins in evoking a prolonged facilitation of the flexor reflex in the rat. Neuroscience 6:1433–1442, 1986.

170. Wyke B: The neurology of joints: A review of general principles. Clin Rheum Dis 7:223–239, 1981.

171. Yaksh TL: Behavioural and autonomic correlates of the tactile evoked allodynia produced by spinal glycine inhibition: Effects of modulatory receptor systems and excitatory amino acid antagonist. Pain 37:111–123, 1989.

172. Yelin EH, and Felts WR: A summary of the impact of musculoskeletal conditions in the United States. Arthritis Rheum 33:750–755, 1990.

173. Zenz M, Strumpf M, and Tryba M: Long-term oral opioid therapy in patients with chronic nonmalignant pain. Journal of Pain and Symptom Management 7:69–77, 1992.

174. Zimmerman M: Pain mechanisms and mediators in osteoarthritis. Semin Arthritis Rheum 18:22–29, 1989.

CHAPTER 9

PAIN SYNDROMES IN PATIENTS WITH CANCER

Kathleen M. Foley, M.D.

TYPES OF PAIN SYNDROMES
ASSESSMENT OF CANCER PAIN
Principles of Assessment
PAIN SYNDROMES ASSOCIATED WITH
   TUMOR INVOLVEMENT
Headache From Intracranial Tumors
Cranial Neuralgias
Pain Syndromes Resulting From Bony
   Infiltration of the Skull
Tumor Infiltration of Nerve, Nerve Root,
   Plexus, Meninges, and Spinal Cord
Tumor Infiltration of Hollow Viscus
PAIN SYNDROMES ASSOCIATED WITH
   CANCER THERAPY
Postsurgical Pain Syndromes
Pain Syndromes After Chemotherapy
Pain Syndromes After Radiation Therapy

A scientifically based approach to the evaluation and treatment of cancer pain requires knowledge of the common pain syndromes in this population, as well as their postulated neurophysiologic and neuropharmacologic mechanisms.[30,47,94] This information is complemented by other classifications of patients with pain,[48,94] methodologies to measure pain, and algorithms for the use of analgesic drug therapy and adjunctive anesthetic, neurosurgical, and behavioral approaches.[69,99] Several studies confirm that pain can be treated effectively in a large majority of patients,[49] and patients must be reassured that pain control is usually possible.

Cancer pain is prevalent and extremely heterogeneous. Chronic pain occurs in one-third of patients in active therapy and in two-thirds of patients with advanced disease.[50,61] Pain usually results from tumor infiltration of pain-sensitive structures, such as bone, soft tissue, muscle, nerve, viscera, and blood vessels.* Less often, pain is caused by surgery, chemotherapy, or radiation therapy. Approximately 15 percent of patients with cancer develop neurologic complications,[36,56,102] and, among those requiring neurologic assessment, pain is the most common symptom.

The broad categorization of inferred pain mechanisms into nociceptive and neuropathic types (see Chapters 1 and 5) has been useful in the assessment of cancer pain.[47,94] Patients with cancer commonly have multiple pain complaints and mixed types of pain. Many patients experience pain that has both nociceptive and neuropathic components.[5,31,57,128,132] Neuropathic cancer pain may be produced by neural injury related to the neoplasm or by antineoplastic therapy. For example, nerve or plexus may be compressed or infiltrated by tumor or transected during surgery. Chemotherapy may produce axonal injury or changes in axoplas-

---

*References 71, 77, 84, 98, 100, 102, 107, 116, 118.

191

mic flow, and radiation injury can produce gliosis, fibrosis, and late vascular compromise.

TYPES OF PAIN SYNDROMES

Many pain syndromes are unique to the cancer population and are often misdiagnosed because health care professionals are unfamiliar with their clinical presentations. These syndromes can be categorized into three major groups. The first and most important is pain associated with direct tumor involvement. From studies at Memorial Sloan-Kettering Cancer Center (MSKCC), 78 percent of pain problems in an inpatient cancer population and 62 percent of pain problems in an outpatient cancer pain clinic population related directly to the neoplasm.[50] Metastatic bone disease, nerve compression or infiltration, and involvement of the viscera by either obstruction of the hollow viscus or diffuse peritoneal seeding are the most important causes.[65,77,107]

The second group of pain syndromes occurs during the course of, or as a result of, chemotherapy, surgery, or radiation therapy. Nineteen percent of pain problems in an inpatient cancer pain population and 25 percent of pain problems referred to an outpatient cancer pain clinic are due to cancer therapy.[50] Each syndrome has a characteristic clinical presentation that needs to be carefully differentiated from tumor-induced pain.

The third group of pain syndromes consists of pains that are not related to the cancer or the cancer therapy. Although figures vary, the MSKCC experience suggests that 3 percent of cancer inpatients with pain have such an etiology. This figure increases to 10 percent in an outpatient cancer pain population.[32,50] Accurate diagnosis in this group of patients can alter both therapy and prognosis.

ASSESSMENT OF CANCER PAIN

The management of cancer pain requires a careful neurologic assessment.[32] A survey of 851 patients evaluated for neurologic symptoms found that the three most common syndromes were back pain (18.2 percent), altered mental status (17.1 percent), and headache (15.4 percent) (Table 9–1, Figs. 9–1 and 9–2).[32] Of 133 patients with undiagnosed back and neck pain, 44 (33 percent) had epidural extension or metastases from tumor and 40 (30 percent) had pain associated with vertebral metastases only. In 15 patients (11 percent), the cause for the back pain was unrelated to metastatic disease. In contrast, of the 97 patients with undiagnosed headache, 59 (61 percent) had a nonstructural cause. This survey highlights the important role of the neurologic assessment in distinguishing cancer-related pain problems from those unrelated to the neoplasm.

Another study that assessed the impact of a comprehensive evaluation in the management of cancer pain further confirmed the importance of a neuro-oncologic evaluation in such patients.[57] Gonzales et al surveyed 276 consecutive inpatient consultations performed by a cancer pain service. This consultation identified a previously undiagnosed etiology for the pain in 64 percent of patients. Metastatic tumor was the most common lesion, and neurologic symptoms and signs were the most common presentation.

Principles of Assessment

Lack of attention to the principles of assessment (Table 9–2)[47] is the major cause of misdiagnosis. The physician must establish a trusting relationship with the patient and elicit a complete history of the pain complaint. The history should include the site, quality, and temporal pattern of the pain, exacerbating and relieving factors, and the degree to which pain interferes with activities of daily living, work, social life, and psychologic functioning. Multiple pain complaints are common, particularly in patients with advanced disease, and each pain must be prioritized and classified. In some instances, it may be necessary to acquire additional history from a family member because the patient is either unable or unwilling to detail the pain or its impact.

After a careful history, medical and neurologic examinations are needed to clarify a provisional diagnosis of the etiology and pathophysiology of the pain. Knowledge of pain referral patterns and the common cancer pain syndromes can direct the examination.[76]

Table 9–1. **NEUROLOGIC COMPLAINTS IN 851 PATIENTS WITH CANCER REFERRED TO THE MEMORIAL SLOAN-KETTERING CANCER CENTER NEUROLOGY SERVICE**

Complaint	No.	Percentage of Patients
Pain		
Back pain	155	18.2
Headache	131	15.4
Pain in a limb	112	13.2
Neck pain	23	2.7
Other Neurologic Complaints		
Altered mental status	146	17.2
Leg weakness	84	9.9
Ataxia or gait disturbance	75	8.8
Sensory disturbance	53	6.2
Visual disturbance or diplopia	49	5.8
Arm weakness	47	5.5
Seizures	46	5.4
Speech or language disturbance	36	4.2
Hemiparesis	32	3.8
Movement disorder	24	2.8
Syncope	21	2.5
Vertigo	20	2.4
Sphincter disturbance	18	2.1
Other	91	10.7
Total	*1,163*	

Source: Clouston PD, De Angelis L, and Posner JB: The spectrum of neurological disease in patients with systemic cancer. Reprinted with permission from Ann Neurol 31:269, 1992.

Figure 9–1. Principal neurologic diagnoses of 133 patients with cancer and undiagnosed back or neck pain. (From Clouston PD, De Angelis L, and Posner JB: The spectrum of neurological disease in patients with systemic cancer. Reprinted with permission from Ann Neurol 31:269, 1992.)

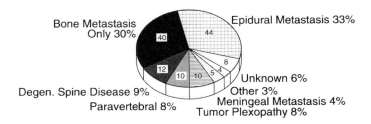

Figure 9–2. Principal neurologic diagnoses of 97 patients with cancer and undiagnosed headache. (From Clouston PD, De Angelis L, and Posner JB: The spectrum of neurological disease in patients with systemic cancer. Reprinted with permission from Ann Neurol 31:270, 1992.)

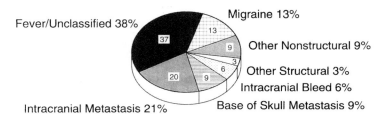

For example, the postmastectomy pain syndrome presents so characteristically that its recognition can help define the site and nature of the nerve injury responsible for the pain.[58]

Each pain requires a specific diagnostic approach designed to establish the underlying cause and clarify its relationship to the disease. Plain radiographs, bone scintigraphy, computed tomography (CT), and magnetic resonance imaging (MRI) all have their place in helping to define the nature of the pain in this population.[66] In some instances, algorithms have been developed to assist in targeting the evaluation. For example, in the patient with back pain (Fig. 9–3), the differential diagnosis of vertebral body collapse includes both osteoporosis and vertebral body metastasis, with or without associated epidural disease. The lesion can usually be distinguished by the history and the characteristic appearance of bony changes on CT and MRI scans. In all cases, the physician ordering the diagnostic procedures should personally review them with the radiologist to correlate pathologic changes with the site of pain.

No patient should be inadequately evaluated because of an uncontrolled pain. Early management of the pain while its cause is being investigated will markedly improve the patient's ability to participate in the necessary diagnostic procedures.

By clarifying the relationship between the pain and the underlying neoplasm, it is usually possible to identify recurrence or progression of disease. For example, in a patient with carcinoma of the lung, the presence of recurrent disease is closely associated with the appearance of a late postthoracotomy pain following initial resolution of postoperative pain in the surgical site.[73]

The patient's psychologic state also should be evaluated carefully. The psychiatric history, current level of anxiety or depression, suicidal ideation, and degree of functional incapacity are all critical in developing an appropriate management plan. Depression occurs in as many as 25 percent of patients,[20,67] and uncontrolled pain is a major factor in cancer-related suicide.

PAIN SYNDROMES ASSOCIATED WITH TUMOR INVOLVEMENT

Detailed description of cancer-related pain syndromes, both acute and chronic, can be found in recent reviews and textbooks.[30,48,94] Common syndromes are described in the following sections.

Table 9–2. **CLINICAL ASSESSMENT OF PAIN**

1. Believe the patient's complaint of pain.
2. Take a careful history of the pain complaint to place it temporally in the patient's cancer history.
3. Assess the characteristics of each pain, including its site, its pattern of referral, and its aggravating and relieving factors.
4. Clarify the temporal aspects of the pain: acute, subacute, chronic, episodic, intermittent, breakthrough, or incident.
5. List and prioritize each pain complaint.
6. Evaluate the response to previous and current analgesic therapies.
7. Evaluate the psychologic state of the patient.
8. Ask if the patient has a history of alcohol or drug dependence.
9. Perform a careful medical and neurologic examination.
10. Order and personally review the appropriate diagnostic procedures.
11. Treat the patient's pain to facilitate the necessary work-up.
12. Design the diagnostic and therapeutic approach to suit the individual.
13. Provide continuity of care from evaluation to treatment to ensure patient compliance and to reduce patient anxiety.
14. Reassess the patient's response to pain therapy.
15. Discuss advance directives with the patient and the family.

Source: Foley KM: Pain assessment and cancer pain. In Doyle D, Hanks GW, and MacDonald RN (eds): Oxford Textbook of Palliative Medicine. Oxford University Press, Oxford, 1933, p 156, with permission.

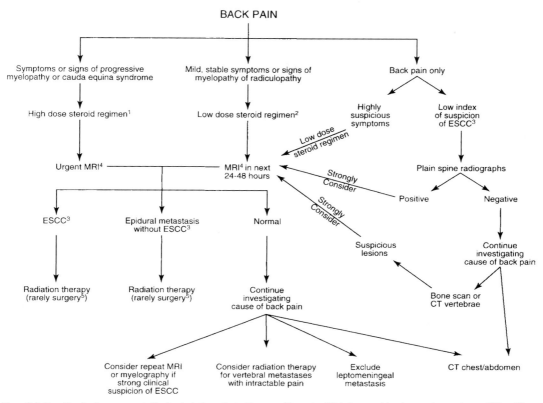

Figure 9–3. Algorithm for the assessment of back pain in the patient with cancer. [1]Example of high-dose steroid regimen = dexamethasone 100 mg IV stat followed by dexamethasone 24 mg 96h, with slow taper over weeks. [2]Example of low-dose steroid regimen = dexamethasone 16 mg followed by dexamethasone 4 mg 96h, with slow taper over weeks. [3]ESCC = epidural spinal cord compression. [4]In patients with known metastatic disease, a complete spinal MRI is recommended because of data indicating that additional epidural lesions will be discovered in > 10% of cases. [5]Surgery is considered in select circumstances; see text.(Adapted from Portenoy RK, Lipton RB, and Foley KM: Back pain in the cancer patient: An algorithm for evaluation and management. Neurology 37:135, 1987.)

Headache From Intracranial Tumors

Head pain in the patient with cancer can result from traction, inflammation, or infiltration of pain-sensitive vascular or neural structures. Pain can be experienced in the distribution of the trigeminal, glossopharyngeal, vagus, and other cervical nerves.[31,52,96]

Estimates of the incidence of headache in patients with brain tumors range from 36 to 80 percent.[32,103] In a recent study, Forsyth and Posner elicited a complaint of headache from 48 percent of 111 patients with brain tumors (Table 9–3).[52] Prevalence was similar in patients with primary tumors or metastatic disease,[52] and most headaches were "mild to moderate" in severity. Tension-type headaches were described by 75 percent of patients, migraine by about 10

percent, and other types of headaches by 15 percent. The typical headache was an ache, pressure, or "sinus headache," located bifrontally, and worse ipsilaterally. Among those with headache, it was the worst symptom in 45 percent.

In 85 percent of patients, brain tumor headache is different from headaches experienced previously. Knowledge of the specific features of brain tumor headaches, therefore, may help the clinician differentiate benign headache from those requiring further investigation. Usually, however, it is not the quality of the headache but its course or the appearance of other symptoms or signs that suggest a brain tumor. In the study by Clouston et al,[31] headaches represented 15.4 percent of the requests for neurologic consultation, and nonmetastatic causes were more common than metastatic causes.[31,96]

Table 9–3. **FREQUENCY OF HEADACHE IN PATIENTS WITH BRAIN TUMORS ACCORDING TO LOCATION OF TUMOR**

Type	Number of Patients With Headaches	Number of Patients Without Headaches
Supratentorial tumors	25 (39%)	39 (61%)
Infratentorial tumors	9 (82%)	2 (18%)
Tumors that are both supratentorial and infratentorial	8 (47%)	9 (53%)
Dural-based tumors	5 (45%)	6 (55%)
Leptomeningeal without structural tumors	6 (75%)	2 (25%)
Total	53 (48%)	58 (52%)

Source: Forsyth PA, and Posner JB: Intracranial neoplasm. In Olesen J, Tfelt-Hansen P, and Welch KMA (eds): The Headaches. Raven Press, New York, 1993, p 712, with permission.

Cranial Neuralgias

PAINFUL TRIGEMINAL NEUROPATHY

A pain syndrome that mimics classical trigeminal neuralgia can herald middle or posterior fossa tumors.[28] Trigeminal neuralgia also has been reported as a presentation of lymphomatous meningitis.[35] Continuous facial pain, which may be dysesthetic, can also occur with nerve involvement outside the skull or at its base.[40] For example, squamous carcinomas of the face can cause pain mediated by perineural spread along the trigeminal nerve and invasion of the base of the skull.[3,10,23,32,37,39,86]

REFERRED FACIAL PAIN SYNDROME

Facial pain can result from tumor involvement of the lung (Table 9–4).[9,13,17,92] Most patients describe a constant, aching, sometimes sharp pain, which may have a paroxysmal component. This pain is usually located in the ear and temporal region, and occasionally in the jaw. In the largest series, 12 of the 16 patients had right-sided predominance. The etiology of the pain referral pattern is thought to be vagal in origin, which may also explain the right-sided predominance because of the close anatomic relationship of the right vagus to the trachea and mediastinal lymph nodes. Surgery (vagotomy, or resection of the neoplasm and nodes) or radiation therapy to the lung may relieve the pain.[9]

PAINFUL GLOSSOPHARYNGEAL NEUROPATHY

Glossopharyngeal neuralgia associated with syncope and hypotension has been reported in patients with leptomeningeal metastases, the jugular foramen syndrome, and head and neck malignancies.[85,120,137] In the latter group of patients, severe pain in the neck or temporal area that can radiate to the ear and mastoid may be the prodrome to a syncopal episode. Evaluation of this syndrome can lead to the diagnosis of a head and neck tumor.

Pain Syndromes Resulting From Bony Infiltration of the Skull

The syndromes associated with neoplastic invasion of the base of the skull are well recognized.[60] They are common in patients with nasopharyngeal tumors but may occur with any type of tumor that metastasizes to bone. Pain is usually the first complaint, often preceding neurologic signs and symptoms by weeks or months. The lesion may be difficult to identify even with CT or MRI. Early treatment is associated with the greatest improvement of neurologic function.

ORBITAL SYNDROME

The first symptom of the orbital syndrome is progressive, continuous pain in the supraorbital area of the affected eye. Blurred vision is followed by diplopia. Examination reveals proptosis of the involved eye and

Table 9–4. **REFERRED FACIAL PAIN: CLINICAL FEATURES IN 16 CASES***

Age/Sex	Duration/Type of Pain	Location of Pain	CT of Brain	Type of Lung Carcinoma	Left/Right	Treatment	Effect on Pain
45/M	4 mo/constant, deep, boring	Maxilla; later, face and neck	Normal	Adeno	R	Vagotomy	Good
60/M	4 mo/vague aching and shooting	Lower jaw and ear; later, oropharynx	NP	Adeno	R	Vagotomy	—
53/F	10 wk/"pain"	Temporal, ear	Normal	Poorly differentiated	L	—	—
62/F	3 yr/aching	Ear, jaw	Normal	Small-cell	R	RT	Good
59/F	4 yr/aching	Temporomandibular; later, face and ear	Normal	Squamous cell	R	RT	Good
39/F	4 mo/—	Ear and throat; later, face	NP	Undifferentiated	R	RT	Good
54/M	4 wk/sharp, lasting hours	Eye, face	Normal	No histology	L	RT	Good
48/M	4 mo/aching	Ear and jaw; later, face	NP	Squamous cell	R	RT	Good
34/M	9 mo/constant, nagging ache	Teeth and jaws; later, ear	Normal	Adeno	R	Chemo/RT	Good
69/F	16 mo/aching, episodes of sharp pain	Lower jaw, forehead, ear	NP	Adeno	R	RT	Good
78/M	12–18 mo/aching	Ear and eye; later, face	NP	Adeno	R	Lobectomy	Moderate
53/F	12 mo/constant, severe aching	Teeth, ear, nostrum	Normal	Adeno	R	RT	Good
38/F	8 mo/dull aching	Teeth, ear	Normal	Poorly differentiated	R	RT	Good
40/M	2 mo/long-lasting bouts of severe pain	Cheek, ear	Normal	Adeno	L	Lobectomy plus nodectomy	Good
60/F	8 mo/sharp pain	Temporal, ear	Normal	Small-cell	L†	Chemo	Good
47/F	3 mo/continuous burning	Jaw, ear, temporal	Normal	Adeno	R	None	—

*Chemo = chemotherapy; L = left; NP = not performed; R = right; RT = radiation therapy.
†Later, bilateral.
Source: Bongers KM, Willigers MM, and Koehler PJ: Referred facial pain from lung carcinoma. Neurology 42:1841, 1992, with permission.

external ophthalmoparesis. Decreased sensation may occur in the ophthalmic division of the trigeminal nerve.

PARASELLAR SYNDROME

Parasellar syndrome usually presents as unilateral supraorbital and frontal headache. Pain is followed by diplopia without proptosis. There may be associated papilledema.

MIDDLE FOSSA SYNDROME

As noted, patients with neoplastic invasion of the middle fossa present with numbness, paresthesias, and pain referred to the second or third divisions of the trigeminal nerve. Most patients experience a dull ache in the cheek or jaw, but some patients experience a pain that is similar to trigeminal neuralgia, without trigger points. With growth of the tumor, sensory symptoms may be accompanied by other disturbances, including diplopia, headache, dysarthria, and dysphagia. The neurologic signs include sensory loss in the trigeminal nerve distribution as well as weakness of pterygoids and masseters, abducens palsy, and other ocular palsies.

JUGULAR FORAMEN SYNDROME

Occipital pain referred to the vertex of the head and ipsilateral shoulder and arm is an early symptom of the jugular foramen syndrome. Head movement often exacerbates the pain, and local tenderness may be present over the occipital condyle. The development of signs and symptoms consistent with dysfunction of cranial nerves IX, I, and XI localizes the lesion. These signs may include hoarseness, dysarthria, dysphagia, and neck and shoulder weakness. Involvement of adjacent structures may lead to a Horner's syndrome and tongue weakness (involvement of cranial nerve XII at the hypoglossal canal).

CLIVUS METASTASES

Vertex headache exacerbated by neck flexion is the most common presentation of tumor involving the clivus. Lower cranial nerve dysfunction (VI to XII) usually begins unilaterally and progresses to involve both sides.

SPHENOID SINUS METASTASES

Severe bifrontal headache that radiates to both temples and may be associated with intermittent retro-orbital pain suggests sphenoid sinus metastases. The patient may complain of nasal stuffiness or a sense of fullness in the head. Diplopia may occur, usually as a result of either unilateral or bilateral sixth nerve palsies.

ODONTOID FRACTURE

Occipital and nuchal pain can result from pathologic fracture of the odontoid process. Secondary subluxation can result in spinal cord or brainstem compression. Initially, patients report severe neck pain and stiffness. The pain characteristically radiates over the posterior aspect of the skull to the vertex and is exacerbated by neck movement, particularly flexion. The examination may be normal at first. If sensory and motor dysfunctions occur, they may begin in the upper extremities and be associated with autonomic signs. In the evaluation of these patients, neck radiographs in flexion and extension may be helpful but must be performed cautiously. MRI may be necessary to confirm the diagnosis.

OTHER SKULL LESIONS

Lesions of the calvarium can produce localized pain. These lesions usually have exophytic growth but can invade and spread to the meninges (dural deposits or leptomeningeal spread) and can cause saggital sinus occlusion, intracranial hypertension, and seizures.

Jaw metastases can be locally painful and are often heralded by a painless "numb chin" syndrome.[15,21,88] Although the numb chin is usually due to a lesion in the jaw at the mental foramen, it can also be associated with disease at the base of the skull, leptomeningeal tumor, or local perineural spread of a squamous lip carcinoma.

Tumor Infiltration of Nerve, Nerve Root, Plexus, Meninges, and Spinal Cord

PERIPHERAL NERVE

Peripheral nerves are most commonly infiltrated by tumors that invade the chest wall or the paravertebral or retroperitoneal spaces.[86,87] These lesions typically produce unilateral pain in a radicular distribution. A careful sensory examination can delineate the site of nerve compression. CT and MRI scanning are most helpful to document the anatomic region of nerve compression and exclude extension into the intervertebral foramen or epidural space.[73,80]

Peripheral nerve compression in the buttock, thigh, or more distally in a limb occurs more rarely. For example, femoral and sciatic neuropathies can occur from a tumor, often a sarcoma, that involves the anterior or posterior region of the thigh, and peroneal mononeuropathy can occur with lesions of the head of the fibula or popliteal fossa sarcomas. Rogers reported six patients with obturator mononeuropathy as the sole clinical manifestation of new or recurrent pelvic cancer (Table 9–5).[110] Diagnosis was delayed in four patients because the clinical signs were confused with lumbar radiculopathy, plexopathy, or inguinal hernia. The pain was typically in the groin and anterior or medial thigh, and weakness occurred in flexion and adduction. Patients with cancer who present with these symptoms should undergo a pelvic CT or MRI to exclude pelvic tumor.

Tumor-related mononeuropathies usually produce constant dysesthesias in the area of sensory loss.

PAINFUL PERIPHERAL NEUROPATHIES

Paraneoplastic painful peripheral neuropathy can be the initial manifestation of an underlying malignancy (see Chapter 5).[84,102] With the exception of the neuropathy associated with myeloma, the course of these neuropathies is usually independent of the primary tumor.

Sensory Neuronopathy. A paraneoplastic sensory neuronopathy is characterized by tingling sensations in the extremities, burning paresthesias, sensory ataxia (with marked impairment of joint position sense), and, occasionally, lancinating pains. The syndrome results from an inflammatory lesion of the dorsal root ganglion, which may be part of a more generalized process that affects the limbic region, brainstem, and spinal cord. The course of this dorsal root ganglionitis is independent of the primary tumor and does not appear to improve with treatment of the underlying malignancy. It is most often associated with small-cell carcinoma of the lung and occasionally with other carcinomas, including breast, ovary, and colon.[102]

Sensorimotor Peripheral Neuropathy. The sensorimotor peripheral neuropathy associated with cancer may produce dysesthesias and sensory loss, muscle wasting and weakness, or both. Rarely, this disorder presents as a Guillain-Barré syndrome.

Neuropathy is prevalent among those with multiple myeloma. Clinical evidence of peripheral neuropathy occurs in 10 to 15 percent of these patients, and electrophysiologic evidence can be found in 40 percent. The neuropathy precedes detection of the myeloma in 80 percent of the patients.[102]

NERVE ROOT

Malignant radiculopathy usually results from tumor infiltration of the vertebrae or paraspinal space. Leptomeningeal disease may present similarly but typically has polyradicular symptoms or signs. A root lesion can produce focal back pain or pain in a radicular distribution. At times, it is difficult to distinguish radiculopathy from a plexus lesion.[111] Electrodiagnostic studies, CT scanning, and MRI can be helpful in localizing the lesion. MRI is necessary to fully image the epidural space.[80]

C-7 to T-1 Radiculopathy. Metastatic disease to the C-7 to T-1 vertebral bodies may produce dull, aching pain that is localized to the adjacent paraspinal area and radiates to the shoulders. There is often tenderness over the spinous process at this level. Radicular pain may occur in the posterior arm, elbow, and ulnar aspect of the hand. The pain usually precedes other symptoms or signs for weeks to months. In the absence of local pathology, the development of progressive pain in the elbow, shoulder, or hand should

Table 9–5. CLINICAL AND PELVIC CT FEATURES IN SIX PATIENTS WITH OBTURATOR MONONEUROPATHY CAUSED BY PELVIC CANCER

Patient	Tumor Type and Status	Location of Pain	Weakness on Examination	Leg Edema	Location of Tumor on Pelvic CT
1	Bladder TCC, recurrent*	Groin	Hip flexion and adduction	Absent	Right anterior lower pelvis with erosion of the superior pubic ramus
2	Bladder TCC, recurrent[†]	Groin and anterior upper thigh	Hip flexion and adduction	Present	Left posterolateral midpelvis, anterior lower pelvis, and extrinsic to the bony pelvis in the external obturator and pectineus muscles
3	Bladder TCC, progressive[‡]	Groin and medial thigh	Hip adduction	Present	Left posterolateral midpelvis in the region of the psoas and iliacus muscles
4	Pelvic papillary adenocarcinoma, new	Groin and anterior upper thigh	Hip flexion	Absent	Right posterolateral midpelvis in the region of the psoas and iliacus muscles
5	Carcinoma of unknown origin, new	Hip, groin, and anterior upper thigh	Hip adduction	Absent	Left posterolateral upper, mid, and lower pelvis in the region of the psoas and iliacus muscles
6	Non-Hodgkin's lymphoma, new	Groin and lower pelvis	Hip adduction	Present	Left posterolateral upper, mid, and lower pelvis in the region of the psoas and iliacus muscles

Key: TCC = Transitional-cell carcinoma.
*Cystectomy 9 months before diagnosis.
[†]Cystectomy and radiation 2 years before diagnosis.
[‡]Cystectomy 2 months before diagnosis; receiving radiation.
Source: Rogers LR, Borkowski GP, Albers JW, et al: Obturator mononeuropathy caused by pelvic cancer: Six cases. Neurology 43:751, 1993, with permission.

lead to investigation of possible root disease. Obviously, an evolving plexopathy is the most important alternative diagnosis, because disk disease at this level is rare.

L-1 Metastases. L-1 nerve root compression may lead to pain referred to the paraspinal region, iliac crest, or sacroiliac joint. These pains may occur without associated focal bony pain. Any of these pains may be exacerbated by moving from a lying to a sitting position or by twisting.

TUMOR INFILTRATION OF NERVE PLEXUS

In patients with cancer, cervical, brachial, or lumbosacral plexopathy can be due to local or metastatic spread of tumor, transient or permanent radiation injury, radiation-induced secondary tumors, new primary neoplasms, infection or other inflammatory lesions, or trauma (e.g., during surgery). All of these clinical syndromes have been reported, but metastatic spread of tumor, radiation injury to the plexus, and radiation-induced second primaries are the most common causes of plexus dysfunction and pain.[79,83] Early and accurate diagnosis is critical to prevent irreversible nerve damage, which may be associated with chronic neuropathic pain, and to determine both prognosis and treatment of the tumor.

Cervical Plexopathy. Cervical plexopathy may result from direct compression by head and neck neoplasms or from metastases to cervical nodes.[89,130] The most important differential diagnosis is a postsurgical pain syndrome.[124] Symptoms usually include local pain with lancinating or other dysesthetic components referred to the retroauricular and nuchal areas, the shoulder, and the jaw. Changes on sensory examination may define the affected nerves (e.g., greater auricular or greater occipital nerves). In patients with head and neck cancer, occult infection can contribute to pain and potentially respond to antibiotic treatment.[18]

Brachial Plexopathy. Malignant brachial plexopathy is most common in patients with breast cancer (see Table 9–6) or lung cancer.[24,29,79] Pain often precedes neurologic signs or symptoms for several months. By the time of diagnosis of a brachial plexus lesion, 98 percent of patients have pain, which is most often severe.

The pain distribution depends on the site of plexus involvement. Of patients with malignant plexopathy due to a neoplasm arising from the superior sulcus of the lung (Pancoast tumor), 85 percent experience pain that begins in the shoulder girdle and radiates to the elbow, medial forearm, and the fourth and fifth fingers.[79] In some patients, pain is localized to the posterior aspect of the arm or the elbow, and some patients complain of a burning or freezing sensation and hypersensitivity of the skin along the ulnar aspect of the arm. This distribution of pain is consistent with involvement of the lower plexus (C-7 to C-8, T-1). Pain restricted to the shoulder girdle or extending to the first and second finger may be due to infiltration of the upper plexus (C-5 to C-6). This lesion may originate from neoplasm in the supraclavicular fossa.

Although the pain of brachial plexopathy is often the only symptom of tumor recurrence,[79] other symptoms or signs occasionally present first. Paresthesias, most commonly affecting the ulnar distribution, are the presenting symptom in 15 percent of patients, and lymphedema occurs in about 10 percent of patients who had previous radiation therapy to the plexus and who subsequently have developed recurrent tumor.

The neurologic signs of malignant brachial plexopathy include focal weakness, atrophy, and sensory changes in the distribution of the affected nerves. Neurologic signs can be found in more than 75 percent of patients by the time of diagnosis. In one series, 25 percent of patients presented with whole plexus motor weakness (panplexopathy); this lesion was associated with epidural deposits. Horner's syndrome, which occurs in over 50 percent of patients with tumor infiltration of the plexus, is also an ominous sign because it suggests paraspinal and, potentially, epidural extension.

Radiologic studies such as CT, MRI, and myelography can be helpful in determining the extent of the lesion causing a brachial plexopathy. Both CT scan and MRI represent the diagnostic procedures of choice for evaluating this anatomic site.[24,45,80]

Pancoast syndrome is the most common malignant brachial plexopathy and illustrates the range of findings associated with plexus injury.[72,79,93] Both primary and meta-

Table 9–6. CLINICAL FEATURES OF BRACHIAL PLEXUS SYNDROMES IN PATIENTS WITH BREAST CANCER

Feature	Tumor Infiltration	Radiation Fibrosis	Reversible Radiation Injury	Acute Ischemic Brachial Plexopathy	Radiation-Induced Second Primary Tumor
Incidence of pain	89%	18%	40%	Painless	90%
Location of pain	Shoulder, upper arm, elbow, radiating to 4th and 5th fingers	Shoulder, wrist, hand	Hand, forearm	Hand, forearm	At site of enlarging mass in supraclavicular fossa
Nature of pain	Dull aching in shoulder; lancinating pain in elbow and ulnar aspect of hand; occasional dysesthesias, burning or freezing sensations	Aching pain in shoulder; paresthesias in C-5 to C-6 distribution in hand	Aching pain in shoulder; paresthesias in hand and forearm	Paresethesias in hand and forearm	Aching pain in shoulder and arm with positive Tinel's sign
Severity of pain	Moderate to severe (severe in 98% of patients)	Mild to moderate; severe in 35% of patients	Mild	—	Moderate to severe
Course	Progressive neurologic dysfunction; atrophy and weakness with C-7 to T-1 distribution; persistent pain; Horner's syndrome	Progressive weakness with C-5 to C-6 distribution; stabilizing pain with appearance of weakness	Transient weakness and atrophy affecting C-6 to C-7, T-1; complete resolution of motor findings	Acute nonprogressive weakness and sensory changes	Progressive neurologic dysfunction with panplexopathy
CT scan findings	Circumscribed mass with diffuse infiltration of tissue planes	Diffuse infiltration of tissue planes	Normal	Normal; angiography shows subclavian artery segmental obstruction	Diffuse infiltration of tissue planes
MRI	High signal intensity in circumscribed mass on T_2-weighted images; may enhance with gadolinium	Diffuse low signal intensity of T_2-weighted images; no change with gadolinium	No data	Normal	Diffuse low signal intensity on T_2-weighted images; no change with gadolinium
EMG Findings	Segmental slowing; no myokymia	Myokymia	Segmental slowing; no myokymia	Segmental slowing; no myokymia	Segmental slowing and myokymia

Source: Adapted from Cherny NI, and Foley KM: Brachial plexopathy in patients with breast cancer. In Harris JR, Helman S, Henderson IC, et al (eds): Breast Diseases, ed 2. JB Lippincott, Philadelphia, 1995, pp 796–808.

static tumor in the apex of the lung can produce the characteristic symptoms. Pain is the initial symptom in 95 percent of patients and usually begins as an aching sensation in the elbow.[79] Twenty-five percent of patients present with burning paresthesias in the fourth and fifth fingers of the hand as their major symptom. Pain progresses to involve the medial hand and arm and often the shoulder. In a series of 30 patients studied at MSKCC, 20 had been initially diagnosed as having cervical osteoarthritis or shoulder bursitis; the delay between onset of the pain and diagnosis ranged from 2 to 7 months.

At the time of presentation, the neurologic examination is commonly abnormal. As many as 50 percent have a Horner's syndrome. The muscles innervated by the lower plexus are weak, and atrophy of the hand may be severe. Sensory loss begins in an ulnar distribution.

Of patients with Pancoast tumor, 50 percent develop epidural spinal cord compression during the course of their illness.[72] This complication is usually characterized by worsening pain, with or without neurologic signs. Early diagnosis, followed by aggressive treatment with radiation therapy and surgery, may prevent the development of myelopathy.

In Patients With Lymphoma. Tumor infiltration of the brachial plexus by lymphoma occurs in 5 to 15 percent of patients with Hodgkin's disease. A common feature of lymphoma is that it tracks along the nerve itself into the epidural and intradural space. This may result in spinal cord compression and/or leptomeningeal disease without any bony changes in the adjacent vertebrae.[63] This observation should lead clinicians to careful assessment of the epidural space concurrent with evaluation of the brachial plexus, and it supports the need for combinations of CT and MRI scanning as the appropriate diagnostic tests.

From Radiation-Induced Second Primaries. Both second primary tumors and radiation-induced malignant peripheral nerve tumors are in the differential diagnosis of a progressive plexopathy in a patient previously treated for cancer.[51] Pain is typically the presenting symptom, with signs of an enlarging mass in an irradiated port. Because of their long survivals, patients with breast cancer and lymphoma are at increased risk to develop these tumors.

Lumbosacral Plexopathy. In a cancer center, lumbosacral plexopathy represents 15 percent of the consultations for low back pain, leg pain, and leg weakness, and 3 percent of all neurologic consultations.[56,70] In these patients, pain is followed weeks to months later by numbness, paresthesias, and weakness. In rare patients, lumbosacral plexopathy can present as a red, burning foot.

In Jaeckle et al's prospective series, one-third of patients demonstrated a lag of at least 3 months between pain and the appearance of other neurologic symptoms or signs.[70] The pain was usually aching or pressurelike and seldom burning or dysesthetic. In most patients, the pain was located focally in the back or pelvis or described in a radicular distribution; it was referred outside this distribution in one-third of patients. Almost all patients with lymphoma, breast carcinoma, and sarcoma complained of posteriorly located pain. Patients with colorectal tumor experienced pain in a posterior radicular distribution, whereas patients with lymphoma described pain that radiated laterally. Although many patients reported pain in more than one distribution, only two-thirds of patients with radiologically documented bilateral plexus involvement complained of bilateral pain.

In the Jaeckle et al series,[70] the evolution of findings followed a predictable pattern. Initial mild weakness, sensory signs, and reflex asymmetry progressed to focal paralysis during a median of 8 months (range, 1 to 24 months) following diagnosis. In most patients, reflexes became focally absent early in the course. The upper plexus (L-1 to L-4) was involved in one-third of patients, whereas one-half had lower plexopathy (L-5 to S-3), and fewer than one-fifth had a panplexopathy (L-1 to S-3). Incontinence was unusual, occurring in fewer than 10 percent of patients, and was associated with massive intrapelvic tumor.

Patients with low pelvic tumors, usually colorectal or genitourinary, may develop a predominant sacral plexopathy. This plexopathy results from direct extension of a presacral mass that may invade the sacrum. The clinical signs include prominent sphincter dysfunction and a perineal ("saddle") sensory loss.[123]

Patients with a suspected lumbosacral plexopathy can undergo electrodiagnostic studies to define further the extent of neurologic injury. The radiologic diagnostic test of choice is the CT scan. MRI can further define bony or epidural extension.[80] The use of serum markers, such as CEA, CA-125, and CA-15, as well as monoclonal antibodies as diagnostic scanning tools, are under study to improve early diagnosis.[100]

The evaluation of patients with suspected malignant lumbosacral plexopathy must include distinguishing this lesion from leptomeningeal metastases, which can cause low back pain or leg pain with subacute motor and sensory involvement, and epidural cord or root compression. Epidural neoplasm can usually be distinguished on the basis of intense back pain, bowel/bladder dysfunction, and the symmetric nature of the findings. The differential diagnosis also includes other causes of plexopathy—for example, retroperitoneal or iliopsoas hemorrhage and tumor infiltration of the psoas muscle—the latter of which can produce the so-called "malignant psoas syndrome."[122] This is characterized by signs of an upper plexopathy, with pain on hip flexion and on stretching the psoas muscle. Tumor is adjacent to the L-1 vertebral body and may injure the iliohypogastric, ilioinguinal, or genitofemoral nerves; pain and paresthesias may radiate into the inguinal region.

Similar to other tumor-related pain syndromes, the pain due to malignant lumbosacral plexopathy can be influenced by primary antitumor modalities. In one series of 65 patients interviewed 1 month after primary therapy,[70] 10 had experienced improved pain and 13 reported stabilization of pain; 42 patients worsened. The syndrome is commonly associated with advanced disease, and the overall prognosis is poor. The median survival in the Jaeckle et al series,[70] for example, was 5.5 months.

LEPTOMENINGEAL METASTASES

Pain occurs in 40 percent of patients with leptomeningeal tumor infiltration.[74,111,119,134] The pain is generally of two types: a dull, constant headache, with or without neck stiffness, and back pain, which is usually localized to the lower back and buttocks.[32] The pain results from traction on tumor-infiltrated nerves and meninges.

Lumbar puncture is the procedure of choice to detect neoplastic cells in the cerebrospinal fluid of these patients. An elevated cerebrospinal fluid protein and low glucose concentration are often associated findings.[74] In patients with low back or buttock pain, single-dose or double-dose contrast MRI can be helpful to delineate tumor nodules along the nerves and cauda equina.[111] Myelography can be performed as an alternative procedure to define the presence or absence of nodules on nerve roots. The differential diagnosis of this disorder varies with the site of neurologic involvement. Most typically, signs and symptoms indicate neurologic dysfunction at several levels of the neural axis.

EPIDURAL SPINAL CORD OR CAUDA EQUINA COMPRESSION

Back pain is the initial symptom in more than 95 percent of patients with epidural spinal cord or cauda equina compression.[53,56,101] It may be the only neurologic symptom or sign, even in the 10 percent of patients who are discovered to have high-grade epidural lesions at presentation. The pain may be local, radicular, referred, or funicular.[33] Local pain over the involved vertebral body, which results from disruption of the vertebral periosteum, is dull and exacerbated by recumbency. Radicular pain from compressed or damaged nerve roots is usually unilateral in the cervical and lumbosacral regions and bilateral in the thorax, where it is experienced as a tight band across the chest or abdomen. Referred pain in the mid-scapular region or in both shoulders may accompany cervical/thoracic epidural disease, and bilateral sacroiliac and iliac crest pain may be observed with L-1 vertebral compression. A so-called funicular pain is uncommon and presumably results from compression of the sensory tracts in the spinal cord. This central pain (see Chapter 5) occurs some distance from the site of the compression and is typically described as a hot or cold pain in a poorly localized nondermatomal distribution.

Progressive pain is usually associated with progressive weakness, sensory loss, autonomic dysfunction, and reflex abnormalities. The weakness may be segmental from nerve root damage or pyramidal if myelopathy develops. Sensory abnormalities include ascending paresthesias, a sensory level or complete loss of all sensory modalities below a dermatomal level in paraplegic patients. The upper level of sensory findings may correspond to the location of the epidural tumor or may be below it by many segments. Bladder and bowel dysfunction are less common presenting symptoms but may appear after sensory symptoms have developed. The exception to this occurs with compression of the conus medullaris, which can present as acute urinary retention or progressive constipation without preceding motor or sensory symptoms.

An early diagnosis is critical to prevent the development of irreversible neurologic deficits.[95,97,99,108] Clinical studies have tried to discern differences between patients with cancer who have back pain predominantly from bony vertebral body disease and those who have vertebral body and epidural disease.[72] Neurologic and radiographic findings are used to select patients for definitive imaging of the epidural space (Fig. 9–3).[99] For example, in patients with back pain and a normal neurologic examination, the presence of greater than 50 percent collapse of the vertebral body on plain radiographs is associated with an 87 percent chance of epidural disease.[59] Therefore, many patients with back pain and abnormal plain radiographs require further evaluation for epidural extension. At the present time, MRI is the procedure of choice for the study of patients with potential epidural disease.

The usual treatment of epidural spinal cord or cauda equina compression includes corticosteroids and radiation therapy.[14] Surgery is strongly considered in the following settings: an unknown primary tumor, recurrent symptoms after radiation therapy, neurologic progression during radiation therapy, and spinal instability. Surgical resection (laminectomy for posterior lesions and vertebrectomy for the more common anterior lesions) is also considered for high-grade epidural tumors from relatively radioresistant primary neoplasms, such as renal-cell cancer or melanoma. The functional outcome for the individual patient with epidural spinal cord compression is clearly related to functional status at the time of diagnosis.[6,62]

Patients who are paraplegic at presentation do not become ambulatory, whereas ambulatory patients will remain so with prompt treatment. More than 85 percent of patients will obtain pain relief, at least transiently, from high-dose steroid therapy.

Tumor Infiltration of Hollow Viscus

Obstruction of hollow viscus including the intestine, biliary tract, and ureters is the most common cause of tumor-induced visceral pain.[30] The pain typically results from stretching or compression and is referred to cutaneous sites in well-defined dermatomal patterns. Distention of the parietal pleura, as well as of the hepatic capsule, produces pain usually at the site of tumor infiltration. Retroperitoneal infiltration in the region of the celiac plexus (e.g., with pancreatic cancer) is typically associated with diffuse abdominal and back pain. Peritoneal carcinomatosis is associated with inflammation, mesenteric tethering, adhesions,and secondary ascites, all of which cause pain. Management of these common syndromes includes decompression, the use of anesthetic blocks, and combinations of analgesic drugs concurrent with the use of appropriate antitumor approaches.

PAIN SYNDROMES ASSOCIATED WITH CANCER THERAPY

Many pain syndromes occur in the course of, or subsequent to, surgery, chemotherapy, or radiation therapy. Acute pain syndromes occur within weeks after the specific therapy. Examples include postoperative pain syndromes, mucositis following chemotherapy, and esophagitis induced by radiation therapy.[19,106] These syndromes are readily recognized, and the associated pain is self-limited. In contrast, most chronic pain syndromes begin weeks to months—and in some circumstances, years—after the completion of treatment. The occurrence of these late pains usually suggests recurrent disease and requires a detailed evaluation. The incidence of these late pain syndromes is not fully known.

Postsurgical Pain Syndromes

Postsurgical pain is characterized by either persistent pain following a surgical procedure or recurrent pain after the initial surgical pain has cleared. The major syndromes occur after common surgical procedures and result from changes in musculoskeletal structures and injury to peripheral nerves.

PAIN AFTER RADICAL NECK DISSECTION

Surgical injury or interruption of the cervical nerves at the time of radical neck dissection may produce a chronic neuropathic pain.[89] This pain is usually characterized as a burning sensation in an area of sensory loss. Intermittent, shocklike pain often accompanies the continuous dysesthesia. This pain becomes evident as incisional pain fades and intensifies in an area of sensory loss. A second type of pain can result from a "droopy shoulder" syndrome, which is caused by musculoskeletal imbalance. Thoracic outlet symptoms and signs of suprascapular nerve entrapment can occur.[124]

The diagnostic approach to neck and shoulder pain following radical neck dissection includes a CT or MRI scan through the area of pain, with a repeat head and neck examination to exclude the presence of recurrent tumor. In addition to pharmacotherapy, treatment may include physical therapy, exercise, trigger point injections, and appropriate bracing of the shoulder and back.

PAIN AFTER MASTECTOMY

Postmastectomy pain syndrome occurs in 4 to 6 percent of women undergoing any surgical procedure on the breast, from lumpectomy to radical mastectomy[129,131] or axillary dissection for lymph node removal. The pain may occur immediately following the surgical procedure or many months later. It is characterized as a tight, constricting, burning pain in the posterior aspect of the arm and axilla, which may radiate across the anterior chest wall. The pain is exacerbated by movement of the arm and relieved by immobilization. There is typically a trigger point in the axilla or at the anterior chest wall. Patients often posture the arm in a flexed position, close to the chest wall, and are at risk for developing a frozen shoulder if adequate pain management and postsurgical rehabilitation are not implemented. The nature of the pain and the clinical symptoms should readily distinguish it from tumor infiltration of the brachial plexus.[136]

Postmastectomy pain results from interruption of the intercostobrachial nerve, a cutaneous sensory branch of T-1 to T-2 (Fig. 9–4). The marked anatomic variation in the size and distribution of the intercostobrachial nerve may explain the variable incidence of this syndrome in patients undergoing surgery of the breast. The pain appears to occur more commonly in patients with postoperative complications; its incidence is not altered by breast reconstruction. As in any patient with peripheral nerve injury and pain, management includes the use of physical therapy, trigger point injections, and a wide range of treatment with analgesic drugs.

PAIN AFTER THORACOTOMY

Persistent pain in the distribution of a thoracotomy incision, with or without local autonomic changes, may occur as a result of surgical damage to intercostal nerves. This nonmalignant pain syndrome is probably very uncommon and must be distinguished from recurrent or persistent pain due to neoplasm. Kanner et al[73] studied 126 patients undergoing thoracotomy at MSKCC to define the pattern of pain following thoracotomy. Group 1 consisted of patients whose immediate postoperative pain resolved within 2 months of surgery but then recurred. In all cases, the pain was due to recurrence of tumor. Group 2 had pain that persisted following the thoracotomy and then increased during the follow-up period. Local recurrence of disease was again the most common cause of this pain. Group 3 had stable or decreasing pain, which gradually resolved over an 8-month period. Tumor recurrence was noted in less than half this group. Thus, postthoracotomy pain usually heralds recurrent tumor,[86,87,135] unlike chronic postmastectomy pain, which is rarely, if ever, associated with recurrent tumor.

Chest radiographs are insufficient to evaluate postthoracotomy pain. A CT scan or

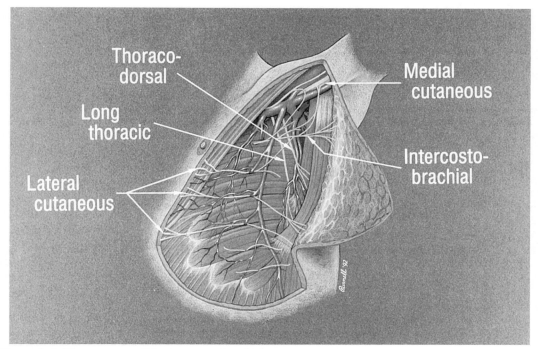

Figure 9–4. The anatomy of the intercostobrachial nerve.

MRI of the chest is the diagnostic procedure of choice. MRI scan also may be necessary to define the presence of epidural disease if tumor is noted to be adjacent to the spine. Such studies should be undertaken before an intercostal nerve block is administered.

Persistent pain in these patients may lead to a frozen shoulder and secondary reflex sympathetic dystrophy involving the arm on the side ipsilateral to the thoracotomy incision. Early and aggressive physical therapy should be used to prevent these complications.

PHANTOM PAIN

Phantom pain syndromes have been described following surgical procedures for cancer. Phantom breast pain after mastectomy may occur in as many as 15 to 30 percent of patients.[16,81,82] It typically presents in the area of the nipple and then spreads to include the entire breast. Like other phantom pains, it occurs more commonly in patients with preoperative breast pain. The character of the pain is variable and may be lancinating, continuous, or intermittent.

A phantom anus pain syndrome occurs in approximately 15 percent of patients who undergo abdominoperineal resections.[11,12] Phantom anus pain may develop either in the early postoperative period or after a latency of months to years. Late-onset pain is almost always associated with tumor recurrence. Rare cases of phantom bladder pain after cystectomy have also been reported.

After limb amputation, phantom limb pain may initially magnify and then slowly fade over time.[75] The pain may have paroxysmal or continuous, often burning qualities and may be associated with bothersome paresthesias in the limb. The phantom limb often assumes painful and unusual postures; over time, it may "telescope" and approach the stump. The incidence of phantom pain is significantly lower in patients with short-lasting preamputation pain and in patients who do not have pain in the limb the day before the amputation. Preoperative epidural blockage has been reported to be useful in reducing the incidence of phantom limb pain in the first years after the amputation.[44] Numerous therapies have been used for this pain, with limited success (see Chapter 5).

STUMP PAIN

Stump pain may occur several months to years following amputation.[38] It results from the development of a traumatic neuroma at the site of the nerve section (see Chapter 5). The pain is usually a burning dysesthesia and may have a lancinating or paroxysmal component. It is often exacerbated by movement or contact with the stump and may be relieved by the injection of a local anesthetic at the site of the trigger point. Careful assessment will help to distinguish stump pain from phantom pain. Stump pain is treated by identifying the trigger-point site and treating it locally, readjusting the prosthesis, and using drugs to suppress neuronal firing, such as anticonvulsants and antidepressants.

Recurrence of pain in a phantom limb is an ominous sign and should alert the physician to reassess the patient for proximal tumor recurrence.[38] For example, the onset of phantom leg pain several years after leg resection for a primary bone tumor has been observed to herald recurrent disease in the pelvis.

PAIN AFTER NEPHRECTOMY

Postnephrectomy pain may occur following surgical procedures on the kidney or ureter. It is characterized by pain in the area of sensory loss. The pain is burning, with intermittent paroxysmal features. It is often exacerbated by movement and relieved by immobility. The surgical scar often leads to disruption of normal muscles and may produce secondary motor weakness in the posterior and lateral abdominal wall.

POSTSURGICAL PELVIC FLOOR MYALGIA

A persistent deep pelvic pain may occur following abdominoperineal resection for carcinoma of the colon or pelvic exenteration procedures. The pain is absent when the patient is sitting or lying and begins with standing or walking. It has been described as "tension myalgia of the pelvic rim"[123] and should be distinguished by history from phantom anus syndrome. Careful assessment is needed to exclude recurrent disease, particularly if this syndrome occurs long after surgery. It is very difficult to treat because of its unique association with standing.

Pain Syndromes After Chemotherapy

A variety of acute and chronic pain syndromes occur following chemotherapy.[1,4,27,30,36,38,121,127] Arterial, intravenous, and intraperitoneal chemotherapy are each associated with acute pain syndromes.[30] For example, intravenous chemotherapy infusion may produce painful venous spasm, chemical phlebitis, or vesicant extravasation; anthracycline-associated local flares may also be painful.[1] Both hepatic artery infusion and intraperitoneal infusion are associated with transient abdominal pains.[78] With intraperitoneal infusion, 25 percent of patients have a transient mild abdominal pain, and an additional 25 percent report moderate or severe pain necessitating opioid analgesia or discontinuation of the therapy.

PAINFUL CHEMOTHERAPY-RELATED TOXICITIES

Chemotherapy also produces painful toxicities, including oral mucositis and both focal and diffuse pains.[1,27,36,68,106,117] For example, *trans*-retinoic acid therapy can produce acute bone pain, 5-fluorouracil can cause anginal chest pain, and interferon can produce myalgias and arthralgias.[68,71] Jaw pain is a specific syndrome occurring acutely following vincristine administration.[25]

There are also specific pain syndromes associated with other neurologic manifestations.[38] Patients receiving intrathecal or intraventricular methotrexate can develop headache due to an acute meningeal syndrome hours after treatment for leukemia or leptomeningeal metastases.[138] This syndrome occurs in 5 to 50 percent of patients treated. The incidence increases with the number of intrathecal injections. It is commonly associated with vomiting, nuchal rigidity, fever, irritability, and lethargy. The symptoms usually resolve in a few days and do not interfere with further treatment. Headache also occurs in patients treated with L-asparaginase, a chemotherapeutic agent used in combination therapy for the treatment of acute lymphoblastic leukemia.[43] Because L-asparaginase depletes L-asparagine and leads to depletion of plasma proteins involved in coagulation and fibrinolysis, either central nervous system hemorrhage or thrombotic infarction occurs in 1 to 2 percent of patients. Headache is the most common initial symptom and may occur in more than 40 percent of patients. Seizures, hemiparesis, altered mental status, vomiting, and cranial nerve palsies may also occur.

PAINFUL POLYNEUROPATHY

Some chemotherapeutic agents produce a painful peripheral neuropathy. The drugs most commonly responsible are the *Vinca* alkaloids (especially vincristine), cisplatin, and paclitaxel; procarbazine, misonidazole, and hexamethylmelamine may also cause this syndrome.[22,25,26,90,113]

Dysesthesias and paresthesias occur in up to 100 percent of patients treated with *Vinca* alkaloids.[116] The painful sensations are usually localized to the hands and the feet, are burning in quality, and are frequently exacerbated by cutaneous stimulation of the distal extremities. Many patients develop associated autonomic changes.

PAINFUL PLEXOPATHY FROM INTRA-ARTERIAL CHEMOTHERAPY

Lumbosacral plexopathy or mononeuropathies may result from infusion of chemotherapeutic agents, such as cisplatin, into the iliac artery.[54] Patients develop symptoms within 48 hours of the procedure. Acute pain, weakness, and paresthesias occur in the distribution of the lumbosacral plexus. This syndrome is thought to be due to small-vessel damage and infarction of the plexus at the site of injection. The prognosis for neurologic recovery has not been fully established.

CORTICOSTEROID-ASSOCIATED PAIN SYNDROMES

Perineal Pain. A severe burning sensation in the perineum is described by patients receiving intravenous doses of 100 mg of dexamethasone, which is usually administered as part of a protocol for the treatment of epidural compression.[101] Patients should be warned that such symptoms may occur. No

treatment is available, and none is usually required because of the transient nature of this complaint. The etiology of this syndrome is unknown.

Steroid Pseudorheumatism. A second pain syndrome associated with the use of corticosteroids manifests as diffuse arthralgias and myalgias, with muscle and joint tenderness, following withdrawal from these drugs.[112] These symptoms occur with rapid or slow withdrawal and may occur in patients who have been receiving steroids for long or short periods. The pathogenesis of this syndrome is poorly understood, but it has been speculated that steroid withdrawal may sensitize joint and muscle mechanoreceptors and nociceptors. Treatment consists of reinstituting the steroids at a higher dose and withdrawing them more slowly.

Aseptic Necrosis of the Femoral and Humeral Head. A third pain syndrome that may follow steroid use is due to necrosis of the femoral or humeral head.[41] Aseptic necrosis may occur after intermittent or continuous steroid therapy. It may be unilateral or bilateral and usually presents as pain in the shoulder, hip, or knees, which is exacerbated by movement and relieved by rest. If progressive bone destruction and poorly controlled pain occur, joint replacement can provide dramatic pain relief.

POSTHERPETIC NEURALGIA

Acute herpes zoster and postherpetic neuralgia represent important painful neuropathies in patients with cancer who are undergoing immunosuppressive therapies (see Chapter 5).[30,38,114] Antiviral therapy for acute zoster is essential in this setting.

Pain Syndromes After Radiation Therapy

Pain is an uncommon late complication of radiation therapy.[8] It may result from damage to peripheral nerves or the spinal cord. This damage may be due to changes in the microvasculature, to fibrosis and chronic inflammation in adjacent connective tissues, or to demyelinization and focal necrosis of white and gray matter in the spinal cord. The differential diagnosis always includes recurrent tumor. In all instances, pain is not as prominent a complaint as when the syndrome is associated with recurrent tumor.

RADIATION INJURY TO THE BRACHIAL PLEXUS

Radiation to the brachial plexus is associated with three distinct pain syndromes: (1) radiation fibrosis, (2) reversible or transient brachial plexopathy, and (3) acute ischemic brachial plexopathy. All are rare clinical entities, each with a characteristic clinical presentation and course (see Table 9–6).

Radiation Fibrosis. Radiation fibrosis of the brachial plexus results in progressive and irreversible neurologic dysfunction.[2,7,79,125,126] Pain is the presenting symptom in fewer than 20 percent of patients but is experienced by 65 percent at some point during the course of the disease. Pain is commonly described as mild aching in the shoulder or hand; it is reported to be severe in 35 percent of patients. Other symptoms include paresthesias in the lateral fingers or entire hand, which occur in more than 50 percent of affected patients; lymphedema and heaviness of the arm, which are also noted in 50 percent of patients; and proximal weakness of the arm (C-5 to C-6 distribution), which occurs in almost all patients.[42,46,53,64] When symptoms occur in the hand, the syndrome may be confused with carpal tunnel syndrome.

The syndrome of radiation fibrosis begins a median of 4 years and a mean of 5.5 years after radiation treatment. Radiation injury has been reported to occur at doses greater than 6000 cGy, but numerous factors appear to alter susceptibility, including patient age, the site of the port, and the premorbid state of the irradiated nerve.[79,104]

The evaluation of the patient with suspected radiation fibrosis requires CT or MRI.[24,45,80] These studies usually demonstrate diffuse infiltration. MRI scans do not show enhancement with gadolinium, and T_2-weighted images suggest radiation change by low signal intensity.[45] Electrodiagnostic studies typically demonstrate myokymic discharges and signs of denervation.[42,46,53,64,91,105] Radiation-induced bony changes in the ribs or clavicle can provide additional evidence of the diagnosis.

The current management of patients with pain from radiation injury begins with establishment of an accurate diagnosis. There are no proven methods of reversing neurologic damage but splinting the arm at the chest wall, preventing subluxation of the shoulder joint, and aggressive lymphedema management are all approaches.

Reversible or Transient Radiation Injury. Transient radiation injury was reported in 8 patients (1.4 percent of those treated) who received moderate doses of supervoltage radiation therapy for breast cancer.[115] The clinical symptoms included paresthesias in the arm and hands, weakness, and pain. The onset of symptoms was 3 to 14 months following irradiation, with a median of 4.5 months. Seven of the eight patients received adjuvant chemotherapy, and, in six, symptoms began after drug treatment. There was temporal clustering of these cases, which also suggested a possible neurotropic viral component. A second study[29] reported radiation-induced plexopathies in 19 of 63 patients treated with radiation therapy to the chest wall and adjacent nodal areas. Of these patients, 14 had a transient plexopathy and 5 had a permanent plexopathy.

Acute Ischemic Brachial Plexopathy. Acute ischemic brachial plexopathy is another rare postradiation syndrome. In one case, subclavian artery occlusion occurred 19 years after a patient with breast cancer received 400 cGy to the breast and axillary area.[55] The syndrome occurred acutely after she carried a heavy object and held her left arm outstretched above the shoulder. Weakness, atrophy, and fasciculation rapidly progressed in a C-5 to T-1 distribution, and angiography showed segmental occlusion of the left subclavian artery. The pathophysiology of this injury remains in question.

RADIATION FIBROSIS OF THE LUMBOSACRAL PLEXUS

Radiation fibrosis of the lumbosacral plexus may present 1 to 30 years following radiation treatment.[70] The use of intracavitary radium implants with pelvic radiation for carcinoma of the cervix may be a risk factor. Presenting symptoms include weakness of the legs, associated with sensory symptoms, numbness, and paresthesias. Pain occurs in only 10 percent of patients. Symptoms and signs are usually bilateral in presentation, and weakness starts distally in the L-5 to S-1 segments and slowly progresses. Radiation necrosis of the pelvic bone commonly accompanies this disorder and can help in making the diagnosis.

RADIATION MYELOPATHY

L'Hermitte's sign has been reported as an early acute pain syndrome in patients receiving radiation therapy to an area that includes the cervical or thoracic spinal cord.[133] Persistent pain may be an early symptom of chronic radiation-induced myelopathy. It is usually burning in quality and may be part of a Brown-Séquard's syndrome. MRI scan may demonstrate an area of hypointensity in the spinal cord. The pathology is characterized by changes in the vascular supply with fibrinoid degeneration and demyelination with gliosis.

RADIATION-INDUCED PERIPHERAL NERVE TUMORS

Malignant peripheral nerve tumors and second primary tumors in a previously radiated site may present as a painful expanding mass in a patient with a history of previously treated cancer.[51] Patients with neurofibromatosis have an increased risk of developing malignant peripheral nerve tumors following radiation therapy. The diagnosis may be difficult in a patient presumed cured of the original malignancy. The use of CT or MRI scan can be helpful, particularly if there is evidence of gadolinium enhancement, but often the diagnosis is made by surgical exploration and pathologic confirmation.[80]

SUMMARY

One-third of patients with cancer in active therapy and two-thirds with advanced disease have pain severe enough to require analgesic drugs. Both nociceptive and neuropathic pains are common. Metastatic bone disease, nerve compression and infiltration, and involvement of the viscera by either obstruction of hollow viscus or diffuse peritoneal seeding are the most prevalent pain syndromes related directly to the tumor. Treatment-related pain syndromes may follow surgery, chemotherapy, or radiation therapy. These syndromes have a characteristic clinical presentation that may allow delineation from tumor-induced pain. Patients with cancer also develop pain syndromes that are unrelated to their cancer or cancer treatment.

The heterogeneity of cancer pain syndromes and the possibility of effective primary therapy in some cases support the need for a careful medical and neurologic assessment to define the pain etiology. This assessment relies on history-taking, medical and neurologic examination, and review of relevant radiologic procedures. Technologic advances in neuroradiology have facilitated assessment of these common neurologic syndromes in cancer. Knowledge of common pain syndromes, coupled with this improving technology, greatly enhances the ability to make an accurate and timely diagnosis.

The increasing number of patients with cancer who survive for long periods after medical treatment has focused attention on the need to further define the posttreatment syndromes and their natural history. For example, knowledge of the specific and sensitive radiologic diagnostic procedures for assessing a collapsed vertebral body to differentiate tumor from radiation necrosis, coupled with information on the clinical presentation of this type of bone pain, facilitates early and accurate diagnosis and treatment. Similarly, the progressive, painless loss of neurologic function in a patient treated with radiation therapy to the brachial plexus is most commonly radiation fibrosis.

Clarifying the diagnosis of a specific pain syndrome and its neurophysiologic mechanism is only the first step in the development of a pain treatment strategy. For patients with tumor-induced pain, antitumor approaches combined with analgesic drug therapy are the most common first-line approach. The use of combinations of nonopioids, opioids, and adjuvant analgesic drugs can provide adequate pain relief in as high as 90 to 95 percent of patients. Understanding the indications, use, side effects, and risk-benefit ratios of drug therapy is critical to provide patients with adequate pain relief to function as they choose and, for the dying patient, to die pain free. Other chapters review these principles of drug therapy.

Cancer pain can be treated and the large population of patients with heterogeneous pain syndromes can benefit from the extensive knowledge now available to better diagnose and treat their clinical pain states.

REFERENCES

1. Almadrones L, and Yerys C: Problems associated with the administration of intraperitoneal therapy using the Port-A-Cath system. Oncology Nursing Forum 17:75–80, 1990.
2. Bagley FH, Walsh JW, Cady B, et al: Carcinomatous versus radiation induced brachial plexus neuropathy in breast cancer. Cancer 41:2154–2157, 1978.
3. Ballantyne AJ, McCarten AB, and Ibanez ML: The extension of cancer of the head and neck through peripheral nerves. Am J Surg 106:651–667, 1963.
4. Balmer CM: Clinical use of biologic response modifiers in cancer treatment: A overview. Part II. Colony-stimulating factors and interleuken-2. DICP 25:490–498, 1991.
5. Banning A, Sjogren P, and Henriksen H: Pain causes in 200 patients referred to a multidisciplinary cancer pain clinic. Pain 45:45–48, 1991.
6. Barcena A, Lobato RD, and Rivas JJ: Spinal metastatic disease: Analysis of factors determining functional prognosis and choice of treatment. Neurosurgery 15:820–827, 1984.
7. Basso-Ricci S, della Costa C, Viganotti G, et al: Report on 42 cases of post-irradiation lesions of the brachial plexus and their treatment. Tumori 66:117–122, 1980.
8. Ben Yosef R, and Kapp DS: Persistent and/or late complications of combined radiation therapy and hyperthermia. Int J Hyperthermia 8:733–745, 1992.
9. Bindoff LA, and Heseltine D: Unilateral facial pain in patients with lung cancer: A referred pain via the vagus. Lancet 1:812–815, 1988.
10. Bingas B: Tumors of the base of the skull. In Vinken PJ, and Bruyn GW (eds): Handbook of Clinical Neurology. Elsevier, Amsterdam, 1974, 136–233.
11. Boas RA: Phantom anus syndrome. In Bonica JJ, Lindblom U, and Iggo A (eds): Proceedings of the Third World Congress on Pain. Raven Press, New York, 1983, pp 947–951.
12. Boas RA, Schug SA, and Acland RH: Perineal pain after rectal amputation: A 5-year follow-up. Pain 52:67–70, 1993.
13. Bongers KM, Willigers MM, and Koehler PJ: Referred facial pain from lung carcinoma. Neurology 42:1841–1842, 1992.
14. Boogerd W, and van der Sande JJ: Diagnosis and treatment of spinal cord compression in malignant disease. Cancer Treat Rev 19:129–150, 1993.
15. Brazis PW, Vogler JB, and Shaw KE: The "numb cheek-limb lower lid" syndrome. Neurology 41:327–328, 1991.
16. Bressler B, Cohen SI, and Magnussen S: The problem of phantom breast and phantom pain. J Nerv Ment Dis 123:181–187, 1955.
17. Broux R, Moonen G, and Schoenen J: Unilateral facial pain as the first symptom of lung cancer, report

of three cases. Cephalalgia 11(Suppl 11):319–320, 1991.
18. Bruera E, and McDonald N: Intractable pain in patients with advanced head and neck tumors: A possible role of local infection. Cancer Treatment Report 70:691–692, 1986.
19. Buchi K: Radiation proctitis: Therapy and prognosis. JAMA 265:1180–1184, 1991.
20. Bukberg J, Penman D, and Holland J: Depression in hospitalized cancer patients. Psychosom Med 43:199–212, 1984.
21. Burt RK, Sharfam WH, Karp BI, et al: Mental neuropathy (numb chin syndrome). A harbinger of tumor progression or relapse. Cancer 70:877–881, 1992.
22. Byfield JE: Ionizing radiation and vincristine: Possible neurotoxic synergism. Radiologica Clinica et Biologia 41:129–138, 1972.
23. Carter RL, Pittam MR, and Tanner NSB: Pain and dysphagia in patients with squamous carcinomas of the head and neck: The role of perineural spread. J R Soc Med 75:598–606, 1982.
24. Cascino TL, Kori S, Krol G, et al: CT scan of brachial plexus in patients with cancer. Neurology 33:1553–1557, 1983.
25. Casey EB, Jellife AM, LaQuesne PM, et al: Vincristine neuropathy: Clinical and electrophysiological observations. Brain 96:69–86, 1973.
26. Cassady JB, Tonnesen GL, Wolfe LC, et al: Augmentation of vincristine neurotoxicity by irradiation of peripheral nerves. Cancer Treat Rep 64:963–965, 1980.
27. Chapko MK, Syrjala KL, Schilter L, et al: Chemoradiotherapy toxicity during bone marrow transplantation: Time course and variation in pain and nausea. Bone Marrow Transplant 4:181–186, 1990.
28. Cheng TM, Cascino TL, and Onofrio BM: Comprehensive study of diagnosis and treatment of trigeminal neuralgia secondary to tumors. Neurology 43:2298–2302, 1993.
29. Cherny NI, and Foley KM: Brachial plexopathy in patients with breast cancer. In Harris JR, Hellman S, Henderson IC, et al (eds): Breast Diseases, ed 2. JB Lippincott, Philadelphia, 1995, 796–808.
30. Cherny NI, and Portenoy RK: Cancer pain pathophysiology, assessment and syndromes. In Wall PD, and Melzack R (eds): Textbook of Pain. Churchill Livingstone, Edinburgh, 1994, pp 787–823.
31. Clouston PD, De Angelis L, and Posner JB: The spectrum of neurological disease in patients with systemic cancer. Ann Neurol 31:268–273, 1992.
32. Clouston PD, Sharpe DM, Corbett AJ, et al: Perineural spread of cutaneous head and neck cancer. Its orbital and central neurologic complications. Arch Neurol 47:73–77, 1990.
33. Constans JP, DeVitis E, Donzelli R, et al: Spinal metastases with neurological manifestations: Review of 600 cases. J Neurosurg 59:111–118, 1983.
34. Dalmau J, Graus F, and Marco M: "Hot and dry foot" as initial manifestation of neoplastic lumbosacral plexopathy. Neurology 39:871–872, 1989.
35. DeAngelis LM, and Payne R: Lymphomatous meningitis presenting as atypical cluster headache. Pain 30:211–216, 1987.
36. Delattre JY, and Posner JB: Neurological complications of chemotherapy and radiation therapy. In

Aminoff MJ (ed): Neurology and General Medicine. Churchill Livingstone, New York, 1989, pp 365–387.

37. Des Prez RD, and Freeman FR: Facial pain associated with lung cancer: A case report. Headache 23:43–44, 1983.

38. Elliott K, and Foley KM: Neurologic pain syndromes in patients with cancer. Neurol Clin 7:333–360, 1989.

39. Eng CT, and Vasconez LO: Facial pain due to perineural invasion by basal cell carcinoma. Ann Plast Surg 12:374–377, 1984.

40. Epstein JB, Schubert MM, and Scully C: Evaluation and treatment of pain in patients with orofacial cancer. The Pain Clinic 4:3–20, 1991.

41. Epstein JB, Wong FLW, and Stephenson-Moore P: Osteoradionecrosis: Clinical experience and a proposal for classification. J Oral Maxillofac Surg 45:104–110, 1987.

42. Fardin P, Lelli S, Negrin P, et al: Radiation-induced brachial plexopathy: Clinical and electromyographical (EMG) considerations in 13 cases. Electromyogr Clin Neurophysiol 30:277–282, 1990.

43. Feinberg WM, and Swenson MR: Cerebrovascular complications of L-asparaginase therapy. Neurology 38:127–133, 1988.

44. Fisher A, and Meller Y: Continuous postoperative regional analgesia by nerve sheath block for amputation surgery—a pilot study. Anesth Analg 72:300–303, 1991.

45. Fishman EK, Campbell JN, Kuhlman JE, et al: Multiplanar CT evaluation of brachial plexopathy in breast cancer. J Comput Assist Tomog 15:790–795, 1991.

46. Flaggman PD, and Kelly JJ: Brachial plexus neuropathy: An electrophysiological evaluation. Arch Neurol 37:160–164, 1980.

47. Foley KM: Pain assessment and cancer pain. In Doyle D, Hanks GW, and MacDonald RN (eds): Oxford Textbook of Palliative Medicine. Oxford University Press, Oxford, 1993, pp 148–166.

48. Foley KM: Pain syndromes in patients with cancer. Med Clin North Am 71:169–184, 1987.

49. Foley KM: The management of pain of malignant origin. In Tyler HD, and Dawson PM (eds): Current Neurology, Vol 2. Raven Press, New York, 1979, pp 279–302.

50. Foley KM: Pain syndromes in patients with cancer. In Bonica JJ, and Ventafridda V (eds): Advances in Pain Research and Therapy, Vol 2. Raven Press, New York, 1979, pp 59–75.

51. Foley KM, Woodruff JM, and Ellis FT: Radiation-induced malignant and atypical peripheral nerve sheath tumors. Arch Neurol 7:311–318, 1980.

52. Forsyth PA, and Posner JB: Intracranial neoplasm. In Olesen J, Tfelt-Hansen P, and Welch KMA (eds): The Headaches. Raven Press, New York, 1993, pp 705–714.

53. Freilich RJ, and Foley KM: Epidural metastases. In Harris JR, Hellman S, Henderson IC, et al (eds): Breast Diseases, ed 2. JB Lippincott, Philadelphia, 1995, 779–789.

54. Gebbia V, Testa A, Valenza R, et al: Acute pain syndrome at tumor site in neoplastic patients treated with vinorelbine: Report of unusual toxicity. Eur J Cancer 30A:889, 1994.

55. Gerard JM, Franck N, Moussa Z, et al: Acute ischemic brachial plexus neuropathy following radiation therapy. Neurology 39:450–451, 1989.

56. Gilbert MR, and Grossman SA: Incidence and nature of neurologic problems in patients with solid tumors. Am J Med 81:951–956, 1986.

57. Gonzales GR, Elliott KJ, Portenoy RK, et al: The impact of a comprehensive evaluation in the management of cancer pain. Pain 47:141–144, 1991.

58. Granek I, Ashikari R, and Foley KM: Postmastectomy pain syndrome: Clinical and anatomic correlates. Proc ASCO 3: Abstract 122, 1983.

59. Graus F, Krol G, and Foley KM: Early diagnosis of spinal epidural metastasis: Correlation with clinical and radiological findings. Proceedings of the American Society of Clinical Oncology 5: Abstract 1047, 1986.

60. Greenberg HS, Deck MDF, Vikram B, et al: Metastasis to the base of the skull: Clinical findings in 43 patients. Neurology 31:530–537, 1981.

61. Greenwald HP, Bonica JJ, and Bergner M: The prevalence of pain in four cancers. Cancer 60: 2563–2569, 1987.

62. Hacking HG, Van AH, and Lankhorst GJ: Factors related to the outcome of inpatient rehabilitation in patients with neoplastic epidural spinal cord compression. Paraplegia 31:367–374, 1993.

63. Haddad P, Thaell JF, Kiely JM, et al: Lymphoma of the spinal epidural space. Cancer 38:1862–1866, 1976.

64. Harper CM, Thomas JE, Cascino TL, et al: Distinction between neoplastic and radiation-induced brachial plexopathy, with emphasis on EMG. Neurology 39:502–506, 1989.

65. Healey J: The mechanism and treatment of bone pain. In Arbit E (ed): Management of Cancer-Related Pain. Futura, Mt Kisco, 1993, pp 515–526.

66. Hewitt DJ, and Foley KM: Neuro-Imaging. In Greenberg J (ed): A Companion to Adams and Victors Principles of Neurology. McGraw-Hill, New York, 1995, pp 41–82.

67. Holland J, and Rowland JH (eds): Handbook of Psychooncology: Psychological Care of the Patient. Oxford University Press, New York, 1989.

68. Huang ME, Ye YC, Chen SR, et al: Use of all-trans retinoic acid in the treatment of acute promyelocytic leukemia. Blood 72:567–572, 1988.

69. Jacox A, Carr DB, Payne R, et al: Management of cancer pain. Clinical practice guidelines No. 9. AHCPR Publication N 94-0592. Agency for Health Care Policy and Research, US Department of Health and Human Services, Public Health Service, Rockville, MD, 1994.

70. Jaeckle KA, Young DF, and Foley KM: The natural history of lumbrosacral plexopathy in cancer. Neurology 35:8–15, 1985.

71. Jonsson OG, Sartain P, Ducore JM, et al: Bone pain as an initial symptom of childhood acute lymphoblastic leukemia: association with nearly normal hematologic indexes. J Pediatr 117:233–237, 1991.

72. Kanner RM, Martini N, and Foley KM: Epidural spinal cord compression (ESCC) in Pancoast (superior pulmonary sulcus) tumor: Clinical presentation and outcome. Trans Am Neurol Assoc 106:75–77, 1981.

73. Kanner RM, Martini N, and Foley KM: Nature and incidence of postthoracotomy pain. Proceedings of the American Society of Clinical Oncology 1: Abstract 590, 1982.

74. Kaplan JG, DeSouza TG, Farkash A, et al: Leptomeningeal metastases: Comparison of clinical features and laboratory data of solid tumors, lymphomas and leukemias. J Neurooncol 9:225–229, 1990.

75. Katz J, and Melzack R: Pain 'memories' in phantom limbs: Review and clinical observations. Pain 43:319–336, 1990.

76. Kellgren JG: On distribution of pain arising from deep somatic structures with charts of segmental pain areas. Clin Sci (Colch) 4:35–46, 1939.

77. Kelsen DP, Portenoy RK, Thaler HT, et al: Pain and depression in patients with newly diagnosed pancreas cancer. J Clin Oncol, 13:748–755, 1995.

78. Kemeny N, Cohen A, Bertino J, et al: Continuous intrahepatic infusion of floxuridine and leucovorin through an implantable pump for the treatment of hepatic metastases from colorectal carcinoma. Cancer 65:2446–2450, 1990.

79. Kori SH, Foley KM, Posner JB, et al: Brachial plexus lesions in patients with cancer: 100 cases. Neurology 31:45–50, 1981.

80. Krol G: Evaluation of neoplastic involvement of brachial and lumbar plexus: Imaging aspects. Journal of Back and Musculoskeletal Rehabilitation 3:35–43, 1993.

81. Kroner K. Knudsen UB, Lundby L, et al: Long-term phantom breast syndrome after mastectomy. Clin J Pain 8:346–350, 1992.

82. Kroner K, Krebs B, Skov J, et al: Immediate and long-term phantom breast syndrome after mastectomy: Incidence, clinical characteristic relationship to premastectomy breast pain. Pain 36:327–335, 1989.

83. Lederman RJ, and Wilbourn AJ: Brachial plexopathy: Recurrent cancer or radiation. Neurology 34:1331–1335, 1984.

84. Lipton RB, Galer BS, Dutcher JP, et al: Large and small fibre type sensory dysfunction in patients with cancer. J Neurol Neurosurg Psychiatry 54:706–709, 1991.

85. MacDonald DR, Strong E, Nielson S, et al: Syncope from head and neck cancer. Journal of Neurological Oncology 1:257–267, 1983.

86. Marangoni C, Lacerenza M, Formaglio F, et al: Sensory disorder of the chest as presenting symptom of lung cancer. J Neurol Neurosurg Psychiatry 56: 1033–1034, 1993.

87. Marino C, Zoppi M, Morelli F, et al: Pain in early cancer of the lungs. Pain 27:57–62, 1986.

88. Massey EW, Moore J, and Schold SC: Mental neuropathy from systemic cancer. Neurology 31:1277–1281, 1981.

89. Molinari R: Problems of cancer pain in the head and neck. In Bonica JJ, and Ventafridda V (eds): Advances in Pain Research and Therapy, Vol 2. Raven Press, New York, 1979, pp 519–531.

90. Mollman JE, Glover DJ, Hogan WM, et al: Cisplatin neuropathy: Risk factors. Prognosis and protection by WR-2721. Cancer 61:2192–2195, 1988.

91. Mondrup K, Olsen NK, Pfeiffer P, et al: Clinical and electrodiagnostic findings in breast cancer patients with radiation-induced brachial plexus neuropathy. Acta Neurol Scand 81:153–158, 1990.

92. Nestor J, and Ngo L: Incidence of facial pain caused by lung cancer. Otolaryngol Head Neck Surg 111:155–156, 1994.

93. Pancoast HK: Importance of careful roentgen ray investigations of apical chest tumor. JAMA 83: 1407–1411, 1923.

94. Portenoy RK: Cancer pain: Pathophysiology and syndromes. Lancet 339:1026–1031, 1992.

95. Portenoy RK: Evaluation of back pain caused by epidural neoplasm. Journal of Back and Musculoskeletal Rehabilitation 3:44–52, 1993.

96. Portenoy RK, Abissi CJ, Robbins J, et al: Increased intracranial pressure with normal ventricular size due to superior vena cava obstruction. Arch Neurol 40:598, 1983.

97. Portenoy RK, Galer BS, Salamon O, et al: Identification of epidural neoplasm. Radiography and bone scintigraphy in the symptomatic and asymptomatic spine. Cancer 64:2207–2213, 1989.

98. Portenoy RK, Kornblith AB, Wong G, et al: Pain in ovarian cancer patients. Prevalence, characteristics, and associated symptoms. Cancer 74:907–915, 1994.

99. Portenoy RK, Lipton RB, and Foley KM: Back pain in the cancer patient: An algorithm for evaluation and management. Neurology 37:134–138, 1987.

100. Portenoy RK, Miransky J, Thaler HT, et al: Pain in ambulatory patients with lung and colon cancer. prevalence and characteristics. Cancer 70:1616–1624, 1992.

101. Posner JB: Back pain and epidural spinal cord compression. Med Clin North Am 71:185–206, 1987.

102. Posner JB: Paraneoplastic syndromes. Neurol Clin 9:919–936, 1991.

103. Posner JB, and Chernik NL: Intracranial metastases from systemic cancer. Adv Neurol 19:575–587, 1978.

104. Powell S, Cooke J, and Parsons C: Radiation induced brachial plexus injury: Folllow-up of two different fractionation schedules. Radiother Oncol 18:213–220, 1990.

105. Rappaport S, Stacy C, and Foley KM: Median nerve somatosensory-evoked potentials are useful in the diagnosis of metastases to the brachial plexus and adjacent spinal roots and epidural space. Ann Neurol 14:143, 1983.

106. Rider CA: Oral mucositis. A complication of radiotherapy. New York State Dental Journal 56:37–39, 1990.

107. Ripamonti C: Malignant bowel obstruction in advanced terminal cancer patients. European Journal of Palliative Care 1:16–19, 1994.

108. Rodichock LD, Ruckdeschel JC, Harper GR, et al: Early detection and treatment of spinal epidural metastases: The role of myelography. Ann Neurol 20:696–702, 1986.

109. Rogers LH, Cho ES, Kempin S, et al: Cerebral infarction from non-bacterial thrombotic endocarditis. A clinical and pathological study including the effects of anticoagulation. Am J Med 83:746–756, 1987.

110. Rogers LR, Borkowski GP, Albers JW, et al: Obturator mononeuropathy caused by pelvic cancer: Six cases. Neurology 43:1489–1492, 1993.

111. Rogers L, and Foley KM: Leptomeningeal metastases. In Harris JR, Hellman S, Henderson IC, et al (eds): Breast Diseases, ed 2. JB Lippincott, Philadelphia, in press.

112. Rotstein J, and Good RA: Steroid pseudorheumatism. Arch Intern Med 99:545–555, 1957.

113. Rowinski EK, Chaudhry V, Cornblath D, et al: Neurotoxicity of taxol. Monogr Natl Cancer Inst 15: 107–115, 1993.

114. Rusthoven JJ, Ahlgren P, Elhakim T, et al: Risk factors for varicella zoster disseminated infection among adult cancer patients with localized zoster. Cancer 62:1641–1646, 1988.

115. Salner AL, Botnick L, Hertzog AG, et al: Reversible transient plexopathy following primary radiation therapy for breast cancer. Cancer Treat Rep 65: 797–801, 1981.

116. Saltzburg D, and Foley KM: Management of pain in pancreatic cancer. Surg Clin North Am 69:629–649, 1989.

117. Siegal T: Muscle cramps in the cancer patient: Causes and treatment. Journal of Pain and Symptom Management 6:84–91, 1991.

118. Siegal T, and Haim N: Cisplatin-induced peripheral neuropathy. Frequent off-therapy deterioration, demyelinating syndromes, and muscle cramps. Cancer 66:1117–1123, 1990.

119. Siegal T, Lossos A, and Pfeffer MR: Leptomeningeal metastases. Analysis of 31 patients with sustained off-therapy response following combined-modality therapy. Neurology 44:1463–1469, 1994.

120. Sozzi C, Marotta P, and Piatti L: Vagoglossopharyngeal neuralgia with syncope in the course of carcinomatous meningitis. Italian J Neurol Sci 8: 271–276, 1987.

121. Stark DB, and Fletcher WS: Severe tumor pain with intravenous injection of vinblastine sulfate (NSC-49842). Cancer Chemotherapy Reports 50: 281–282, 1966.

122. Stevens MJ, and Gonet YM: Malignant psoas syndrome: Recognition of an oncologic entity. Australas Radiol 34:150–154, 1990.

123. Stillman M: Perineal pain: Diagnosis and management, with particular attention to perineal pain of cancer. In Foley KM, Bonica JJ, and Ventafridda V (eds): Second International Congress on Cancer Pain, Vol 16. Raven Press, New York, 1990, pp 359–377.

124. Swift TR, and Nichols FT: The droopy shoulder syndrome. Neurology 34:212–215, 1984.

125. Thomas JE, Cascino TL, and Earl JD: Differential diagnosis between radiation and tumor plexopathy of the pelvis. Neurology 35:1–7, 1985.

126. Thomas JE, and Colby MY: Radiation-induced or metastatic brachial plexopathy: A diagnostic dilemma. JAMA 222:1392–1395, 1972.

127. Thompson IM, Zeidman EJ, and Rodriguez FR: Sudden death due to disease flare with luteinizing hormone-releasing hormone agonist therapy for carcinoma of the prostate. J Urol 144:1479–1480, 1990.

128. Twycross RG, and Fairfield S: Pain in far-advanced cancer. Pain 14:303–310, 1982.

129. Vecht CJ: Arm pain in the patient with breast cancer. Journal of Pain and Symptom Management 5:109–117, 1990.

130. Vecht CJ, Hoff AM, Kansen PJ, et al: Types and causes of pain in cancer of the head and neck. Cancer 70:178–184, 1992.

131. Vecht CJ, Van de Brand HJ, and Wajer OJ: Post-axillary dissection pain in breast cancer due to a lesion of the intercostobrachial nerve. Pain 38:171–176, 1989.

132. Ventafridda V, and Caraceni A: Cancer pain classification: A controversial issue. Pain 46:1–2, 1991.

133. Ventafridda V, Caraceni A, Martini C, et al: On the significance of Lhermitte's sign in oncology. J Neurooncol 10:133–137, 1991.

134. Wasserstrom WR, Glass JP, and Posner JB: Diagnosis and treatment of leptomeningeal metastasis from solid tumors: Experience with 90 patients. Cancer 49:759–772, 1982.

135. Watson CPN, and Evans RJ: Intractable pain with lung cancer. Pain 29:163–173, 1987.

136. Watson CPN, Evans RJ, and Watt VR: The postmastectomy pain syndrome and the effect of topical capsaicin. Pain 38:177–186, 1989.

137. Weinstein RE, Herec D, and Friedman JH: Hypotension due to glossopharyngeal neuralgia. Arch Neurol 40:90–92, 1986.

138. Weiss HD, Walker MD, Wiernik PH, et al: Neurotoxicity of commonly used antineoplastic agents. N Engl J Med 291:75–81, 1974.

PART 3

Therapeutic Interventions

CHAPTER 10

NONOPIOID AND ADJUVANT ANALGESICS

Russell K. Portenoy, M.D., and Ronald M. Kanner, M.D.

NONOPIOID ANALGESICS
Mechanism of Action
Clinical Pharmacology
Clinical Applications
ADJUVANT ANALGESICS
Multipurpose Adjuvant Analgesics
Adjuvant Analgesics for Neuropathic Pain
Other Adjuvant Analgesics

Rapid advances in basic and clinical pharmacology have yielded a very large and diverse group of clinically useful analgesic drugs. These drugs can be divided into three broad categories: the nonopioid analgesics, the opioid analgesics, and the so-called "adjuvant analgesics." Most of the nonopioid analgesics and the opioids have been formally approved for the treatment of pain. The adjuvant analgesics can be defined as drugs that have been approved for the treatment of other conditions but are analgesic in selected circumstances.

NONOPIOID ANALGESICS

The nonopioid analgesics are among the most widely prescribed drugs. This group includes acetaminophen and the nonsteroidal anti-inflammatory drugs (NSAIDs), three of which (aspirin, ibuprofen, and naproxen) are available without prescription.

The "aspirin-like" NSAIDs came into the analgesic armamentarium as a by-product of the search for effective antipyretic agents. Extracts from willow bark were first found to be both antipyretic and analgesic, presumably because of their salicin content. In the late 19th century, the pyrazole derivatives aminopyrine and antipyrine were introduced as antipyretics, then discovered to be analgesic. Sodium salicylate was the first synthetic salicylate, and aspirin was brought into popular use in 1899. Phenylbutazone was marketed in 1949, after it had been used for many years as a solubilizing agent for aminopyrine.

During the past quarter-century, numerous NSAIDs have been developed in a variety of drug classes. Aspirin remains the prototype, but the newer NSAIDs offer the potential of reduced side effects and more convenient dosing schedules.* Individual variability in response to different NSAIDs, combined with the potential advantages of tailored dosing schedules, justifies the panoply of drugs currently available.

Mechanism of Action

The precise mechanism by which NSAIDs produce analgesia is unknown. NSAIDs in-

---

*References 8,18,21,37,42,86,91,176.

219

hibit the enzyme cyclooxygenase and thereby reduce prostaglandin synthesis.[185] Prostaglandins are key components in the inflammatory cascade and sensitize nociceptors to the actions of other compounds, such as bradykinin and histamine. Reduction in the tissue concentration of prostaglandins could potentially explain both the anti-inflammatory and analgesic activities of the NSAIDs.

Although the analgesic effects of the NSAIDs are usually ascribed to this reduction of peripheral prostaglandin production, there is considerable evidence that a central mechanism may also be involved in NSAID analgesia. Support for the existence of this putative central mechanism derives from studies in animals that have demonstrated analgesic efficacy from intraspinal administration,[115] a study in humans that investigated NSAID modulation of nociceptive reflexes in paraplegic patients,[195] and the observed disparity between the anti-inflammatory and analgesic potencies of these drugs in clinical use.[123]

The relative importance of central NSAID mechanisms in analgesia is unknown and theoretically could vary with the individual or the predominating mechanism of the pain. Regardless, the existence of such effects underscores the clinical observation that NSAIDs may provide analgesia even without a peripheral focus of inflammation. Future research may expand clinical opportunities with these drugs by yielding agents with stronger central actions or by establishing the efficacy of intraspinal administration.

Clinical Pharmacology

NSAIDs may be administered by the oral, rectal, and parenteral routes. All these drugs are readily absorbed after oral administration and usually reach peak plasma levels within 2 hours after a dose. Simultaneous ingestion of food decreases abdominal discomfort and slows absorption but does not change the ultimate bioavailability of most agents. There is conflicting evidence that rectal administration decreases the incidence of gastric ulceration.

Elimination half-lives vary from less than 4 hours for some of the propionic acid derivatives to nearly 45 hours for piroxicam (Table 10-1). Some NSAIDs, such as meclofenamate and sulindac, have active metabolites that prolong clinical efficacy far beyond the half-life of the parent drug. The salicylates are metabolized by a saturable enzyme system, which results in dose-dependent increases in half-life. At doses in the anti-inflammatory range, dose increments produce nonlinear increases in plasma concentrations; as a result, large loading doses can achieve adequate plasma levels quickly and steady state can be reached in less than 1 day. The salicylates also undergo an enterohepatic cycle, further increasing half-life.

Most of the NSAIDs undergo hepatic conjugation and renal excretion. Only a small percentage of the drug can be found unchanged in the urine. With the exception of the salicylates, elimination follows first-order kinetics, with rapidity of elimination dependent on drug concentration. Impaired renal function is only a relative contraindication to the use of these drugs. Patients with renal insufficiency should be managed with lower doses and close monitoring of kidney function.

Acetaminophen is also readily absorbed after oral or rectal administration. It is approximately equianalgesic with aspirin on a milligram basis. Although its mechanism of action is unknown, its primary action appears to be in the central nervous system. It does not inhibit peripheral cyclooxygenase but may not be entirely devoid of anti-inflammatory activity.[6] In contrast to the NSAIDs, acetaminophen has little gastrointestinal toxicity and no effect on platelet function.

The dose-response relationship for the NSAIDs is characterized by a minimal effective dose and a ceiling dose for analgesia. Doses higher than the ceiling do not provide additional analgesia but presumably increase the risk of dose-related toxicity. There is large individual variation in the minimal effective dose, toxic dose, and ceiling dose. Consequently, the recommended therapeutic doses for each drug, which have been developed from dose-ranging studies in relatively healthy populations, should be viewed as broad guidelines and not absolute requirements. This individual variation suggests the potential value of dose titration in the clinical setting (see following).

Table 10–1. **PHARMACOLOGY OF NONSTEROIDAL ANTI-INFLAMMATORY DRUGS**

Group and Drug	Total Daily Dose (mg)	Dosing Interval	Half-Life (hours)	Cost/Month ($)
Salicylates				
Salsalate	3000	q12h	16	30
Diflunisal*	1000–1500	q12h	8–12	30–45
Choline Mg†† trisalicylate	1500–4000	q12h	9–17	40–120
Propionic Acids				
Ibuprofen*	1200–3200	q4–6h	2	30–80
Flurbiprofen	100–300	q12h	5.7	50–150
Fenoprofen*	900–2400	q8h–q6h	3	50–125
Ketoprofen*	150–300	q8h–q6h	2–4	90–180
Naproxen*	500–1025	q12h	13	44–80
Naproxen Na*	275–1375	q12h	13	44–80
Indoles				
Indomethacin	50–150	q8h–q6h	4.5	35–100
Sulindac	200–400	q12h	8†	45–90
Tolmetin	600–1800	q8h	2–5	30–90
Etodolac*	600–1600	q4–6h	3–11‡	70–175
*Fenamates**				
Mefenamic acid	1000†	q6h	2†	—
Meclofenamate	200–600	q4–6h	2†	54–162
Others				
Piroxicam	20–40	daily	50	80–160
Nabumetone	1000–2000	daily–q12h	24	60–120
Ketorolac*	10–40†	q6h	4–7	60–120
Diclofenac	100–150	q8h–q6h	2	45–60

Cost (in dollars/month) reflects approximate retail cost, based on prices for bottles of 100 pills of the most common strengths. Prices vary with pharmacies, and some of the agents are available as generics, costing 20% to 50% less.

*Drugs that have primary indications as analgesics.

†These drugs are not recommended for prolonged use because of increased risk of gastrointestinal toxicity.

‡Metabolites are active and their half-life is long enough to allow less frequent dosing.

Extensive pharmacokinetic and pharmacodynamic interactions exist between NSAIDs and other drugs.[186] Although the administration of other drugs can change NSAID metabolism, the effects are rarely clinically important. Antacids can decrease NSAID absorption and increase excretion, cimetidine can inhibit NSAID metabolism, and aspirin can decrease plasma NSAID concentration. None of these changes, however, produces clinically significant effects.

In contrast, the consequences of NSAID administration for the pharmacokinetics or pharmacodynamics of other drugs can be clinically important.[88] Coadministration of an NSAID can reduce methotrexate clearance to such an extent that potentially toxic levels can be reached within 10 days.[58] The risk of gastric ulceration is increased fourfold when an NSAID is coadministered with a corticosteroid.[141] NSAID-induced changes in warfarin levels can result in a serious coagulopathy, with increased risk of hemorrhage. Lithium clearance is decreased by concurrent administration of an NSAID; thus, lithium plasma concentration should be monitored every 4 or

5 days after an NSAID is added.[148] Careful monitoring is also required when an NSAID is added to a therapeutic regimen containing phenytoin or other anticonvulsants, sulfonylureas, some diuretics, and some antihypertensives.[16,88]

Clinical Applications

The use of the NSAIDs is largely based on empirical knowledge of indications and dosing guidelines. Information about the pharmacology of the group as a whole and specific drugs within it influences clinical decision making.

INDICATIONS

Although relatively few of the NSAIDs are formally approved for pain as an indication (see Table 10–1), all are analgesic. The major use of these drugs is in the treatment of pain associated with inflammatory conditions, particularly osteoarthritis and autoimmune arthritides. Most NSAIDs have received formal approval for the treatment of rheumatoid arthritis. Selected drugs have also been formally approved for other conditions, such as painful shoulder (indomethacin and sulindac), dysmenorrhea (mefenamic acid, meclofenamate, and others), and postoperative pain (ketorolac).

The NSAIDs may also be useful in pains associated with noninflammatory conditions. Thus, empirical trials of one or more of these drugs should be considered for any patient with chronic pain, including those with neuropathic or idiopathic pain. Therapeutic trials are also appropriate for patients with chronic or frequently recurrent headache; indeed, indomethacin is considered to be the drug of choice in several specific headache syndromes, such as chronic paroxysmal hemicrania (see Chapter 4). NSAIDs are also an integral part of the World Health Organization's "analgesic ladder" approach for the management of cancer pain.[60,198] Although comparative controlled trials are lacking, these drugs appear to be particularly useful in cancer-related bone pain or pain associated with a grossly inflammatory lesion.[137]

ADVERSE EFFECTS

As a group, the NSAIDs share numerous side effects. There are, however, important drug-specific differences that may have clinical relevance in some circumstances.

Clinically important adverse gastrointestinal (GI) symptoms occur in about 10 percent of patients treated with NSAIDs[21,110]; ulcers occur in about 2 percent.[114,165] Adjusted for age and sex, the relative risk for ulceration is two to three times that of the general population.[13] Although some epidemiologic data suggest that the risk of ulceration is limited to gastric lesions, other data implicate both gastric and duodenal lesions. It is also likely that the complications that ensue following duodenal ulceration are greater in patients receiving NSAIDs. Acetaminophen does not appear to increase the risk of ulceration, although chronic use can cause dyspepsia. Rare GI complications of the NSAIDs include colitis and the formation of membranous sheets (diaphragms) in the small and large bowel.[168]

The common adverse GI effects of the NSAIDs, including ulceration, are presumably related to inhibition of prostaglandins that play a role in protecting the gastric mucosa from acid damage. GI toxicity does not require a local action, although there also may be a direct irritative effect on the stomach wall. A direct effect can also be seen endoscopically in the esophagus.[34,129]

Numerous studies have attempted to clarify the risk factors for major GI toxicity (ulceration and bleeding). Although nausea and abdominal pain raise concern about the potential for ulceration, these symptoms are actually poor predictors. As many as two-thirds of NSAID users have no symptoms before bleeding or perforation. Some studies,[114,194] but not others,[102] demonstrate an increased risk of ulcer associated with advanced age, the use of higher NSAID doses, concomitant administration of a corticosteroid, and a history of either ulcer disease or previous GI complications from NSAIDs; other risk factors may include alcohol and cigarette consumption. In contrast to the established role for chronic infection with the bacterium *Helicobacter pylori* in peptic ulcer disease unrelated to NSAID therapy, a contribution of this organism to NSAID-related gastropathy has been suggested but never proved.[167]

The risk of GI toxicity varies among NSAIDs.[93,102,104,163,196] The most consistent findings from epidemiologic studies indicate that the prototype NSAID, aspirin, is relatively more toxic than ibuprofen and relatively less toxic than piroxicam. A recent study evaluating the outcome of bleeding ulcer associated with a specified group of NSAIDs observed that the risk of this complication was lowest for ibuprofen and diclofenac; intermediate for indomethacin, naproxen, and piroxicam; and highest for ketoprofen and azapropazone.[102] This study could not identify different risks for gastric versus duodenal ulcer or for short-term versus long-term NSAID use. Risk of bleeding ulcer was dose related, however.

The effort to prevent serious GI complications has included empirical trials with antacids, sucralfate, H_2 blockers, omeprazole, and misoprostol. With the exception of misoprostol, a prostaglandin analog, no convincing evidence exists that any of these approaches reduces the risk of serious GI toxicity associated with NSAID use.

Misoprostol reduces the incidence of NSAID-induced ulcers without reversing the desired anti-inflammatory and analgesic effects.[134] Given the cost of long-term therapy with this drug, it is reasonable to limit treatment to patients with significant risk factors for GI complications. Specifically, therapy should be considered in the elderly, in patients with a history of peptic ulcer disease or concurrent corticosteroid use, and in those who could not tolerate a GI hemorrhage (such as those who are severely debilitated by intercurrent disease and those who are receiving anticoagulants). Patients at high risk of GI morbidity but unable to afford or tolerate misoprostol treatment may be given an alternative, albeit unproven treatment, such as sucralfate, an H_2 blocker, regular use of antacids, or some combination of these approaches.

Although there is relatively little risk of renal toxicity when NSAIDs are used at the usual therapeutic doses in normal subjects,[132] occasional patients develop serious complications. The risk of renal toxicity also accompanies long-term acetaminophen therapy.[162] The claim that some drugs, such as sulindac and etodolac, are relatively "renal sparing" should not be assumed to have clinical relevance, given the lack of adequate comparative studies at appropriate doses.

Renal impairment can present in a number of ways. Acute renal failure from NSAIDs is far less common than the more slowly progressive forms. Acute renal failure usually occurs only in rare susceptible individuals, such as binge drinkers or patients with preexisting renal dysfunction or hypovolemia.[33,168] Renal blood flow and glomerular filtration drop rapidly, and renal ischemia results in a sharp rise in creatinine and urea nitrogen. This acute syndrome is usually reversible with cessation of the NSAID.

Acute interstitial nephritis with glomerulopathy is another reversible NSAID-induced syndrome characterized by proteinuria and mild renal failure. It is more common in elderly women, is not allergic in nature, and does not respond to steroid therapy.[142]

In contrast to the acute forms, irreversible renal failure may result from prolonged NSAID use at high levels. Indeed, end-stage renal disease may be the presenting sign of analgesic abuse. While diminishing in frequency, analgesic nephropathy is still the most common cause of toxic nephropathy.[77] The mechanism is not known but may represent a combination of medullary ischemia and direct toxic effects of NSAID metabolites.[132]

NSAID-induced inhibition of platelet aggregation may also result in adverse effects. Aspirin, which is the strongest inhibitor, irreversibly alters exposed platelets; a single dose can double the bleeding time for up to 1 week. Other NSAIDs have reversible effects on platelet function and, therefore, affect bleeding time only when circulating in the plasma. There are drug-specific differences in these platelet effects (e.g., the nonacetylated salicylates, such as choline magnesium trisalicylate and salsalate, have minimal platelet effects), but the clinical implications of these differences have not been evaluated. Acetaminophen, which does not inhibit platelet function, is preferred if a nonopioid analgesic is indicated in a patient with a bleeding diathesis.

The potential for other adverse effects may limit NSAID therapy in some patients. Vague complaints of dizziness and confusion occur more commonly in the elderly than in younger patients. Headache appears to be somewhat more common during treatment with indomethacin than with other NSAIDs. Tinnitus is a frequent side effect of the salicylates and may even occur at therapeutic levels. Rarely, an NSAID causes an aseptic meningitis, presumably on an allergic basis.

Hypersensitivity reactions to the NSAIDs, which may be severe, are fortunately rare. Given the potential for serious morbidity and the possibility of cross-sensitivity among NSAIDs, a history of aspirin sensitivity or hypersensitivity to one NSAID is a relative contraindication to the use of others.

COST CONSIDERATIONS

The cost of drugs is a major issue for many patients. High drug costs may reduce compliance and place a substantial burden on the patient's family. Unfortunately, physicians are rarely aware of drug prices and typically prescribe without considering this factor. House officers are less likely than attending staff to consider the cost of a drug before prescribing it.[161] This situation must change to optimize prescribing practices.

The newer NSAIDs are relatively costly drugs, particularly when compared with aspirin (see Table 10–1). Given the lack of evidence that any NSAID has better efficacy than any other in the population overall, the use of a relatively expensive drug is not appropriate without a clear justification.[76] Such a justification may be convenience of dosing or, more likely, the need to identify an agent with better efficacy or fewer side effects for a given patient.

The total cost of NSAID therapy must also consider the potential burden produced by adverse effects and the cost of prophylactic measures. Although misoprostol therapy adds a substantial additional cost to long-term treatment with an NSAID, this choice becomes cost-effective in those populations with a relatively increased risk of ulceration, such as the elderly and those with a history of gastric bleeding.[50,66] It is probably not cost-effective in the young and has its own set of undesirable side effects, such as diarrhea.

DOSING GUIDELINES

Drug selection and dosing guidelines are derived from clinical observation and the known pharmacology of the NSAIDs. The value of dose titration and the potential utility of sequential trials are the most important considerations.

The observation that the minimal effective dose, ceiling dose, and toxic dose in the individual patient may be actually higher or lower than the standard recommended dosing range justifies the use of dose titration in selected patients. This approach, which involves gradual dose escalation from a relatively low starting dose, is most appropriate for patients with mild to moderate pain and for those with a relatively increased risk of NSAID toxicity (such as the elderly). Conventional starting doses can be used in most other patients, and occasional patients with acute severe pain should be considered for an initial loading dose of 1½ to 2 times the conventional starting dose. The use of such a loading dose is standard practice when ketorolac is administered to treat postoperative pain.

If dose titration is used, a brief period of observation is needed between dose changes. Generally, this period should be at least 1 week; several weeks are optimal. The occurrence of increased analgesia after a dose change implies that the ceiling dose has not been reached.

Dose escalation can continue until analgesia is adequate, the ceiling dose is reached, side effects occur, or the dose approaches a conventionally accepted maximum. This maximal dose is usually considered to be in the range of 1½ to 2 times the average recommended starting dose. If a satisfactory balance between analgesia and side effects cannot be attained at a dose below the maximal safe dose, the drug should be discontinued and consideration given to a trial of an alternative NSAID.

In most patients, long-term NSAID therapy should be accompanied by regular monitoring for adverse effects. This monitoring, which should include a test for occult fecal blood and an evaluation of hemoglobin, renal function, and hepatic function, may be appropriate every few months. Patients who are predisposed to adverse effects and those who are receiving relatively high doses should be monitored more frequently.

ADJUVANT ANALGESICS

Adjuvant analgesics are drugs that have a primary indication other than pain but are analgesic in selected circumstances. This category comprises an extremely diverse group of drug classes, most of which contain more than one putative analgesic (Table 10–2).

Like the traditional analgesics (NSAIDs and opioids), the adjuvant analgesics should not be administered without a comprehensive assessment that clarifies the nature of the pain, the medical status of the patient, and the concomitant need for other therapies. To optimize therapy with any selected drug, the clinician must be knowledgeable about its relevant clinical pharmacology when it is administered as an analgesic. Dosing regimens and pharmacokinetic-pharmacodynamic relationships for analgesic effects may be different than for the primary indication of the drug. The clinician must be aware of common side effects and potentially serious adverse effects as well as factors that may increase the risk of therapy, such as advanced age, disease of the liver or kidney, or preexisting encephalopathy.

Large interindividual and intraindividual variability characterizes the response to all of the adjuvant analgesics. Neither favorable effects nor side effects can be reliably predicted at the time a therapeutic trial is initiated, even if the proposed drug is pharmacologically similar to drugs used in the past. Accordingly, the clinician must consider the potential value of sequential drug trials. A rational plan for a series of trials should be developed based on the nature of the target pain and the perceived risk-benefit ratio of the various drugs.

To improve compliance, reduce distress, and increase the likelihood of salutary outcomes during sequential trials with the adjuvant analgesics, patients should be informed about the difficulties inherent in this therapeutic approach. Specifically, patients should be told that drug selection is largely by trial and error; that multiple trials are often necessary; and that each trial is usually characterized by ineffective starting doses, gradual dose escalation, and side effects.

Multipurpose Adjuvant Analgesics

Some of the adjuvant analgesics have established utility in diverse pain syndromes (Table 10–3). These drugs may be considered multipurpose analgesics, potentially useful in the management of any chronic pain.

Table 10–2. ADJUVANT ANALGESICS: MAJOR CLASSES

Antidepressants
α_2-Adrenergic agonists
Neuroleptics
Local anesthetics
Anticonvulsants
GABA agonists
Sympatholytics
Muscle relaxants
Benzodiazepines
Corticosteroids

Table 10–3. MULTIPURPOSE ADJUVANT ANALGESICS

Antidepressants
Tricyclic antidepressants
　Tertiary amine drugs
　　Amitriptyline
　　Doxepin
　　Imipramine
　　Clomipramine
　Secondary amine drugs
　　Nortriptyline
　　Desipramine
"Newer" antidepressants
　Trazodone
　Maprotiline
　Paroxetine
Monoamine oxidase inhibitors
　Phenelzine

α_2-Adrenergic Agonists
　Clonidine

Neuroleptics
　Methotrimeprazine
　Fluphenazine
　Haloperidol

ANTIDEPRESSANT DRUGS

Compelling evidence indicates that antidepressant drugs are analgesic in a heterogeneous group of pain syndromes.[22,62,127,143] Controlled clinical trials have demonstrated the efficacy of amitriptyline in migraine and other types of headache,[36,46,135] arthritis,[63] chronic low back pain,[188] postherpetic neuralgia,[189,190] central pain,[109,136] fibromyalgia,[29,47] painful diabetic neuropathy,[120] and psychogenic pain.[140] Imipramine was beneficial in studies of arthritis,[70] headache,[101] painful diabetic neuropathy,[100] and low back pain.[2] Doxepin was effective in coexistent pain and depression,[56] headache,[135] and low back pain.[79] Controlled trials of desipramine in postherpetic neuralgia,[96] nortriptyline (combined with fluphenazine) in painful diabetic neuropathy,[74] and clomipramine in both neuropathic and nonneuropathic pain syndromes[49,103] have produced similarly favorable outcomes.

Although there have been many fewer studies of the "newer" antidepressants, evidence exists that some of these drugs are analgesic as well. Paroxetine, a selective serotonergic reuptake inhibitor (SSRI), was analgesic in a controlled trial that evaluated patients with painful polyneuropathy.[170] Similarly convincing evidence of analgesic efficacy is lacking for other SSRIs, such as fluoxetine and sertraline. Although a study of trazodone, which is also relatively serotonergic, suggested benefit in cancer pain, a well-controlled trial in patients with dysesthetic pains due to traumatic myelopathy failed to demonstrate a favorable effect from this drug.[39] The analgesic efficacy of maprotiline, a relatively selective noradrenergic drug, was suggested in controlled studies that evaluated patients with idiopathic pain[49] and postherpetic neuralgia.[189]

Monoamine oxidase inhibitors have also been evaluated in limited clinical settings. A placebo-controlled trial of phenelzine demonstrated efficacy in patients with atypical facial pain.[106] Several uncontrolled trials of either phenelzine or tranylcypromine have also been reported, usually for pain complicated by depression. An uncontrolled survey of patients with severe migraine suggested very favorable effects from phenelzine.[4]

Mechanism of Action. In contrast to an early hypothesis that linked the analgesic effects of antidepressant drugs to their mood-elevating properties,[56] there is now strong evidence that these drugs have primary analgesic effects. In animal models of nociception, antidepressant drugs have actions that mimic primary analgesics.[172] In clinical use, the analgesic dose is lower than that required to treat depression, and the onset of analgesia is more rapid than for antidepressant effects. Most important, analgesia can occur without an effect on mood.[120,190] Although it is certainly true that the patient with pain and depression may benefit additionally from resolution of the mood disturbance during antidepressant therapy, analgesia is not dependent on a primary effect on mood.

The analgesic actions of antidepressant drugs are most likely related to effects on monoamine-mediated endogenous pain-modulating pathways.[80,199] The efficacy of both serotonin-selective and norepinephrine-selective antidepressants suggests that actions on pathways that use either of these transmitters may contribute to analgesia. The tricyclic antidepressants are not highly selective, however, and also interact with other types of receptors (e.g., acetylcholine and histamine) that may be important in the development of analgesia.[153]

Clinical Applications. Useful dosing guidelines can be developed from the extensive clinical experience with these drugs and their known pharmacology.

Indications. Trials of antidepressants may be appropriate in the management of virtually any patient with chronic pain or frequently recurring pains, including headache. The only potential exception is the population with pure lancinating neuropathic pain, such as those with trigeminal neuralgia; clinical observation suggests that the response of these patients to the antidepressants is variable and less certain than their response to anticonvulsant therapy.

Adverse Effects. The occurrence of serious adverse effects during antidepressant therapy is rare, particularly at the relatively low doses typically used to treat pain. Nonetheless, low doses can sometimes produce relatively high plasma concentrations,[145] and some patients develop toxicity even at relatively low concentrations. Hence, the risk of adverse effects must be considered whenever therapy is considered. Advanced age may predispose to toxicity.

Although adverse cardiac effects are very uncommon during treatment with the tricyclic antidepressants,[71] these drugs are contraindicated in patients with significant cardiac conduction abnormalities or heart failure. Cardiologic evaluation may be helpful when such a decision is not clear cut. Most patients who have no known heart disease but are older than 50 years should have a baseline electrocardiogram (ECG) prior to therapy. Older patients should undergo repeated ECG if doses are increased to relatively high levels (e.g., amitriptyline above 150 mg per day). Plasma drug concentration can also be monitored for some drugs, further reducing the risk of adverse effects associated with unexpectedly high levels. Monitoring should include both the drug and its primary metabolite, when appropriate (e.g., amitriptyline and its metabolite, nortriptyline, or imipramine and its metabolite, desipramine).

Orthostatic hypotension is the most frequent adverse cardiovascular event ascribed to the tricyclic antidepressants. The elderly are at particular risk, and orthostasis probably contributes to the increased incidence of hip fracture sustained by elderly patients when they are treated with these drugs.[151] The newer antidepressants and the secondary amine tricyclic drugs are both less likely to produce orthostasis than is the tertiary amine tricyclic group (see Table 10–3); of the secondary amine drugs, nortriptyline is the least likely to produce this effect. Consequently, patients who are predisposed to orthostatic hypotension should be considered for a trial of nortriptyline or one of the newer antidepressants as initial therapy for pain.

Somnolence is a common side effect of antidepressant drugs, particularly the tricyclic antidepressants. This effect is variable, however, and many patients develop tolerance within several weeks after treatment is instituted. Of the tricyclic antidepressants used in pain management, desipramine is generally considered to be the least sedating. The newer antidepressants are usually less sedating than the tricyclic compounds. Indeed,

the SSRIs are actually activating in a substantial proportion of patients and should be taken early in the day to avoid insomnia.

Weight gain and anticholinergic effects may also be problematic during treatment with the tricyclic antidepressants. Weight gain is variable and often does not occur. If marked, however, it can contraindicate continued therapy.

Dry mouth is very common, and many patients who receive a tricyclic antidepressant note blurred vision or constipation. Serious anticholinergic toxicity, including precipitation of acute angle-closure glaucoma, obstipation, urinary retention, or delirium, is rare. Acute angle-closure glaucoma is a largely preventable ophthalmologic emergency, which may be induced by the administration of an anticholinergic compound to a patient who has a shallow anterior chamber of the eye. Bedside evaluation of the depth of the anterior chamber should be considered prior to the start of therapy with tricyclic antidepressants.[111] It is prudent to seek ophthalmologic evaluation if the patient is suspected of having a narrow anterior chamber or is under treatment for open-angle glaucoma, which can be worsened by anticholinergic drugs. Other patients at significant risk for anticholinergic effects, such as those with symptoms of prostatism or encephalopathy of some other cause (e.g., an early dementia) should be considered for treatment with an antidepressant that has relatively little anticholinergic action, such as a secondary amine tricyclic (desipramine or nortriptyline) or one of the SSRIs.

Dosing Guidelines. The most extensive data from controlled clinical trials support the analgesic efficacy of the tricyclic antidepressants, particularly amitriptyline. Consequently, a trial of amitriptyline should be considered for first-line therapy, unless relatively contraindicated by its side effect profile. If treatment with amitriptyline has failed or is not indicated because of concerns about toxicity, desipramine is an appropriate substitute, given the good evidence of analgesia[96] and a favorable side effect profile. In any individual case, however, the response may be more favorable to one of the other tricyclic compounds, and trials of other antidepressants in this class, including imipramine, doxepin, and nortriptyline, can be considered in refractory cases. Patients who cannot tolerate any tricyclic compound or who have a contraindication to these drugs may be candidates for a therapeutic trial with one of the newer antidepressants. Paroxetine is presently preferred on the basis of data that demonstrate analgesic effects.[170] Sequential trials of antidepressants are often justified.

The starting dose of the tricyclic antidepressants should be low. For example, treatment with amitriptyline should be initiated with 10 mg in the elderly and 25 mg in younger patients. The initial dosing increments are usually the same size as the starting dose. The usual effective daily dose for amitriptyline is 50 to 150 mg; occasional patients will have substantial benefit with a dose lower or higher than this range. Although most patients can be treated with a single nighttime dose, some patients have less morning "hangover" and some report less late afternoon pain if doses are divided.

Given the suggestion of dose dependent analgesic effects in some clinical trials,[120] it is reasonable to continue upward dose titration beyond the usual analgesic doses in patients who fail to achieve benefit and have no limiting side effects. This course should be undertaken even in patients with no evidence of clinical depression. Those with depression have an independent reason to escalate the dose into the antidepressant range.

Although no studies have systematically evaluated the relationship between plasma drug concentration and analgesia, monitoring of drug concentration, if available, can help guide dosing decisions. Low plasma concentration in patients with inadequate analgesia and no intolerable side effects suggests either a problem with compliance or atypical pharmacokinetics (the patient may absorb the drug poorly or metabolize it rapidly). In the latter situation, further dose escalation may be useful. Relatively high levels compared with the established antidepressant range does not prove that analgesia could not occur at yet higher doses, but the likelihood of benefit is probably low and the risks of toxicity are increased. In most cases, therefore, the clinician is justified in stopping dose escalation even in the absence of adverse effects when the plasma concentra-

tion is near the upper limit of the antidepressant range. It may be also useful to measure plasma levels in patients who develop analgesia; should pain recur, the plasma level can be measured again and a change in pharmacokinetics can be identified or excluded as a cause for the clinical findings.

Both favorable and unfavorable effects must be carefully monitored during dose escalation. The possibility of a therapeutic window for the analgesic effects produced by some tricyclic antidepressants has been suggested from anecdotal observation but does not alter the recommended dosing regimen for pain. If both effectiveness and side effects are carefully monitored, the dose can be reduced (or the drug discontinued) if adverse effects exceed benefits or analgesia declines following a dose increment.

A favorable analgesic effect is usually observed within a week after an effective dosing level is achieved. Antidepressant effects may require a longer period to evolve. Of course, days or even weeks may be required before the dose is gradually increased to the level associated with either analgesia or antidepressant effects. As noted, this delay, which is often accompanied by side effects such as dry mouth and somnolence, may undermine the patient's mood or compromise compliance with the therapy. These negative outcomes may be tempered by appropriate explanations to the patient about the expected course of the treatment.

No systematic studies have evaluated the long-term outcomes associated with antidepressant therapy for pain. Anecdotally, some patients who initially benefit from a tricyclic antidepressant can later discontinue the drug without a recurrence of the baseline pain, at least for a period of time. Following sustained analgesia for a period of months, gradual dose reduction can be attempted and can continue until the drug is discontinued if neither pain nor any other rebound effects occur. In contrast, some patients develop a gradual recurrence of pain over a period of weeks to months. This phenomenon could be related to tolerance, progression of the underlying disorder, or some intercurrent process (such as depression). If the breakthrough occurs very quickly (within weeks after obtaining analgesia), the possibility of a placebo effect should be considered. Evaluation of these possibilities is needed whenever pain worsens.

α₂-ADRENERGIC AGONISTS

Clonidine, the best-studied α_2-adrenergic agonist, has antinociceptive activity when administered intrathecally or epidurally in animals.[51] Both controlled and uncontrolled trials in humans have demonstrated analgesic effects in diverse pain syndromes, including migraine, postoperative pain, painful diabetic neuropathy, postherpetic neuralgia, and cancer pain.[14,15,121,180]

Mechanism of Action. The analgesic effects produced by an α_2-adrenergic agonist are presumably related to enhanced activity in endogenous pain-modulating pathways that use norepinephrine as a neurotransmitter. The specific function of the α_2-receptor in enhancing this activity is not known. Peripheral actions could be important, particularly in those patients whose pain is at least partly maintained by sympathetic efferent function (see Chapter 2).

Clinical Application. Although numerous studies support the conclusion that clonidine is a nonspecific analgesic, long-term clinical experience in populations with chronic pain is limited.

Indications. Chronic pain of any type, including migraine and neuropathic pain states, may be considered a potential target of treatment with clonidine. Given the limited empirical information and clinical experience, however, clonidine should be considered a second-line agent for patients with pain that has been refractory to trials of NSAIDs, antidepressants, and perhaps other drugs.

Adverse Effects. In the published reports, hypotension and sedation were the major side effects. In clinical practice, dry mouth and sedation have been the major limiting toxicities. Clearly, clonidine must be used cautiously in the elderly and in patients who are predisposed to hypotensive effects, including those who are receiving other drugs with additive effects on blood pressure and those with concurrent diseases such as neuropathy or heart failure. In the younger patient without a significant associated medical disorder, the risk of serious adverse cardiovascular effects appears to be low.

Dosing Guidelines. Clonidine can be administered via the oral or transdermal route. Currently, no data suggest better analgesic efficacy from one or the other, and the choice is based on patient preference. To limit the risk of adverse effects, starting doses should be low (e.g., 0.1 mg orally per day). Monitoring of both pain and adverse effects is necessary during gradual dose escalation. Neither dose-dependent effects nor the potential for a ceiling dose has been evaluated during systemic therapy. Consequently, gradual dose escalation should continue until side effects occur or a significant effect on blood pressure is noted.

NEUROLEPTICS

Although neuroleptic drugs can produce antinociceptive effects in animal studies,[201] few empirical data support the clinical analgesic potential of this class. Unequivocal analgesic effects have been demonstrated for one of the phenothiazines, methotrimeprazine, in several single-dose studies.[7,40,105,128] Although the analgesic efficacy of methotrimeprazine 10 to 20 mg approximates morphine 10 mg intramuscularly, the clinical utility of the drug is limited by the sole availability of a parenteral formulation and the common adverse effects of orthostatic hypotension and somnolence.

Other single-dose controlled studies have not demonstrated analgesic effects from chlorpromazine,[85] promethazine,[94] or haloperidol.[89] A controlled multiple-dose trial of fluphenazine (1 mg per day) did, however, demonstrate significant pain reduction in 50 patients with chronic tension headache.[78] Recently, a double-blind crossover trial that compared pimozide (4 to 12 mg per day) with carbamazepine in the treatment of trigeminal neuralgia indicated greater efficacy during pimozide treatment[108]; unfortunately, more than 83 percent of patients experienced dose-dependent side effects from pimozide, including physical and mental slowing, tremor, and slight parkinsonian symptoms.

A large number of uncontrolled reports have suggested the potential for analgesia during the administration of trifluoperazine, chlorprothixene, haloperidol, and fluphenazine in a variety of pain syndromes, including chronic headache and several types of neuropathic pain.[41,118] Other uncontrolled reports have purported to show that the addition of a neuroleptic to another analgesic, such as a tricyclic antidepressant or an opioid, augments pain relief.[17,97,183]

Mechanism of Action. The mechanism of methotrimeprazine analgesia is unknown. Dopaminergic pathways may be involved in endogenous pain modulation,[201] but there is no direct evidence that the well-known effects on dopamine receptors of the neuroleptic drugs underlie their analgesic effects in man.

Clinical Applications. The clinical utility of neuroleptic drugs in the management of chronic pain is limited. Nonetheless, occasional patients should be considered for trials of these drugs.

Indications. Although the available data suggest that the analgesic effects associated with neuroleptic drugs are nonspecific, the availability of safer alternatives has limited the use of these drugs to some patients with neuropathic pain refractory to other drugs and occasional patients with cancer pain. In patients with neuropathic pain, neuroleptic drugs are generally considered for continuous dysesthesias that have not responded to sequential trials of antidepressants, oral local anesthetics, and other drugs (e.g., anticonvulsants and baclofen).

Anecdotally, methotrimeprazine has been found useful in patients with advanced cancer, whose pain is accompanied by nausea, anxiety, or terminal agitation. In this setting, its sedative and anxiolytic effects can be highly favorable.

Adverse Effects. Common side effects of neuroleptic drugs include sedation, orthostatic dizziness, and anticholinergic effects. Phenothiazines, such as chlorpromazine and fluphenazine, are more likely to produce these effects than other subclasses. The sedation produced by the neuroleptics can be additive to other central nervous system depressants. Rare idiosyncratic reactions include blood dyscrasias, dermatoses (including photosensitivity), and hepatic damage.

Neuroleptic drugs can induce a spectrum of extrapyramidal effects that includes acute dystonic reactions, akathisia, parkinsonism, and tardive movement disorders (dyskinesia, dystonia, tic, and myoclonus). Acute dystonic reactions can usually be reversed promptly with an anticholinergic drug such as benztropine. Akathisia may be manageable with a benzodiazepine but also usually impels the discontinuation of neuroleptic therapy.

When neuroleptic treatment continues for a period of months, the greatest concern is the development of a tardive syndrome.[3] At the first signs of any tardive syndrome, the drugs should be tapered and discontinued. Rarely, tapering of the neuroleptic will be accompanied by the development of worsening dyskinesias (so-called "withdrawal emergent dyskinesias"), which are usually transient; this phenomenon should not prevent a trial of a drug-free period.

Neuroleptic therapy also predisposes to another serious extrapyramidal reaction, the neuroleptic malignant syndrome. This rare syndrome is characterized by rigidity, autonomic instability, and encephalopathy. Successful management requires prompt diagnosis, discontinuation of the neuroleptic, and intensive supportive measures (including intravenous hydration and fever control). The use of dantrolene and bromocriptine has been suggested in severe cases.[155]

Dosing Guidelines. For long-term oral therapy in patients with chronic pain (usually those with refractory neuropathic pain), clinical experience is greatest with fluphenazine and haloperidol. Pimozide is preferred, however, for patients with refractory neuropathic pain characterized by lancinating or paroxysmal dysesthesia. Methotrimeprazine is often considered for the patient with pain from advanced cancer who has some other indication for a neuroleptic, is largely bedridden, and has continuous subcutaneous or intravenous access.

For the treatment of refractory neuropathic pain, the doses of neuroleptic drugs associated with analgesia have generally been low. In the absence of data suggesting either a dose-response relationship or a clear benefit from dose escalation in patients who fail to respond to low doses, it is prudent to limit dosing to the parameters generally defined by published reports. Thus, a trial of fluphenazine should generally be limited to 1 to 2 mg three times a day, and a trial of haloperidol usually goes no higher than 2 to 5 mg two to three times a day. The use of lower initial doses, which can then be increased to these levels, is particularly important in the elderly. A trial of several weeks is reasonable, given experience with other adjuvant analgesics, and the failure to obtain a clear-cut analgesic response should be followed by discontinuation of the drug. Combination therapy with either a tricyclic antidepressant or an anticonvulsant drug has been described repeatedly and suggests that the addition of either fluphenazine or haloperidol to a partially effective regimen that includes one or more of these other agents may have value in selected patients with neuropathic pain.

Methotrimeprazine has been given by repetitive intramuscular or intravenous dosing or by continuous subcutaneous infusion. If intravenous bolus doses are used, a brief infusion (e.g., more than 30 minutes) reduces the risk of acute hypotension. A prudent dosing schedule begins with 5 mg every 6 hours, which is gradually increased as needed. Most patients will not require more than 20 mg every 6 hours to gain the desired effects.

Adjuvant Analgesics for Neuropathic Pain

The neuropathic pain syndromes are among the most challenging for the clinician. These syndromes are extremely heterogeneous and almost certainly involve numerous distinct pathophysiologic processes (see Chapter 5). Ultimately, scientific advances may be able to link specific mechanisms with identifiable clinical phenomena or disease states and then provide drugs that can be targeted specifically to these processes. Such specificity is largely lacking at the present time. Although there are currently a few indicators that suggest one or another pharmacologic approach, the clinician usually selects a series of therapies on a trial-and-error basis.

On the basis of clinical experience, the heterogeneous drugs that comprise the adjuvant analgesics are often considered in three overlapping groups. One group is preferred for neuropathic pains predominantly characterized by continuous dysesthesias. These drugs are typically selected early in the treatment of neuropathic pains described as burning, aching, or tingling, irre-

spective of the specific etiology. A second group is preferred for the treatment of neuropathic pains characterized by a predominant lancinating or paroxysmal component. These pains may occur as a component of virtually any neuropathic pain syndrome and are the sole element in some well-known disorders, such as trigeminal neuralgia. The third group includes drugs that have been used specifically in the treatment of sympathetically maintained pain. Sympathetically maintained pain refers to those syndromes (also known as reflex sympathetic dystrophy and causalgia) that are believed to be sustained by efferent activity in the sympathetic nervous system.

This categorization is used clinically in the selection of adjuvant analgesics for neuropathic pain. It has a limited empirical basis and should be considered only a guideline that may be helpful in organizing therapeutic drug trials. Experienced clinicians have observed many exceptions, and studies have suggested an overlapping response for at least some drugs, including the antidepressants.[120] Nonetheless, the use of clinical criteria to select drugs that may be somewhat more likely to be effective is a reasonable strategy, which could potentially reduce the burden and costs to the patient.

ADJUVANT ANALGESICS FOR CONTINUOUS DYSESTHESIA

The patient with a neuropathic pain syndrome that is experienced predominantly as a continuous dysesthesia is usually offered one or more therapeutic trials of an analgesic antidepressant first, as described previously. Several other drug classes are considered after these trials, including the oral local anesthetics (usually mexiletine) and the α_2-adrenergic agonist clonidine (Table 10–4). Trials of drugs usually preferred for the management of lancinating or paroxysmal pains, such as anticonvulsant drugs, are usually considered after failure of these therapies.

Local Anesthetics. Intravenous administration of local anesthetic has been reported to be analgesic in many acute and chronic pain syndromes, including neuropathic pains.[38,72,92,117,158] Although durable effects occasionally can be observed after a brief in-

Table 10–4. **ADJUVANT ANALGESICS PREFERRED FOR CONTINUOUS NEUROPATHIC PAIN**

Oral Local Anesthetics
Mexiletine
Tocainide

Topical Agents
Capsaicin
Local anesthetic (EMLA)
Anti-inflammatory drugs

Other Drugs for Continuous Neuropathic Pain
Calcitonin
Antidepressants
Neuroleptics

---

fusion, analgesia is usually not prolonged. Several oral local anesthetic drugs are now commercially available and provide an opportunity for long-term therapy.

Tocainide was demonstrated to be effective in a controlled study of patients with trigeminal neuralgia,[112] and mexiletine was effective in patients with painful diabetic neuropathy[44] and painful peripheral nerve injury.[30] Anecdotal reports have also suggested benefit from oral flecainide therapy. These studies confirm the potential analgesic efficacy of oral local anesthetic drugs in at least some types of neuropathic pain. Like the tricyclic antidepressants, the available data suggest that both continuous and lancinating dysesthesias may respond favorably.

Mechanism of Action. Local anesthetics block sodium channels and impose a non-depolarizing conduction block of the action potential. If they are placed adjacent to peripheral nerves at adequate concentration, a profound conduction block of both unmyelinated and myelinated axons can be produced. This peripheral effect, however, is unlikely to explain the analgesia produced by systemic administration of the oral local anesthetics. When systemically administered at nontoxic doses, local anesthetics do not block the peripheral action potential. In experimental models, systemic administration can suppress the activity of neurons in the dorsal horn of the spinal cord that are activated by C-fiber input[197] and then spontaneous firing of fibers in a 7-day-old neu-

roma.[31] It may thus be hypothesized that these drugs produce analgesia by suppressing aberrant electrical activity generated by central neurons, damaged peripheral axons, or both.

Clinical Applications. Although many published surveys describe the treatment of pain with brief intravenous infusions of a local anesthetic, many practitioners have no personal experience with the technique and no studies have assessed the nature of the dose-response relationship or the factors that determine the optimal dosing regimen. Similarly, there is still relatively little experience with the use of oral local anesthetics in the treatment of pain. Clinical recommendations, therefore, derive from limited data.

INDICATIONS. Systemic administration of a local anesthetic should be considered for the treatment of neuropathic pains. The available data suggest that patients with diverse types of neuropathic pain, including those with prominent continuous dysesthesias and those with lancinating pain, may respond. A trial with one of the oral local anesthetic drugs is warranted in patients with continuous dysesthesias who do not benefit from analgesic antidepressants and patients with lancinating pains that have been refractory to anticonvulsant drugs and baclofen (see following).

The utility of brief intravenous local anesthetic infusions is less well defined. Although it is reasonable to conjecture that the analgesic response to oral local anesthetic treatment may predict the outcome of an intravenous infusion and, likewise, that the response to an infusion may predict oral therapy, neither of these relationships has been demonstrated. A trial of a local anesthetic infusion is sometimes implemented in patients with refractory neuropathic pain who have failed to benefit from an oral formulation and, conversely, a trial of oral therapy is appropriate even though an intravenous infusion has been ineffective.

ADVERSE EFFECTS. The dose-dependent adverse effects of the local anesthetics are well known. The central nervous system effects generally occur at a lower concentration than the cardiovascular effects.[35] Dizziness, perioral numbness and other paresthesias, and tremor usually occur first; at higher plasma concentrations, progressive encephalopathy develops and seizures may occur.

Although mexiletine and tocainide are generally well tolerated at the doses used in the management of neuropathic pain, side effects are common and serious adverse effects have been described.[99,131] A survey of patients administered tocainide for arrhythmia noted nausea in 34 percent, dizziness in 31 percent, lightheadedness in 24 percent, tremors in 22 percent, palpitations in 17 percent, vomiting in 16 percent, and paresthesias in 16 percent.[84] Rare serious adverse effects have included interstitial pneumonitis, severe encephalopathy, blood dyscrasia, hepatitis, and dermatologic reactions[99,174,187]; of these, the lung disorder appears to be most frequent.

Mexiletine is generally considered to be a safer drug than tocainide. Side effects are also common, however, and may impel discontinuation of the drug in as many as 40 percent of the patients who receive it.[25,99] Nausea and vomiting (which is diminished by ingesting the drug with food), tremor, dizziness, unsteadiness, and paresthesias may occur. Serious side effects, including liver damage and blood dyscrasias, are rare.

All local anesthetic drugs must be used cautiously in patients with preexisting heart disease. It is prudent to avoid the analgesic use of these drugs in patients with severe heart failure or cardiac rhythm disturbances and in those on antiarrhythmic drugs. Patients with other significant cardiac disease should be appropriately monitored with repeated electrocardiograms; consultation with a cardiologist prior to treatment is reasonable in this setting.

DOSING GUIDELINES. In the United States, mexiletine has been the preferred drug for the treatment of neuropathic pain. No comparative trials have been undertaken, however, and it is possible that drug-specific differences may exist or that substantial intraindividual variability exists in the response to the various drugs.

As with the oral local anesthetics, there have been no controlled comparisons of the effects produced by brief intravenous infusions of the various parenteral anesthetics. The published experience is greatest with procaine and lidocaine, and it is reasonable to consider these drugs first.

Treatment with the oral local anesthetics should generally begin with low initial doses. Dose titration is warranted and, in the absence of contrary information, overall dosing levels should conform to those used in the treatment of cardiac arrhythmias. For example, mexiletine should usually be started at 150 mg per day. If intolerable side effects do not occur, the dose can be increased every few days until the usual maximum dose of 300 mg three times per day is reached. Plasma drug concentrations, if available, can provide guidance during dose escalation.

Neither the safety nor efficacy of the combination of an oral local anesthetic with either a tricyclic antidepressant or an anticonvulsant has been demonstrated in clinical trials. Nonetheless, trials of such combinations, undertaken with close clinical monitoring, can be justified in patients with refractory neuropathic pain. If a therapeutic trial with one of these adjuvant analgesics yields meaningful partial analgesia, it should be continued while a trial with another drug is initiated. If there is a risk of drug interactions, or additive toxicities, dosing must be very cautious and monitoring must be intensified.

Dosing guidelines for local anesthetic infusion are empirical, derived from the large experience described previously but complicated by the great variety of drugs and regimens reported. The doses used in lidocaine infusion, for example, have varied widely below a maximum dose of 5 mg/kg infused over 30 minutes.[67] Most experienced clinicians would select a dose of lidocaine in the range 2 to 5 mg/kg, which is administered over 20 to 30 minutes.

Topical Therapies. Topical approaches to the management of neuropathic pain have generally been applied to those syndromes characterized by both a predominating peripheral mechanism and continuous dysesthesia. Available topical therapies include capsaicin preparations, aspirin/nonsteroidal anti-inflammatory preparations, and local anesthetic preparations.[156]

Surveys of patients with postherpetic neuralgia or postmastectomy pain syndrome suggest that up to one-third of patients achieve partial relief of symptoms from topical capsaicin.[10,191,192] A controlled trial also suggested benefit in painful diabetic neuropathy.[28,181] These data support a trial of capsaicin in both painful mononeuropathy and painful polyneuropathy. Recent controlled trials also suggest that topical capsaicin may relieve the pain associated with osteoarthritis of the finger joints.[122] The latter finding suggests that some painful somatic disorders related to ongoing activation of nociceptors surrounding joints or other structures may also be amenable to this therapy.

Numerous anti-inflammatory drugs have been investigated for topical use, including aspirin, indomethacin, diclofenac, and benzydamine.[156] One small controlled trial demonstrated efficacy greater than placebo for topical aspirin, indomethacin, and diclofenac in patients with acute herpetic neuralgia or postherpetic neuralgia.[43] Another controlled trial found no efficacy whatsoever for topical treatment with a benzydamine cream in a similar patient population.[124] The results of surveys, which have also generally been conducted in patients with postherpetic neuralgia, have been mixed.[156] On the basis of these limited data, topical anti-inflammatory drugs appear to be safe, but efficacy in neuropathic pain states is questionable.

A eutectic mixture of local anesthetics (EMLA) is now commercially available in the United States. This compound, a 1:1 mixture of prilocaine and lidocaine, is capable of penetrating the skin and producing a dense cutaneous anesthesia. Limited studies of this drug[175] and a topical lidocaine gel[157] in patients with postherpetic neuralgia yielded favorable results, and a controlled trial of topical lidocaine in the same population was confirmatory.[156]

Mechanisms of Action. The topical agents are presumed to have different mechanisms of action. Capsaicin releases, then depletes, small peptides from primary afferent neurons. Presumably, local reduction in the neurotransmitters involved in the transfer of nociceptive information into the central nervous system accounts for the analgesic effects of this drug.[48] Topical anti-inflammatory preparations probably reduce tissue levels of prostaglandins, thereby diminishing the impact of these compounds on the peripheral activation of nociceptive primary afferent neurons. Local anesthetic compounds presumably block local nerve conduction or activation of receptor organs at a peripheral level. Although these putative mechanisms are supported by the known pharmacology of each of these drugs, no studies have adequately investigated the mode of analgesic action in human pain states and, consequently, all potential mechanisms are conjectural.

Clinical Applications. As noted, there have been few controlled studies of these drugs, and clinical experience is limited. Nonetheless, the potential advantages of the topical route for some patients is substantial, and empirical trials of topical drugs are reasonable in selected cases.

INDICATIONS. A trial of a topical analgesic drug can be considered for those patients with neuropathic pain presumed to be sustained, at least in part, by peripheral input. Topical agents should be considered particularly for those who are predisposed to side effects from systemically administered drugs, such as the elderly or those with comorbid conditions such as dementia.

There have been no comparative trials of the different topical drugs. The available data for the topical anti-inflammatory drugs are somewhat more equivocal than the others, and it would be reasonable to first undertake trials with capsaicin and local anesthetics.

ADVERSE EFFECTS. The reported adverse effects associated with topical analgesic therapy have been minimal. Capsaicin-containing preparations can cause local burning, which is presumably related to the initial release of peptides, such as substance P, in the periphery. It is not related to tissue damage and appears to pose no risk to the patient. Burning may be transitory, disappearing with repeated administrations over days to weeks, or more persistent. Some patients are able to tolerate the drug if administration is preceded by application of a local anesthetic or ingestion of an analgesic. When severe and poorly responsive to these measures, the burning may necessitate cessation of the drug.

With the exception of rare allergy, the topical anti-inflammatory drugs do not appear to be associated with serious toxicity. Presumably, the systemic absorption of the drugs administered by this route is minimal. Similarly, the systemic absorption of the topical local anesthetics, including EMLA, is limited,[175] and side effects are unlikely. The metabolites of the prilocaine contained in EMLA have been associated with the development of methemoglobinuria in predisposed patients. This is a rare event but does suggest that the drug should be used cautiously in infants, patients with prior histories of methemoglobinemia, and those who are coadministered drugs that may also cause this complication, such as sulfonamides.[64]

DOSING GUIDELINES. Based on clinical experience and survey data, a trial of capsaicin cream should be undertaken with the available 0.075 percent formulation. Four weeks of treatment with four applications per day is required to judge the value of this approach.

Guidelines for a trial of EMLA or other local anesthetic preparation are not well defined. EMLA is currently the only commercially available product that can produce an area of dense cutaneous anesthesia, but this effect requires that a relatively thick application remain in contact with the skin under an occlusive dressing for at least 1 hour. This mode of administration may be difficult if the area of pain is large or proximate to the face or a mobile area of the body.

It has not been established that cutaneous anesthesia is necessary to gain benefit from a topical local anesthetic, and the patient should be encouraged to try various modes of administration in an effort to identify an approach that is salutary. If possible, the initial trials should include an occlusive dressing of some type (ordinary plastic wrap can be used for large areas, and a product such as Tegaderm can be applied to smaller areas) and a duration of application of at least 1 hour.

A trial of a topical anti-inflammatory drug is usually implemented by application on the painful area of a solution in which aspirin (or other drugs in published reports) is dissolved in ether or chloroform. The solvent evaporates, leaving the drug in contact with the skin.

ADJUVANT ANALGESICS FOR LANCINATING OR PAROXYSMAL PAIN

Patients with neuropathic pain characterized by lancinating or paroxysmal pains should be offered empirical trials of anticonvulsant drugs as the first-line therapy

(Table 10–5). Baclofen is also considered for this indication. Antidepressant drugs and mexiletine can be effective for lancinating pains, and trials of these drugs are reasonable if the response to an anticonvulsant and baclofen is poor. As noted, the neuroleptic pimozide has demonstrated efficacy in trigeminal neuralgia and, on this basis, is now also considered among those agents attempted in patients with refractory neuropathic pain of this type.

Anticonvulsant Drugs. Some anticonvulsant drugs, specifically carbamazepine, phenytoin, clonazepam, and valproate, are useful in the management of lancinating neuropathic pains.[177] Controlled trials have demonstrated the efficacy of phenytoin in the painful neuropathies associated with Fabry's disease[113] or diabetes,[32] and favorable responses have been described in patients with trigeminal neuralgia, glossopharyngeal neuralgia, tabetic lightning pains, central pain, and the lancinating pains associated with postherpetic neuralgia.[27,75,178]

Data from controlled studies have established the utility of carbamazepine in trigeminal neuralgia, postherpetic neuralgia, and painful diabetic neuropathy.[12,24,83,95,154,159] Benefit has been reported anecdotally in patients with a variety of other lancinating dysesthesias, including glossopharyngeal neuralgia, tabetic lightning pains, paroxysmal pain in multiple sclerosis, postsympathectomy pain, lancinating dysesthesias in spinal cord–injured patients, stabbing pains following laminectomy, and lancinating pains due

Table 10–5. ADJUVANT ANALGESICS PREFERRED FOR LANCINATING NEUROPATHIC PAIN

Anticonvulsants
Carbamazepine
Phenytoin
Valproate
Clonazepam

Other Drugs
Baclofen
Pimozide
Oral local anesthetics (mexiletine)
Antidepressants

to cancer and posttraumatic mononeuropathy.[52–54,130,150,178,184]

Empirical support for the efficacy of clonazepam and valproate derives from uncontrolled surveys and case reports. A favorable response to clonazepam was reported in patients with trigeminal neuralgia, paroxysmal postlaminectomy pain, and posttraumatic neuralgia.[23,119,178] Valproate was effective in patients with trigeminal neuralgia and postherpetic neuralgia.[139,147]

The newer anticonvulsants, felbamate and gabapentin, have not been evaluated in the management of chronic pain. Felbamate interacts with the *N*-methyl-D-aspartate receptor,[152] which has been implicated in the disturbed neurophysiology that accompanies painful nerve injury (see Chapter 2).[200] Unfortunately, this theoretical justification for an empirical trial must be balanced by the potential for a serious complication, aplastic anemia. A trial of felbamate should be pursued only in extreme cases.

Mechanism of Action. The mechanism of the analgesia produced by the anticonvulsant drugs is not known but is presumably related to the actions that underlie their anticonvulsant effects. These may include suppression of paroxysmal discharges and their spread from the site of origin, as well as a reduction of neuronal hyperexcitability.[193] Aberrant electrical activity has been recorded from various sites along the neuraxis in humans with neuropathic pain and experimental models of nerve injury (see Chapter 2), and it may be postulated that this activity underlies the pain and is the target for anticonvulsant activity.

Clinical Applications. The optimal administration of anticonvulsants as analgesics has not been studied. Consequently, guidelines are extrapolated from the use of these drugs in the treatment of seizures.

INDICATIONS. An anticonvulsant trial should be considered early in the treatment of neuropathic pain syndromes characterized by lancinating or paroxysmal pain. In patients with neuropathic syndromes characterized by predominating continuous dysesthesias, these drugs are second-line or third-line agents, which may be appropriate after failure of other adjuvant analgesics, including antidepressants and oral local anesthetics.

ADVERSE EFFECTS. Carbamazepine commonly causes somnolence, dizziness, nausea, and unsteadiness. These effects are often transient and can be minimized by low initial doses and gradual upward titration. Of greater concern, leukopenia and/or thrombocytopenia occurs in approximately 2 percent of patients and aplastic anemia is a rare complication.[82] To monitor this potential hematologic toxicity, a complete blood count should be obtained prior to the start of therapy, after 2 to 3 weeks, again after 2 to 3 months, then periodically thereafter. A leukocyte count below 4000 is a contraindication to treatment. After therapy is begun, the drug should be discontinued if the white blood cell count falls below 3000, the absolute neutrophil count declines below 1500, or other blood elements become abnormal. Rare adverse effects of carbamazepine include hepatotoxicity, inappropriate secretion of antidiuretic hormone, and congestive heart failure.[59] Baseline liver and renal function tests should be obtained prior to therapy.

The common dose-dependent side effects of phenytoin include somnolence or mental clouding, dizziness, unsteadiness, and diplopia.[149] These effects usually occur at plasma concentrations above the usual therapeutic range, but some patients develop them at lower concentrations. Ataxia, progressive encephalopathy, and even seizures can occur at toxic levels. Idiosyncratic effects include hepatoxocity and exfoliative dermatitis. A maculopapular rash can be the harbinger of a life-threatening Stevens-Johnson syndrome and indicates the need to discontinue the drug. A rare permanent cerebellar degeneration has been reported in patients with chronic phenytoin intoxication.[68]

The common side effects of valproate include somnolence, nausea, tremor, and, sometimes, increased appetite; idiosyncratic reactions are hepatotoxicity, encephalopathy, dermatitis, alopecia, and a rare hyperammonemia syndrome.[166] Evaluation of an encephalopathy in a patient who is receiving valproate should include measurement of serum ammonia, which can be elevated without abnormalities in the liver function tests.

Drowsiness is the most common and troubling side effect of clonazepam but is transitory in many patients. Anxiolytic effects may accompany early somnolence and be perceived very favorably. Occasional patients develop ataxia, particularly at higher doses. Idiosyncratic reactions, including dermatitis, hepatotoxicity, and hematologic effects, appear to be very rare. As with other benzodiazepine drugs, a withdrawal syndrome may occur with abrupt discontinuation of relatively high doses.

DOSING GUIDELINES. No studies have compared the relative efficacy of the anticonvulsant drugs in patients with various types of neuropathic pain. In the absence of a contraindication, most practitioners begin with carbamazepine in recognition of the abundant data supporting analgesic actions. Individual variation in the response to these drugs is great, however, and trials with alternative drugs should be considered if the patient fails to respond or is unable to tolerate any particular anticonvulsant. Patients with chronic pain associated with anxiety or insomnia might be considered for an early trial of clonazepam, which may also be effective for these symptoms.

With the exception of phenytoin, which is usually well tolerated during a cautious oral or intravenous loading regimen, all anticonvulsant drugs are best initiated at low doses when used in the treatment of pain. Carbamazepine, for example, is usually initiated at a dose of 100 mg twice daily. Doses are then gradually increased, during which the patient and the plasma concentration are monitored. Dose escalation typically continues until favorable effects occur, intolerable side effects supervene, or some arbitrary plasma concentration is reached. Although the relationship between plasma concentration and analgesic effects has not been assessed, clinical experience does not support the utility of plasma concentrations substantially above the upper limit of the therapeutic range for seizures. Given the additional risk of toxicity, it is prudent to discontinue the therapeutic trial at doses associated with a plasma concentration at, or just above, this upper limit.

Other Adjuvant Analgesics for Lancinating Pain. Patients with neuropathic pain of any type that is characterized by a prominent lancinating or paroxysmal component may also benefit from drugs in other classes. As discussed previously, antidepressant drugs and oral local anesthetics may both be useful in this setting. Before implementing the latter trials, however, a therapeutic trial with baclofen should be considered. Baclofen is a GABA agonist that has established efficacy in trigeminal neuralgia[65] and is used empirically for lancinating or paroxysmal neuropathic pains of other types. In the treatment of pain, the typical starting dose, 5 mg three times daily, is gradually increased until favorable effects occur or side effects supervene. The principal side effects are nausea, confusion, and drowsiness.

Patients with refractory lancinating or paroxysmal neuropathic pain can also be considered for a trial of pimozide.[108] Given the risks associated with long-term neuroleptic therapy, a trial of this drug should generally await the failure of drugs in several other classes.

ADJUVANT ANALGESICS USED FOR SYMPATHETICALLY MAINTAINED PAIN

The diagnosis of sympathetically maintained pain is suggested by focal autonomic dysregulation and, at times, trophic changes (see Chapter 5). Although appropriate sympathetic nerve blocks are usually considered to be the first line of treatment, pharmacotherapy should be considered if nerve blocks are contraindicated or fail.[138] Drug treatments have not been systematically studied, however, and most of the evidence supporting their use comes from single cases or small series of patients.

In addition to the nonspecific use of the adjuvant analgesics described previously, pharmacotherapy for sympathetically maintained pain has focused on several drugs that influence sympathetic function (Table 10–6). None of these drugs has been investigated in a controlled fashion, and the supporting data are meager. Phenoxybenzamine, administered at a dose of 60 to 120 mg per day, was reported to be effective in a series of patients with causalgia of recent onset.[69] The most troubling side effect of this sympatholytic drug is orthostatic hypotension, which is especially problematic in the elderly. Prazosin was found to be effective in a small series of patients with causalgia,[1] and propranolol has been reported to be effective in patients with causalgia.[164,169] Corticosteroids,[98] nifedipine,[146] and guanethidine[179] have both been beneficial in a small se-

Table 10–6. **ADJUVANT ANALGESICS PREFERRED FOR SYMPATHETICALLY MAINTAINED PAIN**

Calcitonin
Phenoxybenzamine
Nifedipine
Prazosin
Corticosteroid
Propranolol

Table 10–7. **ADJUVANT ANALGESICS FOR MUSCULOSKELETAL PAIN**

Muscle Relaxants
Carisoprodol
Methocarbamol
Chlorzoxazone
Cyclobenzaprine

Benzodiazepines
Diazepam

ries of patients. Recently, a small controlled trial suggested that calcitonin may be effective in sympathetically maintained pain.[73] This fascinating finding cannot presently be explained on the basis of any known mechanism of action. Another recent controlled trial suggests that calcitonin may also be useful in the management of acute phantom pain.[87] A therapeutic trial, which may gradually increase from a starting dose of 25 IU daily to 100 to 150 IU once or twice daily, is appropriately considered for patients with refractory neuropathic pain, including sympathetically maintained pain.

ADJUVANT ANALGESICS USED FOR MUSCULOSKELETAL PAIN

A careful assessment of the patient with chronic musculoskeletal pain often suggests the need for a multimodality treatment approach that emphasizes physiatric and psychologic approaches rather than pharmacotherapy (see Chapter 7). Patients with acute musculoskeletal pain, however, are commonly managed with analgesic drugs, including the NSAIDs, opioids, so-called muscle relaxants, and benzodiazepines (Table 10–7). The long-term use of all but the NSAIDs remains controversial and should not be undertaken without a clear understanding of goals of the therapy and the method for appropriate monitoring. The issues related to the long-term use of opioid drugs are discussed in Chapter 11.

Muscle Relaxants. In the United States, the so-called muscle relaxant drugs include carisoprodol, chlorzoxazone, methocarbamol, orphenadrine, and cyclobenzaprine. These drugs are marketed alone and in combination with other compounds, usually as-

pirin or acetaminophen. The benefits, compared with placebo, of each of these drugs for common musculoskeletal pains have been established in controlled studies.[5,9,11] Some studies have demonstrated analgesic effects that are superior to either aspirin or acetaminophen, and others have shown that the combination of a muscle relaxant and one of the latter drugs provides better analgesia than does aspirin or acetaminophen alone. No controlled studies have compared the relative efficacy or side effect profiles of the various muscle relaxant drugs or the efficacy of these agents relative to NSAIDs or opioids. Long-term effects also have not been evaluated. The potential for abuse of these drugs by some patients with chronic nonmalignant pain has been suggested by pain specialists who treat patients referred to multidisciplinary pain management programs.

Mechanism of Action. The muscle relaxant drugs are usually administered for musculoskeletal pains, some of which are characterized by muscle spasm. It should not be assumed, however, that muscle spasm is a necessary condition for the effectiveness of these agents as analgesics. Indeed, with the exception of diazepam,[171] there is no evidence that these drugs actually relax skeletal muscle in the clinical situation. These drugs do inhibit polysynaptic myogenic reflexes in animal models, but the relationship between these actions and analgesic effects is unknown. It is not even clear from the literature that these drugs have analgesic effects that are selective for musculoskeletal pain problems.

Clinical Applications. Guidelines for the clinical use of muscle relaxant drugs are empirical.

INDICATIONS. Notwithstanding limited data from controlled trials, the muscle relaxant drugs have achieved wide acceptance in the treatment of acute musculoskeletal pains. For these indications, the muscle relaxants should be viewed as alternatives to the NSAIDs and opioids or, in more severe cases, potentially useful drugs to combine with these other analgesics.

The use of the muscle relaxant drugs in the treatment of chronic pain is controversial. There is no favorable published experience, and many specialists in pain management express concern about the possibility that the sedative effects of these drugs can hamper rehabilitative efforts and that abuse can occur in some patients. The continued administration of these drugs in patients with acute pain that fails to diminish over time and their use in patients with chronic pain should be undertaken only with careful ongoing assessment and a clear understanding of the therapeutic goals. This assessment should evaluate the durability of favorable effects, monitor side effects, and clarify both the functional status of the patient and the possibility of aberrant drug-related behaviors. Unless the clinician can be assured that the continuing use of these drugs produces benefits that clearly outweigh adverse effects, the therapy should not be continued.

ADVERSE EFFECTS. At the doses used clinically, the muscle relaxant drugs are generally well tolerated. Sedation is the only common side effect.

DOSING GUIDELINES. As noted, the various muscle relaxant drugs have not been compared in clinical trials. Anecdotally, some patients appear to obtain better relief or experience less sedation with one or another, and it is reasonable to switch to an alternative drug if treatment is ineffective. Although the dose-response relationships of the muscle relaxant drugs have not been systematically explored in the clinical setting, there are probably dose-dependent effects within the dosing range usually implemented clinically. Hence, it is reasonable to begin with a low initial dose and then increase it if the response is inadequate and side effects minimal. Although it is possible that dose escalation above the usually recommended doses could yield benefit in some patients, experience is too limited to judge the safety and po-

tential utility of this approach, and it cannot be recommended.

Benzodiazepines. Diazepam is commonly used to treat acute muscle spasm and, as discussed previously, clonazepam is commonly used to manage lancinating or paroxysmal neuropathic pain. Other evidence that benzodiazepines have analgesic effects include a survey that suggests benefit from alprazolam in patients with cancer who have neuropathic pain[57] and studies of diazepam in acute pain.[126,171]

Like the muscle relaxants, benzodiazepines are potentially abusable and could conceivably hamper functional restoration. Consequently, the long-term use of these drugs must be undertaken cautiously. Although treatment with clonazepam is often considered for refractory neuropathic pain, long-term administration of other benzodiazepines for chronic musculoskeletal pain is usually eschewed. Prolonged therapy for intercurrent anxiety may be very appropriate, but ongoing treatment for analgesic purposes is rarely indicated and should be considered only if astute and repeated assessment is planned. As discussed previously, this assessment must include issues related to efficacy, side effects, effect on physical and psychosocial function, and the potential for abuse.

Other Adjuvant Analgesics

Numerous other drugs have been demonstrated to have analgesic effects. Some are commonly used in specific clinical circumstances. The analgesics used to manage headache, for example, include beta blockers, calcium channel blockers, various psychotropics (antidepressants, neuroleptics, and lithium), and others (see Chapter 4). Similarly, trials of several specific drugs, such as naloxone, may be considered in patients with central pain (see Chapter 5).

Adjuvant analgesics are also commonly used to supplement opioid therapy in the cancer population (Table 10–8).[144] Corticosteroids are analgesic and may benefit other cancer-related symptoms, including anorexia, malaise, and nausea.[20,45,55,81,182] Patients with malignant bone pain may undergo trials of a bisphosphonate (e.g., pamidronate), calcitonin, or a bone-seeking

Table 10–8. **ADJUVANT ANALGESICS FOR CANCER PAIN**

Corticosteroids

Drugs for Bone Pain
Pamidronate
Calcitonin
Strontium-89

Drugs for Pain Due to Bowel Obstruction
Anticholinergics (scopolamine)
Octreotide

radionuclide such as strontium-89.[137] Based on anecdotal observation, pain related to bowel obstruction may be addressed with anticholinergic drugs (e.g., scopolamine) or with the somatostatin analog octreotide.[125]

Other drug classes may also be analgesic. There is substantial evidence that antihistamines can relieve pain,[160] but the utility of these drugs has been limited, particularly in the management of chronic pain. These drugs are constituents of many commercially available analgesic combination products, most of which are acquired over the counter. Hydroxyzine, which can clearly have analgesic effects,[173] is sometimes combined with an opioid in the postoperative setting to potentiate analgesic effects while reducing nausea.

Psychostimulant drugs have analgesic properties. Controlled studies have established the analgesic efficacy of dextroamphetamine in postoperative pain[61] and methylphenidate in pain associated with Parkinson's disease[26] and cancer.[19] Numerous single-dose controlled studies of caffeine combined with other analgesics have demonstrated efficacy greater than the analgesic alone.[107] A well-controlled single-dose study found that oral cocaine (10 mg) influenced mood without altering pain,[90] whereas a partially controlled study of intranasal cocaine (delivered by cotton-tip applicators placed in the region of the posterior wall of the nasopharynx) did identify analgesic effects.[116] The latter technique (sphenopalatine ganglion block) remains highly controversial.

Clinically, psychostimulant drugs have two broad uses. Caffeine is commonly added to over-the-counter analgesic compounds as a coanalgesic, particularly those marketed for headache. Dextroamphetamine and ethylphenidate are both used to manage opioid-induced somnolence in the cancer population. Pemoline, a novel stimulant with relatively fewer sympathomimetic effects, has also been used for the latter indication.

Other drugs may have analgesic effects but have not been adopted in clinical practice. For example, studies of the cannabinoids, including the commercially available delta-9-tetrahydrocannabinol, have demonstrated analgesic effects,[133] but the potential for sedation and other central nervous system side effects limits the utility of these drugs.

SUMMARY

Nonopioid analgesics include the NSAIDs and acetaminophen. The analgesic effects produced by the NSAIDs can be attributed, in part, to a reduction in tissue levels of prostaglandins. Central actions are also likely, however, and must be invoked to explain the analgesia produced by acetaminophen, which has minimal peripheral activity. Although the analgesic effects of the nonopioid analgesics are nonspecific, the NSAIDs are presumed to be more effective in inflammatory pain syndromes. All the nonopioid analgesics have a dose-response relationship and a ceiling dose for analgesia. There is large intraindividual and interindividual variability in the efficacy of the various drugs, the potential for side effects, and the actual doses associated with analgesia and toxicity. The selection of an NSAID should be based on the known toxicities of the class as a whole, drug-selective toxicities, prior experience, cost, and convenience. Dose titration is appropriate to identify the minimal effective dose. The potential for GI and renal toxicity should be monitored during therapy. Patients who are predisposed to peptic ulcer disease or who could not tolerate a gastrointestinal hemorrhage should be considered for concurrent misoprostol therapy, which reduces the risk of gastric ulceration.

The adjuvant analgesics are drugs that have primary indications other than pain but are analgesic in selected circumstances. The large number of such drugs currently available has greatly enhanced the therapeutic armamentarium for chronic pain. The tricyclic antidepressants and clonidine have been shown to be nonspecific analgesics, a trial of which should be considered in virtually any chronic pain syndrome. Of the antidepressants, the evidence for analgesic efficacy is best for the tertiary amine compound amitriptyline. The secondary amine desipramine is often better tolerated and has convincing evidence of analgesic efficacy. Although the evidence is less compelling, other tricyclic antidepressants and some of the newer nontricyclic compounds, such as the serotonin-selective reuptake inhibitor paroxetine, are probably analgesic as well.

Adjuvant analgesics for neuropathic pain can be divided into three categories. Drugs that are preferred for the management of continuous dysesthesias include the antidepressants, the local anesthetics (administered orally or parenterally), and various topical drugs, specifically anesthetics, capsaicin, and NSAIDs. Clonidine is also used for this indication. Drugs preferred for the management of lancinating neuropathic pains include the anticonvulsants carbamazepine, phenytoin, valproate, and clonazepam, and the GABA agonist baclofen. The antidepressants and local anesthetics are also administered for this type of pain, and the neuroleptic pimozide can be considered for refractory cases. Adjuvant analgesics specifically used for the management of sympathetically maintained pain include calcitonin, phenoxybenzamine, prazosin, nifedipine, and corticosteroids; in refractory cases, therapeutic trials may also include any of the drug classes used nonspecifically for other types of neuropathic pain.

Muscle relaxants and benzodiazepines are used as adjuvant analgesics for musculoskeletal pain. The muscle relaxants do not actually relax skeletal muscle but, rather, have a nonspecific analgesic effect. These drugs are sedating and, as with the other adjuvant analgesics, their use must be carefully monitored to ensure continued efficacy without adverse effects on functional status.

Many other adjuvant analgesics are used in selected clinical circumstances. In the cancer population, for example, corticosteroids are administered nonspecifically for pain; psychostimulants are used to reverse opioid-induced somnolence; calcitonin, bisphosphonates, and bone-seeking radiopharmaceuticals are used for bone pain; and anticholinergic drugs and the somatostatin analog octreotide are used for pain due to bowel obstruction. Antihistamines and caffeine are commonly added to over-the-counter pain remedies.

REFERENCES

1. Abram SE, Lightfoot RW: Treatment of longstanding causalgia with prozosin. Reg Anesth 6:79–81, 1981.
2. Alcoff J, Jones E, Rust P, et al: A trial of imipramine for chronic low back pain. J Fam Pract 14:841–846, 1982.
3. American Psychiatric Association: Tardive dyskinesia: A task force report of the American Psychiatric Association. American Psychiatric Association, Washington, DC, 1991.
4. Anthony M, and Lance JW: MAO inhibition in the treatment of migraine. Arch Neurol 21:263–268, 1969.
5. Batterman RC: Methodology of analgesic evaluation: Experience with orphenadrine citrate compound. Current Therapeutic Research 7:639–647, 1965.
6. Beaver WT: Nonsteroidal anti-inflammatory analgesics in cancer pain. In Foley KM, Bonica JJ, and Ventafridda V (eds): Advances in Pain Research and Therapy, Vol. 16. Raven Press, New York, 1990, pp 109–131.
7. Beaver WT, Wallenstein SM, Houde RW, et al: A comparison of the analgesic effects of methotrimeprazine and morphine in patients with cancer. Clin Pharmacol Ther 7:436–446, 1966.
8. Benedetti C, and Butler SH: Systemic analgesics. In Bonica JJ (ed): The Management of Pain, ed 2. Lea and Febiger, Malvern, PA, 1990, pp 1640–1675.
9. Bercel NA: Cyclobenzaprine in the treatment of skeletal muscle spasm in osteoarthritis of the cervical and lumbar spine. Current Therapeutic Research 22:462–468, 1977.
10. Bernstein JE, Bickers RR, Dahl MV, et al: Treatment of chronic postherpetic neuralgia with topical capsaicin. A preliminary study. J Am Acad Dermatol 17:93–96, 1987.
11. Birkeland IW, and Clawson DK: Drug combinations with orphenadrine for pain relief associated with muscle spasm. Clin Pharmacol Ther 9:639–646, 1968.
12. Blom S: Tic douloureux treated with new anticonvulsant. Arch Neurol 9:285–290, 1963.
13. Bloom BS: Risk and cost of gastrointestinal side effects associated with nonsteroidal anti-inflammatory drugs. Arch Intern Med 149(5):1019–11022, 1989.
14. Boisen E, Deth S, Hubbe P, et al: Clonidine in the prophylaxis of migraine. Acta Neurol Scand 58: 288–295, 1978.

15. Bonnet F, Boico O, Rostaing S, et al: Clonidine for postoperative analgesia: Epidural vs. I.M. study. [Abstract] Anesthesiology 69:A395, 1988.
16. Brater DC: Drug-drug and drug-disease interactions with non-steroidal anti-inflammatory drug interactions. J Clin Psychopharmacol 10(5):350–354, 1990.
17. Breivik H, and Rennemo F: Clinical evaluation of combined treatment with methadone and psychotropic drugs in cancer patients. Acta Anaesth Scand (Suppl) 74:135–140, 1982.
18. Brogden RN: Nonsteroidal anti-inflammatory analgesics other than salicylates. Drugs 32(Suppl 4):27–45, 1986.
19. Bruera E, Chadwick S, Brenneis C, et al: Methylphenidate associated with narcotics for the treatment of cancer pain. Cancer Treatment Reports 71:67–70, 1987.
20. Bruera E, Roca E, Cedaro L, et al: Action of oral methylprednisolone in terminal cancer patients: A prospective randomized double-blind study. Cancer Treatment Reports 69:751–754, 1985.
21. Brune K, and Lanz R: Non-opioid analgesics. In Kuhar M, and Pasternak G (eds): Analgesics: Neurochemical, Behavioral and Clinical Perspectives. Raven Press, New York, 1984, pp 149–173.
22. Butler S: Present status of tricyclic antidepressants in chronic pain. In Benedetti C, Chapman CR, and Moricca G (eds): Advances in Pain Research and Therapy, Vol 7. Raven Press, New York, 1984, pp 173–198.
23. Caccia MR: Clonazepam in facial neuralgia and cluster headache: Clinical and electrophysiological study. Eur Neurol 13:560–563, 1975.
24. Campbell FG, Graham JG, and Zilkha KJ: Clinical trial of carbamazepine (Tegretol) in trigeminal neuralgia. J Neurol Neurosurg Psychiatry 29:265–267, 1966.
25. Campbell RWF: Mexiletine. N Engl J Med 316:29–34, 1987.
26. Cantello R, Aguggia M, Gilli M, et al: Analgesic action of methylphenidate on parkinsonian sensory symptoms. Mechanisms and pathophysiological implications. Arch Neurol 45:973–976, 1988.
27. Cantor FK: Phenytoin treatment of thalamic pain. British Medical Journal 2:590, 1972.
28. Capsaicin Study Group: Treatment of painful diabetic neuropathy with topical capsaicin. A multicenter, double-blind, vehicle-controlled study. Arch Intern Med 151(11):2225–2229, 1991.
29. Carette S, McCain GA, Bell DA, et al: Evaluation of amitriptyline in primary fibrositis. Arthritis Rheum 29:655–659, 1986.
30. Chabel C, Jacobson L, Mariano A, et al: The use of oral mexiletine for the treatment of pain after peripheral nerve injury. Anesthesiology 76:513–517, 1992.
31. Chabal C, Russell LC, and Burchiel KJ: The effect of intravenous lidocaine, tocainide and mexiletine on spontaneously active fibers originating in rat sciatic neuromas. Pain 38:333–338, 1989.
32. Chadda VS, and Mathur MS: Double blind study of the effects of diphenylhydantoin sodium in diabetic neuropathy. J Assoc Physicians India 26:403–406, 1978.
33. Clive DM, and Stoff JS: Renal syndromes associated with non-steroidal anti-inflammatory drugs. N Engl J Med 310(9):563–572, 1984.
34. Coates AG, Nostrant TT, Wilson JA, et al: Esophagitis caused by nonsteroidal anti-inflammatory medication: Case reports and review of the literature on pill-induced esophageal injury. South Med J 79(9):1094–1097, 1986.
35. Covino BG: Local anesthetics. In Ferrante MF, and VadeBoncouer TR (eds): Postoperative Pain Management. Churchill Livingstone, Edinburgh, 1993, pp 211–254.
36. Couch JR, Ziegler DK, and Hassanein R: Amitriptyline in the prophylaxis of migraine: Effectiveness and relationship of antimigraine and antidepressant effects. Neurology 26:121–127, 1976.
37. Crossley HL, Bergman SA, and Wynn RL: Nonsteroidal anti-inflammatory agents in relieving dental pain: A review. J Am Dent Assoc 106:61–64, 1983.
38. Davar G, and Maciewicz R: Deafferentation pain syndromes. Neurol Clin 7:289–304, 1989.
39. Davidoff G, Guarracini M, Roth E, et al: Trazodone hydrochloride in the treatment of dysesthetic pain in traumatic myelopathy: A randomized, double-blind, placebo-controlled study. Pain 29:151–161, 1987.
40. Davidsen O, Lindeneg O, and Walsh M: Analgesic treatment with levomepromazine in acute myocardial infarction. Acta Med Scand 205:191–194, 1979.
41. Davis JL, Lewis SB, Gerich JE, et al: Peripheral diabetic neuropathy treated with amitriptyline and fluphenazine. JAMA 238:2291–2292, 1977.
42. Davis P: Therapeutic options in the selection of nonsteroidal, anti-inflammatory drugs in the treatment of osteoarthritis: A review. J Rheumatol 14:94–97, 1987.
43. DeBenedittis G, Besana F, and Lorenzettit A: A new topical treatment for acute herpetic neuralgia and postherpetic neuralgia: The aspirin/diethyl ether mixture. An open-label study plus a double-blind controlled clinical trial. Pain 48:383–390, 1992.
44. Dejgard A, Petersen P, and Kastrup J: Mexiletine for treatment of chronic painful diabetic neuropathy. Lancet 1:9–11, 1988.
45. Della Cuna GR, Pellegrini A, and Piazzi M: Effect of methylprednisolone sodium succinate on quality of life in preterminal cancer patients. A placebo-controlled multicenter study. European Journal of Cancer and Clinical Oncology 25:1817–1821, 1989.
46. Diamond S, and Baltes BJ: Chronic tension headache—treatment with amitriptyline—a double blind study. Headache 11:110–116, 971.
47. Dinerman H, Felsen D, and Goldenberg D: A randomized clinical trial of naproxen and amitriptyline in primary fibromyalgia. Arthritis Rheum 159(S):28, 1985.
48. Dubner R: Topical capsaicin therapy for neuropathic pain. Pain 47(3):247–248, 1991.
49. Eberhard G, Von Knorring L, Nilsson HL, et al: A double-blind randomized study of clomipramine versus maprotiline in patients with idiopathic pain syndromes. Neuropsychobiology 19:25–34, 1988.
50. Edelson JT, Tosteson AN, and Sax P: Cost-effectiveness of misoprostol for prophylaxis against nonsteroidal anti-inflammatory drug-induced gastroin-

testinal tract bleeding. [Comment] JAMA 264(1): 83–84, 1990.

51. Eisenach JC, Dewan DM, Rose JC, et al: Epidural clonidine produces antinociception, but not hypotension, in sheep. Anesthesiology 66:496–501, 1987.

52. Ekbom K: Carbamazepine in the treatment of tabetic lightning pains. Arch Neurol 26:374–378, 1972.

53. Elliott F, Little A, and Milbrandt W: Carbamazepine for phantom limb phenomena. N Engl J Med 295:678, 1976.

54. Espir MLE, and Millac P: Treatment of paroxysmal disorders in multiple sclerosis with carbamazepine (Tegretol). J Neurol Neurosurg Psychiatry 33:528–531, 1970.

55. Ettinger AB, and Portenoy RK: The use of corticosteroids in the treatment of symptoms associated with cancer. Journal of Pain Symptom Management 3:99–103, 1988.

56. Evans W, Gensler F, Blackwell B, et al: The effects of antidepressant drugs on pain relief and mood in the chronically ill. Psychosomatics 14:214–219, 1973.

57. Fernandez F, Adams F, and Holmes VF: Analgesic effect of alprazolam in patients chronic, organic pain of malignant origin. J Clin Psychopharmacol 7:167–169, 1987.

58. Fischetti LF: Interaction between nonsteroidal anti-inflammatory drugs and high-dose methotrexate: A literature review. J Pediatr Oncol Nurs 7(1):14–16, 1990.

59. Flegel KM, and Cole CH: Inappropriate antidiuresis during carbamazepine treatment. Ann Intern Med 87:722–723, 1977.

60. Foley KM, and Inturrisi CE: Analgesic drug therapy in cancer pain: Principles and practice. Med Clin North Am 71:207–232, 1987.

61. Forrest, WH Jr, Brown BW Jr., Brown CR, et al: Dextroamphetamine with morphine for the treatment of postoperative pain. N Engl J Med 296:712, 1977.

62. France RD, and Krishnan KRR: Psychotropic drugs in chronic pain. In France RD, and Krishnan KRR (eds): Chronic Pain. American Psychiatric Press, Washington, DC, 1988, pp 322–374.

63. Frank RG, Kashani JH, Parker JC, et al: Antidepressant analgesia in rheumatoid arthritis. J Rheumatol 15:1632–1638, 1988.

64. Frayling IM, Addison GM, Chattergee K, et al: Methaemoglobinaemia in children treated with prilocaine-lignocaine cream. British Medical Journal 301:153–154, 1990.

65. Fromm GH, Terence CF, and Chatta AS: Baclofen in the treatment of trigeminal neuralgia. Ann Neurol 15:240–247, 1984.

66. Gabriel SE, Jaakkimainen RL, and Bombardier C: The cost effectiveness of misoprostol for non-steroidal anti-inflammatory drug-associated adverse gastrointestinal events. Arthritis Rheum 36 (4):447–459, 1993.

67. Galer BS, Miller KV, and Rowbotham MC: Response to intravenous lidocaine differs based on clinical diagnosis and site of nervous system injury. Neurology 43:1233–1245, 1993.

68. Ghatak NR, Santoso RA, and McKinney WM: Cere-

bellar degeneration following long-term phenytoin therapy. Neurology 26:818–820, 1978.

69. Ghostine SY, Comair YG, Turner DM, et al: Phenoxybenzamine in the treatment of causalgia. J Neurosurg 60:1263–1268, 1984.

70. Gingras M: A clinical trial of Tofranil in rheumatic pain in general practice. J Int Med Res 4:41–49, 1976.

71. Glassman AH, and Bigger JT: Cardiovascular effects of therapeutic doses of tricyclic antidepressants. Arch Gen Psychiatry 38:815, 1981.

72. Glazer S, and Portenoy RK: Systemic local analgesics in pain control. Journal of Pain Symptom Management 6:30–39, 1991.

73. Gobelet C, Waldburger M, and Meier JL: The effect of adding calcitonin to physical treatment on reflex sympathetic dystrophy. Pain 48:171–175, 1992.

74. Gomez-Perez FJ, Rull JA, Dies H, et al: Nortriptyline and fluphenazine in the symptomatic treatment of diabetic neuropathy. A double-blind crossover trial. Pain 23:395–400, 1985.

75. Green JB: Dilantin in the treatment of lightning pains. Neurology 11:257–258, 1961.

76. Greene JM, and Winickoff RN: Cost-conscious prescribing of nonsteroidal anti-inflammatory drugs for adults with arthritis. A review and suggestions. Arch Intern Med 152(10):1995–2002, 1992.

77. Gregg NJ, Elseviers MM, DeBroe ME, et al: Epidemiology and mechanistic basis of analgesic-associated nephropathy. Toxicol Lett 46(1-3)141–151, 1989.

78. Hakkarainen, H: Fluphenazine for tension headache: Double-blind study. Headache 17:216–218, 1977.

79. Hameroff SR, Cork RC, Scherer K, et al: Doxepin effects on chronic pain, depression and plasma opioids. J Clin Psychiatry 43:22–27, 1982.

80. Hammond DL: Pharmacology of central pain-modulating networks (biogenic amines and non-opioid analgesics). In Fields HL, Dubner R, and Cervero F (eds): Advances in Pain Research and Therapy, Vol 9. Raven Press, New York, 1985, pp 499–513.

81. Hanks GW, Trueman T, and Twycross RG: Corticosteroids in terminal cancer. Postgrad Med J 59: 702–706, 1983.

82. Hart RG, and Easton JD: Carbamazepine and hematological monitoring. Ann Neurol 11:309–312, 1982.

83. Hatangdi VS, Boas RA, and Richards EG: Postherpetic neuralgia: Management with antiepileptic and tricyclic drugs. In Bonica JJ, and Albe-Fessard D (eds): Advances in Pain Research and Therapy, Vol 1. Raven Press, New York, 1976, pp 583–587.

84. Horn HR, Hadidian Z, Johnson JL, et al: Safety evaluation of tocainide in an American emergency use program. Am Heart J 100:1037, 1980.

85. Houde RW, and Wallenstein SL: Analgesic power of chlorpromazine alone and in combination with morphine. Federal Proceedings [Abstract] 14:353, 1966.

86. Insel PA: Analgesic-antipyretics and anti-inflammatory agents: Drugs employed in the treatment of rheumatoid arthritis and gout. In Goodman LS, Gilman AG, Rall TW, et al (eds): The Pharmaco-

logical Basis of Therapeutics, ed 8. Pergamon Press, New York, 1990, pp 638–681.

87. Jaeger H, and Maier C: Calcitonin in phantom limb pain: A double blind study. Pain 48:21–27, 1992.

88. Johnson AG, Seideman P, and Day RO: Adverse drug interactions with nonsteroidal anti-inflammatory drugs (NSAIDS). Recognition, management and avoidance. Drug Saf 8(2):99–127, 1993.

89. Judkins KC, and Harmer M: Haloperidol as an adjuvant analgesic in the management of postoperative pain. Anaesthesia 37:1118–1120, 1982.

90. Kaiko RF, Kanner R, Foley KM, et al: Cocaine and morphine interaction in acute and chronic cancer pain. Pain 31:35–45, 1987.

91. Kantor TG: New strategies for the use of anti-inflammatory agents. In Dubner R, Gebhart FG, and Bond MR (eds): Proceedings of the Vth World Congress on Pain. Elsevier, New York, 1988, pp 80–86.

92. Kastrup J, Petersen P, Dejgard A, et al: Intravenous lidocaine infusion—a new treatment of chronic painful diabetic neuropathy? Pain 28:69–75, 1987.

93. Kaufman DW, Kelly JP, Sheehan JE, et al: Non-steroidal anti-inflammatory drug use in relation to major upper gastrointestinal bleeding. Clin Pharmacol Ther 53:485–494, 1993.

94. Keats AS, Telford J, and Kurosu Y: Potentiation of meperidine by promethazine. Anesthesiology 22:31, 1961.

95. Killian JM, and Fromm GH: Carbamazepine in the treatment of neuralgia: Use and side effects. Arch Neurol 19:129–136, 1968.

96. Kishore-Kumar R, Max MB, Schafer SC, et al: Desipramine relieves postherpetic neuralgia. Clin Pharmacol Ther 47:305–312, 1990.

97. Kocher R: Use of psychotropic drugs for the treatment of chronic severe pain. In Bonica JJ, and Albe-Fessard D (eds): Advances in Pain Research and Therapy, Vol 1. Raven Press, New York, 1976, pp 279–282.

98. Kozin F, Ryan LM, Carerra GF, et al: The reflex sympathetic dystrophy syndrome (RSDS). III. Scintigraphic studies, further evidence for the therapeutic efficacy of systemic corticosteroids, and proposed diagnostic critiera. Am J Med 70:23–29, 1981.

99. Kreeger W, and Hammill SC: New antiarrhythmic drugs: Tocainide, mexiletine, flecainide, encainide, and amiodarone. Mayo Clin Proc 62:1033–1050, 1987.

100. Kvinsdahl B, Molin J, Froland A, et al: Imipramine treatment of painful diabetic neuropathy. JAMA 251:1727–1730, 1984.

101. Lance JW, and Curran DA: Treatment of chronic tension headache. Lancet 1:1236, 1964.

102. Langman MJS, Well J, Wainwright P, et al: Risks of bleeding peptic ulcer associated with individual nonsteroidal anti-inflammatory drugs. Lancet 343:1075–1078, 1994.

103. Langohr HD, Stohr M, and Petruch F: An open and double-blind cross-over study on the efficacy of clomipramine (Anafranil) in patients with painful mono- and polyneuropathies. Eur Neurol 21:309–317, 1982.

104. Laporte JR, Carne X, Vidal X, et al: Upper gastrointestinal bleeding in relation to previous use of analgesics and non-steroidal anti-inflammatory drugs. Lancet 337:85–89, 1991.

105. Lasagna L, and DeKomfeld TJ: Methotrimeprazine—a new phenothiazine derivative with analgesic properties. JAMA 178:119, 1961.

106. Lascelles RG: Atypical facial pain and depression. Br J Psychiatry 122:651–659, 1966.

107. Laska EM, Sunshine A, Mueller F, et al: Caffeine as an analgesic adjuvant. JAMA 251:1711–1718, 1984.

108. Lechin F, van der Dijs B, Lechin ME, et al: Pimozide therapy for trigeminal neuralgia. Arch Neurol 9:960–962, 1989.

109. Leijon G, and Boivie J: Central post-stroke pain—a controlled trial of amitriptyline and carbamazepine. Pain 36:27–36, 1989.

110. Levy M: Adverse reactions to OTC analgesics—an epidemiological evaluation. In Brune K (ed): Non-opioid (OTC) Analgesics: Risks/Benefits in Perspective. Agents and Actions Supplements, Vol 25. Birkhauser Verlag, Berlin, 1988, pp 21–31.

111. Lieberman E, and Stoudemire A: Use of tricyclic antidepressants in patients with glaucoma. Assessment and appropriate precautions. Psychosomatics 28:145–148, 1987.

112. Lindstrom P, and Lindblom U: The analgesic effect of tocainide in trigeminal neuralgia. Pain 28:45–50, 1987.

113. Lockman LA, Hunninghake DB, Drivit W, et al: Relief of pain of Fabry's disease by dephenylhydantoin. Neurology 23:871–875, 1973.

114. Loeb DS, Ahlquist DA, and Talley NJ: Management of gastroduodenopathy associated with use of nonsteroidal anti-inflammatory drugs. Mayo Clin Proc 67:354–364, 1992.

115. Malmberg AB, and Yaksh TL: Hyperalgesia mediated by spinal glutamate or substance P receptor blocked by spinal cyclooxygenase inhibition. Science 257:1276–1279, 1992.

116. Marbach JJ, and Wallenstein SL: Analgesia, mood and hemodynamic effects of intranasal cocaine and lidocaine in chronic facial pain of deafferentation and myofascial origin. Journal of Pain Symptom Management 3:73–79, 1988.

117. Marchettini P, Lacerenza M, Marangoni C, et al: Lidocaine test in neuralgia. Pain 48:377–382, 1992.

118. Margolis LH, and Gianascol AJ: Chlorpromazine in thalamic pain syndrome. Neurology 6:302–304, 1956.

119. Martin G: The management of pain following laminectomy for lumbar disc lesions. Ann R Coll Surg Engl 63:244–252, 1981.

120. Max MB, Culnane M, Schafer SC, et al: Amitriptyline relieves diabetic neuropathy pain in patients with normal or depressed mood. Neurology 37:589–594, 1987.

121. Max MB, Schafer SC, Culnane M, et al: Association of pain relief with drug side effects in postherpetic neuralgia: A single dose study of clonidine, codeine, ibuprofen and placebo. Clin Pharmacol Ther 43:363–371, 1988.

122. McCarthy GM, and McCarty DJ: Effect of topical capsaicin in the therapy of painful osteoarthritis of the hands. J Rheumatol 19:604–607, 1992.

123. McCormack K, and Brune K: Dissociation between

the antinociceptive and anti-inflammatory effects of the non-steroidal anti-inflammatory drugs. Drugs 41:533–547, 1991.

124. McQuay HJ, Carroll D, Moxon A, et al: Benzydamine cream for the treatment of postherpetic neuralgia: Minimum duration of treatment periods in a cross-over trial. Pain 40:131–135, 1990.

125. Mercadante S: Octreotide in relieving gastrointestinal symptoms due to bowel obstruction. Palliat Med 7:295–299, 1993.

126. Miller R, Eisenkraft JB, Cohen M, et al: Midazolam as an adjunct to meperidine analgesia for postoperative pain. Clin J Pain 2:37–43, 1986.

127. Monks R, and Merskey H: Psychotropic drugs. In Wall PD, and Melzack R (eds): Textbook of Pain, ed 2. Churchill Livingstone, New York, 1989, pp 702–721.

128. Montilla EE, Frederick W, and Cass L: Analgesic effects of methotrimeprazine and morphine. Arch Intern Med 11(1):725, 1963.

129. Moore JG, Bjorkman DJ, Mitchell MD, et al: Age does not influence acute aspirin-induced gastric mucosal damage. Gastroenterology 100(6):1626–1629, 1991.

130. Mullan S: Surgical management of pain in cancer of the head and neck. Surg Clin North Am 53:203–210, 1973.

131. Murray KT, Barbey JT, Kopelman HA, et al: Mexiletine and tocainide: A comparison of antiarrhythmic efficacy, adverse effects, and predictive value of lidocaine testing. Clin Pharmacol Ther 45:553–561, 1989.

132. Murray MD, and Brater DC: Renal toxicity of the nonsteroidal anti-inflammatory drugs. Annu Rev Pharmacol Toxicol 33:435–465, 1993.

133. Noyes R Jr, Bruck SF, Avery DAH, et al: The analgesic properties of delta-9-tetrahydrocannabinol and codeine. Clin Pharamacol Ther 18:84–89, 1975.

134. Numo R: Prevention of NSAID-induced ulcers by the co-administration of misoprostol: Implications of clinical practice. Scand J Rheumatol Suppl 92:25–29, 1992.

135. Okasha A, Ghaleb HA, and Sadeki A: A double-blind trial for the clinical management of psychogenic headache. Br J Psychol 122:181–183, 1973.

136. Panerai AE, Monza G, Movillia P, et al: A randomized, within-patient crossover, placebo-controlled trial on the efficacy and tolerability of the tricyclic antidepressants chlorimipramine and nortriptyline in central pain. Acta Neurol Scand 82:34–38, 1990.

137. Payne R: Pharmacologic management of bone pain in the cancer patient. Clin J Pain 5(Suppl 2):S43–S50, 1985.

138. Payne R: Neuropathic pain syndromes, with special reference to causalgia and reflex sympathetic dystrophy. Clin J Pain 2:59–73, 1986.

139. Peiris JB, Perera GLS, Devendra SV, et al: Sodium valproate in trigeminal neuralgia. Med J Aust 2:278, 1980.

140. Pilowsky I, Hallet EC, Bassett KL, et al: A controlled study of amitriptyline in the treatment of chronic pain. Pain 14:169–179, 1982.

141. Piper JM, Ray WA, Daugherty JR, and Griffin MR:

Corticosteroid use and peptic ulcer disease—role of nonsteroidal anti-inflammatory drugs. Ann Intern Med 114:735–740, 1991.

142. Porile JL, Bakris L, and Garella S: Acute interstitial nephritis with glomerulopathy due to nonsteroidal anti-inflammatory agents: A review of its clinical spectrum and effects of steroid therapy. J Clin Pharmacol 30:468–475, 1990.

143. Portenoy RK: Pharmacologic management of chronic pain. In Fields HL: Pain Syndromes in Neurologic Practice. Butterworth, New York, 1990, pp 257–278.

144. Portenoy RK: Adjuvant analgesics in pain management. In Doyle D, Hanks GW, and MacDonald N (eds): Oxford Textbook of Palliative Medicine. Oxford University Press, Oxford, 1993, pp 187–203.

145. Preskorn SH, and Irwin HA: Toxicity of tricyclic antidepressants—kinetics, mechanism, intervention: A review. J Clin Psychiatry 43:151–156, 1982.

146. Prough DS, McLeskey CH, Borshy GG, et al: Efficacy of oral nifedipine in the treatment of reflex sympathetic dystrophy. Anesthesiology 62:796–799, 1985.

147. Raftery H: The management of postherpetic pain using sodium valproate and amitriptyline. Journal of the Irish Medical Association 72:399–401, 1979.

148. Ragheb M: The clinical significance of lithium–nonsteroidal anti-inflammatory drug interactions. J Clin Psychopharmacol 10(5):350–354, 1990.

149. Ramsay RE, Wilder BJ, Berger JR, et al: A double-blind study comparing carbamazepine and phenytoin as initial seizure therapy in adults. Neurology 33:904–910, 1983.

150. Raskin NH, Levinson SA, Hoffman PM, et al: Postsympathectomy neuralgia: Amelioration with diphenylhydantoin and carbamazepine. Am J Surg 128:75–78, 1974.

151. Ray WA, Griffin MR, Schaffner W, et al: Pyschotropic drug use and the risk of hip fracture. N Engl J Med 316:363–369, 1987.

152. Rho JM, Donevan SD, and Rogawski MA: Mechanisms of the anticonvulsant felbamate: Opposing effects on N-methyl-D-aspartate and gamma-aminobutyric acid-A receptors. Ann Neurol 35:229–234, 1994.

153. Richelson E: Tricyclic antidepressants and neurotransmitter receptors. Psychology Annals 9:186–194, 1979.

154. Rockliff BW, and Davis EH: Controlled sequential trials of carbamazepine in trigeminal neuralgia. Arch Neurol 15:129–136, 1966.

155. Rosenberg MR, and Green M: Neuroleptic malignant syndrome: Review of response to therapy. Arch Intern Med 149:1927–1931, 1989.

156. Rowbotham MC: Topical analgesic agents. In Fields HL, and Liebeskind JC (eds): Pharmacological Approaches to the Treatment of Chronic Pain: New Concepts and Critical Issues. IASP Press, Seattle, 1994, pp 211–229.

157. Rowbotham MC, and Fields HL: Topical lidocaine reduces pain in postherpetic neuralgia. Pain 38:297–302, 1989.

158. Rowbotham MC, Reisner L, and Fields HL: Both i.v. lidocaine and morphine reduce the pain of postherpetic neuralgia. Neurology 41:1024–1028, 1991.

159. Rull JA, Quibrera R, Gonzalez-Milan H, et al: Symptomatic treatment of peripheral diabetic neuropathy with carbamazepine (Tegretol): Double blind cross-over trial. Diabetologia 5:215–218, 1969.

160. Rumore MM, and Schlicting DA: Clinical efficacy of antihistaminics as analgesics. Pain 25:7–22, 1986.

161. Safavi KT, and Hayward RA: Choosing between apples and apples: Physicians' choices of prescription drugs that have similar side effects and efficacies. J Gen Intern Med 7(1):32–37, 1992.

162. Sandler DP, Smith JC, Weinberg CR, et al: Analgesic use and chronic renal disease. N Engl J Med 320:1238–1243, 1989.

163. Savage RL, Moller PW, Ballantyne CL, et al: Variation in the risk of peptic ulcer complications with nonsteroidal anti-inflammatory drug therapy. Arthritis Rheum 36:84–90, 1993.

164. Scadding JW: Clinical trial of propranolol in post-traumatic neuralgia. Pain 14:283–292, 1982.

165. Scheiman JM: Pathogenesis of gastroduodenal injury due to nonsteroidal anti-inflammatory drugs—implications for prevention and therapy. Semin Arthritis Rheum 21:201–210, 1992.

166. Schmidt D: Adverse effects of valproate. Epilepsia (Suppl)25:44–49, 1984.

167. Schubert TT, Bologna SD, Nensey Y, et al: Ulcer risk factors: Interactions between Helicobacter pylori infection, nonsteroidal use, and age. Am J Med 94(4):413–418, 1993.

168. Simon LS: Nonsteroidal anti-inflammatory drug toxicity. Curr Opin Rheumatol 5(3):265–275, 1993.

169. Simson G: Propanolol for causalgia and Sudek's atrophy. JAMA 227:327, 1974.

170. Sindrup SH, Gram LF, Brosen K, et al: The selective serotonin reuptake inhibitor paroxetine is effective in the treatment of diabetic neuropathy symptoms. Pain 42:135–144, 1990.

171. Singh PN, Sharma P, Gupta PK, et al: Clinical evaluation of diazepam for relief of postoperative pain. Br J Anaesth 53:831–836, 1981.

172. Spiegel K, Kalb R, and Pasternak GW: Analgesic activity of tricyclic antidepressants. Ann Neurol 13:462–465, 1983.

173. Stambaugh JE, and Lane C: Analgesic efficacy and pharmacokinetic evaluation of meperidine and hydroxyzine, alone and in combination. Cancer Invest 1:111–117, 1983.

174. Stein MG, Demarco T, Gamsu G, et al: Computed tomography: Pathologic correlation in lung disease due to tocainide. American Review of Respiratory Disease 137:458–460, 1988.

175. Stow PJ, Glynn CJ, and Minor B: EMLA cream in the treatment of post herpetic neuralgia: Efficacy and pharmacokinetic profile. Pain 39:301–305, 1989.

176. Sunshine A, and Olson NZ: Non-narcotic analgesics. In Wall PD, and Melzack R (eds): Textbook of Pain, ed 2. Churchill Livingstone, New York, 1989, pp 670–685.

177. Swerdlow M: Anticonvulsant drugs and chronic pain. Clin Neuropharmacol 7:51–82, 1984.

178. Swerdlow M, and Cundill JG: Anticonvulsant drugs used in the treatment of lancinating pains. A comparison. Anesthesia 36:1129–1132, 1981.

179. Tabira T, Shibasaki H, and Kuroiwa Y: Reflex sympathetic dystrophy (causalgia) treatment with guanethidine. Arch Neurol 40:430–432, 1983.

180. Tan Y-M, and Croese J: Clonidine and diabetic patients with leg pains. Ann Intern Med 105:633–634, 1986.

181. Tandan R, Lewis GA, Krusinski PB, et al: Topical capsaicin in painful diabetic neuropathy. Controlled study with long-term follow-up. Diabetes Care 15(1):8–14, 1992.

182. Tannock I, Gospodarowicz M, Meakin W, et al: Treatment of metastatic prostatic cancer with low-dose prednisone: Evaluation of pain and quality of life as pragmatic indices of response. J Clin Oncol 7:590–597, 1989.

183. Taub A: Relief of postherpetic neuralgia with psychotropic drugs. J Neurosurg 39:235–239, 1973.

184. Taylor PH, Gray K, Bicknell RG, et al: Glossopharyngeal neuralgia with syncope. J Laryngol Otol 91:859–868, 1977.

185. Vane JR: Inhibition of prostaglandin synthesis as a mechanism of action for aspirin-like drugs. Nature 234:231–238, 1971.

186. Verbeeck RK: Pharmacokinetic drug interactions with nonsteroidal anti-inflammatory drugs. Clin Pharmacokinet 19(1):44–66, 1990.

187. Vincent FM, and Vincent T: Tocainide encephalopathy. Neurology 35:1804–1805, 1985.

188. Ward NG: Tricyclic antidepressants for chronic low back pain. Mechanisms of action and predictors of response. Spine 11:661–665, 1986.

189. Watson CPN, Chipman M, Reed K, et al: Amitriptyline versus maprotiline in postherpetic neuralgia: A randomized, double-blind, crossover trial. Pain 48:29–36, 1992.

190. Watson CPN, Evans RJ, Reed K, et al: Amitriptyline versus placebo in postherpetic neuralgia. Neurology 32:671–673, 1982.

191. Watson CPN, Evans RJ, and Watt VR: Postherpetic neuralgia and topical capsaicin. Pain 33:333–340, 1988.

192. Watson CPN, Evans RJ, and Watt VR: The postmastectomy pain syndrome and the effect of topical capsaicin. Pain 38:177–186, 1989.

193. Weinberger J, Nicklas WJ, and Berl S: Mechanism of action of anticonvulsants. Neurology 26:162–173, 1976.

194. Weinblatt ME: Nonsteroidal anti-inflammatory drug toxicity: Increased risk in the elderly. Scand J Rheumatol 91(Suppl):9–17, 1991.

195. Willer JC, De Brouckner T, Bussel B, et al: Central analgesic effect of ketoprofen in humans—electrophysiological evidence for a supraspinal mechanism in a double-blind and cross-over study. Pain 38:1–7, 1989.

196. Willkens RF: The selection of a nonsteroidal anti-inflammatory drug. Is there a difference? J Rheumatol 19(Suppl 36):9–12, 1992.

197. Woolf CJ, and Wiesenfeld-Hallin Z: The systemic administration of local anesthetic produces a selective depression of C-afferent evoked activity in the spinal cord. Pain 23:361–374, 1985.

198. World Health Organization. Cancer pain relief. Geneva: World Health Organization, 1986.
199. Yaksh TL: Direct evidence that spinal serotonin and noradrenaline terminals mediate the spinal antinociceptive effects of morphine in the periaqueductal gray. Brain Res 160:180–185, 1979.
200. Yamamato T, and Yaksh TL: Spinal pharmacology of thermal hyperesthesia induced by constriction injury of sciatic nerve: Excitatory amino acid antagonists. Pain 49:121–128, 1992.
201. Yjritsy-Roy JA, Standish SM, and Terry LC: Dopamine D-1 and D-2 receptor antagonists potentiate analgesic and motor effects of morphine. Pharmacol Biochem Behav 32:717–721, 1989.

CHAPTER 11

OPIOID ANALGESICS

Russell K. Portenoy, M.D.

Although the medicinal value of opioid compounds has been recognized since antiquity, the clinical use of opioid drugs has been problematic. Traditional teaching emphasizes the risks of adverse effects and addiction, suggests that opioid-induced comfort comes only at the high price of function, and recommends that therapy be limited as much as possible. As will be discussed, much of this teaching is influenced by anecdotal experience, conventional wisdom, and a stigma that may derive from the association of opioids with drug abuse. Negative attitudes toward opioid drugs may combine with inadequate

pharmacologic knowledge to undermine the treatment of those conditions, such as cancer pain, for which these drugs are a first-line approach and to impede efforts to investigate more controversial uses, such as the management of chronic nonmalignant pain. The stigma associated with opioids may also undermine patient compliance with needed therapy.[163,166]

Expertise in the use of opioid drugs requires integration of clinically accepted guidelines with a foundation in opioid pharmacology.[41,53] The recommended approach varies across clinical settings, specifically acute pain,[1] chronic cancer pain,[75] and chronic nonmalignant pain.[119] This chapter concerns the major issues encountered in the use of these drugs for the treatment of diverse types of chronic pain.

PRINCIPLES OF OPIOID PHARMACOLOGY

All opioid drugs bind to opioid receptors and produce analgesia and other effects by mimicking the actions of endogenous opioid compounds at multiple types of opioid receptors (see Chapter 2). Those in clinical use include the opium-related alkaloids, morphine and codeine, and a large number of semisynthetic and synthetic drugs. Modification of the radicals on the five-ring morphine molecule yields the semisynthetic opioids, and changes in the basic ring structure yield synthetic opioids (Table 11–1).

Table 11–1. **SELECTED OPIOID COMPOUNDS WITH ANALGESIC PROPERTIES**

Class	Alkaloids	Semisynthetic	Synthetic
Agonists	Morphine	Hydrocodone	Levorphanol
	Codeine	Hydromorphone	Meperidine
		Oxycodone	Fentanyl
		Oxymorphone	Sufentanil
		Dihydrocodeine	Alfentanil
			Methadone
			Propoxyphene
Agonist-Antagonists		Nalbuphine	Pentazocine
		Buprenorphine	Butorphanol
			Dezocine

Mechanisms

Studies of basic opioid mechanisms have progressed rapidly since the discovery of the opioid receptor more than two decades ago[107,143,154] and the subsequent demonstration of multiple receptor types.[88] Opioid receptors have recently been cloned,[25,48] and the application of molecular techniques using probes developed from these nucleotide sequences will further accelerate this work.

Opioid analgesia results from specific drug-receptor interactions in the spinal cord and brainstem.[9] At both the spinal and supraspinal levels, analgesia is mediated by interactions between endogenous endorphinergic systems and multiple subtypes of the so-called mu, kappa, and delta receptors. The opioid drugs most commonly used in clinical practice are morphinelike pure agonists that selectively bind to the mu receptor. The various receptors are functionally independent,[112] however, and delta-selective or kappa-selective drugs could be useful analgesics. Currently available kappa-selective drugs are also weak mu antagonists; these drugs do not appear to have advantages over the pure mu agonists (see following). Novel receptor-selective drugs are under investigation.

Opioid receptors are situated on sensory nerves and cells of the immune system.[146] These peripheral receptors may be the target of endorphinergic compounds released from immune cells. Binding of exogenous opioids to these receptors could contribute a peripheral mechanism to the central nervous system effects of these drugs. The peripheral opioid-mediated antinociception produced in animal models is most prominent in inflammatory conditions.[147] In humans, peripheral opioid mechanisms have been suggested by several controlled trials that demonstrated analgesia following the intra-articular administration of small doses of morphine at the time of knee surgery.[37,78]

In the central nervous system, opioids act both presynaptically and postsynaptically. Binding to presynaptic receptors inhibits the release of transmitters, whereas binding to postsynaptic receptors directly inhibits the firing of neurons in pain pathways. These inhibitory actions occur through the opening of potassium channels or the closing of calcium channels, processes mediated by a second messenger system that uses a G protein (guanine nucleotide-binding protein).[46] Presynaptic inhibition probably predominates at a spinal level, where opioids reduce the release of transmitters from the terminals of the primary afferent neuron. This action, which results in reduced firing of second-order projection neurons in the dorsal horn, could result in analgesia. The specific opioid actions that lead to analgesia supraspinally are not well understood but are likely to involve effects on descending pain modulatory pathways, at least in part (see Chapter 2).

The complexity of the endogenous opioid systems is compounded by their plasticity. These systems may change with disease processes, the type of noxious stimuli, the characteristics of the analgesic drug, and other factors. Changes may be functional or structural and rapid or slowly evolving. They extend to shifts in gene function. Local inflammation, for example, may increase the activity of genes that up-regulate the production of dynorphin in the spinal cord.[45]

Clinically, processes that influence sensitivity to exogenous opioids are most relevant.[41] These include loss of opioid receptors following peripheral nerve axonotmesis,[173] increased activity of "antiopioid" compounds (such as the neurotransmitters cholecystokinin, galanin, or adenosine, or the morphine metabolite morphine-3-glucuronide),[57,167,172] and the development of pain mechanisms that reduce opioid responsiveness as a result of central neuronal sensitization.

The phenomenon of central sensitization induced by noxious afferent input is undergoing intensive investigation (see Chapters 2 and 5). Noxious peripheral input can change the response characteristics of neurons in the spinal cord, yielding patterns that sustain pain perceptions in the absence of additional stimuli or in response to stimuli that are usually nonnoxious. The receptors of excitatory amino acids, specifically the N-methyl-D-aspartate (NMDA) receptor, are fundamental in precipitating or sustaining this hypersensitivity of central neurons.[40,45,169] These NMDA-dependent central neuronal changes produce nociceptive responses that are relatively less sensitive to opioids.[22,173] Accordingly, pain syndromes driven predominantly by NMDA-dependent processes may be less opioid responsive than pains related to other mechanisms. Experimental findings[87,150] suggest that the relatively poorer opioid responsiveness of some types of neuropathic pain,[122] for example, may be explained by mechanisms that involve central sensitization and the NMDA receptor.

Classes

The opioid drugs that produce analgesia all have agonist effects at one or more of the opioid receptor subtypes. These drugs can be classified as pure agonists or agonist-antagonists on the basis of their interactions with opioid receptors.[71,72] Drugs that bind to opioid receptors but have no intrinsic efficacy for analgesia are known as antagonists.

The agonist-antagonist drugs can be divided into a mixed agonist-antagonist subclass and a partial agonist subclass. In the United States, the mixed agonist-antagonist drugs include butorphanol, nalbuphine, pentazocine, and dezocine; the only partial agonist drug is buprenorphine. The mixed agonist-antagonist drugs are weak antagonists at the mu receptor and agonists at the kappa receptor. The partial agonist drugs are selective agonists at the mu receptor but have a limited intrinsic efficacy at this site.

Both agonist-antagonist subclasses have a "ceiling" effect for analgesia and some other opioid effects (e.g., respiratory depression). This effect refers to a plateau in the dose-response curve, which, ultimately, identifies a dose above which further dose increments produce no change in effect. The agonist-antagonists can reverse the effects of pure agonists in patients who are physically dependent, and some of these drugs (most of the mixed agonist-antagonist group) produce psychotomimetic side effects more readily than the pure agonist opioids. Studies in addict populations suggest that these drugs have a lower abuse potential than the pure agonist drugs.

The pharmacologic properties of the agonist-antagonist opioids limit their utility in the management of chronic pain. Patients with severe chronic pain may require analgesic efficacy beyond the ceiling effect of these drugs, and those with substantial prior opioid intake cannot receive them because of their antagonistic effects, which may lead to pain recurrence or an abstinence syndrome. Although the agonist-antagonist opioids may be less abused by those with known substance abuse disorders, the relevance of this property in nonaddicts is debatable.

The only apparent advantage to the use of the agonist-antagonist drugs is the availability of unique routes of administration. For example, a sublingual formulation of buprenorphine, which is not available in the United States, may be useful for patients who cannot swallow or absorb an oral drug. Intranasal butorphanol is available in the United States and may be useful in selected opioid-naive patients with acute pain who cannot tolerate oral administration; for example, this drug has been marketed for use in the ambulatory treatment of acute headache.[39]

The commercially available opioid antagonist drugs include naloxone and naltrexone. These drugs reverse or block the agonist effects of the opioid analgesics. Naloxone is used in the treatment of opioid overdose, and naltrexone has been marketed for the treatment of opioid addiction and alcoholism.

Responsiveness: Efficacy and Potency

In basic research, analgesic response can be quantified precisely, either in graded or quantal terms. Patient outcomes are more complicated, however, and confusion exists about the terminology of response appropriate in the clinical setting.[120] This confusion is most evident in the use of the terms "efficacy," "responsiveness," and "resistance."

The meaning of the term "efficacy" varies with context and should be used only with additional explanation. Pharmacologists refer to *intrinsic efficacy* to depict a property of drugs defined by the proportion of receptors that must be occupied to yield a given effect. The receptor occupancy required for an agonist to produce a response is inversely proportional to its intrinsic efficacy.

In clinical pharmacology, *efficacy* refers to the effect of a given dose of drug or the maximal effect that can be produced by the drug (also called maximal efficacy). This property is often contrasted against *potency*, a term that indicates the dose required to produce a specified effect.

Clinically, opioid potency is less important than efficacy. This principle is exemplified by the differences between the agonist-antagonist opioids such as butorphanol and the pure agonist drugs such as morphine. Butorphanol is five times more potent than morphine (i.e., 2 mg of butorphanol provides analgesia comparable to 10 mg of morphine), but the ceiling effect at higher doses of butorphanol creates a maximal efficacy far lower than that of morphine. If dose escalation is required to treat progressive pain, the analgesic effect of butorphanol plateaus and its effectiveness is lost. In contrast, the analgesia produced by morphine continues to accrue until side effects limit the dose.

Controlled clinical trials have yielded extensive information about the potency of opioid drugs.[74] Standard equianalgesic dose tables have been constructed from these data (Table 11–2). Although the values depicted in these tables should be applied only with appropriate adjustments (see following), they are nonetheless very useful when one is switching opioid drugs or routes of administration. They do not, however, clarify the efficacy of the drug.

Confusion in the use of the term "efficacy" is compounded when clinicians apply it to describe the favorable clinical response to an opioid, by which is meant a favorable balance between analgesia and side effects. In an effort to clarify the nomenclature, the term "responsiveness" has been proposed as a substitute to describe clinical responses.[114,120] *Opioid responsiveness* refers to the probability that adequate analgesia (satisfactory relief without intolerable and unmanageable side effects) can be attained during dose titration. Alternatively, responsiveness can be used to depict the degree of analgesia obtained at dose-limiting toxicity (maximal efficacy from a clinically relevant perspective).

In any specified population of patients with chronic pain, the responsiveness to a specific drug varies remarkably. Some patients achieve excellent pain relief without side effects, whereas others experience intolerable side effects with minimal or no analgesia. Similarly, the responsiveness to different opioids can vary remarkably in any individual patient. For example, a patient may develop dose-limiting somnolence at a morphine dose associated with poor analgesia but then demonstrate dose-limiting nausea without somnolence at a dose of hydromorphone associated with lesser, equal, or better analgesia.

This variability in opioid responsiveness is multifactorial and relates to characteristics of both the patient and the pain syndrome. Among the factors that appear to reduce opioid responsiveness are a neuropathic mechanism for the pain, the presence of incident pain (pain induced by specific maneuvers), a high level of psychologic distress, and the need for rapid dose escalation after the initiation of therapy.[17,97] Any factor that increases the likelihood of dose-limited toxicity, such as advanced age, presumably also reduces responsiveness.

Although the presence or absence of these

Table 11–2. **OPIOID AGONIST DRUGS USED FOR SEVERE PAIN**

Pure Agonist Drug	Dose (mg) Equianalgesic to Morphine (10 mg IM)		Half-Life (hr)	Duration (hr)	Comment
	PO	IM			
Morphine	20–30	10	2–3	2–4	Standard for comparison.
Morphine (controlled-release)	20–30	10	2–3	8–12	Two formulations available; both are long-acting, but they are not bioequivalent.
Oxycodone	20	—	2–3	3–4	Used for moderate pain combined with aspirin or acetaminophen; used as single entity, can be used like oral morphine for severe pain.
Hydromorphone	1.5	7.5	2–3	2–4	Available as high-potency parenteral formulation useful for subcutaneous infusion; controlled-release formulation under development.
Methadone	10	20	12–190	4–12	With long half-life, delayed toxicity can occur because of accumulation at start of therapy and with each dose increment; as a result, treatment should be started with PRN dosing.
Meperidine	75	300	2–3	2–4	No longer preferred for the management of acute or chronic pain due to potential toxicity from active metabolite, normeperidine.
Oxymorphone	1	10 (rectal)	2–3	2–4	Available in rectal and injectable formulations.
Levorphanol	2	4	12–15	4–6	
Fentanyl	—	—	7–12	—	Clinically used as a continuous IV or SQ infusion; based on clinical experience, 100 μg/hr is roughly equianalgesic to morphine 2 mg/hr.
Fentanyl (Transdermal System)	—	—	—	48–72	Patches are available to deliver 25, 50, 75, and 100 μg/hr; based on clinical experience, 100 μg/hr is roughly equianalgesic to morphine 2 mg/hr.

characteristics may increase or decrease opioid responsiveness, there is no evidence that any factor, or group of factors, imparts uniform opioid resistance. The outcome of opioid therapy cannot be accurately predicted, a priori, from any characteristic of the patient or pain.[76,94,114]

The observation that the responsiveness to different opioids varies in the same patient has important clinical implications.[56] It suggests the potential utility of sequential opioid trials to identify the most favorable treatment and further discredits the notion that a particular characteristic, such as a neuropathic mechanism for the pain, produces uniform opioid resistance.

Adverse Pharmacologic Outcomes

The major goal of treatment for most patients is a satisfactory balance between analgesia and side effects. Effective management of adverse drug effects may improve outcome by allowing higher, more effective opioid doses or by reducing uncomfortable symptoms other than pain.

Neither acute nor chronic administration of opioid drugs injures major organ systems. With the exception of isolated reports of pulmonary edema in extremely ill patients with cancer who received very high opioid doses,[19] an extensive clinical experience in the cancer population has been reassuring. In the methadone maintenance population, systematic observations lead to a similar conclusion.[83–85]

Dysimmune effects from opioids are reported, but the clinical implications of these findings are not known. In animal models, acute opioid exposure can alter the immune system by impairing functions that are antigen-nonspecific, such as natural killer cell activity and cytokine production, or antigen-mediated.[6,44,47,99,108,141,164] Prolonged morphine administration (up to 42 days) in a swine model significantly diminished cell-mediated immunity[99] but did not affect humoral immune responses. In other studies, however, lower morphine doses[140] and sustained treatment with methadone[103] had no effect on natural killer cell activity. Although there is a suggestion that opioids may reduce $CD4^+$ T-cell number in humans,[43] clinical data related to this issue of immune suppression are generally lacking. This lack of clinical reports is reassuring but does not exclude the possibility of a small effect that may be relevant in some groups of patients. Although evidence is clearly insufficient to recommend any therapeutic changes, further research in this area is needed.

Side effects, which may be transitory or persistent, are the most important adverse pharmacologic outcomes in practice. Tolerance to most adverse effects, including nausea, somnolence, and mental clouding, occurs within days to weeks after the initiation of therapy. Constipation often persists, however, particularly in those with other predisposing causes, and any of the other adverse effects can potentially continue and limit the utility of therapy. Studies in methadone maintenance patients[83,84] demonstrate that approximately 10 to 20 percent complain of persistent constipation, insomnia, and decreased sexual function, and a somewhat higher percentage report persistent sweating.

Expertise in the management of common side effects is an integral part of opioid pharmacotherapy. Simple approaches usually ameliorate these symptoms (Table 11–3).[118]

Patients and clinicians alike commonly express concern that the long-term use of opioid drugs produces cognitive impairment sufficient to prevent normal functioning. The potential for prolonged impairment has been suggested in surveys of patients referred to multidisciplinary pain management programs[90,93] and several surveys of opioid addicts or methadone maintenance populations.[64,134] These studies must be interpreted cautiously, however, because of the failure to control uniformly for such confounds as prior head trauma, coexistent medical disorders, and concurrent use of sedative or hypnotic drugs. Cognitive impairment was not identified in other methadone-maintained populations,[4,86] and the driving records of methadone-maintained patients have not demonstrated any evidence of increased risk due to this therapy.[7,59] In a small study of chronic pain patients, cognitive effects occurred in those treated with benzodiazepines but not in those treated with opioids alone.[66] A survey of patients with advanced cancer demonstrated cognitive impairment several days but not several weeks following opioid dose escalation.[16] Subtle reaction-time changes measured in patients with cancer receiving long-term systemic or spinal opioid therapy[8,145] have uncertain clinical relevance.[102]

The existing data, combined with extensive clinical experience in both the cancer population and the methadone maintenance population, suggest that long-term opioid therapy is generally compatible with normal functioning. Persistent cognitive impairment is a possible outcome and must be assessed repeatedly during therapy. Normal cognition is the anticipated goal of therapy, however, and patients who have no clinical evidence of impairment should be encouraged to engage in all routine activities.

Table 11–3. **COMMONLY USED PHARMACOLOGIC APPROACHES IN THE MANAGEMENT OF OPIOID SIDE EFFECTS**

Opioid Side Effect	Treatment
Constipation	Several approaches:
	1. Daily contact laxative plus stool softener (e.g., senna plus docusate)
	2. Intermittent use of osmotic laxative (e.g., milk of magnesia)
	3. Chronic lactulose therapy
Nausea	Several approaches:
	1. If associated with vertigo or if markedly exacerbated by movement, antivertiginous drug (e.g., scopolamine, meclizine, dimenhydrinate)
	2. If associated with early satiety, metoclopramide
	3. In other cases, dopamine antagonist drugs (e.g., prochlorperazine, chlorpromazine, haloperidol, metoclopramide)
Sedation	Psychostimulant drug (e.g., methylphenidate, dextroamphetamine)

OPIOID TOLERANCE AND DEPENDENCE

Among the many properties of opioid drugs that influence clinical decision making, the potential for analgesic tolerance and the phenomena related to dependence (physical dependence and addiction) may be the most difficult to grasp. Misconceptions about tolerance and dependence are common and reflect the stigma associated with opioid drugs. To optimize opioid therapy, the nomenclature must be precise and the true risks of these agents be understood.

Tolerance

Tolerance refers to a process defined by the occurrence of decreasing effects at a constant dose or the need for a higher dose to maintain an effect.[54,77,120] Although the term is descriptive and does not imply a specific mechanism, it does connote that exposure to the drug is the primary cause—the "driving force"—for the change in the dose-response relationship. The term does not apply when a decrease in drug effect can be ascribed to increasing pathology rather than drug exposure.

Associative tolerance indicates that the change in the dose-response relationship is related to learning, such as would occur if a decline in drug effect were due to operant conditioning. *Nonassociative* or *pharmacologic tolerance* refers to changes in drug response over time that are unrelated to learning. Pharmacologic tolerance may be *dispositional*—attributable to pharmacokinetic changes—or *pharmacodynamic*. Pharmacodynamic tolerance refers to a decline in drug effect that cannot be attributed to kinetic factors and instead reflects some type of change in the neural systems acted upon by the drug.

In animal models and in vitro preparations used to study opioid drugs, progressive diminution in antinociceptive responses and other opioid effects can be easily induced by repeated opioid exposure.[30,174] This type of pharmacodynamic tolerance is assumed to mirror a similar phenomenon in humans, which diminishes the potential efficacy of long-term therapy with these drugs.

In humans, tolerance to nonanalgesic effects of opioids occurs commonly. After the initiation of dosing, patients often report somnolence, mental clouding, and nausea, all of which diminish within days or weeks. Tolerance to respiratory depressant effects also occurs rapidly and is the basis for safe escalation of the opioid dose. With gradual dose incrementation, doses that would be lethal in the opioid-naive patient can be tolerated without any adverse effects whatsoever. Clinically, tolerance to side effects is beneficial and increases the likelihood that a favorable balance between analgesia and side effects will be attained during dose escalation.

Tolerance to analgesic effects, if sufficiently severe, could become a barrier to effective long-term opioid therapy. To clarify the risk of this phenomenon, the nomenclature must be applied precisely. Clinicians commonly err by referring to any patient who develops a need for dose escalation as tolerant, even if pathology is worsening. This imprecision may reflect the failure to recognize that declining analgesic effects actually have a "differential diagnosis" (Table 11–4).

Increasing activity in nociceptive pathways may occur with progression of a lesion or associated factors, such as evolving inflammation or evolution of peripheral or central neuropathic processes (e.g., the central neuronal sensitization described previously). Worsening pain may also result from psychologic or cognitive processes. Pharmacodynamic tolerance to analgesic effects cannot be imputed to be the "driving force" for loss of analgesia if one or more of these alternative (physical or psychologic) reasons for increasing pain can be discerned.

RISKS ASSOCIATED WITH TOLERANCE

If the definition of pharmacologic tolerance is applied appropriately, a remarkable phenomenon is observed in the clinical setting. In contrast to the findings in experimental paradigms,[73,74,95] loss of analgesia rarely occurs in patients with stable pain syndromes. Patients without progressive disease who are administered an opioid typically achieve stable dosing that extends for a pro-

Table 11–4. A "DIFFERENTIAL DIAGNOSIS" FOR DECLINING ANALGESIC EFFECTS IN THE CLINICAL SETTING

Increased Activity in Nociceptive Pathways
Increasing activation of nociceptors in the periphery
    Due to mechanical factors (e.g., tumor growth)
    Due to biochemical changes (e.g., inflammation)
    Due to peripheral neuropathic processes (e.g., neuroma formation)
Increased activity in central nociceptive pathways
    Due to central neuropathic processes (e.g., sensitization, shift in receptive fields, change in modulatory processes)

Psychologic Processes*
Increasing psychologic distress (e.g., anxiety or depression)
Change in cognitive state leading to altered pain perception or reporting (e.g., delirium)
Conditioned pain behavior independent of the drug

Tolerance
Due to pharmacodynamic processes
Due to pharmacokinetic processes
Due to psychologic processes

*Other than conditioned responses to the drug.

longed period.* When the need for dose escalation occurs, an alternative explanation, typically worsening of the underlying disease, can usually be identified.[58]

Although an explanation for the rare occurrence of analgesic tolerance during opioid treatment of stable pain syndromes is lacking, the observation has important clinical implications. Fear of tolerance should not be used to justify a delay in the initiation of opioid therapy, if otherwise indicated, or the withholding of therapy from those with long life expectancies. Furthermore, tolerance should not be assumed in patients with chronic diseases who experience diminishing analgesia after a period of stable dosing. Progressive pain should trigger an evaluation for progression or recurrence of the disease or the development of a new pathology.

Other observations affirm the complexity of tolerance in the clinical setting. Some patients who appear to be tolerant to adverse opioid effects suddenly develop such effects when an intervention occurs that lessens or eliminates the underlying cause of the pain. For example, a patient who has been administered a high opioid dose to treat pain due to a malignant lesion may develop symptoms and signs of opioid overdose, possibly including respiratory depression, if the dose of the opioid is not promptly reduced after a cordotomy. The treatment of residual pain in such a patient typically requires a small fraction of the dose used prior to the procedure. This evidence of increased responsiveness to analgesic and nonanalgesic opioid actions after the nociceptive focus is blocked would not be expected if the relatively long-lasting changes in receptor function associated with tolerance had actually occurred. Evidently, some of the changes in the dose-response relationship are determined by mechanisms associated with the pain rather than by pharmacodynamic tolerance alone.

Thus, tolerance may not protect the patient from opioid toxicity if the cause of the pain is eliminated. In such cases, the opioid dose must be reduced promptly to minimize risk. Based on an abundant clinical experience, the opioid dose can be reduced by 50 to 75 percent every 2 to 3 days, with a very small likelihood of opioid withdrawal. If faster dose reduction is required, withdrawal can be blocked by the coadministration of the adrenergic blocker clonidine.

Physical Dependence and Addiction

Confusion about the phenomenon described as "dependence" or "addiction" is also common. Confusion results, in part, from the misuse of terms. A discussion about the true risks associated with these outcomes must begin with appropriate definitions.

"Physical dependence" is a physiologic phenomenon characterized by the development of an abstinence syndrome following abrupt discontinuation of therapy, substantial dose reduction, or administration of an antagonist drug.[42,77,89,132] The capacity for withdrawal—that is, physical dependence—is presumed to exist whenever repeated doses of an opioid have been administered for more than a few days.

Clinicians often mistakenly apply the term "addicted" to the patient who may be physically dependent on an opioid. The use of a term with such a negative connotation to describe a physiologic outcome of opioid therapy is an unfortunate error. Patients who are perceived to be at risk of withdrawal should be described only as "physically dependent."

Although early definitions of addiction referred to physical dependence,[170] these two terms are more appropriately defined in a manner that fully distinguishes them. Physical dependence indicates neither the presence nor absence of the behaviors that define addiction (see following), and addiction may exist with or without the capacity for withdrawal that defines physical dependence.

Standard definitions of addiction, which have been developed from clinical experience with substance abusers, must be interpreted cautiously when applied to patients who are receiving opioids as prescribed therapy for an appropriate medical indication. For example, a reference to "relapse after withdrawal" in the definition offered by a major pharmacology text ("a behavioral pattern of drug use, characterized by overwhelming involvement with the use of a drug [compulsive use], the securing of its supply, and the high tendency to relapse after withdrawal")[77] may be difficult to interpret if the

---

*References 12, 54, 55, 70, 80, 104, 110, 121, 138, 156.

drug is prescribed for a medical indication. Similarly, the diagnostic criteria for psychoactive substance dependence developed for the *Diagnostic and Statistical Manual of Mental Disorders-IV* of the American Psychiatric Association[2] includes references to tolerance and physical dependence that have no relevance to clinical populations.[139]

According to a task force of the American Medical Association, addiction is a chronic disorder characterized by "the compulsive use of a substance resulting in physical, psychologic, or social harm to the user and continued use despite that harm."[132] This statement is sufficiently broad but requires operational definitions to be applied to patients who are receiving opioid drugs for painful disorders.

Fundamentally, addiction is a psychologic and behavioral syndrome characterized by (1) loss of control over drug use, (2) compulsive drug use, and (3) continued use despite harm. In operationalizing these criteria for patients who have a clinical indication for the drug in question, the clinician must seek evidence of aberrant drug-related behaviors that cannot be adequately explained by the recognized need for the drug to provide symptomatic relief.[119] Patients may engage in a broad range of aberrant drug-related behaviors (Table 11–5). The diagnostic challenge is to recognize that these behaviors have a "differential diagnosis" and to perform an assessment that clarifies their relationship with the medical disorder and psychosocial condition of the patient. In some cases, the behaviors are sufficiently extreme (e.g., injection of an oral drug formulation or acquisition of illicit opioids to supplement prescribed drugs) to indicate the

Table 11–5. ABERRANT DRUG-RELATED BEHAVIORS THAT RAISE CONCERN ABOUT THE POTENTIAL FOR ADDICTION

Behaviors More Suggestive of an Addiction Disorder

Selling prescription drugs

Prescription forgery

Stealing or "borrowing" drugs from others

Injecting oral formulations

Obtaining prescription drugs from nonmedical sources

Concurrent abuse of alcohol or illicit drugs

Multiple dose escalations or other noncompliance with therapy despite warnings

Multiple episodes of prescription "loss"

Repeatedly seeking prescriptions from other clinicians or from emergency rooms without informing prescriber or after warnings to desist

Evidence of deterioration in the ability to function at work, in the family, or socially that appear to be related to drug use

Repeated resistance to changes in therapy despite clear evidence of adverse physical or psychologic effects from the drug

Behaviors Less Suggestive of an Addiction Disorder

Aggressive complaining about the need for more drug

Drug hoarding during periods of reduced symptoms

Requesting specific drugs

Openly acquiring similar drugs from other medical sources

Unsanctioned dose escalation or other noncompliance with therapy on one or two occasions

Unapproved use of the drug to treat another symptom

Reporting psychic effects not intended by the clinician

Resistance to a change in therapy associated with "tolerable" adverse effects, with expressions of anxiety related to the return of severe symptoms

Source: Portenoy, RK: Opioid therapy for chronic nonmalignant pain: Current status. In Fields HL, and Liebeskind JC (eds): Progress in Pain Research and Management, Vol 1: Pharmacological approaches to the Treatment of Chronic Pain: New Concepts and Critical Issues. IASP Press, Seattle, 1994, p 267, with permission.

diagnosis of an addiction disorder. In other cases, however, the behaviors are less egregious and can reflect other processes, including impulsive behavior driven by unrelieved pain, psychiatric disorder other than an addiction, or mild encephalopathy with confusion about drug intake.

In patients with cancer, this differential diagnosis is reflected in the term "pseudoaddiction." *Pseudoaddiction* refers to drug-seeking behaviors that result from uncontrolled pain.[165] In such cases, improved pain control, which is often achieved by escalation of the opioid dose, eliminates the aberrant behaviors.

The successful long-term management of opioid therapy requires a clear diagnostic formulation through ongoing evaluation of drug-related behaviors. If the patient engages in aberrant behaviors, the clinician must determine whether the problem is transitory and impulsive, perhaps related to a flare of unrelieved symptoms, or more serious and abiding. All such behaviors raise concern about the potential for addiction, and all must be appropriately managed to limit consequences and regain control. Nevertheless, the diagnosis of an addiction disorder should be made only if the criteria for this diagnosis are met and there is no credible alternative diagnosis.

RISKS ASSOCIATED WITH PHYSICAL DEPENDENCE

The major risk associated with physical dependence is abstinence, which is prevented by avoiding abrupt dose reduction and opioid antagonist drugs. Extensive clinical experience has not confirmed that physical dependence, or the fear of withdrawal due to physical dependence, complicates medically indicated dose reduction or discontinuation of opioid therapy.[18,19,80] Although physical dependence has been postulated to drive the development of an addiction disorder in nonpatient substance abusers,[168] experience with patients indicates that physical dependence is neither necessary nor sufficient for addiction. Protracted abstinence[42,89] could produce prolonged physical or psychologic morbidity in patients, but this has not been a problem for either patients with cancer or those with chronic nonmalignant pain.

Physical dependence has been proposed as a factor contributing to persistent pain or a "downhill spiral" in patients with chronic nonmalignant pain who develop functional deterioration.[13,136] In this formulation, subtle abstinence may sustain pain or induce maladaptive behaviors (like drug seeking) that perpetuate disability associated with the pain. A similar process has been suggested to explain "rebound" headache, a syndrome of refractory pain ascribed to frequent use of short-acting analgesics.[135] This phenomenon has not been studied systematically, and headache rebound from opioid therapy has not been confirmed.[176] Nonetheless, the "downward spiral" concept represents a legitimate concern that should be evaluated like other potential adverse effects associated with chronic opioid therapy. Opioid drug use can contribute to global dysfunction in some patients with chronic pain, and the possibility that physical dependence plays a role must be considered.

RISK OF ADDICTION

Iatrogenic addiction is a greater concern than the adverse effects associated with physical dependence. If true addiction were a common outcome of opioid therapy for pain, it would be appropriate to delay the use of this therapy as long as possible in the cancer population and forgo it altogether in virtually all patients with chronic nonmalignant pain. Unfortunately, no systematic studies exist of the addiction liability associated with the long-term medical use of opioid drugs. Information about this outcome derives from limited published surveys that report clinical experience in selected populations.

Concern that the medical use of opioid drugs carries a substantial risk of addiction was heightened by early surveys of addict populations.[128] These data, combined with reports of high recidivism rates among detoxified addicts,[144] stimulated concern that exposure to an opioid drug could induce addiction in previously normal patients. In populations with chronic nonmalignant pain, these data were reinforced by surveys of patients referred to pain clinics, which identified high rates of aberrant drug-related behavior.[19,50,51,120,155]

The portrayal of opioid therapy in other contexts is much more sanguine but also is based on limited data. Addiction is commonly perceived to be extremely rare during chronic opioid therapy for cancer pain.[75] Experienced clinicians generally discount it as a risk unless the patient with cancer pain has a prior history of drug abuse. In one study, addiction was not observed among patients allowed to self-administer an opioid for the treatment of mucositis-related pain following bone marrow transplantation.[23]

Survey data highlight the heterogeneity of nonmalignant pain populations and suggest that patients referred to multidisciplinary pain management programs differ from patients treated in other settings. The addiction rates reported from pain management programs, which range from 3.2 to 18.9 percent,[52] are generally higher than those reported in other types of surveys. For example, a large survey of inpatients, the Boston Collaborative Drug Surveillance Project, identified only 4 cases of addiction among 11,882 hospitalized patients with no history of substance abuse who received at least one dose of an opioid.[127] A national survey of burn units identified no iatrogenic addiction in 10,000 patients who received opioids for burn pain and had no prior history of substance abuse.[106] Only 3 of 2369 patients attending a headache clinic developed a management problem with the opioid analgesics provided to treat intermittent headaches.[96] These data are reassuring, particularly when compared with United States population prevalence rates for alcoholism (3 to 16 percent) and other forms of substance abuse (5 to 6 percent).[130]

The extensive clinical experience reflected in these statistics gives credence to the argument that the risk of addiction does not reside predominantly in the drug. Mere exposure to an opioid, even for prolonged periods, does not produce the aberrant behaviors consistent with an addiction disorder. Extant data suggest that other factors—psychologic,[68,69] situational,[133] and perhaps genetic[63]—must interact with the reinforcing properties of a drug to yield an addiction disorder.

The evidence suggests that the risk of addiction is extremely low in the typical patient with no prior history of drug abuse who is prescribed an opioid for a painful medical condition. The risk probably increases with other factors, such as a prior history of drug abuse, personality disorder, younger age, and chaotic family life, but this remains to be determined. Most patients have received psychoactive drugs through medical or recreational exposure during youth, and older persons with no prior history of substance abuse and a relatively stable psychosocial condition appear to have a very low risk of iatrogenic addiction.

OPIOIDS IN THE MANAGEMENT OF CANCER PAIN

Long-term opioid treatment is now the primary therapeutic approach to cancer pain. It is required by 30 to 50 percent of patients receiving active antineoplastic therapy and more than 75 percent of those with advanced disease.[10,114,171] Although as many as 90 percent of patients benefit from optimally administered opioid therapy,* undertreatment continues in most practice settings[29] despite efforts to identify and redress the barriers to effective management.[117] Improved use of current techniques for opioid therapy is one of the goals of the treatment guidelines for cancer pain published by the US Agency for Health Care Policy and Research.[75]

Basic Approach to Cancer Pain

The management of cancer pain requires a comprehensive patient assessment.[26] This assessment has multiple objectives (Table 11–6), among which is clarification of the goals of care. The predominant goals of care often change during the course of the disease. At varying times, they focus on prolongation of life, maintenance of function, or comfort. Clarification of these goals is essential for the management of pain and other symptoms in patients with life-threatening illness.

The assessment should also clarify the feasibility of primary therapies directed at the

---

*References 10, 100, 113, 114, 137, 149, 158, 159, 162, 171.

Table 11–6. OBJECTIVES OF A COMPREHENSIVE ASSESSMENT OF CANCER PAIN

Characterization of the pain complaint
Severity
Temporal features
Quality
Location
Provocative and palliative factors

*Diagnosis of the pain syndrome**

Inferred pain pathophysiology†
Nociceptive
Neuropathic
Mixed

Evaluation of the extent of disease

Clarification of other processes that contribute to suffering
Other physical symptoms
Psychologic symptoms or disorders
Functional or social disruptions
Financial concerns
Spiritual issues

Clarification of the overriding goals of care

*See Chapter 9.
†See Chapter 1.

lesion or lesions causing the pain. Radiotherapy is used commonly for analgesia, and selected patients may experience pain relief with chemotherapy, surgery, or antibiotic therapy.

Drug Selection

The World Health Organization has developed a simple set of guidelines for the selection and administration of opioid drugs.[171] The high success rates reported for opioid therapy in cancer pain derive from open trials that have evaluated the feasibility and outcomes of this approach.[137,158,159,162] Effective opioid pharmacotherapy for cancer pain is within the purview of all clinicians and, indeed, is the obligation of those caring for patients with cancer.

The approach to the selection of analgesic drugs promulgated by the World Health Or-

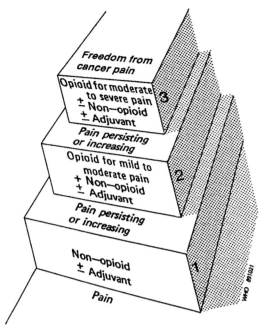

Figure 11–1. Analgesic ladder approach to drug selection for the management of cancer pain, as developed by a committee of the World Health Organization. (Reprinted from World Health Organization: Cancer pain relief and palliative care. World Health Organization, Geneva, 1990, with permission.)

ganization is known as the "analgesic ladder" (Fig. 11–1).[171] Patients with mild to moderate cancer-related pain are first treated with an NSAID. This drug is combined with an adjuvant drug, if indicated. The adjuvant drug can be selected for additional analgesia (i.e., an adjuvant analgesic; see Chapter 10) or for the treatment of a different symptom (either a side effect of the analgesic or a coexisting symptom other than pain).

Pure agonist opioid drugs are recommended for patients with moderate or severe pain. Depending on the usual severity of the pain, patients may begin treatment on the second or third step of the ladder. Those with moderate pain or continued pain, despite treatment with a nonopioid analgesic, are managed with an opioid conventionally used for moderate pain (previously termed a "weak" opioid). This drug is typically combined with an NSAID and may be administered with an adjuvant drug, if indicated. Those with severe pain or continued pain despite administration of an opioid for moderate pain receive an opioid conventionally used for severe pain (previously termed a "strong" opioid). This drug also may be combined with an NSAID or an adjuvant drug, as indicated.

The division of opioid agonist drugs into "weak" and "strong" for the analgesic ladder approach is operational rather than pharmacologic. The prototypic drug in the weak group is codeine; hydrocodone, dihydrocodeine, oxycodone (combined with aspirin or acetaminophen), propoxyphene, and occasionally meperidine are also used in the United States. None of these drugs has a ceiling effect, which would give pharmacologic meaning to the designation "weak." Rather, other considerations support their uses at doses that are capable of treating moderate pain in the relatively nontolerant patient. Meperidine, propoxyphene, and codeine have relatively increased toxicity at higher doses. Hydrocodone and dihydrocodeine are available only in tablets that contain acetaminophen or aspirin and cannot be given in quantities that exceed the maximal safe amount of the nonopioid coanalgesic (e.g., 4 to 6 grams of acetaminophen per day).

The opioids for treating moderate pain that are available in single-entity formulations can potentially be used at higher doses to treat severe pain. Single-entity oxycodone, in particular, is commonly used for this purpose; it is, like morphine, for the third step of the analgesic ladder. Propoxyphene and meperidine are available in single-entity formulations, but dose escalation is not recommended because of the risk of enhanced toxicity from metabolite accumulation. Although a metabolite of propoxyphene, norpropoxyphene, has not been a problem clinically at the usual doses of the parent compound, a metabolite of meperidine, normeperidine, has produced clinical toxicity in the cancer population.[79] Indeed, the risk of normeperidine toxicity, which includes tremulousness, hyperreflexia, myoclonus, and seizures, suggests that meperidine should be avoided during the management of both acute pain and chronic pain.[1,75]

The simplest approach to the management of moderate pain in the patient with cancer who has limited or no prior exposure to opioids involves a combination product containing an opioid and either aspirin or acetaminophen. The opioid may be codeine, oxycodone, hydrocodone, dihydrocodeine, or propoxyphene. The dose of this combination product is increased, if needed, until maximal doses of the coanalgesic are reached (e.g., 2 to 3 tablets every 4 hours of a combination product containing acetaminophen 325 mg per tablet).

The selection of an opioid conventionally used for severe pain (so-called "strong" opioid) is similarly empirical. Morphine is the preferred first-line drug, based on an extensive worldwide experience and the availability of numerous formulations, including a controlled-release form with a duration of up to 12 hours.[123] Any of the other opioid drugs may be better tolerated in the individual patient, however, and may potentially produce a more favorable balance between analgesia and side effects during dose titration.[56]

Morphine effects are produced, in part, by an active metabolite, morphine-6-glucuronide.[126] Accumulation of this metabolite, particularly with renal failure,[105] could lead to unanticipated opioid toxicity. Consequently, morphine should be administered cautiously to patients with renal insufficiency, and the occurrence of morphine toxicity in patients with renal disease should be followed by a trial of an alternative opioid, such as hydromorphone.

The selection of an opioid for the treatment of severe cancer pain is influenced by pharmacokinetic factors, the most salient of which is half-life. Because four to five half-lives are required to approach steady state after dosing is initiated or changed, an opioid with a relatively long half-life requires a prolonged period before the full effect of a new dosing regimen can be judged. Although both levorphanol and methadone have half-lives longer than other opioids (see Table 11–2), only methadone commonly poses clinical difficulty.[49] The half-life of methadone is relatively long and variable (ranging from 12 to 190 hours).[111] After the dose is increased to analgesic levels, plasma concentration can continue to rise for days or even weeks, leading to the delayed onset of adverse effects. Methadone is therefore a second-line drug for patients predisposed to opioid side effects, including the elderly and those with major organ dysfunction, and for patients who are noncompliant or difficult to evaluate. Methadone and levorphanol are most difficult to administer when rapid dose escalation is required, such as during the treatment of acute severe pain.

Controlled-release formulations of opioid drugs, including controlled-release oral morphine and transdermal fentanyl, also require a long period to approach steady state after dosing is initiated or changed. Steady-state concentrations may not be reached for 1 or 2 days with the morphine preparations and for 3 days or longer with the transdermal preparations. Consequently, controlled-release opioids are not optimal if rapid dose titration is required.

Routes of Administration

The oral route is preferred in the management of chronic cancer pain because of its safety, economy, and acceptability to patients. Alternative routes are often required, however, and the clinician must recognize their indications and be familiar with the accepted approaches (Table 11–7).

The transdermal and subcutaneous routes are used most commonly in the long-term management of cancer pain. As noted, the transdermal route of administration is available for the highly lipophilic opioid fentanyl.[61,125] This formulation is indicated for patients who have relatively stable chronic pain and cannot swallow or absorb an orally administered opioid, patients who are noncompliant with oral drugs or would prefer an alternative, and patients who have failed other opioids and may benefit from a trial of fentanyl. The transdermal system is not indicated in acute pain because of its slow onset and prolonged effects after the patch is removed from the skin.

Portable ambulatory infusion devices have enhanced the clinical utility of infusion techniques.[15,148] Patients who are unable to swallow or absorb oral opioids can be managed in the ambulatory setting for long periods when this approach is used. A diverse group of pumps that range considerably in features, complexity, and cost are now available, and the clinician often can select a pump based on the needs and resources of the patient. In the United States, a pump that allows a patient-controlled analgesia mode is typically used; this device is relatively expensive but allows the combination of a continuous infusion with intermittent self-activated bolus injections for the management of breakthrough pains.

Techniques for intraspinal opioid administration have also progressed rapidly.[5,110] Intraspinal administration can provide selective analgesia (analgesia without the motor or sensory block produced by local anesthetics) at doses lower than those required to provide equivalent analgesia systematically. This may reduce the adverse effects mediated by the central nervous system. The strongest indication for a spinal route, therefore, is intolerable somnolence or confusion in patients with otherwise substantial analgesia during systemic treatment.[161]

Many drugs and delivery techniques are now used in long-term spinal therapy.[5,32,160] In the absence of comparative trials, selection is based on clinical experience. The preferred drug continues to be morphine, but others, such as hydromorphone or fentanyl, are used, and there is a growing experience in the long-term administration of an opioid combined with a local anesthetic.

Long-term epidural delivery can be accomplished through a percutaneous catheter, which is usually tunneled to the anterior abdominal wall, or through a totally implanted catheter connected to a subcutaneous portal. The percutaneous catheter or subcutaneous portal may be injected repeatedly or, more commonly in the United States, connected to an ambulatory infusion pump for continuous drug delivery. Compared to long-term intrathecal drug delivery, the epidural approach is simpler to insert, more cost-effective in the short term, and more amenable to combination drug therapy. Intrathecal opioid administration, which is usually accomplished via a totally implanted continuous infusion device, requires less care and is generally more durable. It is more cost-effective if treatment continues for longer than 3 to 6 months.

Guidelines for Administration

Dosing guidelines for cancer pain are widely accepted and highly effective.[27,75] Most patients are treated for the long term with a pure agonist drug selected for severe pain (the third step of the analgesic ladder).

Table 11–7. **ROUTES OF OPIOID ADMINISTRATION**

Route	Comment
Oral	Preferred in cancer pain management.
Buccal	Supporting data meager, and the method is generally unavailable and impracticable.
Sublingual	Buprenorphine effective but not yet available in United States. Efficacy of morphine controversial. No clinical studies of other drugs.
Rectal	Available for morphine, oxymorphone, and hydromorphone. Although few studies available, customarily used as if dose is equianalgesic to oral dose.
Transdermal	Available for fentanyl citrate, with patches delivering 25, 50, 75, and 100 µg/hr. Can provide analgesia for 2- to 3-day period per dose and is indicated for patients who are unable to use oral drug, are noncompliant with repetitive dosing, or have failed other opioids and could potentially benefit from a trial of fentanyl.
Intranasal	Available for butorphanol, a mixed agonist-antagonist not preferred for cancer pain management.
Oral transmucosal	Formulation using fentanyl currently undergoing trials as an approach to the treatment of breakthrough pain.

Subcutaneous
  Repetitive bolus
  Continuous infusion
  Continuous infusion with patient-controlled analgesia (PCA)
	Ambulatory infusion pumps can provide continuous infusion with any parenteral opioid formulation. More advanced pumps can also provide PCA. Clearest indication is inability to tolerate oral route.

Intravenous
  Repetitive bolus
  Continuous infusion
  Continuous infusion with patient-controlled analgesia
	Continuous infusion possible if permanent venous access available.

Epidural
  Repetitive bolus
  Continuous infusion using percutaneous or implanted system
	Clearest indication is pain in lower half of body and dose-limiting side effects from systemic opioid. Often coadministered with local anesthetic.

Intrathecal	Usually administered via a totally implanted infusion pump. May be cost-effective for those patients with clear indication for intraspinal therapy and long life expectancy.
Intracerebroventricular	Rarely indicated. Should be considered investigational.

The usual starting dose with limited prior opioid exposure is equivalent to 5 to 10 mg of intramuscular morphine every 4 hours. A table of equianalgesic doses (see Table 11–2) should be consulted in calculating the specific dose of the drug selected. If the drug is oral morphine, an intramuscular–oral dose ratio of 1:3 should be used. Thus, the starting dose of oral morphine in patients with severe pain and limited prior opioid exposure (such as treatment with an acetaminophen-codeine combination product at a dose of 10 to 12 tablets daily) is usually 15 to 30 mg every 4 hours or 45 to 90 mg of a controlled-release oral morphine preparation every 12 hours.

The starting dose of a new opioid in patients who are already receiving an opioid at higher doses is also calculated from the equianalgesic dose table (see Table 11–2). The total daily dose of the drug is converted to a dose of the new drug or the same drug using a new route that would be theoretically equianalgesic. The dosing regimen based on this calculated dose should be reduced at least 25 to 50 percent to account for inter-patient variability and incomplete cross-tolerance between drugs. A larger reduction, as much as 75 percent, is prudent if the new drug is methadone or if the patient does not have severe pain and is predisposed to opioid side effects, such as occur in the elderly and in those with major organ dysfunction.

Dose adjustment is almost always required. A favorable balance between analgesia and side effects is usually attained during the initial period of dose finding, and this level is typically maintained for a time. Additional dose adjustments are usually necessary as the disease progresses, painful therapeutic interventions are given, or effective primary treatments are administered.

Whenever analgesia is not satisfactory, the dose of the opioid should be increased until acceptable analgesia is produced or intolerable and unmanageable side effects supervene. Ceiling doses for the pure agonist opioids have not been identified. Doses can, therefore, become extremely high as upward titration proceeds. Doses above the equivalent of 35,000 mg of morphine per day have been reported rarely.[33] The absolute dose of the opioid is immaterial as long as the balance between analgesia and side effects remains acceptable.

Patients with continuous pain or frequently recurrent pain should be treated with a fixed schedule of doses ("around the clock"). "As needed" doses are usually provided concurrently to treat breakthrough pains, an approach known as "rescue" dosing. The rescue dose is usually a short–half-life drug offered "as needed" every 2 hours or more frequently at a dose equal to 5 to 15 percent of the total daily opioid requirement.

Adjunctive pharmacologic and nonpharmacologic therapies must be considered on an ongoing basis. Drug treatment for side effects such as nausea, constipation, and somnolence enhances comfort and may allow opioid dose escalation into an effective range.[27,128] Adjuvant analgesics (see Chapter 10) may reduce the opioid requirement and thereby decrease opioid side effects.

OPIOIDS IN THE MANAGEMENT OF CHRONIC NONMALIGNANT PAIN

Long-term opioid administration is usually considered to be inappropriate for chronic nonmalignant pain. In the past, the rationale for this position focused on many of the concerns discussed previously, including tolerance, physical dependence, addiction, the potential for adverse pharmacologic effects, and worsening disability. Beginning a decade ago, however, a critical reappraisal of this rationale began,[101,151] and this has evolved into an ongoing discussion among pain specialists and individuals in regulatory and law enforcement agencies.*

Two sets of observations have encouraged the reevaluation of traditional thinking about the role of opioid drugs. First, the favorable response to opioid therapy in the cancer population has contradicted many commonly held beliefs. Most patients with cancer who are chronically administered opioids attain a favorable balance between analgesia and side effects, which is sustained for prolonged periods (months or years in many cases) and is managed without aberrant drug-related behaviors suggesting addiction.

The second observation is that regulatory policies can negatively affect physician prescribing and lead to undertreatment. Although regulation of controlled drugs is not intended to impede legitimate prescribing for appropriate medical purposes,[28,31,65,67] physician perception of regulatory scrutiny discourages opioid use by inciting concern about the possibility of investigation. In a recent survey, for example, more than 50 percent of physicians admitted that concern about regulation at least occasionally leads to the use of a lower-schedule drug or prescrip-

---

*References 11, 20, 21, 60, 98, 114, 116, 119, 121, 124, 175, 176.

tion of a smaller number of pills or refills than would otherwise be indicated medically.[166] Analyses of the effects of multiple-copy prescription programs also suggests that regulatory scrutiny has a "chilling effect" on legitimate opioid prescribing.[3,31,115,131,142]

Published Experience

Reappraisal of opioid therapy for nonmalignant pain also has been propelled by anecdotal descriptions of successful cases (Table 11–8).* For example, a prospective survey[175] of 100 patients with diverse neuropathic or nociceptive pain syndromes revealed that individualized doses of dihydrocodeine, buprenorphine, or morphine provided greater than 50 percent analgesia to 51 patients and 25 to 50 percent analgesia to 28 patients at 1-month assessment. During this period, average scores on the Karnofsky Performance Status Scale increased from 65 to 79, with the largest increment noted among those with the greatest relief of pain. There were no incidents of serious toxicity or drug-related behaviors suggesting addiction or abuse.

In another survey,[81] 16 patients with intractable daily headache (14 with migraine and 2 with cluster headache) were administered methadone at a total daily dose of 35 to 100 mg for 6 to 36 months. Fifteen of the patients became virtually headache-free during the follow-up period. All patients experienced recurrence of headache when the dose of methadone was lowered and all regained excellent control after the dose was increased. No patient reported serious side effects, and there was no evidence of aberrant drug-related behavior.

In contrast to these favorable reports, some surveys implicate opioid therapy in the multiple problems presented by chronic pain patients referred to multidisciplinary pain management programs. These reports suggest that opioid-treated patients experience greater pain, more functional impairment, mental clouding or somnolence, a tendency to prevaricate about drug use, and, perhaps most important, a poor response to multimodality pain treatment.[19,50,51,90–93,129,155]

Given the potential biases inherent in survey data, including the likelihood of referral bias (clinicians tend to receive referrals that

"fit" their avowed interest) and observer bias, these survey data cannot provide definitive conclusions about the safety or efficacy of opioid therapy. Nonetheless, they offer relevant information about the divergent outcomes possible during opioid therapy. Some patients can evidently attain sustained partial analgesia during long-term administration of an opioid without treatment-limiting toxicity or aberrant drug-related behaviors. Others deteriorate as opioid treatment is administered.

Opioid Therapy for Nonmalignant Pain: Issues and Conclusions

Many of the complex issues discussed previously are among those that must be resolved to assess the safety and efficacy of opioid therapy for nonmalignant pain. These issues include opioid responsiveness, the potential for adverse pharmacologic outcomes and tolerance, and problems associated with physical dependence and addiction.[119]

The impact of opioid therapy on the physical and psychosocial functioning of patients with chronic nonmalignant pain has been a contentious issue for pain specialists.† Therapy for chronic pain is usually guided by the dual goals of comfort and function. Opioid therapy would not be useful if it augmented pain-related disability or undermined the efficacy of rehabilitation efforts, regardless of its effects on the pain.

As noted, the literature describes divergent outcomes of opioid therapy. Some patients who receive opioid drugs can capitalize on enhanced comfort by rapidly improving function. Others experience improved comfort and demonstrate no meaningful changes in other areas. Still others develop global disability.

These disparate observations suggest that the heterogeneous population with chronic pain may contain subgroups that respond differently to opioid therapy. Patients referred to pain clinics, for example, have higher levels of psychosocial distress and functional im-

---

*References 14, 55, 62, 81, 82, 110, 114, 121, 151–153, 157, 175.
†References 21, 50, 51, 55, 60, 93, 98, 114, 119, 121, 136,155.

Table 11–8. **REPRESENTATIVE PUBLISHED SURVEYS OF OPIOID THERAPY FOR THE TREATMENT OF CHRONIC NONMALIGNANT PAIN**

Author	No. Patients	Diagnosis	Opioids	Daily Dose Equivalent	Duration	Analgesic Efficacy	Adverse Effects	Comments
Taub[151]	313	Mixed	Mixed	Mean 10–20 mg (maximum 40 mg) oral methadone	Up to 6 yr	Few details; all said to benefit	No toxicity; abuse in 13	8 of 13 problem cases had prior drug abuse.
Tennant & Uelman[153]	22	Not stated	Not stated	Not stated	Not stated	Not stated	No abuse	All had failed pain clinics; 15 returned to work.
France et al[55]	16	Most, back pain	Mixed	Mean 8 mg (range 3–20) oral methadone	Mean 13 mo (range 6–22)	Pain relief >50% in all; >75% in 13; sustained in 12	No toxicity; no abuse	12 of 16 improved function; higher doses needed in 5 over time.
Portenoy & Foley[121]	38	Mixed; some neuropathic	Mixed	Median 10–20 mg (range <10–60) parenteral morphine	Median 3–4 yr; range 6 mo to 10 yr	Adequate 11; partial 13; inadequate 14	No toxicity; abuse in 2	Both problem cases had prior drug abuse; marked gains in function uncommon but few details.
Urban et al[157]	5	Phantom pain	Methadone	10–20 mg	Mean 22 mo (range 12–26)	At follow-up, all >50% relief	No toxicity; no abuse	Over time, relief waned in 1.
Portenoy[116]	20	Mixed; some neuropathic	Mixed	Median 10–20 mg (range <10–50) parenteral morphine	Median <2 yr; range 6 mo to 10 yr	Adequate 9; partial 10; inadequate 14	Personality change 1; myoclonus 1; abuse in 2	Marked gains in function uncommon but few details; with warning, both problem cases stopped abuse.

Continued on following page

Table 11–8.—*Continued*

Author	No. Patients	Diagnosis	Opioids	Daily Dose Equivalent	Duration	Analgesic Efficacy	Adverse Effects	Comments
Tennant et al[152]	52	Mixed	Mixed	Very variable; range 10–240 mg oral methadone	Duration of program not noted; opioid use averaged >12 yr	Adequate 88%; partial 12%	Constipation 20; edema 12; adrenal insufficiency 1; abuse in 9	Many medically ill, accounting for side effects; no dose increases needed.
Zenz et al[175]	100	Mixed	Morphine; buprenorphine; dihydrocodeine	Variable; morphine range 20–2000 mg	Mean 224 days Range 14–1472 days	Good 51%; partial 28%	Constipation most common; no abuse	Overall improvement in performance status, with significant relationship between analgesia and improvement.

Source: Portenoy RK: Opioid therapy for chronic nonmalignant pain: Current status. In Fields HL, and Liebeskind JC (eds): Progress in Pain Research and Management, Vol 1: Pharmacological Approaches to the Treatment of Chronic Pain: New Concepts and Critical Issues. IASP Press, Seatle, 1994, pp 252–253, with permission.

pairment than patients with chronic pain surveyed in the community,[24,34–36,38,109] and it may be that the characteristics that lead to a pain clinic referral predispose these patients to problems with opioid therapy. Recognition of this variability is necessary to avoid the inappropriate generalization of anecdotal observations.

Although conclusions about the role of long-term opioid therapy for chronic nonmalignant pain will remain tentative until appropriate controlled clinical trials are performed, analysis of these issues supports a balanced perspective. In some cases, opioid therapy becomes part of the problem, contributing to disability or creating independent concerns, such as addiction. In other cases, opioids provide the types of benefits routinely observed in the cancer population. If this perspective is accepted, the clinical stance must shift from the overall acceptability of therapy to patient selection and guidelines for drug administration.

Guidelines for opioid therapy in chronic nonmalignant pain can be developed from clinical experience (Table 11–9). These guidelines highlight several important issues. First, they emphasize the feasibility of a therapeutic opioid trial. If addiction does not occur merely as a result of exposure to an opioid and the likelihood of serious toxicity is low with appropriate dosing, then a treatment trial may be initiated and either continued or discontinued depending on the outcome. Each treatment trial should incorporate dose adjustment and careful monitoring of clinically relevant endpoints, including pain relief, side effects, functional status (including willingness to engage in other components of therapy), and development of aberrant drug-related behaviors.

Second, patients should be informed about the controversial nature of this approach. Some experienced clinicians have adopted formal written consent as standard practice and others opt for a consent discussion that addresses the same issues and is documented in the medical record.

Third, the decision to implement opioid therapy requires knowledge of the pharmacologic techniques described in the cancer pain literature (discussed previously). Although some clinicians recommend specific treatment guidelines for patients with non-malignant pain, none has empirical support. For example, some clinicians believe that only long-acting opioids, such as controlled-release oral morphine or methadone, should be used in patients with nonmalignant pain to reduce dosing frequency and the potential for "rebound" phenomena. This appears reasonable on the surface, but there are no supporting data, and rigid adherence to any recommendation of this type is not justified.

Fourth, a fair therapeutic trial requires individualization of the opioid dose, which should optimize the balance between analgesia and side effects. As observed previously, the absolute dose required to do this is immaterial in the cancer population. In nonmalignant pain populations, however, there are concerns related to the controversial nature of the therapy and the possibility that an intense focus on the dose titration could foster an unrealistic view of the treatment and divert attention from rehabilitative pursuits. If the clinician becomes uncomfortable with the size of the dose, this should be addressed openly with the patient. Consultation with a specialist in pain management may be useful in deciding whether to continue a trial in such cases.

Fifth, the guidelines highlight the need to consider concurrent treatments and continue a therapeutic focus on functional restoration. Opioid therapy is not a substitute for a comprehensive pain management approach that incorporates psychologic and rehabilitative therapies. For well-selected patients who are highly disabled, opioid therapy could be a useful complement to primary rehabilitative therapies.[55]

Finally, the guidelines emphasize the requirement for an appropriate response to aberrant drug-related behaviors, should they occur during therapy. As discussed previously, the assessment of aberrant behavior in patients receiving an opioid for pain is complex and must distinguish an addiction disorder from other phenomena. In some cases, consultation with a specialist in addiction medicine is useful to clarify the nature of the drug-related behavior. If the diagnosis of addiction is tenable, the therapeutic approach must focus on both this problem and the pain.[124] If the assessment suggests less serious pathology, a highly structured response is still

Table 11–9. **PROPOSED GUIDELINES FOR THE MANAGEMENT OF OPIOID THERAPY FOR CHRONIC NONMALIGNANT PAIN**

1. Should be considered only after all other reasonable analgesic therapies have failed.
2. A history of substance abuse, severe character pathology, or chaotic home environment should be viewed as relative contraindications.
3. A single practitioner should take primary responsibility for treatment.
4. Patients should give informed consent before the start of therapy; points to be covered include:
   (a) Recognition of the low risk of true addiction as an outcome
   (b) Potential for cognitive impairment from the drug alone or from the combination of the drug with other centrally acting drugs
   (c) Potential for other side effects
   (d) Likelihood that physical dependence will occur (abstinence syndrome possible with acute discontinuation)
   (e) Need for responsible drug-taking behavior (e.g., no unsanctioned dose escalation, no prescriptions from other physicians, and so on)
5. The use of a written contract to inform patient of his or her responsibilities should be considered but is not mandatory.
6. Except in rare circumstances, therapy should be administered by the oral route.
7. The use of a long-acting opioid (e.g., controlled-release morphine or methadone) may be preferable because of ease of administration, but it is not mandatory.
8. Dosing on a fixed-schedule basis ("around the clock") is preferable if the patient experiences continuous or frequently recurring pain.
9. In addition to the daily dose determined initially, most patients should be permitted to escalate dose transiently on days of increased pain; two methods are acceptable:
   (a) Prescription of an additional 4–6 "rescue doses" to be taken as needed during the month
   (b) Instruction that one or two extra doses may be taken on any day but must be followed by an equal reduction of dose on subsequent days
10. Initially, patients must be seen and drugs prescribed at least monthly; when stable, less frequent visits may be acceptable.
11. Several weeks should be agreed upon as the period of initial dose titration; although improvement in function should be continually stressed, at least partial analgesia should be viewed as the primary goal of therapy.
12. Failure to achieve at least partial analgesia at relatively low initial doses in the patient with limited prior opioid consumption should raise questions about the potential treatability of the pain syndrome with opioids and lead to reassessment.
13. Emphasis should be given to attempts to capitalize on improved analgesia by gains in physical and psychosocial function; opioid therapy should be considered complementary to other analgesic and rehabilitative approaches.
14. Exacerbations of pain not effectively treated by transient and small increases in dose are best managed in the hospital, where dose escalation, if appropriate, can be observed closely and return to baseline doses can be accomplished in a controlled environment.
15. Evidence of drug hoarding, acquisition of drugs from other physicians, uncontrolled dose escalation, or other aberrant behaviors must be carefully assessed. In some cases, tapering and discontinuation of opioid therapy will be necessary. Other patients may appropriately continue therapy with rigid guidelines. Consideration should be given to consultation with an addiction medicine specialist.
16. At each visit, assessment should specifically address:
    (a) Comfort (degree of analgesia)
    (b) Opioid-related side effects
    (c) Functional status (physical and psychosocial)
    (d) Existence of aberrant drug-related behaviors

Continued on following page

Table 11–9.—*Continued*

17. Use of self-report instruments may be helpful in documenting pain relief and functional status but are not mandatory.
18. Documentation is essential; the medical record should specifically address comfort, function, side effects, and the occurrence of aberrant behaviors repeatedly during the course of therapy.

Source: Portenoy RK: Opioid therapy for chronic nonmalignant pain: Current status. In Fields HL, and Liebeskind JC (eds): Progress in Pain Research and Management, Vol 1: Pharmacological Approaches to the Treatment of Chronic Pain: New Concepts and Critical Issues. IASP Press, Seattle, 1994, pp 274–275, with permission.

required to regain control over the therapy. In some cases, the opioid should be discontinued; in others, the response may include new, explicit instructions for dosing (perhaps a written contract), more frequent visits, small prescriptions, and, in some circumstances, occasional urine drug screens. The clinician must be able to address these issues openly with the patient, provide an informed assessment over time, arrive at an appropriate diagnosis, and institute whatever controls are necessary to reestablish appropriate drug use.

SUMMARY

Advances in the clinical use of opioid drugs have paralleled a rapidly growing understanding of opioid mechanisms. Opioid drugs produce analgesia by interacting with subtypes of the mu, kappa, and delta receptors, which are located in the spinal cord and brain, and on primary afferent nerves and immune cells outside the nervous system. In the central nervous system, opioids act both presynaptically and postsynaptically to reduce nociceptive input or transmission. The mechanisms involved may be influenced by numerous physiologic and pathologic processes, which presumably underlie the variability in opioid responsiveness observed in the clinic.

The clinical pharmacology of the opioids is complex. *Potency,* which refers to the dose required to produce a specified effect, is not as relevant as efficacy. The term *efficacy* has multiple meanings, however, and it is clearer to use the term *opioid responsiveness* in the clinical setting. Opioid responsiveness, which is the likelihood of a favorable balance between analgesia and side effects during gradual dose escalation, varies with many characteristics of the patient and pain syndrome, and with the

specific drug tested. There are no clinical characteristics that impart uniform opioid resistance, and sequential opioid trials may be useful for optimizing treatment.

Opioids do not produce major organ toxicity, but the possibility of persistent side effects must always be considered, notwithstanding the development of tolerance to these effects. Analgesic tolerance, which could undermine long-term therapy, can be implicated only if there are no other clinically apparent causes for progressive pain. This occurs rarely. Most patients with stable pain do not require opioid dose escalation, and concerns about the development of analgesic tolerance should not influence the decision to administer an opioid.

Concerns about physical dependence and addiction are profound but complicated by a difficult nomenclature. *Physical dependence* is defined solely by an abstinence syndrome following abrupt dose reduction or administration of an opioid antagonist. Patients who are presumed to be physically dependent should never be described as addicted. *Addiction* is a psychologic and behavioral syndrome characterized by loss of control over drug use, compulsive use, and continued drug use despite harm. Although definitive studies are lacking, the risk of addiction during opioid administration in a population with no prior history of substance abuse appears to be very low. Clinicians who prescribe opioids must develop expertise in the assessment and management of the drug-related behaviors that provide the basis for the diagnosis of addiction.

Opioid therapy is the mainstay approach for the management of cancer pain. Simple methods of drug selection and administration have been codified in the World Health Organization's influential "analgesic ladder" approach. This approach emphasizes the use of oral opioid therapy, which is administered on a fixed schedule at an individualized dosage. Surveys suggest that this approach can be successful in as many as 90 percent of patients with cancer.

The use of opioid therapy for chronic nonmalignant pain continues to be controversial but is no longer uniformly rejected by pain specialists. The population with chronic pain is extremely heterogeneous, and the available survey data suggest that some patients benefit and others deteriorate during opioid treatment. A trial of this approach can be considered in carefully selected patients using clinically derived guidelines that stress a structured approach and ongoing monitoring of efficacy, adverse effects, functional outcomes, and the occurrence of aberrant drug-related behaviors.

REFERENCES

1. Acute Pain Management Guideline Panel: Acute Pain Management. Clinical Practice Guideline. AHCPR Pub No 92-0032. Agency for Health Care Policy and Research, Public Health Service, US Department of Health and Human Services, Rockville, MD, February 1992.
2. American Psychiatric Association, Diagnostic and Statistical Manual of Mental Disorders, ed 4. American Psychiatric Association, Washington, DC, 1994.
3. Angarola RT, and Wray SD: Legal impediments to cancer pain treatment. In Hill CS, and Fields WS (eds): Advances in Pain Research and Therapy, Vol 11. Drug Treatment of Cancer Pain in a Drug-Oriented Society. Raven Press, New York, 1989, pp 213–231.
4. Appel PW, and Gordon NB: Digit-symbol performance in methadone-treated ex-heroin addicts. Am J Psychiatry 133:1337–1340, 1976.
5. Arner S, Rawal N, and Gustafson LL: Clinical experience of long-term treatment with epidural and intrathecal opioids: A nationwide survey. Acta Anaesthsiol Scand 32:253–259, 1988.
6. Arora PK, Fride E, Petitto J, et al: Morphine-induced immune alterations in vivo. Cell Immunol 126:343–353, 1990.
7. Babst DV, Newman S, Gordon NB, et al: Driving records of methadone maintained patients in New York State. New York State Narcotic Control Commission, 1973.
8. Banning A, and Sjogren P: Cerebral effects of long-term oral opioids in cancer patients measured by continuous reaction time. Clin J Pain 6:91–95, 1990.
9. Besson J-M, and Chaouch A: Peripheral and spinal mechanisms of nociception. Physiol Rev 67:67–186, 1987.
10. Bonica JJ: Treatment of cancer pain: Current status

and future needs. In Fields HL, Dubner R, and Cervero F (eds): Advances in Pain Research and Therapy, Vol 9, Raven Press, New York 1985, pp 589–616.
11. Brena SF, and Sanders SH: Opioids in nonmalignant pain: Questions in search of answers. Clin J Pain 7:342–345, 1991.
12. Brescia FJ, Portenoy RK, Ryan M, et al: Pain, opioid use and survival in hospitalized patients with advanced cancer. J Clin Oncol 10:149–155, 1992.
13. Brodner RA, and Taub A: Chronic pain exacerbated by long-term narcotic use in patients with nonmalignant disease: Clinical syndrome and treatment. Mt Sinai J Med 45:233–237, 1978.
14. Brookoff D, and Palomano R: Treating sickle cell pain like cancer pain. Ann Intern Med 116:364–368, 1992.
15. Bruera E: Subcutaneous administration of opioids in the management of cancer pain. In Foley KM, Bonica JJ, and Ventafridda V (eds): Advances in Pain Research and Therapy, Vol 16. Second International Congress on Cancer Pain. Raven Press, New York, 1990, pp 203–218.
16. Bruera E, Macmillan K, Hanson J, et al: The cognitive effects of the administration of narcotic analgesics in patients with cancer pain. Pain 39:13–16, 1989.
17. Bruera E, Macmillan K, Hanson J, et al: The Edmonton staging system for cancer pain: Preliminary report. Pain 37:203–210, 1989.
18. Buckley FP, Sizemore WA, and Charlton JE: Medication management in patients with chronic nonmalignant pain. A review of the use of a drug withdrawal protocol. Pain 26:153–166, 1986.
19. Bruera E, and Miller MJ: Non-cardiogenic pulmonary edema after narcotic treatment for cancer pain. Pain 39:297–300, 1989.
20. Chabal C, Jacobson L, Chaney EF, et al: Narcotics for chronic pain: Yes or no? A useless dichotomy. APS Journal 1:276–281, 1992.
21. Chabal C, Jacobson L, Chaney EF, et al: The psychosocial impact of opioid treatment. APS Journal 1:289–291, 1992.
22. Chapman V, and Dickenson AH: The combination of NMDA antagonism and morphine produces profound antinociception in the rat dorsal horn. Brain Res 573:321–323, 1992.
23. Chapman CR, and Hill HF: Prolonged morphine self-administration and addiction liability: Evaluation of two theories in a bone marrow transplant unit. Cancer 63:1636–1644, 1989.
24. Chapman CR, Sola AE, and Bonica JJ: Illness behavior and depression in pain center and private practice patients. Pain 6:1–7, 1979.
25. Chen Y, Mestek A, Liu J, et al: Molecular cloning and functional expression of a mu-opioid receptor from rat brain. Mol Pharmacol 44:8–12, 1993.
26. Cherny NI, and Portenoy RK: Cancer pain: Principles of assessment and syndromes. In Wall PD, and Melzack R (eds): Textbook of Pain, ed 3. Churchill Livingstone, Edinburgh, 1994, pp 787–824.
27. Cherny NI, and Portenoy RK: Practical management of cancer pain. In Wall PD, and Melzack R (eds): Textbook of Pain, ed 3. Churchill Livingstone, Edinburgh, 1994, pp 1437–1467.

28. Clark HW, and Sees KL: Opioids, chronic pain and the law. Journal of Pain and Symptom Management 8:297–305, 1993.

29. Cleeland CS, Gonin R, Hatfield AK, et al: Pain and its treatment in outpatients with metastatic cancer. N Engl J Med 330:592–597, 1994.

30. Cochin J, and Kornetsky C: Development and loss of tolerance to morphine in the rat after single and multiple injections. J Pharmacol Exp Ther 145:1–20, 1964.

31. Cooper JR, Czechowicz CJ, Petersen RC, et al: Prescription drug diversion control and medical practice. JAMA 268;1306–1310, 1992.

32. Cousins MJ, and Mather LE: Intrathecal and epidural administration of opioids. Anesthesiology 61:276–310, 1984.

33. Coyle N, Adelhardt J, Foley KM, et al: Character of terminal illness in the advanced cancer patient: Pain and other symptoms in the last 4 weeks of life. Journal of Pain and Symptom Management 5:83–93, 1990.

34. Crook J, and Tunks E: Defining the 'chronic pain syndrome': An epidemiological method. In Fields HL, Dubner R, and Cervero R (eds): Advances in Pain Research and Therapy, Vol 9: Proceedings of the Fourth World Congress on Pain. Raven Press, New York, 1985, pp 871–878.

35. Crook J, Tunks E, Rideout E, et al: Epidemiologic comparison of persistent pain sufferers in a specialty pain clinic and in the community. Arch Phys Med Rehabil 67:451–455, 1986.

36. Crooks J, Weir R, and Tunks E: An epidemiological follow-up survey of persistent pain sufferers in a group family practice and specialty pain clinic. Pain 36:49–61, 1989.

37. Dalsgaard J, Flesby S, Juelsgaard P, et al: Low-dose intra-articular morphine analgesia in day-case knee arthroscopy: A randomized, double-blinded, prospective study. Pain 56:151–154, 1994.

38. Deyo RA, Bass JE, Schoenfeld NE, et al: Prognostic variability among chronic pain patients: Implications for study design, interpretation, and reporting. Arch Phys Med Rehabil 69:174–178, 1988.

39. Diamond S, Freitag FG, Diamond ML, et al: Transnasal butorphanol in the treatment of migraine headache pain. Headache Quarterly 3:164–171, 1992.

40. Dickenson AH: A cure for wind-up: NMDA receptor antagonists as potential analgesics. Trends Pharmacol Sci 11:307–309, 1990.

41. Dickenson AH: Where and how do opioids act? In Gebhart FG, Hammond DL, and Jensen TS (eds): Progress in Pain Research and Management, Vol 2. Proceedings of the 7th World Congress on Pain. IASP Press, Seattle, 1994, pp 525–552.

42. Dole VP: Narcotic addiction, physical dependence and relapse. N Engl J Med 286:988–992, 1972.

43. Donohoe RM, and Falek A: Neuroimmunomodulation by opiates and other drugs of abuse: Relationship to HIV infection and AIDS. Adv Biochem Psychopharmacol 44:145–158, 1988.

44. Donohoe RM, Madden JJ, Hollingsworth F, et al: Morphine depression of T cell E-rosetting: Definition of the process. Federal Proceedings 44:95–99, 1985.

45. Dubner R, and Ruda MA: Activity dependent neuronal plasticity following tissue injury and inflammation. Trends Neurosci 15:96–103, 1992.

46. Duggan AW, and North RA: Electrophysiology of opioids. Pharmacol Rev 35:219–281, 1984.

47. Einstein TK, Meissler JJ, Geller EB, et al: Immunosuppression to tetanus toxoid induced by implanted morphine pellets. Ann NY Acad Sci 594:377–379, 1990.

48. Evans CJ, Keith DE, Morrisson H, et al: Cloning of a delta receptor by functional expression. Science 258:1952–1955, 1992.

49. Fainsinger R, Schoeller T, and Bruera E: Methadone in the management of cancer pain: A review. Pain 52:137–147, 1993.

50. Finlayson RD, Maruta T, and Morse BR: Substance dependence and chronic pain: Profile of 50 patients treated in an alcohol and drug dependence unit. Pain 26:167–174, 1986.

51. Finlayson RD, Maruta T, Morse BR, et al: Substance dependence and chronic pain: Experience with treatment and follow-up results. Pain 26:175–180, 1986.

52. Fishbain DA, Rosomoff HL, and Rosomoff RS: Drug abuse, dependence, and addiction in chronic pain patients. Clin J Pain 8:77–85, 1992.

53. Foley KM: Opioid analgesics in clinical pain management. In Herz A, Akil H, and Simon EJ (eds): Handbook of Experimental Pharmacology. Springer-Verlag, New York, 1993, pp 697–762.

54. Foley KM: Changing concepts of tolerance to opioids: What the cancer patient has taught us. In Chapman CR, and Foley KM (eds): Current and Emerging Issues in Cancer Pain: Research and Practice. Raven Press, New York, 1993, pp 331–350.

55. France RD, Urban BJ, and Keefe FJ: Long-term use of narcotic analgesics in chronic pain. Soc Sci Med 19:1379–1382, 1984.

56. Galer BS, Coyle N, Pasternak GW, et al: Individual variability in the response to different opioids: Report of five cases. Pain 49:87–91, 1992.

57. Gong QL, Hedner J, Bjorkman R, et al: Morphine-3-glucuronide may functionally antagonize morphine-6-glucuronide induced antinociception and ventilatory depression in the rat. Pain 48:249–255, 1992.

58. Gonzales GR, Elliot KJ, Portenoy RK, et al: The impact of a comprehensive evaluation in the management of cancer pain. Pain 47:141–144, 1991.

59. Gordon NB: Influence of narcotic drugs on highway safety. Accid Anal Prev 8:3–7, 1976.

60. Gourlay GK, and Cherry DA: Can opioids be successfully used to treat severe pain in nonmalignant conditions? Clin J Pain 7:347–349, 1991.

61. Gourlay GK, Kowalski SR, Plummer JL, et al: The efficacy of transdermal fentanyl in the treatment of postoperative pain: A double-blind comparison of fentanyl and placebo systems. Pain 40:21–27, 1990.

62. Green J, and Coyle M: Methadone use in the control of nonmalignant chronic pain. Pain Management Sept/Oct:241–246, 1989.

63. Grove WM, Eckert ED, Heston L, et al: Heritability of substance abuse and antisocial behavior: A study of monozygotic twins reared apart. Biol Psychiatry 27:1293–1304, 1990.

64. Haertzen CA, and Hooks NT: Changes in personality and subjective experience associated with the

chronic administration and withdrawal of opiates. J Nerv Ment Dis 148:606–614, 1969.

65. Haislip GR: Impact of drug abuse on legitimate drug use. In Hill CS and Fields WS (eds): Advances in Pain Research and Therapy, Vol 11: Drug Treatment of Cancer Pain in a Drug-Oriented Society. Raven Press, New York, 1989, pp 205–211.

66. Hendler N, Cimini C, Ma T, et al: A comparison of cognitive impairment due to benzodiazepines and to narcotics. Am J Psychiatry 137:828–830, 1980.

67. Hill CS: Influence of regulatory agencies on the treatment of pain and standards of medical practice for the use of narcotics. Pain Digest 1:7–12, 1991.

68. Hill HE, Haertzen CA, and Davis H: An MMPI factor analytic study of alcoholics, narcotic addicts and criminals. Quarterly Journal of Studies on Alcohol 23:411–431, 1962.

69. Hill HE, Haertzen CA, and Glaser R: Personality characteristics of narcotic addicts as indicated by the MMPI. J Gen Psychol 62:127–139, 1960.

70. Hill HF, Chapman CR, Kornell JA, et al: Self-administration of morphine in bone marrow transplant patients reduces drug requirement. Pain 40: 121–129, 1990.

71. Hoskin PJ, and Hanks GW: Opioid agonist-antagonist drugs in acute and chronic pain states. Drugs 41:326–344, 1991.

72. Houde RW: Analgesic effectiveness of narcotic agonist-antagonists. Br J Clin Pharmacol 7:297–308, 1979.

73. Houde RW, and Nathan B. Eddy Memorial Lecture: The analgesic connection. In Harris LS (ed): NIDA Research Monograph: Problems of Drug Dependence 55. Natl Inst Drug Abuse, Rockville, MD, 1985, pp 4–13.

74. Houde RW, Wallenstein SL, and Beaver WT: Evaluation of analgesics in patients with cancer pain. In Lasagna L (ed): International Encyclopedia of Pharmacology and Therapeutics, Section 6, Vol 1. Clinical Pharmacology. Pergamon Press, Oxford, 1966, pp 59–98.

75. Jacox A, Carr DB, Payne R, et al: Management of Cancer Pain. Clinical Practice Guideline No. 9. AHCPR Publication No. 94-0592. Agency for Health Care Policy and Research, US Department of Health and Human Services, Public Health Service, Rockville, MD, March 1994.

76. Jadad AR, Carroll D, Glynn CJ, et al: Morphine responsiveness of chronic pain: Double-blind randomised crossover study with patient-controlled analgesia. Lancet 339:1367–1371, 1992.

77. Jaffe JH: Drug addiction and drug abuse. In Gilman AG, Goodman LS, Rall TW, and Murad F (eds): The Pharmacological Basis of Therapeutics, ed 7, Macmillan, New York, 1985, pp 532–581.

78. Joshi GP, McCarroll SM, O'Brien TM, et al: Intraarticular analgesia following knee arthroscopy. Anesth Analg 76:33–336, 1993.

79. Kaiko RF, Foley KM, Grabinski PY, et al: Central nervous system excitatory effects of meperidine in cancer patients. Ann Neurol 13:180–185, 1983.

80. Kanner RM, and Foley KM: Patterns of narcotic drug use in a cancer pain clinic. Ann NY Acad Sci 362:161–172, 1981.

81. Kell MJ, and Musselman DL: Methadone prophylaxis of intractable headaches: Pain control and serum opioid levels. American Journal of Pain Management 3:7–14, 1993.

82. Krames ES, and Lanning RM: Intrathecal infusional analgesia for nonmalignant pain: Analgesic efficacy of intrathecal opioid with or without bupivacaine. Journal of Pain and Symptom Management 8:539–548, 1993.

83. Kreek MJ: Medical safety and side effects of methadone in tolerant individuals. JAMA 223:665–668, 1973.

84. Kreek MJ: Medical complications in methadone patients. Ann NY Acad Sci 311:110–134, 1978.

85. Kreek MJ, Dodes S, Kne S, et al: Long-term methadone maintenance therapy: Effects on liver function. Ann Intern Med 77:598–602, 1972.

86. Lombardo WK, Lombardo B, and Goldstein A. Cognitive functioning under moderate and low dose methadone maintenance. Int J Addict 11:389–401, 1976.

87. Mao J, Price DD, Hayes RL, et al: Intrathecal treatment with dextrophan or ketamine potently reduces pain-related behaviours in a rat model of peripheral mononeuropathy. Brain Res 605:164–168, 1993.

88. Martin WR, Eades CG, Thompson JA, et al: The effects of morphine- and nalorphine-like drugs in non-dependent and morphine-dependent chronic spinal dogs. J Pharmacol Exp Ther 197:517–532, 1976.

89. Martin WR, and Jasinski DR: Physiological parameters of morphine dependence in man-tolerance, early abstinence, protracted abstinence. Journal of Psychiatric Research 7:9–17, 1969.

90. Maruta T: Prescription drug-induced organic brain syndrome. Am J Psychiatry 135:376–377, 1978.

91. Maruta T, and Swanson DW: Problems with the use of oxycodone compound in patients with chronic pain. Pain 11:389–396, 1981.

92. Maruta T, Swanson DW, and Finlayson RE: Drug abuse and dependency in patients with chronic pain. Mayo Clin Proc 54:241–244, 1979.

93. McNairy SL, Maruta T, Ivnik RJ, et al: Prescription medication dependence and neuropsychologic function, Pain 18:169–177, 1984.

94. McQuay HJ, Bullingham RES, and Moore RA: Acute opiate tolerance in man. Life Sci 28:2513–2517, 1981.

95. McQuay HJ, Jadad AR, Carroll D, et al: Opioid sensitivity of chronic pain: A patient-controlled analgesia method. Anaesthesia 47:757–767, 1992.

96. Medina JL, and Diamond S: Drug dependency in patients with chronic headache. Headache 17:12–14, 1977.

97. Mercadante S, Maddaloni S, Roccella S, et al: Predictive factors in advanced cancer pain treated only by analgesics. Pain 50:151–155, 1992.

98. Merry AF, Schug SA, Richards EG, et al: Opioids in chronic pain of nonmalignant origin: State of the debate in New Zealand. European Journal of Pain 13:39–43, 1992.

99. Molitor TW, Morilla A, Risdahl JM, et al: Chronic morphine administration impairs cell-mediated immune responses in swine. J Pharmacol Exp Ther 260:581–586, 1992.

100. Moulin DE, and Foley KM: A review of a hospital-based pain service. In Foley KM, Bonica JJ, and Ventafridda V (eds): Advances in Pain Research and Therapy, Vol 16. Second International Congress on Cancer Pain. Raven Press, New York, 1990, pp 413–428.
101. Newman RG: The need to redefine addiction. N Engl J Med 18:1096–1098, 1983.
102. O'Neill WM: The cognitive and psychomotor effects of opioid drugs in cancer pain management. In Hanks GW (ed): Cancer Surveys, Vol 21. Palliative Medicine: Problem Areas in Pain and Symptom Management. Cold Spring Harbor Laboratory Press, Plainview, NY, 1994, pp 67–84.
103. Ochshorn M, Novick DM, and Kreek MJ: In vitro studies of the effect of methadone on natural killer cell activity. Isr J Med Sci 26:421–425, 1990.
104. Onofrio BM, and Yaksh TL: Long-term pain relief produced by intrathecal morphine infusion in 53 patients. J Neurosurg 72:200–209, 1990.
105. Osborne RJ, Joel SP, and Slevin ML: Morphine intoxication in renal failure: The role of morphine-6-glucuronide. British Medical Journal 292:1548–1549, 1986.
106. Perry S, and Heidrich G: Management of pain during debridement: A survey of U.S. burn units. Pain 13:267–280, 1982.
107. Pert CB, and Snyder SH: Opiate receptor: Demonstration in nervous tissue. Science 179:1011–1014, 1973.
108. Peterson PK, Sharp B, Gekker G, et al: Opioid-mediated suppression of interferon-δ production by cultured peripheral blood mononuclear cells. J Clin Invest 80:824–831, 1987.
109. Pilowsky I, Chapman CR, and Bonica JJ: Pain, depression, and illness behavior in a pain clinic population. Pain 4:183–192, 1977.
110. Plummer JL, Cherry DA, Cousins MJ, et al: Long-term spinal administration of morphine in cancer and non-cancer pain: A retrospective study. Pain 44:215–220, 1991.
111. Plummer JL, Gourlay GK, Cherry DA, et al: Estimation of methadone clearance: Application in the management of cancer pain. Pain 33:313–322, 1988.
112. Porreca F, Mosberg HI, Hurst R, et al: Roles of mu, delta, and kappa opioid receptors in spinal and supraspinal mediation of gastrointestinal transit effects and hot plate analgesia in the mouse. J Pharmacol Exp Ther 230:341–348, 1984.
113. Portenoy RK: Cancer pain: Epidemiology and syndromes. Cancer 63:2298–2307, 1989.
114. Portenoy RK: Opioid therapy in nonmalignant pain. Journal of Pain and Symptom Management 5:S46–S62, 1990.
115. Portenoy RK: The effect of drug regulation on the management of cancer pain. NYS J Med Suppl 91:13S–18S, 1991.
116. Portenoy RK: Chronic opioid therapy for nonmalignant pain: From models to practice. APS Journal 1:285–288, 1992.
117. Portenoy RK: Inadequate outcome of cancer pain treatment: Influences on patient and clinician behavior. In Patt RB (ed): Problems in Cancer Pain Management: A Comprehensive Approach. JB Lippincott, Philadelphia, 1992, pp 119–128.
118. Portenoy RK: Management of common opioid side effects during long-term therapy of cancer pain. Ann Acad Med Singapore 23:160–170, 1994.
119. Portenoy RK: Opioid therapy for chronic nonmalignant pain: Current status. In Fields HL, and Liebeskind JC (eds): Progress in Pain Research and Management, Vol 1: Pharmacological Approaches to the Treatment of Chronic Pain: New Concepts and Critical Issues. IASP Press, Seattle, 1994, 247–288.
120. Portenoy RK: Opioid tolerance and responsiveness: Research findings and clinical observations. In Gebhart GF, Hammond DL, and Jensen TS (eds): Progress in Pain Research and Management, Vol 2: Proceedings of the 7th World Congress on Pain. IASP Press, Seattle, 1994, pp 95–619.
121. Portenoy RK, and Foley KM: Chronic use of opioid analgesics in non-malignant pain: Report of 38 cases. Pain 25:171–186, 1986.
122. Portenoy RK, Foley KM, and Inturrisi CE: The nature of opioid responsiveness and its implications for neuropathic pain: New hypotheses derived from studies of opioid infusions. Pain 43:273–286, 1990.
123. Portenoy RK, Maldonado M, Fitzmartin R, et al: Controlled-release morphine sulfate: Analgesic efficacy and side-effects of a 100 mg tablet in cancer pain patients. Cancer 63:2284–2287, 1989.
124. Portenoy RK, and Payne R: Acute and chronic pain. In Lowinson JH, Ruiz P, and Millman RB (eds): Substance Abuse: A Comprehensive Textbook. Williams & Wilkins, Baltimore, 1992, pp 691–721.
125. Portenoy RK, Southam M, Gupta SK, et al: Transdermal fentanyl for cancer pain: Repeated dose pharmacokinetics. Anesthesiology 28:36–43, 1993.
126. Portenoy RK, Thaler HT, Inturrisi CE, et al: The metabolite, morphine-6-glucuronide, contributes to the analgesia produced by morphine infusion in pain patients with normal renal function. Clin Pharmacol Ther 51:422–431, 1992.
127. Porter J, and Jick H: Addiction rare in patients treated with narcotics. N Engl J Med 302:123, 1980.
128. Rayport M: Experience in the management of patients medically addicted to narcotics. JAMA 156:684–691, 1954.
129. Ready LB, Sarkis E, and Turner JA: Self-reported vs. actual use of medications in chronic pain patients. Pain 12:285–294, 1982.
130. Regier D, Meyers JK, Kramer M, et al: The NIMH epidemiologic catchment area program. Arch Gen Psychiatry 41:934–958, 1984.
131. Reidenberg MM: Effect of the requirement for triplicate prescriptions for benzodiazepines in New York State. Clin Pharmacol Ther 50:129–131, 1991.
132. Rinaldi RC, Steindler EM, Wilford BB, et al: Clarification and standardization of substance abuse terminology. JAMA 259:555–557, 1988.
133. Robins LN, Davis DH, and Nurco DN: How permanent was Vietnam drug addiction. Am J Public Health 64:38–43, 1974.
134. Rounsaville BH, Novelly RA, Kleber HD, et al: Neuropsychological impairment in opiate addicts: Risk factors. NY Acad Sci 362:79–90, 1981.
135. Saper JR: Daily chronic headache. Neurol Clin 8:891–902, 1990.

136. Schofferman J: Long-term use of opioid analgesics for the treatment of chronic pain of nonmalignant origin. Journal of Pain and Symptom Management 8:279–288, 1993.

137. Schug SA, Zech D, and Dorr U: Cancer pain management according to WHO analgesic guidelines. Journal of Pain and Symptom Management 5:27–32, 1990.

138. Schug SA, Zech D, Grond S, et al: A long-term survey of morphine in cancer pain patients. Journal of Pain and Symptom Management 7:259–266, 1992.

139. Sees KL, and Clark HW: Opioid use in the treatment of chronic pain: Assessment of addiction. Journal of Pain and Symptom Management 8:257–264, 1993.

140. Shavit Y, Martin FC, Yirmiya R, et al: Effects of a single administration of morphine or footshock on natural killer cell cytotoxicity. Brain Behav Imun 1:318–328, 1987.

141. Shavit Y, Lewis JW, Terman WG, et al: Opioid peptides mediate the suppressive effect of stress on natural killer cell cytotoxicity. Science 223:188–190, 1984.

142. Sigler KA, Guernsey BG, Ingim MB, et al: Effects on a triplicate prescription law on prescribing of Schedule II drugs. Am J Hosp Pharm 41:108–111, 1984.

143. Simon EJ, Hiller JM, and Edelman I: Stereospecific binding of the potent narcotic analgesic (^{3}H)etorphine to rat brain homogenates. Proc Natl Acad Sci USA 70:1947–1949, 1973.

144. Simpson DD, Savage LJ, and Lloyd MRP: Follow-up evaluation of treatment of drug abuse during 1969 to 1972. Arch Gen Psychiatry 36:772–780, 1979.

145. Sjogren P, and Banning A: Pain, sedation and reaction time during long-term treatment of cancer patients with oral and epidural opioids. Pain 39:5–12, 1989.

146. Stein C: Interaction of immune-competent cells and nociceptors. In Gebhart GF, Hammond DL, and Jensen TS (eds): Progress in Pain Research and Management, Vol 2. Proceedings of the 7th World Congress on Pain. IASP Press, Seattle, 1994, pp 285–297.

147. Stein C, Hassan AHS, Lehrberger K, et al: Local analgesic effect of endogenous opioid peptides. Lancet 342:321–324, 1993.

148. Swanson G, Smith J, Bulich R, et al. Patient-controlled analgesia for chronic cancer pain in the ambulatory setting: A report of 117 patients. J Clin Oncol 7:1903–1906, 1989.

149. Takeda F: Results of field testing in Japan of the WHO draft interim guidelines on relief of cancer pain. Pain Clinic 1:83–89, 1986.

150. Tal M, and Bennett GJ: Dextrophan relieves neuropathic heat-evoked hyperalgesia in the rat. Neurosci Lett 151:107–110, 1993.

151. Taub A: Opioid analgesics in the treatment of chronic intractable pain of non-neoplastic origin. In Kitahata LM, and Collins D (eds): Narcotic Analgesics in Anesthesiology. Williams & Wilkins, Baltimore, 1982, pp 199–208.

152. Tennant FS, Robinson D, Sagherian A, et al: Chronic opioid treatment of intractable non-malignant pain. Pain Management Jan/Feb:18–36, 1988.

153. Tennant FS, and Uelman GF: Narcotic maintenance for chronic pain: medical and legal guidelines. Postgrad Med 73:81–94, 1983.

154. Terenius L: Stereospecific interaction between narcotic analgesics and a synaptic plasma membrane fraction of the rat cerebral cortex. Acta Pharmacologica et Toxicologica 32:317–320, 1973.

155. Turner JA, Calsyn DA, Fordyce WE, et al: Drug utilization pattern in chronic pain patients. Pain 12:357–363, 1993.

156. Twycross RG: Clinical experience with diamorphine in advanced malignant disease. Int J Clin Pharmacol Ther Toxicol 9:184–198, 1974.

157. Urban BJ, France RD, Steinberger DL, et al: Long-term use of narcotic-antidepressant medication in the management of phantom limb pain. Pain 24:191–197, 1986.

158. Ventafridda V, Tamburini M, Caraceni A, et al: A validation study of the WHO method for cancer pain relief. Cancer 59:859–856, 1987.

159. Ventafridda V, Tamburini M, and DeConno F: Comprehensive treatment in cancer pain. In Fields HL, Dubner R, and Cervero F (eds): Advances in Pain Research and Therapy, Vol 9: Proceedings of the Fourth World Congress on Pain. Raven Press, New York, 1985, pp 617–628.

160. Waldman SD: Implantable drug delivery systems: Practical considerations. Journal of Pain and Symptom Management 5:169–175, 1990.

161. Waldman SD: The role of spinal opioids in the management of cancer pain. Journal of Pain and Symptom Management 5:163–169, 1990.

162. Walker VA, Hoskin PJ, Hanks GW, et al: Evaluation of WHO analgesic guidelines for cancer pain in a hospital-based palliative care unit. Journal of Pain and Symptom Management 3:145–149, 1988.

163. Ward SE, Goldberg N, Miller-McCauley V, et al: Patient-related barriers to management of cancer pain. Pain 52:319–324, 1993.

164. Weber RJ, Ikejiri B, Rice KC, et al: Opiate receptor mediated regulation of the immune response in vivo. NIDA Res Monogr 76:341–348, 1987.

165. Weissman DE, and Haddox JD: Opioid pseudoaddiction—an iatrogenic syndrome. Pain 36:363–366, 1989.

166. Weissman DE, Joranson DE, and Hopwood MB: Wisconsin physicians' knowledge and attitudes about opioid analgesic regulations. Wis Med J 90:671–675, 1991.

167. Wiesenfeld-Hallin Z, Xu X-J, Villar MJ, et al: Intrathecal galanin potentiates the spinal analgesic effect of morphine: Electrophysiological and behavioural studies. Neurosci Lett 109:217–221, 1990.

168. Wikler A: Opioid dependence: Mechanisms and treatment. Plenum Press, New York, 1980.

169. Woolf CJ, and Thompson SWN: The induction and maintenance of central sensitization is dependent on N-methyl/D-aspartic acid receptor activation: Implications for the treatment of post-injury hypersensitivity states. Pain 44:293–299, 1991.

170. World Health Organization. Technical report no. 516: Youth and drugs. World Health Organization, Geneva, 1973.

171. World Health Organization. Cancer pain relief and palliative care. World Health Organization, Geneva, 1990.

172. Xu X-J, Puke MJC, Verge VMK, et al: Up-regulation of cholecystokinin in primary sensory neurons is associated with morphine insensitivity in experimental neuropathic pain in the rat. Neurosci Lett 152:129–132, 1993.

173. Xu X-J, and Wiesenfeld-Hallin Z: The threshold for the depressive effect of intrathecal morphine on the spinal nociceptive flexor reflex is increased during autotomy after sciatic nerve section in rats. Pain 46:223–229, 1991.

174. Yaksh TL: Tolerance: Factors involved in changes in the dose-effective relationship with chronic drug exposure. In Basbaum AI, and Besson J-M (eds): Towards a New Pharmacotherapy of Pain. John Wiley & Sons, New York, 1991, pp 157–180.

175. Zenz M, Strumpf M, and Tryba M: Long-term opioid therapy in patients with chronic nonmalignant pain. Journal of Pain and Symptom Management 7:69–77, 1992.

176. Ziegler DK: Opiate and opioid use in patients with refractory headache. Cephalalgia 14:5–10, 1994.

CHAPTER 12

ANESTHETIC TECHNIQUES FOR PAIN CONTROL

Ian R. Sutton, M.D., F.R.C.P.C., and
Michael J. Cousins, M.B., B.S., M.D.(Sydney),
F.A.N.Z.C.A., F.R.C.A.

Pain treatment usually relies on the systemic administration of centrally acting drugs, the utility of which is determined by the balance between analgesic efficacy and side effects mediated by the central nervous system (CNS). Nonetheless, the potential for regionalized pain control as an alternative to this systemic approach has been recognized since the demonstration of nerve conduction block by Koller in 1884. This observation led to an explosion of anesthetic techniques that target with varying degrees of selectivity any region of the nervous system to provide pain relief with less risk of CNS side effects. This is the major advantage of anesthetic approaches in the management of chronic pain.[19]

ROLE OF THE ANESTHETIST AND ANESTHETIC TECHNIQUES IN PAIN MANAGEMENT

In the past, conduction blockade of peripheral nerves and of sympathetic ganglia were the major tasks of the anesthesiologist. The potential exists, however, for profound analgesia from the delivery of diverse agents to various sites of the nervous system. The experimental[87] and clinical[77] use of spinally administered drugs has shifted the focus to regional administration of agents that modulate neuronal transmission. Anesthetic approaches to pain control now comprise techniques that are designed to deliver drugs that:

1. Interact with nociceptive receptors (local anesthetics and NSAIDs)

277

2. Block axonal transmission (local anesthetic or neurolytic blockade)
3. Block sympathetic function (local anesthetic or neurolytic blockade)
4. Decrease CNS transmission of nociceptive information (e.g., opioids)

The approaches selected in any individual case may involve one site or multiple sites of the nervous system.

The anesthesiologist provides both technical skills and knowledge of the indications, contraindications, and management strategies used in the application of these techniques. The appropriately trained anesthesiologist can, therefore, make a considerable number of contributions to the management of the patient with chronic pain.

TECHNIQUES FOR PAIN CONTROL: THE CENTRAL NERVOUS SYSTEM

Spinal Opioid Administration

The spinal application of opioids provides analgesia in the setting of acute pain,[21] cancer pain,[58] and selected cases of non–cancer-related chronic pain.[51] This technique developed rapidly after the description by Yaksh and Rudy[87] of the analgesia produced in rats by the subarachnoid administration of morphine. Supportive evidence was provided by Calvillo[11] and Duggan.[28] This led to the first human application of spinal opioids in 1979.[77] Since then, the number of cases treated with spinal opioids has steadily increased. Despite the potential for side effects,[31] techniques of spinal administration have gained a firm position in the clinical management of severe pain.

SPINAL ACTION OF OPIOIDS

In the spinal cord, opioid receptors are present predominantly in the dorsal horn of the gray matter.[3,86] They are located both presynaptically and postsynaptically at the site of interaction between primary afferent A-delta and C-fiber nociceptors and second-order spinal neurons. Activation of these receptors exerts an inhibitory effect on neuronal transmission.[79]

Brain and spinal opioid receptors probably contribute to pain relief following the administration of opioids by any route. Systemically administered opioids likely provide analgesia by effects on spinal opioid receptors[39] and, conversely, spinally administered opioids may spread to receptors beyond those in the spinal cord. Following epidural injection, for example, systemic absorption and cephalad spread within the CSF result in opioid delivery to the brain and medullary receptors, which may contribute to analgesia and side effects.[33,49] Nonetheless, spinal administration of opioids has the advantage of enhanced delivery to spinal receptors. This may allow greater efficacy at far lower doses than those required by systemic administration. Consequently, if systemic opioids fail to provide adequate analgesia or if the patient develops intolerable side effects, spinal administration can enhance analgesia.[58]

PHARMACOKINETIC MODEL OF SPINAL OPIOIDS

The pharmacokinetics of different opioids vary when administered spinally, largely in relation to variation in lipid solubility.[84] After *epidural* administration (Fig. 12–1), opioid must transfer across the dura, spread within the CSF, and penetrate the spinal cord to reach opioid receptors. An opioid like morphine, which is hydrophilic and, therefore, less absorbed into epidural fat or blood vessels, may be best suited for chronic epidural administration. Only a small proportion of morphine is in the nonionized, lipid-soluble form. Because the ionized moiety crosses membranes slowly, the movement of morphine is prolonged and peak CSF levels occur 90 minutes following epidural injection. The resultant slow onset of analgesic effect, which can be a disadvantage, is usually balanced by a long duration of pain relief. Prolonged pain relief occurs because egress from the spinal cord is inhibited by the persistence of morphine in the aqueous CSF.[33] In comparison, the lipophilic opioid fentanyl is rapidly transferred across the dura, leading to rapid onset of analgesia and a short duration of action.[34,35]

Subarachnoid injection is similar to epidural administration once the opioid is present in the CSF. The drug is not subject to the initial uptake by epidural fat or blood

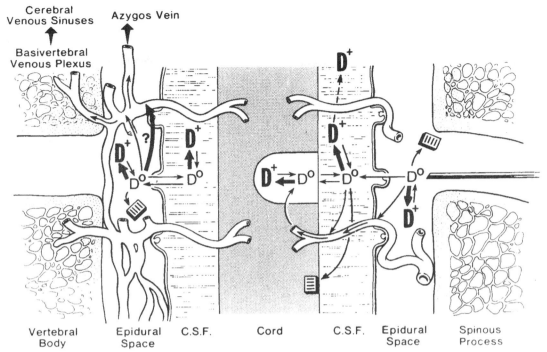

Figure 12–1. Pharmacokinetic model of spinal opioid administration. An epidural needle (right) is shown delivering a hydrophilic opioid, such as morphine, to the epidural space. Within the epidural space, cerebrospinal fluid (CSF), and spinal cord, equilibria of $D°$ (non-ionized moiety of drug) and D^+ (ionized, hydrophilic moiety) are shown. Nonspecific lipid binding sites are indicated by the shaded squares. The role of spinal arteries, in proximity to arachnoid granulations, in drug delivery is speculative. Epidural veins are the major point of clearance of an epidural drug. (From Cousins MJ, Cherry DA, and Gourlay GK: Acute and chronic pain: Use of spinal opioids. In Cousins MJ, and Bridenbaugh PD [eds]: Neural Blockade in Clinical Anesthesia and Management of Pain, ed 2. JB Lippincott, Philadelphia, 1988, p 987, with permission.)

vessels, however, and consequently the doses required are generally 1 to 10 percent of the epidural dose. The time to onset of analgesia is decreased and analgesia is prolonged compared with epidural administration.[19] The prolonged elevation of the morphine concentration in the CSF increases the likelihood of cephalad migration due to the normal CSF circulation.[54] The migration to other segments and, to some extent, to supraspinal structures may extend the level of analgesia and increase the utility of intrathecal morphine in chronic pain.[33,34,54]

CLINICAL APPLICATION OF SPINAL OPIOIDS

Spinal administration of opioids is most commonly used in the treatment of severe cancer-related pain. It can also be useful in otherwise intractable non–cancer-related pain. Alternative settings include pain due to (1) severe inoperable peripheral vascular disease,[45,58] (2) vertebral crush fractures,[51,58] (3) inoperable myocardial ischemia,[43] and (4) various conditions such as postherpetic neuralgia, phantom limb pain, reflex sympathetic dystrophy, and inoperable spinal stenosis.[38,48,51,58] In general, the indications for a trial of this approach include (1) pain that cannot be controlled with systemic opioids because dose escalation is limited by toxicity and (2) effective pain relief with systemic opioids but with intolerable side effects such as nausea, vomiting, or clouding of consciousness (see Chapter 11).

Before the spinal route is implemented, the nature of the underlying disease, the character of the pain, and the overall prognosis must be considered. In cancer pain, the best response is obtained in patients who complain of deep, constant somatic pain. The responses vary with cutaneous pain, intermittent visceral or intermittent somatic pain, and coexistent noncancer pain.[2] Although neuropathic pain may be less sensitive to opioid drugs than nociceptive pain, a good result is possible in selected cases.[38,60] In all patients a trial of epidural opioid may be useful before embarking on long-term therapy.[14]

Contraindications to the use of spinal opioids are similar to those of any regional technique. They include (1) bleeding diathesis (increasing the risk of epidural hematoma), (2) septicemia (increasing the risk of infection), and (3) local cutaneous infection. The approach should be undertaken cautiously in immunocompromised patients and those with insulin-dependent diabetes mellitus, who may have a higher risk of infection. Treatment should not be started in any patient unless support is available for ongoing management of spinal opioid administration. Anticipation of prolonged therapy is not a contraindication to the spinal route. Because epidural fibrosis may develop with epidural catheters within 2 to 6 months of placement, however, the anticipation of prolonged therapy should suggest the use of the subarachnoid route using a totally implanted programmable pump (see following).

SIDE EFFECTS AND COMPLICATIONS OF SPINAL OPIOIDS

The chronic use of the spinal route is generally well tolerated. Side effects and complications may relate to either the pharmacology of opioids or the devices and techniques required to deliver these preparations.[19] Most side effects result from known opioid actions: respiratory depression, nausea and vomiting, urinary retention, dysphoria, and pruritus. These are fortunately rare and, should they occur, are often self-limited or controllable by dosage adjustments.[19] The migration of morphine within the CSF appears to explain the potential for delayed respiratory depression (onset 3 to 20 hours after injection),[31,33–35] which has been observed most often following the administration of morphine in opioid-naive patients. Respiratory depression has not been reported with the more lipophilic opioid

fentanyl. This effect can be reversed with the opioid antagonist naloxone.

Very high subarachnoid doses of morphine can produce convulsions, intense generalized motor rigidity, and myoclonic jerks.[19,53] In patients with cancer, high spinal doses of morphine also can produce dysesthetic pain and hyperalgesia.[85] These effects are not reversible with naloxone and may result from receptor interactions unrelated to those that mediate analgesia.[86]

The incidence of complications related to the delivery system is not clearly known. The majority of patients have no clinically significant problems with the delivery system, regardless of type.[58] Localized fibrous reaction to epidural catheters and superficial infections are the most common encountered.

As mentioned, a sheath of fibrous scar, which appears 2 to 6 months after insertion, has been documented with chronically implanted epidural catheters. This may account for the observed variability in CSF concentrations and decreased analgesic efficacy of long-term epidural opioids. Fibrosis does not occur with subarachnoid catheter systems.

Infectious complications vary with the different delivery systems. Implanted epidural catheters connected to injection portals have an 8 percent incidence. If treated promptly, such infections are limited to the subcutaneous tissues and epidural catheter track. Meningitis can occur with involvement of the subarachnoid systems.[61] Fortunately, this is a rare complication. Serious infections associated with any delivery system must be managed aggressively with removal of the delivery system and appropriate antibiotics.[13]

TECHNICAL CONSIDERATIONS IN THE EFFICACY OF SPINAL OPIOIDS

Before any spinal approach is undertaken, consideration first must be given to patient and social factors. For example, all patients must have access to trained nurses.

To minimize the risk of infection and reduce the likelihood of epidural fibrosis, totally implanted subarachnoid delivery systems have been recommended.[47,55] These systems are expensive, however, and a range of more economical alternatives exists. At the lower end of cost and technical complexity, simple percutaneous epidural catheters can deliver intermittent bolus doses of opioid. Without modifications, such percutaneous systems have a relatively high risk of infection. Infusion devices range in cost and sophistication from totally implanted, programmable pumps to simple, externally applied mechanical syringe drivers. All infusion systems are more expensive than intermittent dosing into a percutaneous or subcutaneous injection portal.

A subcutaneously tunneled epidural catheter with an implanted injection portal is a reasonable compromise between cost and infection (Fig. 12–2). This can be inserted under local anesthesia[74] and has proven effective in a variety of clinical settings. Continuous infusion of agents can be performed with an external infusion pump if intermittent bolus proves ineffective.

Patients' ability to participate in their care can be an overriding factor in deciding on the type of therapy. Percutaneous injection two to four times daily can be managed by most patients and families. Totally implanted, programmable pumps are easy for patients to manage but require refilling, usually in a hos-

pital setting, every 2 to 4 weeks. In all cases, trained nursing support is needed to provide ongoing assessment, whether in the patient's home, the pain clinic, or the hospital.[6]

MANAGEMENT OF PAIN RESISTANT TO SPINAL OPIOIDS

Some patients undergo dose escalation of the spinal opioid but fail to attain adequate analgesia before side effects supervene. The initial approach to resistant pain should be to reevaluate the patient for the possibility of progression of the underlying disease, change in type of pain (e.g., change to a neuropathic pathophysiology), or malfunction of the delivery system. If neuropathic pain develops from either progression of the underlying disease or treatment-related nerve injury, a variety of adjuvant drugs may be useful, including tricyclic antidepressants, anticonvulsant medications, and oral[24] or systemic local anesthetics[8] (see Chapter 10). To ensure adequate functioning of the spinal delivery system, radiographs following injection of contrast may be needed to verify the appropriate placement of the catheter. If pain control continues to be a

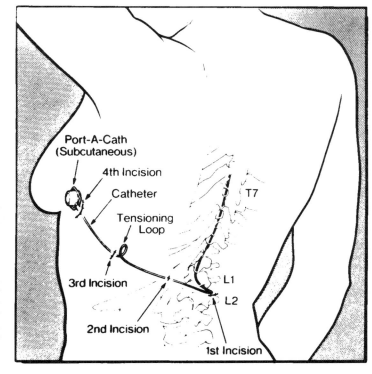

Figure 12–2. Epidural catheter tunneled subcutaneously to an implanted portal (Port-A-Cath, Pharmacia Deltec, St. Paul, MN) for chronic epidural access. (From Cousins MJ, Cherry DA, and Gourlay, GK: Acute and chronic pain: Use of spinal opioids. In Cousins MJ, and Bridenbaugh PD [eds]: Neural Blockade in Clinical Anesthesia and Management of Pain, ed 2. JB Lippincott, Philadelphia, 1988, p 1008, with permission.)

problem, the use of other regional techniques should be considered.

Spinal Local Anesthetics. The addition of a local anesthetic to the opioid may provide significant analgesia when spinal opioids alone are inadequate. Low doses of epidural local anesthetic can achieve excellent analgesia without motor or sensory blockade. The epidural route is more advantageous than the subarachnoid route for this differential blockade of pain.[52]

Recently, two local anesthetic agents (veratridrine and *n*-butyl-*p*-aminobenzoate [BAB]) with apparent selectivity for nociceptive sensory afferents have been developed.[44,63] Veratridrine, a steroidal alkaloid, is unique in that it produces conduction blockade while maintaining open sodium channels.[63] BAB is a highly lipid-soluble congener of benzocaine that produces prolonged pain relief in both animals and humans.[44] BAB toxicity appears not to be a problem; however, additional research is required before widespread clinical application can be considered. If toxicity is limited and preferential nociceptive fiber blockage occurs, these agents may provide a useful tool for epidural and peripheral analgesia.

Subarachnoid Opioid Peptides. The endogenous opioid pentapeptide, D-Ala^2-D-Leu^5-enkephalin (DADLE), is a stable leu-enkephalin analog that is 20-fold more selective for the delta opioid receptor than for the mu receptor. Intrathecal administration of DADLE produces antinociceptive effects that have limited cross-tolerance to those produced by relatively pure mu agonists, such as morphine.[70] In clinical studies, this compound has produced profound analgesia in patients who have developed tolerance to intrathecal morphine.[50] Side effects appear to be similar to those of morphine, with drowsiness the most common. DADLE is only one of several opioid pentapeptides that may have a role in chronic pain management. Further evaluation is required before widespread clinical use of these agents can be considered in patients with chronic pain.

Nonopioid Spinal Analgesics. Recent advances in the neurophysiology of nociception demonstrated the potential for analgesic effects following spinal administration of nonopioid drugs (Fig. 12–3). Nonopioid analgesics might be used synergistically with opioid and nonopioid agents. If so, this approach could potentially reduce the incidence of side effects and improve pain management in patients resistant or tolerant to opioid therapy alone.[68] Agonists of adrenergic (noradrenaline), cholinergic (carbachol), serotoninergic (5-hydroxytryptamine), and adenosine (NECA) receptors, as well as the NMDA-receptor antagonists (e.g., ketamine and MK-801), have antinociceptive effects following intrathecal administration.

Clonidine, an α_2-adrenergic agonist, has been the most studied nonopioid analgesic. Activation of the α_2-adrenergic receptor inhibits neurotransmission between primary afferent nociceptive fibers and second-order dorsal horn neurons.[29] Spinal clonidine has analgesic efficacy in animals[27] and in humans.[15,30] Epidural analgesia requires doses similar to those used systemically, and side effects, including sedation and hypotension, are reported.[30] Although cross-tolerance exists between spinal opioids and α_2-adrenergic agonists,[66,69] animal studies suggest a synergy between the antinociceptive effects produced by intrathecal clonidine and morphine over a rather narrow dose range.[59] Further examination of the safety and efficacy of clonidine alone and in combination with other agents is required before widespread spinal use is recommended.

Baclofen (β-4-chlorophenyl-γ-aminobutyric acid) is a GABA$_B$ agonist that inhibits the release of excitatory neurotransmitters, reduces the flexor reflex, and possibly alters pain transmission. Several studies have documented benefit from spinal administration in the treatment of spasticity.[56] Further research is needed to evaluate analgesic effects.

Neurolytic Blockade

Neurolytic blocks are generally best suited for patients with short life expectancy and well-localized pain. These techniques are most effective in nociceptive pain.[17] Deafferentation pain[9] responds poorly despite initial temporary relief.

Ethyl alcohol and phenol are the most frequently used neurolytic agents. Glycerol, which also has been used, can be advantageous in trigeminal ganglion block. Phenol has local anesthetic properties that can re-

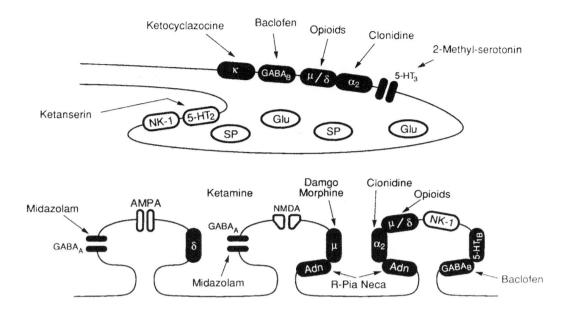

Post Synaptic Element

Figure 12–3. Summary of neurotransmission from primary afferent sensory fibers to second-order spinal neurons (postsynaptic element) in the spinal dorsal horns. Neurotransmitters (open circles) include the excitatory amino acid transmitters (glutamate = Glu) and neurokinins (substance P = SP). Activation of postsynaptic, excitatory amino acid receptors (classified by their response to N-methyl-D-aspartate [NMDA] and α-amino-3-hydroxy-5-methyl-4-isoxazolepropionic acid [AMPA]), as well as neurokinin receptors (NK-1), results in depolarization of the postsynaptic membrane. Excitatory receptors (open ovals) are also located presynaptically, where activation results in enhanced transmitter release (5-HT_2 = excitatory serotonin receptors). Activation of inhibitory receptors (filled ovals), located both presynaptically and postsynaptically, decreases the release and effectiveness of transmitters (k, μ, δ = opioid; GABA = gamma-aminobutyric acid; 5-HT_3 = inhibitory serotonin receptor; α_2 = alpha$_2$-adrenergic; Adn = adenosine). The drugs shown affect pain transmission, at least experimentally, and are believed to be active at the sites indicated (arrows). (From Wilcox GL: Excitatory neurotransmitters and pain. In Bond MR, Charlton JE, and Woolf CJ [eds]: Proceedings of the VIth World Congress on Pain. Elsevier, Amsterdam, 1991, p 99, with permission.)

sult in painless injection. Like local anesthetics, however, phenol may produce convulsions followed by CNS depression if injected intravascularly. Few data presently exist to demonstrate an advantage of one agent over others.

Subarachnoid neurolytic block can be an effective method of pain relief for patients with advanced malignancy. The pain should be unilateral and limited to a few segments. The aim is to produce a posterior rhizotomy to relieve pain in the affected region.

The progressive nature of the underlying disease complicates assessment of spinal neurolytic blockade for cancer pain. In experienced hands, 60 percent of patients experience pain relief for more than 1 month.

Complications have been reported in the range of 1 to 14 percent, with the lowest complication rate following injection into the thoracic region.[16]

Subdural or epidural neurolytic blockade can also be effective. Although no studies have compared the effects of subarachnoid blocks with subdural or epidural blocks, the latter approach is preferable in the cervical segments. The reason is that subarachnoid injection at this site can be followed by rapid dilution of neurolytic agents in the CSF from the rapid circulation of adjacent intracranial CSF.[16] This dilution makes it difficult to limit the spread of the neurolytic agent to the desired segments. Cervical subdural block has been used for pain in the region of the ear, nose and throat, as well as for tumors in the cervical region.

Neurolytic trigeminal nerve block can be effectively used in the management of chronic pain, particularly trigeminal neuralgia (see Chapter 4). Injection of the Gasserian ganglion with ethyl alcohol was widely used in the past, but newer drug therapies, balloon compression, glycerol injection,[36] surgical rhizotomy, and thermogangliolysis[65] have superseded this technique. Gasserian ganglion blockade is usually achieved via the foramen ovale approach using fluoroscopic control.[32]

TECHNIQUES FOR PAIN CONTROL: THE PERIPHERAL NERVOUS SYSTEM

Local anesthetic blockade of the peripheral nervous system is probably most important in the management of severe somatic pain, such as pathologic fractures. Nonetheless, standard techniques, perhaps modified to allow continuous infusion of local anesthetic, also have analgesic benefit.

Neurolytic somatic neural blockade occasionally has a role, despite concern about neuralgia or motor blockade. Examples of such neurolytic blocks include intercostal, infraorbital, facial, and obturator nerve blocks, brachial plexus block, and intralesional neurolytic injection for bony metastases.[26] The incidence of inadequate analgesia can be lessened with the use of a nerve stimulator to identify the proper target.[16]

TECHNIQUES FOR PAIN CONTROL: THE SYMPATHETIC NERVOUS SYSTEM

Visceral afferent nociceptive fibers traverse the efferent sympathetic fibers and sympathetic ganglia without synapsing. Sympathetic blockade can disrupt either the sympathetic efferent or the visceral nociceptive afferent fibers. Stellate ganglion block is the most common approach for pain in the head, neck, or upper extremity; celiac plexus block can be used for upper abdominal visceral pain; and lumbar sympathetic block can be used for lower abdominal visceral pain and lower extremity pain.

Recent work has drawn attention to the central, spinal component of sympathetically maintained pain, as well as the peripheral effect of sympathetic activity on nociceptors (see Chapter 5).[78] α-Adrenergic receptors can be expressed on nociceptors[12] after nerve or soft tissue injury, and activity in the sympathetic nervous system can activate those nociceptors. Increased activity in nociceptors can sensitize and enlarge the receptive fields of neurons in the dorsal horn (see Chapter 5). This, in turn, can lead to a reflex increase in sympathetic discharge, creating a vicious cycle of sympathetically maintained pain. In addition, ephapses may form between the sympathetic nervous system and nociceptive fibers.[64] To abort or lessen these processes, sympathetic nerves may be blocked with local anesthetic or neurolytic techniques.

Local Anesthetic Sympathetic Blockade

Local anesthetic sympathetic block can be used for both diagnostic and therapeutic purposes. Relief of neuropathic pain by sympathetic blockade may presage a favorable response to further sympathetic blockade or suggest benefit from neurolytic sympathetic blockade. Sympathetic blockade with local anesthetic can also improve the management of acute exacerbations of chronic problems, such as ischemic crises in Raynaud's disease and other obliterative arteriopathies.[46] Local anesthetic sympathetic block can help to manage the pain of acute herpes zoster[71] and can assist in the management of established postherpetic neuralgia.[83]

Neurolytic Celiac Plexus Blockade

Celiac plexus block can interrupt visceral nociceptive afferent fibers from the upper abdomen. Neurolytic celiac plexus blockade (NCPB) is helpful in managing severe upper abdominal pain of malignant origin, especially carcinoma of the pancreas.[62] NCPB can provide 70 to 80 percent of patients with good immediate relief (Table 12–1) and 60 to 75 percent with good relief until death.

Table 12–1. **RESULTS OF "CLASSIC" CELIAC PLEXUS BLOCK WITH ALCOHOL**

Author	Indication	Number of cases	Results (%)		
			Good	Fair	Poor
Brown[10]	Pancreatic cancer	136	85*	—	15
Black[5]	Pancreatic cancer	20	70	30	0
	Other abdominal malignancy	37	70	17	13
Bridenbaugh[7]	Upper abdominal cancer	41	73	24.5	2.5
Ischia[37]	Pancreatic cancer	18	72	—	28†
		43	37	—	63‡

*In 75% of patients, good relief lasted through remaining life.
The success of repeated blocks was also 85%.
†Patients with duration of pain ≤2 months.
‡Patients with duration of pain ≥2 months.

Chronic pancreatitis is not improved by NCPB, partly because of the limited duration of analgesia.

NCPB is associated with temporary orthostatic hypotension and increased gastrointestinal motility. These side effects are usually mild and self-limiting. Fortunately, the incidence of more severe complications is low (Table 12–2). The true incidence and etiology of catastrophic complications are unknown, but in view of the several thousand patients who are reported to have safely undergone NCPB, the incidence appears to be extremely low. The most important factors in the application of NCPB are careful patient selection and meticulous technique

Table 12–2. **COMPLICATIONS OF CELIAC PLEXUS BLOCKADE**

Complication	Percent
Weakness or numbness T = 10, L = 2	8
Lower chest pain	3
Failure of ejaculation	2
Urinary retention	1
Postural hypotension*	1
Diarrhea, pneumothorax, paraplegia	Uncertain

*Temporary postural hypotension occurs in 30–60% of patients.[5]
Source: Data from Black A, and Dwyer B: Coeliac plexus block. Anaesthesia and Intensive Care 1:315–318, 1973.

with radiographic imaging to verify needle placement.[72]

Neurolytic Lumbar Sympathetic Blockade

Ischemia due to peripheral vascular disease (PVD) is often associated with severe pain. This may lead to increased sympathetic discharge, resulting in sensitization of nociceptors. Neurolytic lumbar sympathetic block may cause vasodilatation and interrupt the cycle of pain and reflex sympathetic discharge. Sympathetic blockade reduces ischemic rest pain, increases blood flow, and enhances healing of chronic ulceration in inoperable PVD.[20,76] Chemical sympathetic blockade is as efficacious as surgical sympathetic block but is less invasive and is associated with lower morbidity, mortality, and cost.[20] It is also more easily repeated.[46] Similar to surgical sympathetic blocks, chemical sympathectomy has an average duration of effect of approximately 6 months.

Lumbar sympathetic block interrupts pelvic visceral afferent fibers and relieves the pain associated with pelvic cancers. Bilateral blocks may be useful in pain caused by tumors of the sigmoid colon, rectum, or urogenital organs, if the disease is confined to those viscera. Lumbar sympathetic blocks in combination with NCPB may provide pain relief for extensive intra-abdominal spread of neoplasm.

Neurolytic superior hypogastric plexus

block is also effective in the management of pelvic cancer pain.[57] This provides a more selective block of afferent visceral fibers than lumbar sympathectomy. The role of superior hypogastric block in pelvic pain management requires further evaluation of benefits and side effects.

RECENT ADVANCES AND FUTURE DIRECTIONS

Elucidation of the neurophysiology and neurochemistry of nociception, including the complex processes in the dorsal horn (as depicted in Fig. 12–3), holds the potential for greater and more fundamental advances in pain management. Because of the plasticity of the nervous system (i.e., alteration of function in response to previous neural activity), nociception modifies spinal cord function and may facilitate further pain transmission, leading to the development of severe, intractable pain. Profound changes in the dorsal-horn processing of afferent input range from temporal and spatial summation of nociceptive input to shifts in gene regulation. Long-term changes in response to noxious and nonnoxious stimuli result from these processes.* Anesthetic interventions, including drug delivery to the spinal cord, may offer innovative techniques to reverse or prevent these changes.

Uncontrolled pain is a severe physiologic stress with effects on many body systems. Prompt, consistent, adequate pain relief is not simply a humane endeavor: There is now evidence detailing the potential medical consequences of unrelieved pain.[18] The importance of these recent developments and improved pain management is confirmed by respiratory, cardiovascular, immune, neurophysiologic, psychologic, and other adverse consequences of unrelieved pain.

Early or prophylactic analgesic therapy can reduce or eliminate some chronic pain.[4,22,80] Tolerance is not an integral characteristic of chronic systemic or spinal opioid analgesia[58]; rather, failure to provide adequate pain control may contribute to the development of severe opioid-resistant pain. The availability of appropriate early man-

agement strategies, including anesthetic techniques, has the potential for reducing the incidence, severity, and consequences of acute and chronic pain.

SUMMARY

Numerous anesthetic techniques have been developed for the management of acute and chronic pain. These techniques are designed to deliver drugs that interact with nociceptor receptors, block axonal transmission, block sympathetic function, or decrease CNS transmission of noxious input. Nerve blocks may be temporary (local anesthetic) or more prolonged (neurolytic drugs, such as phenol or alcohol). Local anesthetic blocks of somatic nerves or sympathetic nerves are applied in the treatment of many painful conditions, most notably sympathetically maintained pain. Neurolytic blocks are usually limited to patients with refractory pain due to advanced cancer. Techniques of spinal opioid administration are varied and involve epidural or subarachnoid drug delivery. These techniques are used in patients who are unable to tolerate systemic opioids because of side effects. The anesthesiologist who is trained in pain management plays an important role in the interdisciplinary approach to chronic pain, potentially providing needed technical skills and knowledge of the indications for these invasive therapies.

REFERENCES

1. Almay BG, Johansson F, Von Knorring L, et al: Substance P in CSF of patients with chronic pain syndromes. Pain 33:3–9, 1988.
2. Arner S, and Arner B: Differential effects of epidural morphine in the treatment of cancer-related pain. Acta Anaesth Scand 29:32–36, 1985.
3. Atweh SF, and Kuhar MJ: Autoradiographic localization of opiate receptors in rat brain. I. Spinal cord and lower medulla. Brain Res 124:53–67, 1977.
4. Bach S, Noreng MF, and Tjellden NU: Phantom limb pain in amputees during the first 12 months following limb amputation, after preoperative lumbar epidural blockade. Pain 33:297–301, 1988.
5. Black A, and Dwyer B: Coeliac plexus block. Anaesthesia and Intensive Care 1:315–318, 1973.
6. Blue CL, and Purath G: Continuing education. Home care of the epidural analgesia patient: The nurse's role. Home Health Nurse 7:23–32, 1989.
7. Bridenbaugh LD, Moore DC, and Campbell DD: Management of upper abdominal cancer pain.

*References 1, 23, 25, 40–42, 67, 73, 81, 82.

Treatment with celiac plexus block with alcohol. JAMA 190:877–880, 1964.

8. Brose WG, and Cousins MJ: Subcutaneous lidocaine for treatment of neuropathic cancer pain. Pain 45:145–148, 1991.

9. Brown AS: Current views on the use of nerve blocking in the relief of chronic pain. In Swerdlow M (ed): The Therapy of Pain. JB Lippincott, Philadelphia, 1981, pp 111–134.

10. Brown DL, Bulley CK, and Quiel EL: Neurolytic celiac plexus block for pancreatic cancer pain. Anesth Analg 66:869–873, 1987.

11. Calvillo O, Henry JL, and Neuman RS: Effects of morphine and naloxone on dorsal horn neurones in the cat. Canadian Journal of Physiology and Pharmacology 52:1207–1211, 1974.

12. Campbell JN, Raja SN, and Meyer A: Painful sequelae of nerve injury. In Dubner R, Gebhart GF, and Bond MR (eds): Proceedings of the Vth World Congress on Pain. Elsevier, Amsterdam, 1988, pp 114–128.

13. Cherry DA, Gourlay GK, Cousins MJ, et al: A technique for the insertion of an implantable portal system for the long term epidural administration of opioids in the treatment of cancer pain. Anaesth Intensive Care 13:145–152, 1985.

14. Cherry DA, Gourlay GK, McLachlan M, et al: Diagnostic epidural opioid blockade and chronic pain: Preliminary report. Pain 21:143–152, 1985.

15. Coombs DW, Saunders AL, LaChance D, et al: Intrathecal morphine tolerance: Use of intrathecal clonidine, DADLE, and intraventricular morphine. Anesthesiology 62:358–363, 1985.

16. Cousins MJ: Chronic pain and neurolytic neural blockade. In Cousins MJ, and Bridenbaugh PO (eds): Neural Blockade in Clinical Anesthesia and Management of Pain, ed 2. JB Lippincott, Philadelphia, 1988, pp 1053–1084.

17. Cousins MJ: Introduction to acute and chronic pain: Implications for neural blockade. In Cousins MJ, and Bridenbaugh PO (eds): Neural Blockade in Clinical Anesthesia and Management of Pain, ed 2. JB Lippincott, Philadelphia, 1988, pp 739–790.

18. Cousins MJ: Prevention of postoperative pain. In Bond MR, Charlton JE, and Woolf CJ (eds): Proceedings of the VIth World Congress on Pain. Elsevier, Amsterdam, 1991, pp 41–52.

19. Cousins MJ, Cherry DA, and Gourlay GK: Acute and chronic pain: Use of spinal opioids. In Cousins MJ, and Bridenbaugh PO (eds): Neural Blockade in Clinical Anesthesia and Management of Pain, ed 2. JB Lippincott, Philadelphia, 1988, pp 955–1029.

20. Cousins MJ, Reeve TS, Glynn CJ, et al: Neurolytic lumbar sympathetic blockade: Duration of denervation and relief of rest pain. Anaesth Intensive Care 7:121–135, 1979.

21. Crews JC: Epidural opioid analgesia. Crit Care Clin 6:315–342, 1990.

22. Davar G, and Maciewicz R: MK-801 blocks thermal hyperalgesia in a rat model of neuropathic pain. Brain Res 553:327–330, 1991.

23. Davies SN, and Lodge D: Evidence for involvement of N-methylaspartate receptors in 'wind up' of class 2 neurones in the dorsal horn of the rat. Brain Res 424:402–406, 1987.

24. Dejgard A, Petersen P, and Kastrup J: Mexiletine for treatment of chronic painful diabetic neuropathy. Lancet 1:9–11, 1988.

25. Dickenson AH, and Sullivan AF: Evidence for a role of the NMDA receptor in the frequency dependent potentiation of deep rat dorsal horn nociceptive neurones following C-fiber stimulation. Neuropharmacology 26:1235–1238, 1987.

26. Doyle D: Nerve blocks in advanced cancer. Practitioner 226:539–544, 1982.

27. Drasner K, and Fields HL: Synergy between the antinociceptive effects of intrathecal clonidine and systemic morphine in the rat. Pain 32:309–312, 1988.

28. Duggan AW, Hall JG, and Headley PM: Morphine, enkephalin, and the substantia gelatinosa. Nature 264:456–458, 1976.

29. Fleetwood-Walker SM, Mitchell R, Hope PJ, et al: An alpha-2 receptor mediates the selective inhibition by noradrenaline of nociceptive responses of identified dorsal horn neurones. Brain Res 334:243–254, 1985.

30. Germain H, Neron A, and Lamssy A: Analgesic effect of epidural clonidine. In Dubner GF, and Bond MR (eds): Proceedings of the Vth World Congress on Pain. Elsevier, Amsterdam, 1988, pp 472–476.

31. Glynn CJ, Mather LE, Cousins MJ, et al: Spinal narcotics and respiratory depression. Lancet 2:356–357, 1979.

32. Gomori JM, and Rappaport ZH: Transovale trigeminal cistern puncture: Modified fluoroscopically guided technique. American Journal of Neuroradiology 6:93–94, 1985.

33. Gourlay GK, Cherry DA, and Cousins MJ: Cephalad migration of morphine in CSF following lumbar epidural administration in patients with cancer. Pain 23:317–326, 1985.

34. Gourlay GK, Cherry DA, Plummer JL, et al: The influence of drug polarity on the absorption of opioid drugs into CSF and subsequent cephalad migration following lumbar epidural administration: Application to morphine and pethidine. Pain 31:297–305, 1987.

35. Gourlay GK, Murphy TM, Plummer JL, et al: Pharmacokinetics of fentanyl in lumbar and cervical CSF following lumbar epidural and intravenous administration. Pain 38:253–259, 1989.

36. Hakanson S: Trigeminal neuralgia treated by the injection of glycerol into the trigeminal cistern. Neurosurgery 9:638–646, 1981.

37. Ischia S, Ischia A, Polati E, et al: Three posterior percutaneous celiac plexus block techniques. A prospective, randomized study in 61 patients with pancreatic cancer pain. Anesthesiology 76:534–540, 1992.

38. Jacobson L, Chabal C, Brody MC, et al: A comparison of the effects of intrathecal fentanyl and lidocaine on established postamputation stump pain. Pain 40:137–141, 1990.

39. Johnson SM, and Duggan AW: Evidence that opiate receptors at the substantia gelatinosa contribute to depression by intravenous morphine of the spinal transmission of impulses in the unmyelinated primary afferents. Brain Res 207:223–228, 1981.

40. Jorum E, Holin E, Lundberg L, et al: Temporal summation in nociceptive systems. Pain Supplement 5:S314, 1990.

41. Katz J, Vaccarino AL, Coderre TJ, et al: Injury prior to neurectomy alters the pattern of autonomy in rats: Behavioral evidence of central neural plasticity. Anesthesiology 75:876–883, 1991.

42. Kehl LJ, Basbaum AI, Pollock CM, et al: The NMDA antagonist MK-801 reduces noxious stimulus evoked Fos expression in the spinal dorsal horn. Pain Suppl 5:S165, 1990.

43. Kock M, Blomberg S, Emanuelsson H, et al: Thoracic epidural anesthesia improves global and regional left ventricular function during stress-induced myocardial ischemia in patients with coronary artery disease. Anesth Analg 71:625–630, 1990.

44. Korsten HH, Ackerman EW, Grouls RJE, et al: Long-lasting epidural sensory blockade by n-butyl-p-aminobenzoate in the terminally ill intractable cancer pain patient. Anesthesiology 75:950–960, 1991.

45. Layfield DJ, Lemberger RJ, Hopkinson BR, et al: Epidural morphine for ischemic rest pain. British Medical Journal 282:697–698, 1981.

46. Lofstrom JB, and Cousins MJ: Sympathetic neural blockade of upper and lower extremity. In Cousins MJ, and Bridenbaugh PO (eds): Neural Blockade in Clinical Anesthesia and Management of Pain, ed 2. JB Lippincott, Philadelphia, 1988, pp 461–502.

47. Madrid JL, Fatela LV, Lobato RD, et al: Intrathecal therapy: rationale, technique, clinical results. Acta Anaesth Scand 31(Suppl 85):60–67, 1987.

48. Magora C, Olshwang D, Eimerl D, et al: Observations of extradural morphine analgesia in various pain conditions. Br J Anaesth 52:247–252, 1980.

49. Max MB, Inturrisi CE, Kaiko RF, et al: Epidural and intrathecal opiates: Cerebrospinal fluid and plasma profiles in patients with chronic cancer pain. Clin Pharmacol Ther 38:631–641, 1985.

50. Moulin DE, Max MB, Kaiko RF, et al: The analgesic efficacy of intrathecal D-ala^2-D-leu^5-enkephalin in cancer patients with chronic pain. Pain 23:213–221, 1985.

51. Murphy TM, Hinds S, and Cherry DA: Intraspinal narcotics: Non-malignant pain. Acta Anaesth Scand 31(Suppl 85): 75–76, 1987.

52. Nitescu P, Appelgren L, Linder LE, et al: Epidural versus intrathecal morphine-bupivacaine: Assessment of consecutive treatments in advanced cancer pain. Journal of Pain and Symptom Management 5:18–26, 1990.

53. Parkinson SK, Bailey SL, Little WL, et al: Myoclonic seizure activity with chronic high-dose spinal opioid administration. Anesthesiology 72:743–745, 1990.

54. Payne R, and Inturrisi CE: CSF distribution of morphine, methadone and sucrose after intrathecal injection. Life Sci 37:1137–1144, 1985.

55. Penn RD, and Paice JA: Chronic intrathecal morphine for intractable pain. J Neurosurg 67:182–186, 1987.

56. Penn RD, Savoy SM, Corcos D, et al: Intrathecal baclofen for severe spasticity. N Engl J Med 320:1517–1521, 1989.

57. Plancarte R, Amescua C, Patt RB, et al: Superior hypogastric plexus block for pelvic cancer pain. Anesthesiology 73:236–239, 1990.

58. Plummer JL, Cherry DA, Cousins MJ, et al: Long-term spinal administration of morphine in cancer and non-cancer pain: A retrospective study. Pain 44:215–220, 1991.

59. Plummer JL, Cmielewski PL, Gourlay GK, et al: Antinociceptive and motor effects of intrathecal morphine combined with intrathecal clonidine, noradrenaline, carbachol or midazolam in rats. Pain 49:145–152, 1992.

60. Portenoy RK, Foley KM, and Inturrisi CE: The nature of opioid responsiveness and its implications for neuropathic pain: New hypothesis derived from studies of opioid infusions. Pain 43:273–286, 1990.

61. Ready LB, and Helfer D: Bacterial meningitis in parturients after epidural anesthesia. Anesthesiology 71:988–990, 1989.

62. Saltzburg D, and Foley KM: Management of pain in pancreatic cancer. Surg Clin North Am 69:629–649, 1989.

63. Schneider M, Datta S, and Strichartz G: A preferential inhibition in C-fibers of the rabbit vagus nerve by Veratridine, an activator of sodium channels. Anesthesiology 74:270–280, 1991.

64. Seltzer Z, and Devor M: Ephaptic transmission in chronically damaged peripheral nerves. Neurology 29:1061–1064, 1979.

65. Shapshay SM, Scott RM, McCann CF, et al: Pain control in advanced and recurrent head and neck cancer. Otolaryngol Clin North Am 13:551–560, 1980.

66. Solomon RE, and Gebhart GF: Intrathecal morphine and clonidine: Antinociceptive tolerance and cross tolerance and effects on blood pressure. J Pharmacol Exp Ther 245:444–454, 1988.

67. Sonnenberg JL, Rauscher FR III, Morgan JI, et al: Regulation of proenkephalin by Fos and Jun. Science 246:1622–1625, 1989.

68. Sosnowski M, and Yaksh TL: Spinal administration of receptor selective drugs as analgesics: New horizons. Journal of Pain and Symptom Management 5:204–213, 1990.

69. Stevens CW, Monasky MS, and Yaksh TL: Spinal infusion of opiate and alpha-2 agonists in rats: Tolerance and cross-tolerance studies. J Pharmacol Exp Ther 224:63–70, 1988.

70. Stevens CW, and Yaksh TL: Studies of morphine and D-ala^2-D-leu^5-enkephalin (DADLE) cross-tolerance after continuous intrathecal infusion in the rat. Anesthesiology 76:596–603, 1992.

71. Tenicela R, Lovasik D, and Eaglestein W: Treatment of herpes zoster with sympathetic blocks. Clin J Pain 1:63–67, 1985.

72. Thompson GE, and Moore DC: Celiac plexus, intercostal and minor peripheral blockade. In Cousins MJ, and Bridenbaugh PO (eds): Neural Blockade in Clinical Anesthesia and Management of Pain, ed 2. JB Lippincott, Philadelphia, 1988, pp 503–532.

73. Tolle TR, Castro-Lopes JM, Evans G, et al: C-fos induction in the spinal cord following noxious stimulation: Prevention by opiates but not NMDA antagonists. In Bond MR, Charlton JE, and Woolf CJ (eds): Proceedings of the VIth World Congress on Pain, Elsevier, Amsterdam, 1991, pp 249–305.

74. Van Diejen D, Driessen JJ, and Kaanders JHAM: Spinal cord compression during chronic epidural morphine administration in a cancer patient. Anaesthesia 42:1201–1203, 1987.

75. Waldman SD: The role of spinal opioids in the management of cancer pain. Journal of Pain and Symptom Management 5:163–168, 1990.

76. Walsh JA, Glynn CJ, Cousins MJ, et al: Bloodflow, sympathetic activity and pain relief following lumbar sympathetic blockade or surgical sympathectomy. Anaesth Intensive Care 13:18–24, 1985.

77. Wang JK, Nauss LA, and Thomas JE: Pain relief by intrathecally applied morphine in man. Anesthesiology 50:149–151, 1979.

78. Wiesenfeld-Hallin Z, and Hallin RG: The influence of the sympathetic system on mechanoreception and nociception: A review. Human Neurobiology 3:41–46, 1984.

79. Wilcox GL: Excitatory neurotransmitters and pain. In Bond MR, Charlton JE, and Woolf CJ (eds): Proceedings of the VIth World Congress on Pain. Elsevier, Amsterdam, 1991, pp 97–117.

80. Woolf CJ: Recent advances in the pharmacology of acute pain. Br J Anaesth 63:139–146, 1989.

81. Woolf CJ, Shortland P, and Coggesall RE: Peripheral nerve injury triggers central sprouting of myelinated afferents. Nature 2:75–78, 1992.

82. Woolf CJ, and Wall PD: Morphine sensitive and morphine insensitive actions of C-fibre input on the rat spinal cord. Neurosci Lett 64(2):221–225, 1986.

83. Yaksh TL: Spinal opiate analgesia: Characteristics and principles of action. Pain 11:293–346, 1981.

84. Yaksh TL, Harty GJ, and Onofrio BM: High dose of spinal morphine produces a non-opiate receptor-mediated hyperesthesia: Clinical and theoretical implications. Anesthesiology 64:590–597, 1986.

85. Yaksh TL, and Noueihed R: The physiology and pharmacology of spinal opiates. Annu Rev Pharmacol Toxicol 25:443–462, 1985.

86. Yaksh TL, and Rudy TA. Analgesia mediated by a direct spinal action of narcotics. Science 192:1357–1358, 1976.

87. Yanagida H, Suwa K, and Corssen G: No prophylactic effect of early sympathetic blockade on postherpetic neuralgia. Anesthesiology 66:73–76, 1987.

CHAPTER 13

SURGICAL APPROACHES TO CHRONIC PAIN

Ronald R. Tasker, M.D., F.R.C.S.(C)

The accumulation of literature describing the indications, techniques, and results associated with surgery for chronic pain is daunting. The poor consensus on a taxonomy of pain syndromes makes it difficult to compare the experiences of different authors. This is, in part, the result of imperfect knowledge of underlying pathophysiology, which, in turn, interferes with the effort to tailor surgery scientifically and thereby correct specific pain-producing malfunctions. Lack of uniform criteria for assessing surgical outcome and variation in the intervals of postoperative follow-up further the confusion. While it is im-

possible to review all the relevant information in a single chapter, I will attempt to propose a rational consideration of procedures for the relief of chronic pain based upon a pathophysiologic framework derived from clinical experience (and rarely scientific study). I will cite common clinical examples and mention available techniques that have been reasonably successful.

INDICATIONS FOR SURGERY AND AN APPROACH TO CLASSIFICATION

When a patient with chronic pain is being considered for a surgical procedure, the questions outlined in Table 13–1 need to be honestly addressed. Questions 5 and 7 are easier to answer when pathophysiology is understood, allowing selection of procedures that are known to reverse that particular abnormality of function. In many patients, however, the pathophysiology can only be guessed at, and worse, this ignorance may be obscured under a mantle of confusing diagnostic terms for which there is little agreement or understanding (see Chapter 1). Nonetheless, pain classification must be addressed before one embarks on a discussion of surgery.

Table 13–1. INDICATIONS FOR SURGICAL TREATMENT OF CHRONIC PAIN

1. Is the pain amenable to primary treatment of the causative disease?
2. Have all means of simpler therapy been exhausted?
3. Is the cause of the pain known?
4. Is the patient's disability, for which relief is sought, the result of the pain? What are the patient's expectations for surgery?
5. What is the likely chance the procedure being considered will relieve the patient's pain, to what degree, and for how long?
6. What are the risks?
7. Is the procedure being considered the most cost-effective available in terms of the expected success and risk compared with the degree of disability from pain?

It would seem logical, as in the motor system, to assume that there is a final common path that, when activated by whatever means, results in pain. Intuitively, this path likely resides in cerebral cortex, though possibly not in any constant site within it. Accepting this assumption, Table 13–2 lists possible ways this final common path might be triggered.

Although the mechanisms suggested in the first part of Table 13–2 are speculative, they are not difficult to accept. Allodynia, hyperpathia, and hyperesthesia are reasonably comprehensible if one accepts Lindblom's suggestion[40] that these conditions depend on normal receptor stimulation with perverted central processing. Of course, the specific mechanisms involved are obscure. For example, there never has been an adequate explanation for the pain such as that of sciatica that arises from stimulation of a nerve or root; activation of nervi nervorum or nervi arteriorum has been suggested but never proved.[59] The concept of ectopic impulse generation at a neural injury site or "upstream" from it has often been suggested[91] as a process that results in pain, and it seems a reasonable explanation for the shooting neuralgic pain that accompanies some types of nerve injury. The dependence upon transmission in nociceptive pathways of the pain that results from direct mechanical stimulation of nerves or roots or from impulses generated spontaneously at an ectopic site, as well as the induced discomfort of allodynia, hyperpathia, and hyperesthesia, is suggested from clinical observations

Table 13–2. CHRONIC PAIN SYNDROMES

Chronic Pain Syndromes Dependent on Transmission	Chronic Pain Independent of Transmission	Chronic Pain Related to Sympathetic Function

Through Stimulation of Peripheral Receptors
With normal processing:
  Cancer, osteoarthritis, pancreatitis, migraine
With abnormal processing:
  Hyperpathia, allodynia, hyperesthesia
 	
Without Stimulation of Peripheral Receptors
Normal nerves:
  Neuralgia, cancerous neural compression
Injured nerves:
  (1) Induced—neuroma compression, Tinel's sign
  (2) Spontaneous—lancinating element of neuropathic pain
	Psychogenic
	Steady Element in Neuropathic Pain
		Sympathetically Maintained Pain(SMP)
		Reflex Sympathetic Dystrophy (RSD)

that show relief of these types of pain by interruption of nociceptive transmission.[90]

The mechanisms suggested for chronic pain independent of transmission are also speculative. For psychogenic pain, the concept is intuitive, whereas for neuropathic pain it is based on the clinical observation that the usually burning, dysesthetic, and sometimes aching pain referred to an area of sensory alteration after neurologic injury responds poorly to interruption of sensory transmission.[91] The role of the sympathetic system has been proposed for generations, first by means of ephapses at injury sites[65] and more recently in the construct of sympathetically maintained pain (SMP).[13,67] Parenthetically, the pain is being considered here and not the sympathetic malfunction seen in reflex sympathetic dystrophy (RSD). Finally, tic douloureux (trigeminal neuralgia) is in a class by itself; whatever the pathophysiology, it is cured by, among other strategies, denervation of the part of the head in which the pain is felt, notwithstanding the observation that, with the exception of "triggering," the pain occurs in the absence of peripheral receptor stimulation.

This type of classification, which is fundamentally similar to previous descriptions in this volume (see Chapter 5), will not be acceptable to all. It is doubtlessly flawed, and I hope it will be updated, corrected, and fine-tuned as more information is gathered. It does, however, serve as a rational basis upon which to consider surgery for chronic pain. Current knowledge is such that imperfect results are to be expected even after the most careful matching of pain syndrome against a surgical technique that is performed in an exemplary manner. At present, only tic douloureux can be expected to be treated with a high degree of success.

SURGICAL TREATMENT OF SELECTED PAIN SYNDROMES

Nociceptive Pain

Nociceptive pains may depend on stimulation of nociceptors and transmission in nociceptive pathways, or on direct stimulation of nerves or roots. Some clinical examples of chronic nociceptive pain are listed in Table 13–2. The surgical treatments that arrest transmission of the nociceptive messages presumed to underlie these pains comprise procedures that actually interrupt a pain pathway and procedures that modulate transmission (e.g., morphine infusion or chronic electrical stimulation of the nervous system) (Table 13–3). Pain that arises from direct stimulation of nociceptors is exemplified by cancer in a long bone. A large number of common pain syndromes do not depend on stimulation of peripheral receptors, however, such as the pain caused by compression of a sciatic nerve root by a sequestrated disk, the pain of neuralgia, and that produced by cancerous involvement of the lumbosacral or brachial plexus. The exact mechanism of these types of pain remains elusive, though activation of nervi arteriorum[59] has been implicated. Whatever the cause, the process appears to set up transmission in pain pathways as though peripheral nociceptors had been stimulated. Surgical treatment is identical to that used for

Table 13–3. PROCEDURES THAT ARREST NOCICEPTIVE TRANSMISSION

Interruptive
Neurectomy
Excision or relocation of neuromas
Rhizotomy
Cordotomy
Trigeminal tractotomy
Commissurotomy
Dorsal root entry zone (DREZ) lesions
Stereotactic tractotomy
    Pontine
    Mesencephalic
    Hassler's parvocellularis ventrocaudal nucleus
    Medial thalamus
Sympathectomy

Modulatory
Morphine infusion
    Epidural
    Spinal intrathecal
    Intraventricular
Chronic stimulation
    Periventricular-periaqueductal gray
      (PVG-PAG)

pain caused by peripheral nociceptor stimulation. In fact, the most common indication for cordotomy is malignant lumbosacral plexopathy. All these types of pain are usually considered examples of nociceptive pain.

DESTRUCTIVE PROCEDURES

The use of destructive procedures to manage refractory nociceptive pains is limited largely to the cancer population.[89] Pain related to cancer usually results from stimulation of nociceptors.

Neurectomy and Rhizotomy. Although neurectomy and rhizotomy are conceptually simple, they are seldom useful, because the nonselective neural deficits produced are often unacceptable and nociceptive lesions rarely respect the territories of single or a few nerves or roots. When neurectomy or rhizotomy is indicated, either is best performed with percutaneous rather than open techniques because of the lesser impact on the patient and by radiofrequency lesioning rather than chemical neurolysis. Radiofrequency lesioning avoids the unpredictable spread and penetration of tissues that may occur with the injection of neurolytic solutions and takes advantage of the ease of physiologic guidance and control of lesion size possible with the radiofrequency technique.[84]

In a few patients, percutaneous radiofrequency neurectomy is feasible. This procedure is helpful in patients with cancerous involvement restricted to trigeminal territory (assuming that the anatomy necessary for the procedure has not been destroyed) and those with cancerous involvement of the chest wall. The technique involves an electronic backup unit, which uses electrodes specifically designed for the particular application.

For trigeminal neurectomy, the patient is briefly anesthetized, and a straight electrode, insulated except for 5 mm at its tip, is introduced under radiologic control into Meckel's cave through the foramen ovale. Return of cerebrospinal fluid confirms location among the preganglionic rootlets rather than within nerve or ganglion. In this location, 2-Hz stimulation may induce contractions in the masticatory muscles. The needle should be positioned so that 100-Hz stimulation produces paresthesias in the part of the face afflicted by the pain. A radiofrequency lesion is then made. The size of the lesion is determined by the length of time current flows (usually 90 seconds), the temperature produced at the electrode tip (usually over 80°C), and the current used to make the lesion. In cases of cancer pain, an attempt is made to destroy the entire nerve, making a maximum lesion by gradually increasing current until it "falls off," signaling vaporization and an accompanying rise of impedance.

There are few reports of trigeminal neurectomy in patients with lesions other than tic douloureux. Effective pain relief has been described in 40 to 89 percent of such patients, with complications similar to those listed when the operation is performed for tic (see following).[75,84,92] Percutaneous radiofrequency neurectomy of the lower cranial nerves can also be performed to treat pain due to head and neck cancer.[11,63]

Intercostal neurectomy can relieve refractory chest wall pain. The patient is anesthetized and an electrode with a curved, bare 8- to 10-mm tip is slipped under the trailing edge of each rib. Its position is adjusted until intercostal muscle contractions are produced at 2 Hz using the lowest possible voltage, whereupon a maximum radiofrequency lesion is made.[94]

Migrainous head pain that always affects the same region and is intractable to other therapy is another example of nociceptive-dependent pain that can occasionally be treated by neurectomy.[45] In this condition, the receptors probably reside in the arteries. If the pain occurs in trigeminal territory, trigeminal rhizotomy can be used; otherwise, occipital or superficial artery transection or occipital neurectomy can be considered. Arteriotomy presumably denervates nociceptors directly, and neurectomy presumably denervates areas to which pain is referred.[4]

Another opportunity for neurectomy to treat nociceptor-mediated pain is splanchnicectomy for pain of pancreatic origin. The nociceptive somesthetic fibers, which use the splanchnic nerves and sympathetic trunk as a scaffold to reach the spinal cord, can be interrupted by bilateral exposure and resection of the greater and lesser splanchnic nerves, and section of the sympathetic trunk and adjacent ganglia extrapleurally through the 11th rib bed.[25,69] Up to 70 percent incidence of pain relief has been reported, with some degree of recurrence in 41 percent; a 7 percent mortality rate is the major risk. Percutaneous alcohol blockade of the celiac ganglion may achieve the same effect (see Chapter 12). Moore[51] reported significant pain relief in 94 percent of cases, with a variety of complications such as hypotension, postoperative pain, nerve damage, and subarachnoid injection.

As an alternative to neurectomy, percutaneous radiofrequency dorsal rhizotomy can be considered.[41,95] This procedure has largely replaced open rhizotomy. Under radiologic control, an electrode similar to that used for trigeminal rhizotomy is introduced into the dorsal portion of the appropriate intervertebral foramen. Appropriate position is confirmed by the induction of appropriate paresthesias at minimal threshold, without motor effects. A maximal radiofrequency lesion is then made. The lowermost and uppermost thoracic roots are avoided for fear of concomitant damage to end arteries supplying the spinal cord. Compared with a review of 585 patients with cancer pain who underwent open dorsal rhizotomy and experienced a 59 percent success rate and a 0 to 20 percent mortality rate,[76] the percutaneous technique is without significant mortality and yields up to 70 percent relief. The major morbidity is the risk of temporary paresis, presumably from interference with segmental arteries.[62]

Receptor-dependent nociceptive pain is rarely treated by these methods, and there are no reliable outcome data. One procedure for which abundant experience exists, however, is so-called "facet rhizotomy." This technique is most frequently applied in the patient with chronic low back pain that is specifically aggravated by extension, relieved by local anesthetic facet nerve blocks, and unexplained by pathology capable of treatment by other means. It can be used equally well at any level in the spine. Under radiologic control, large-bore hollow needles are introduced to the sites at which dorsal rami diverge from the anterior rami just beyond the intervertebral foramina and possibly also at sites in which the facet nerves approach the joints. Electrodes with a 5-mm bare tip are then introduced through the needles, which are then partially withdrawn to clear the electrode tips. The location is confirmed physiologically. In the conscious patient,

100-Hz stimulation should induce paresthesias in more or less the same distribution as the patient's pain; in the anesthetized patient, muscular contraction in paravertebral muscles should occur at 2 Hz at a low threshold. No responses should be seen in the sensory or motor distribution of anterior rami. Maximum radiofrequency lesions are then made at each site. Since all posterior rami except those at the C-1 and L-4 to L-5 levels have sensory branches, facet rhizotomy induces clinically detectable sensory loss in a paravertebral strip. This is often temporarily accompanied by postoperative dysesthesias and allodynia. At the upper end of the spine, the sensory distribution of the posterior rami expands enormously to include the territory of the occipital nerves, while those from L-1, L-2, and L-3 expand to supply the rather extensive territory of the cluneal nerves.

Oudenhaven[61] reported the results of facet rhizotomy in 66 patients. Among those who had not undergone previous spinal surgery, outcome was excellent in 74 percent and good in 15 percent. Among those who had earlier surgery, excellent results were achieved by 35 percent and good results, by 24 percent. Both Burton[12] and McCulloch[46] reported 67 percent success in unoperated patients, while Dunsker et al[18] observed favorable results in only 20 percent of patients overall and 40 percent after previously successful local anesthetic facet blocks.

Procedures Performed on the Spinal Cord. A variety of percutaneous procedures directed toward the spinal cord have been described, including trigeminal tractotomy[16,28]; commissurotomy[29]; and cordotomy by the low anterior cervical,[39] high dorsal cervical,[27] and high lateral cervical approaches.[53] Percutaneous cordotomy appears to be most often employed.

Percutaneous Cordotomy. Incorporating all the advantages of open cordotomy—selective interruption of pain and temperature pathways—the percutaneous technique exposes the patient to less impact and offers easily incorporated physiologic localization and a precisely tailored radiofrequency lesion.[2] For these reasons, percutaneous cordotomy is the most successful pain operation other than those for tic douloureux. It is usually the procedure of choice, because it is not often that nociceptor-based pain falls within the range of a single or a few peripheral nerves or roots with expendable sensory or motor function. The selective elimination of pain transmission that spares other sensory and motor functions achieved by cordotomy is the ideal alternative.

The favored lateral high cervical approach has been perfected by the use of impedance recording,[21] radiofrequency lesioning,[68] and positive contrast imaging.[60] With the patient heavily sedated or briefly anesthetized, the cord is impaled to a depth of 2 mm with a special cordotomy electrode. The cord is entered at its equator in the occipital C-1 or, usually, the C1-2 interspace (Fig. 13–1). Myelographic and impedance control is maintained, and penetration is confined to 2 mm by the electrode's Teflon tubing insulation, which leaves a projecting 2-mm sharpened bare tip. Stimulation at 2 Hz should induce ipsilateral motor responses confined to neck, upper limb, or both; 100-Hz stimulation should produce no motor response but a contralateral sensory effect, usually of warmth or cold. If the latter

occurs in the lower limb, the tip is likely in the distal part of the spinothalamic homunculus. A lesion here tends to produce a lower level of dissociated sensory loss. If paresthesias occur in the hand, the tip is more centrally located and more extensive contralateral sensory loss results.

Cordotomy is effective for pain below the C-5 dermatome—the highest level at which analgesia consistently persists—and is contraindicated if the only effective lung (the only one not impaired, for example, by diaphragmatic paralysis, partial or complete pneumonectomy, or other disease) is ipsilateral to the proposed cordotomy. The strictly ipsilateral reticulospinal tract responsible for unconscious respiration lies adjacent to the proximal part (upper limb fibers) of the spinothalamic homunculus,[31,57] and its loss will result in inadequate unconscious respiration in patients dependent on the ipsilateral lung alone. For this reason, bilateral cordotomy in patients with two healthy lungs must also be approached with caution. A high level of analgesia must be avoided on at

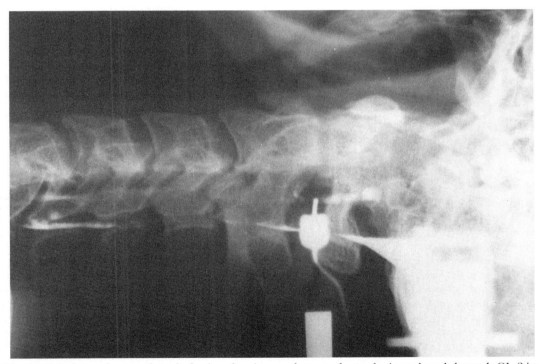

Figure 13–1. Lateral x ray of cervical spine showing cordotomy electrode, introduced through C1–2 interspace, impinging upon cord just anterior to the dentate ligament, visualized with positive contrast medium. The dorsal meninges and anterior margin of the cord are also outlined.

least one side to avoid damaging the reticulospinal tract alongside spinothalamic fibers from the upper limb. Bilateral cordotomy, although sometimes necessary, is also somewhat unsatisfactory for the relief of midline (especially pelvic-perineal) pain, possibly because such pain is often accompanied by a deafferentation element immune to relief by cordotomy.[48]

With experience, unilateral cordotomy can be accomplished with technical success, defined by the expected levels of analgesia in 99 percent of patients. Technical success is even likely among those who are uncooperative and must be placed under general anesthesia, which forecloses the guidance provided by 100-Hz–induced contralateral sensory effects.[85,87]

Complications from unilateral cordotomy include mortality (0.3 percent), temporary respiratory suppression (0.5 percent), significant persistent (0.5 percent) and transient (16.8 percent) paresis, significant bladder dysfunction (2.9 percent), and significant postcordotomy dysesthesias (3 percent). Bilateral procedures carry a 1 percent mortality and a 20 percent risk of bladder dysfunction.

Success in producing adequate contralateral analgesia during cordotomy does not ensure pain relief. About 41 percent of patients develop significant pain on the opposite side of the body, including 2.6 percent with recurrent pain from a falling or inadequate level of analgesia, 5 percent from upward advancement of cancer, and 34 percent with a usually lesser degree of persistent or recurrent pain below an adequate level of analgesia. The latter phenomenon is presumably caused by a component of deafferentation pain accompanying the nociceptive pain caused by the cancer. In my series,[85,87] unilateral cordotomy yielded long-term freedom from the pain to which the cordotomy had been directed in 72 percent of patients, and 84 percent experienced no significant residual pain; after bilateral surgery, significant pain relief was reported by 72 percent.

Alternatives to Cordotomy. Alternatives to cordotomy are limited when respiratory function is at risk, pain is midline in lower trunk, or pain extends above C-5. There is no procedure as effective as cordotomy. Procedures to be considered are commissurotomy,[29] Sindou's dorsal root entry zone procedure,[76] destructive procedures aimed at the brain, or modulatory operations.

COMMISSUROTOMY. Commissurotomy, introduced by Armour,[3] was originally performed by open means. Recently, the open technique has been supplanted by the percutaneous technique introduced by Hitchcock,[29] which is performed percutaneously through the occipital C-1 interspace dorsally in a similar fashion to percutaneous cordotomy. Pain relief was originally believed to result from interruption of decussating spinothalamic fibers but is now thought to occur through interruption of an unknown pain pathway other than the spinothalamic tract. Pain relief, reported in 78 to 100 percent of cases, is not related to the unpredictably located and often transient analgesia that the lesion produces and may occur at sites that are apparently somatotopographically remote from the lesion site.[15,73] Occasional adverse consequences include dysmetria and gait ataxia.

THE SINDOU PROCEDURE. Lesions of Lissauer's tract in the dorsal root entry zone were originally added by Hyndman[34] during open cordotomy to cut spinothalamic fibers missed by the cordotomy lesion while in the process of decussating and thereby raise the level of analgesia by a segment or two. Sindou[76,77] advocated making a series of 1-mm incisions angled at 45° in the cord just lateral to the sites of entry of cervical dorsal roots somatotopographically related to the patient's pain, thus avoiding risk of respiratory function and achieving analgesia more rostral than that achieved at C-5. He cautioned, however, against making lesions at C-4, lest phrenic function be compromised. He reported 65 percent pain relief with a 5 percent mortality; a 15 percent incidence of leg weakness was the chief complication.

Procedures Performed on the Brain. Most destructive procedures in brain attempt to interrupt the spinoreticulothalamic tract.

Spinothalamic Tractotomy. For patients unsuited to cordotomy and those with appropriate types of pain in the head or neck, stereotactic procedures in the brain can be considered. Four operations are apparently in regular use, three of them rostral extensions of cordotomy, plus medial thalamotomy.

As the spinothalamic tract passes rostrally through the brainstem, it traverses the pons and midbrain and comes to lie on the inferolateral margin of the sensory relay nucleus in thalamus—Hassler's parvocellularis ventrocaudal nucleus (VCpc).[26] Hitchcock[30] has advocated stereotactic interruption of the pain pathway at the pontine level using a radiofrequency lesion; he has reported promising results, but the technique has not been widely employed. A number of authors have made lesions in Hassler's VCpc,[23,32] also with favorable results.

The most popular procedure, however, is stereotactic mesencephalic tractotomy. Introduced by Spiegel and Wycis[78] as a safer and physiologically controlled replacement of the original open tractotomy, it has a much lower incidence of postoperative dysesthetic effects than the latter. Performed like any other functional stereotactic procedure, it begins with the application of a suitable stereotactic frame to the head. CT or MRI imaging is then carried out to derive the stereotactic coordinates of anterior (AC) and posterior commissures (PC) (Figs. 13–2 and 13–3). With reference to a brain atlas (Fig. 13–4), the expected location of the mesencephalic spinothalamic tract is extrapolated from the positions of these structures, and its position is confirmed

relative to the medial lemniscus by stimulation. Stimulation of the medial lemniscus produces contralateral somatotopographically organized paresthesias, whereas stimulation of the spinothalamic tract produces contralateral, somatotopographically organized, usually warm or cold effects. When suitable positioning is obtained, a radiofrequency lesion is made with a specially designed thalamotomy electrode (Fig. 13–5). The lesion includes the spinothalamic tract and structures immediately medial to it; it extends as far as the periaqueductal gray and is thought to include the nonsomatotopographically organized pain fibers that project to medial thalamus and cannot be easily recognized physiologically (Fig. 13–6).

Relief of nociceptive-dependent pain has been reported in 67 to 100 percent of patients who have undergone mesencephalic tractotomy. There has been a 6.5 to 38 percent mortality, and complications have included dysesthesia (5 percent), paresis (7 percent), oculomotor disturbances (13 to 88 percent), ataxia (4 percent), and hearing loss (50 percent).[1,6,19, 55, 78, 97]

Medial Thalamotomy. An alternative to the

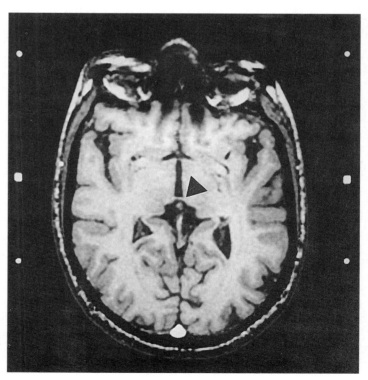

Figure 13–2. Axial magnetic resonance imaging (MRI) scan of brain showing posterior commissure (arrowhead).

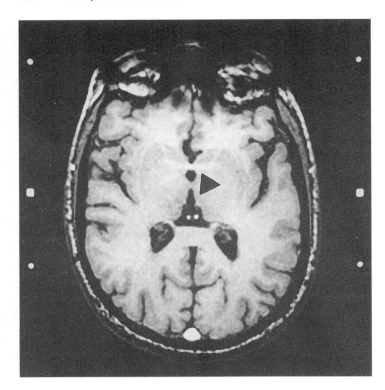

Figure 13–3. Axial MRI scan of brain showing anterior commissure (arrowhead).

foregoing procedure is medial thalamotomy, which is directed at the parafascicular (PF)-intralaminar region and is thought to destroy the projection sites of the nonsomatotopographically arranged pain pathway mentioned previously (Fig. 13–7). As Frank et al[19] and others[70,71,83] have shown, this procedure achieves results similar to those achieved with mesencephalic tractotomy, with the possible exception of lower incidence of adequate pain relief. In the series of Frank et al, 51.9 percent of patients reported pain relief, compared with 83.5 percent after mesencephalic tractotomy; pain recurrence was also more frequent following thalamotomy. On the other hand, mortality was zero with medial thalamotomy, compared with 1.8 percent with mesencephalic tractotomy, and morbidity with medial thalamotomy consisted of a 10 to 20 percent risk of usually transient cognitive problems, compared with the more serious problems after tractotomy.

Recognition of the medial thalamus by microelectrode recording has been described but, in my experience, is not reliable. The area does not yield recognizable responses to stimulation and usually must be located on anatomic grounds by extrapolation based on the position of the sensory relay nucleus and the AC-PC line.

Other Destructive Techniques. Psychosurgical procedures, particularly cingulotomy, have been advocated to alleviate the suffering that accompanies pain. It is difficult to know the usefulness of this procedure today. Bouckoms[8] suggests a 50 to 75 percent short-term incidence of pain relief at the expense of a 0.1 percent mortality and 0.3 percent morbidity.

Manipulation of the hypothalamo-hypophyseal axis has also been extensively employed as an analgesic procedure. Hypothalamotomy[70] has had limited application, but hypophyseal ablation for the relief of cancer pain, particularly pain associated with endocrine-dependent tumors, is well known. Open hypophysectomy has apparently been largely replaced by the injection of alcohol into the pituitary gland,[52] which is accomplished transphenoidally through a transnasal approach using image intensification. This is

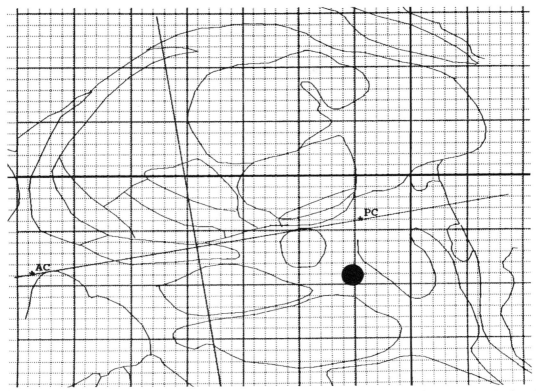

Figure 13–4. 9-mm lateral sagittal brain diagram from atlas by Schaltenbrand and Bailey, stretched and redrawn by computer to match the patient's AC-PC distance and reading in stereotactic frame coordinates. Site of medial lemniscus marked with black dot. (Adapted from Schaltenbrand G, Bailey P: Introduction to Stereotaxis with an Atlas of the Human Brain. Georg Thieme, Stuttgart, 1959.)

a simple procedure that has received wide application, particularly for the pain of cancer. Moreover, although most effective in hormone-dependent cancer, it also appears to relieve to a somewhat lesser extent the pain of non–hormone-dependent disease. The mechanism of pain control is elusive[14,81,82] and does not depend upon hormonal or endorphin-related activity. Unfortunately, the procedure is fraught with a number of usually transient side effects, and pain relief may be short-lived. Pain relief has been reported in 41 to 95 percent of patients with hormone-dependent cancer and 69 percent of those with non–hormone-dependent cancer; these results are achieved at the expense of mortality in 2 to 6.5 percent, rhinorrhea in 3 to 20 percent, meningitis in 0.3 to 1 percent, oculomotor disturbances in 2 to 10 percent, and diabetes insipidus in 5 to 66 percent.[37,50,52]

MODULATORY PROCEDURES

Modulation of pain by nociceptive-dependent processes can be accomplished in two ways. Chronic stimulation of periventricular gray (PVG),[66] which presumably activates a descending serotoninergic pathway, is thought to inhibit access of nociceptive information into the spinothalamic tract and has been used widely in the treatment of the pain associated with chronic degenerative lumbar disk disease. Although it is generally believed that the PVG is part of a midline system that is involved in pain modulation and extends from the rostral third ventricle to the periaqueductal gray (PAG) and that chronic stimulation at sites other than PVG induces unpleasant effects, some authors claim that this is not so and that either PVG or PAG stimulation is practical and effective.[98–100] Moreover, not all au-

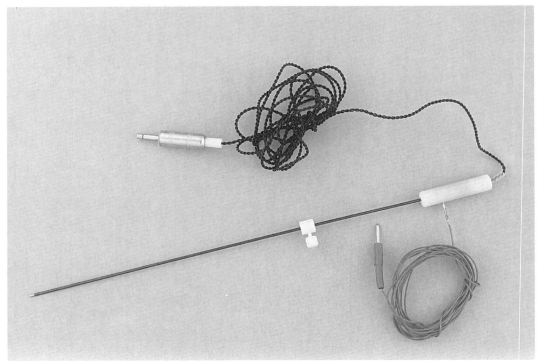

Figure 13–5. Thalamotomy lesion-making electrode from Diros Technology, Inc, Toronto, Ontario, Canada, 1.1-mm diameter with a 3-mm bare tip and fitted with a temperature monitoring probe. (From Arbit E: Anterolateral cordotomy. In Arbit E [ed]: Management of Cancer-Related Pain. Futura Publishing, Mount Kisco, NY, 1993, p 247, with permission.)

thors agree that stimulation of PVG is effective only for the control of nociceptive pain; some believe that stimulation at these sites can be effective for neuropathic pains as well. In contrast to PVG and PAG stimulation, chronic hypothalamic stimulation[70] has been used infrequently.

The usual target for stimulation is thought to consist of the medial portion of PF, which is usually located stereotactically on anatomic grounds—approximately 2 mm from the wall of the third ventricle and 5 mm rostral to PC on the AC-PC line. Physiologic confirmation is elusive. Although some patients experience a diffuse, pleasant, warm effect, a sense of satiety, and pain relief with stimulation of PVG sites, others report no detectable effect other than possibly paresthesias from volume conduction. Even in the absence of physiologic confirmation, however, institution of chronic stimulation may still prove effective.

Long-term stimulation of brain sites is usually effected by attaching the appropriately located electrode to either a totally implantable battery-powered programmable stimulator or to a radiofrequency-coupled receiver. Long-term transcutaneous PVG stimulation also can be effectively used in treating patients with cancer. Pain relief has been quoted at 60 to 80 percent, with 11 percent neurologic complications, 4 to 5 percent infection rate, and 3 to 9 percent incidence of device failure.[38,66,86,98,99]

Another type of modulatory surgery employs spinal epidural or intrathecal opioid infusion (see Chapter 12), or intraventricular opioid infusion. Although these infusion techniques can be performed with a cannula and injectable reservoir, they are more elegantly accomplished when injection is made into the cerebrospinal fluid by programmable pumps. Spinal injections take advantage of the fact that opioids can inhibit access of nociceptive information to the spinothalamic tract at the cord level. Opioid infusion into the third ventricle is widely used in Eu-

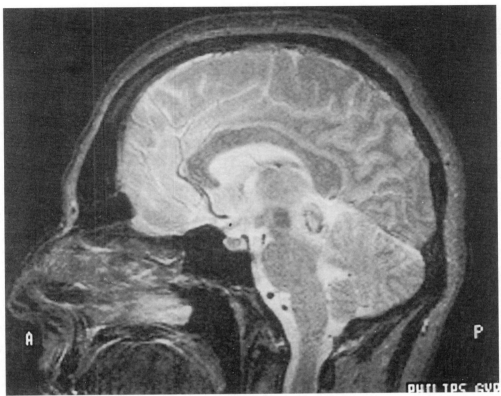

Figure 13–6. Sagittal MRI scan of the brain showing a mesencephalotomy lesion 2 days postoperatively that produced reduction of pain and temperature appreciation in the contralateral upper quarter of the body in a patient with intractable pain from a neurofibrosarcoma of the brachial plexus.

rope. That it remains an experimental procedure in North America is unfortunate, because it appears to be a safe and effective means of controlling nociceptor-based pain untreatable by simpler measures.[17,22]

Modulatory surgery, though attractive by virtue of its reversibility and avoidance of the risks of destructive lesions, does introduce other complications, including equipment failure and, in the case of opioid infusion, drug toxicity. It requires the use of expensive equipment that may be difficult to acquire and may not be cost-effective in the patients who need it most—those with terminal cancer.

The Problem of Neuropathic Pain

The discussion thus far has involved the Cartesian concept of pain dependent upon the stimulation of nociceptors in an apparently normal way (the "normal processing" part of Table 13–2). Pain can also result from aberrant processes established following injury to the nervous system at the level of peripheral nerve, root, plexus, cord, or the brain itself.[91] These neuropathic pains include causalgia, brachial plexus avulsion, postherpetic neuralgia, prolonged incisional pain, phantom and stump pain, postcordotomy dysesthesia, pain associated with cord trauma, stroke-induced pain, and others (see Chapter 5). These conditions tend to be associated with injury to sensory pathways and result in sensory loss that may be subclinical, transient, severe, or even complete. The associated pain is usually referred to the area of sensory change and may consist of steady, intermittent, and evoked elements. The words patients use to describe these pains are pathophysiologically signifi-

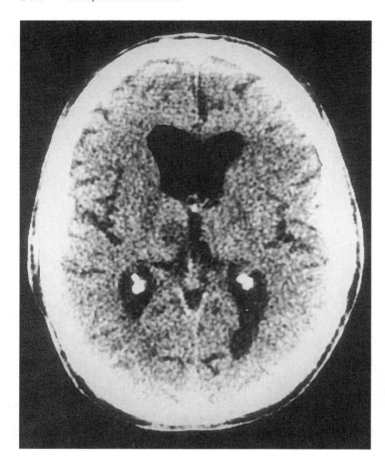

Figure 13–7. Axial computed tomography (CT) scan performed 3 days postoperatively showing a medial thalamic stereotactic lesion centered on parafascicular nucleus that produced no clinically detectable neurologic effect in a patient with metastatic pharyngeal cancer in the brachial plexus.

cant, as suggested by the work of Boureau et al[9] and others. Steady pain is most frequent, occurring in almost every case of neural injury pain and usually reported using descriptors consistent with a dysesthesia, such as burning, tingling, or electrical. Intermittent neuralgic pain is less frequent, as is evoked pain, the incidence of which varies with the type of injury. Both these latter elements can occur in isolation but usually accompany steady pain; in some cases all three are present.

Pain Dependent Upon Stimulation of Receptors With Abnormal Processing

When evoked pain is a component of a neuropathic pain syndrome, it usually consists of an unnatural, unpleasant sensation, which is often associated with temporal or spatial spreading elicited when the skin in the affected area is stimulated. Although taxonomy is difficult, such unpleasant effects, which can occur in areas of both increased and clinically normal sensory threshold (by definition they cannot occur in areas of anesthesia) are designated by the terms *allodynia*, *hyperpathia*, and *hyperesthesia*. They are thought to be dependent upon perverted central processing of incoming sensory information caused by changes wrought by the original neural injury.[40] If this is how evoked pain comes about, then allodynia, hyperpathia, and hyperesthesia (see Table 13–2) might be expected to respond to the same techniques as does nociceptive pain. This expectation is borne out to some extent by experience. Neurectomy or rhizotomy or retransection of spinal cord above a level of damage abolishes these effects at the original site. Because of regeneration or reinnervation from adjacent structures, however, they may persist or recur at the margins of the denervation. In my experience with central pain caused by cord or brain lesions, destructive procedures such as cordotomy, stereotactic mesencephalic tractotomy, and medial thalamotomy appear to have been effective in treating at least small numbers of patients with evoked pain.[90] Three patients with stroke-induced central pain, in which evoked pain was the most prominent element, were relieved by chronic stimulation of PVG. These observations suggest that the spinothalamic tract is involved in evoked pain, though it is still unclear to what extent nonnociceptive pathways may also be implicated.

Pain Dependent Upon Transmission in the Damaged Nervous System

Although it is not difficult to understand a neuralgic component (intermittent, lancinating pain) in neuralgia, sciatica, or cancerous compression of the lumbosacral plexus, all of which have an obvious stimulus source, similar pain may also occur in other types of neuropathic pain without stimulating peripheral receptors (see Table 13–2). The simplest examples are those in which pain is elicited by mechanical stimulation of a site of nerve damage, often in amputation stumps. This is usually attributed to the presence of neuromas. Presumably, such pain depends on a similar mechanism to that entrained by a ruptured disk or cancerous plexopathy and is susceptible to the same surgical treatment. Usually, however, peripheral resections and burial of neuromas are used, with variable degrees of success because neuromas tend to recur.

Not all intermittent neuralgic pain in neuropathic syndromes has such an obvious mechanism, however. As mentioned previously, pain associated with injury to peripheral nerve, plexus, root, cord, or brain may be associated with spontaneous neuralgic elements, which rarely occur alone and are usually accompanied by steady pain, the incidence of which varies with the syndrome.

This neuralgia seems to occur unrelated to any obvious manipulation. When present, it is usually the most severe problem. It is rare in stroke-induced central pain but very common in the pain of spinal cord injury, particularly with incomplete lesions in the conus/cauda region. The incidence is variable with more peripheral lesions.[90]

There is considerable published experience with surgical treatment of this intermittent pain (which often occurs in a radicular distribution) in patients with spinal cord injury.[7,64] This experience indicates that destructive lesions such as cordotomy and "cordectomy"[36] (i.e., retransection of spinal cord above the level of injury) are very effective, as is the dorsal root entry zone (DREZ) operation advocated by Nashold. In contradistinction to Sindou, Nashold advocated making rows of small radiofrequency lesions in the exposed spinal cord at the sites of dorsal rootlets that are somatotopographically related to the patient's pain. This lesion, used to treat certain pain syndromes caused by neurologic damage, has proved very effective for the pain that results from avulsion of the brachial and lumbosacral plexus (where lesions are actually made in the pits out of which the rootlets were avulsed) and the pain that may follow injury to the spinal cord. The patients with cord injury who achieve the best results appear similar to those who respond to cordectomy and cordotomy[20]—that is, those with neuralgic lancinating pain. Nashold and colleagues have also advocated a trigeminal DREZ procedure,[56] a series of small radiofrequency lesions made in the exposed trigeminal caudal nucleus, for pain syndromes involving the fifth nerve, especially postherpetic neuralgia. This may also be an example of interruption of nociceptive transmission to relieve essentially intermittent and evoked pain.

My colleagues and I[90] have shown that destructive procedures aimed at interrupting pain pathways are generally selectively effective for the intermittent, lancinating element of central pain caused both by cord and brain lesions. This further suggests that intermittent lancinating pain may be considered an indicator of potential response to neuroablative procedures, regardless of the underlying pathophysiology of the pain syndrome of which it is part. Such clinical observations also suggest that spontaneous intermittent and evoked pains associated with neuropathic pain syndromes are dependent on nociceptive transmission, though clearly not upon stimulation of receptors. Ectopic impulses instituted at an injury site or at a site proximal to it may explain neuropathic pain and may be the basis of the neuralgic component.

Pain Involving the Sympathetic Nervous System

The role of the sympathetic nervous system in chronic pain is confusing. The striking sympathetic dysfunction manifest by swelling, color, and temperature change, and by the dystrophic phenomena that accompany the pain of reflex sympathetic dystrophy (RSD) are well known, and RSD sometimes complicates neuropathic pain syndromes. The relief of such sympathetic effects by sympathetic blockade led to the application of sympathectomy, not only for the treatment of the associated manifestations but also for the pain itself. Sympathetic blockade has even been used for neuropathic pain without the classical findings of RSD. Terms such as "causalgia," "RSD," and "deafferentation pain syndrome" came to be used interchangeably, and the notion was advanced that neuropathic pain may result from sympathetic activation of nociceptive transmission via ephapses at the injury site. Although sympathetic blockade has usually been effective in relieving sympathetic hyperfunction, it has often failed to relieve the pain associated with neural injury, whether or not accompanied by other sympathetic signs.

Sympathetic blockade does succeed in some cases, most notably in patients with so-called "major causalgia" as defined by Bonica.[5] Nathan and co-workers[42,43] pointed out that proximal or distal sympathetic blockade sometimes abolished the pain caused by injury in either the peripheral or the central nervous system; relief was more likely if allodynia or hyperpathia was present. Roberts[67] suggested that the term "sympathetically maintained pain" (SMP) be applied to neural injury pain that is reduced by sympathetic blockade; he

proposed that the pain in these cases results from sympathetically stimulated mechanoreceptors, which activate sensitized central projection neurons. Sympathetic involvement in neural injury pain has been vigorously pursued by Campbell and coworkers,[13] who feel that SMP in some cases of nerve injury may result from sympathetic drive of nociceptors rendered susceptible by injury. Such an injury may sensitize central neurons, producing an enhanced response to low-threshold mechanoreceptors and an increase in adrenergic receptors in the periphery, which may then be activated further by norepinephrine release from sympathetic fibers. All this may produce a vicious cycle. Whatever the actual mechanisms, there appear to be patients in whom pain depends on impulse transmission driven by the sympathetic nervous system. These patients may be candidates for sympathectomy in carefully selected circumstances.

Tic Douloureux

Peculiar to cranial nerves, nearly always the fifth, and diagnosable only by history, tic douloureux (trigeminal neuralgia) stands in a class by itself (Table 13–2). The pain is intermittent, lancinating, and referred to a consistent portion of trigeminal (occasionally other cranial nerve) territory. Hypotheses too numerous to mention have been proposed to explain its occurrence, the most popular being irritation of the proximal portion of the root by the pulsation of an artery. Other etiologies, however, such as a plaque of multiple sclerosis or a schwannoma, may cause identical pain. Whatever the mechanism, tic apparently does not depend on stimulation of peripheral receptors (except for "triggering") but depends on transmission, perhaps in pain fibers in the nerve whose source of activation remains a mystery. Antidromic activation was proposed long ago by Turnbull and colleagues[93] on the basis of laboratory models.

As noted previously, the pain of tic douloureux is always completely and permanently stopped by complete interruption of those fibers of the nerve that serve the area of the face in which the pain is felt; recurrence after such interruption occurs only if there is nerve regeneration. Thus, tic surgery is the most successful pain surgery. The pain also may be relieved by less-than-complete nerve interruption and possibly by selective interruption of pain fibers upon which it may be dependent. Instillation of glycerol[24] in Meckel's cave, partial sensory loss from radiofrequency coagulation,[92] and surgical traumatization of the roots in Meckel's cave (by open means, as advocated by Taarnhoj,[80] or by balloon cannula, as suggested by Mullan and Lichtor[54]) all may arrest the pain. Finally, pain may be alleviated by microvascular decompression in the posterior fossa,[35] in which an artery or, occasionally, a vein, that is usually found compressing the root near the pons is dissected away from the nerve and separated from it by some type of insulating material.

The plethora of surgical procedures (Table 13–4) suggested for the relief of medically intractable tic douloureux makes the choice of operation difficult. The final decision depends on the age, health, and personal preferences of the patient, and the location of the pain. The most conservative approach consists of infraorbital, mental, or supraorbital nerve avulsion, accomplished by open means or alcohol block for pain confined to the territories of these nerves. Unfortunately, nerve regeneration results in pain recurrence within a year or two, which requires repetition of the procedure. Nevertheless, the mortality is low and dysesthetic complications are rare. Somewhat less conservative is glycerol injection or radiofrequency coagulation of the gasserian ganglion and/or preganglionic rootlets in

Meckel's cave. Long-term relief is produced in 60 to 70 percent of patients after either procedure. These are relatively low-impact operations performed percutaneously through the foramen ovale under image intensification. Either glycerol is layered into the cerebrospinal fluid in Meckel's cave or analgesia in the area of pain is produced by the radiofrequency technique described earlier in this chapter. Mortality is low, perhaps 1 in 1000 from intracranial hemorrhage caused by blood pressure escalations or direct damage to the internal carotid artery, both of which are avoidable. Meningitis and abscess can occur. Other side effects include usually transient auditory phenomena, unilateral masticatory weakness from motor root damage (occurring in up to 25 percent of patients after the radiofrequency technique), and usually temporary diplopia (2 percent risk). Both procedures may result in sensory loss. This is inevitable after the radiofrequency technique and is a nuisance in itself; it is also associated with a 14 to 27 percent incidence of dysesthesia, which is significant in 5 percent. This complication is more common in older patients, after dense sensory loss, and following V_1 involvement.

There is little experience with Mullan's compression procedure, and Taarnhoj's operation is probably rarely performed today. Microvascular decompression, however, has become very popular, particularly by virtue of the usual but not inevitable avoidance of sensory loss and dysesthetic effects. It can cer-

Table 13–4. **SURGICAL PROCEDURES FOR TIC DOULOUREUX (TRIGEMINAL NEURALGIA)**

```
   I. Neurectomy
  II. Rhizotomy
      A. Middle fossa
         1. Open
         2. Percutaneous
            a. Alcohol
            b. Glycerol
            c. Radiofrequency (RF)
      B. Posterior fossa
 III. Compression/Decompression
      A. Middle fossa
         1. Open
         2. Percutaneous balloon
      B. Posterior fossa
```

tainly be offered to any fit patient and is particularly valuable for V_1 pain, for which it provides a good chance of relief while avoiding
corneal anesthesia and the high risk of anesthesia dolorosa after V_1 denervation. However, the mortality is 10 times that of the percutaneous procedures, it has its own peculiar
severe complications, and the incidence of
long-term pain relief is similar to that of the
percutaneous procedures.

Pain Apparently Not Dependent Upon Transmission

At first glance, it may be difficult to con-
ceive of pain that does not depend upon
transmission in pain pathways, other than
the rare purely psychogenic pain seen occasionally in schizophrenics and hysterics,
which is presumably fed into the final common path by cortical input (see Table 13–2).
But other pains behave clinically as if they
are independent of transmission in sensory
pathways, such as the spontaneous, steady,
often burning (causalgic) or dysesthetic
pain that may accompany damage to any
level of the nervous system. In my experience, this constant pain, which has been
termed "deafferentation pain" (see Chapter
5), is usually felt in the same part of the body
as that affected by damage to the sensory
pathways, responds poorly to opioids and
better to drugs such as thiopental sodium
and amitriptyline, and is transiently relieved
by proximal or distal local anesthetic blockade. This pain is not usually permanently relieved by interruption of somatosensory
pathways.[91] This dichotomy of response between the constant and the intermittent and
evoked elements of neuropathic pain[90] is
clearest in central pain following spinal cord
injury.

TREATMENT WITH CHRONIC STIMULATION

A new era in the treatment of the so-called
deafferentation pains appeared when
chronic stimulating techniques came into
service. Their development followed the
proposal of the gate control theory.[47] Paradoxically, however, constant dysesthetic pain
that is refractory to interruption of nocicep-

tive transmission responds best, not the nociceptive pain that is suggested by the gate
control theory. Furthermore, such neuropathic pains appear to be treated best by
chronic stimulation that induces paresthesias in the patient's area of pain.[88] A commonly held view is that constant dysesthetic
pain is centrally generated by perverted
function, the result of deafferentation, in
much the same way as epileptic foci are established, and that chronic stimulation in
some way suppresses this abnormal activity
(Table 13–5).

Chronic stimulation is usually preceded by
temporary implantation of an electrode on
nerve, cord, or in brain so as to produce
paresthesias in the painful area. After a trial of
several days, a decision is made about permanent stimulation on the basis of the pain relief achieved during the trial. If permanent
stimulation is warranted, either a battery-powered, totally implantable programmable or a
radiofrequency-coupled stimulating device is
attached to the electrode.

Although, conceptually, the simplest stimulation technique applies current to peripheral nerves,[96] this procedure usually requires
open exposure of an already damaged nerve,
thus detracting from its usefulness. An exception is chronic stimulation of the trigeminal nerve. Originally undertaken through a
temporal craniotomy, during which an electrode was implanted on Meckel's cave,[49] it is
more readily accomplished percutaneously
through the foramen ovale, as advocated by
Steude et al.[79] The desired position of the
electrode can be established under image intensification with trial stimulation. Such stimulation is useful to treat dysesthetic pain after
denervating surgery, inadvertent iatrogenic
damage, or trauma. In the author's experience, it has not proven useful for posther-

Table 13–5. PROCEDURES THAT TREAT PAIN SYNDROMES INDEPENDENT OF TRANSMISSION

Chronic Stimulation
    Nerve, especially fifth nerve
    Dorsal columns
    Lemniscal pathway in brain
Tractotomy to reestablish input balance?

petic neuralgia and, obviously, it cannot be effective if the portion of the nerve related to the pain has been completely sectioned at, or proximal to, the site of stimulation.

With peripheral nerve stimulation, pain relief has been reported in 30 to 50 percent of patients. Pain tends to recur with time.[84] In one survey of trigeminal stimulation, for example, 56 percent of patients achieved relief during a trial of stimulation and went on to implantation of a permanent system; 75 percent continued to get long-term relief.[49]

Stimulation of the dorsal columns is now a commonplace procedure. Although originally performed by open laminectomy,[74] it is now usually accomplished percutaneously[33] with a monopolar or multipolar wire electrode. Flat electrodes introduced by open laminotomy are also available. Wire electrodes are introduced epidurally under local anesthesia and image intensification. They enter the spine approximately mid-dorsally and are positioned with intermittent stimulation until paresthesias are produced in the patient's area of pain. The electrode is anchored (if not, it will migrate inward or avulse) and tunneled to a lateral incision to minimize infection. The patient is then instructed to engage in trial stimulation for several days to verify that the paresthesias are appropriately located and that significant pain relief is occurring without unpleasant effects.

Dorsal column stimulation is possible only if there has been no previous spinal surgery in the area of the implant, because surgery obliterates the epidural space. It is most effective for pain resulting from peripheral nerve lesions or damage to nerve roots by disk disease and for the pain caused by injury to the cauda equina. My experience has not found it very effective in postherpetic neuralgia, postthoracotomy syndrome, amputation-related pain, and central poststroke pain. Adequate paresthesias can seldom be achieved after severe cord damage and some amputations. Most authors report that 40 to 50 percent of patients obtain success with trial stimulation and that 60 to 84 percent of these patients achieve long-term relief.[84]

Severe complications are rare in dorsal column stimulation. Cord damage, hematoma, and abscess appear to be almost nonexistent; 4 percent of patients develop superficial infections and 25 percent suffer late technical problems, including lead migration. Recent publications suggest that the more versatile the equipment, the more likely the success. Hence, a multipolar lead with a multiprogrammable stimulator, which allows for a variety of choices of stimulation sites in case the electrode migrates,[58] may be preferable.

In patients unable to receive dorsal column stimulation, stereotactic chronic stimulation of medial lemniscus, ventrobasal complex, or internal capsule can be considered.[44] My experience is that, if technically adequate dorsal column stimulation fails, so, usually, does brain stimulation. The stereotactic procedure is carried out as described and the location of the selected target is confirmed by producing paresthesias in the appropriate site. Test stimulation is performed as in dorsal column stimulation, and a successful test period is followed by implantation.

With brain stimulation, the risks are greater. There is a 1 to 2 percent major morbidity/mortality from intracranial hemorrhage and a 10 to 20 percent risk of transient neurologic complications, in additional to the same incidence of infection and technical failure reported for dorsal column stimulation. Levy and colleagues[38] found a 24 percent overall success rate for central pain due to brain injury, a 12.5 percent success rate for central pain due to cord injury, and a 32 percent success rate for peripheral deafferentation pain; there was a 0.7 percent mortality rate, and there were infections in 12.1 percent, intracranial infection in 3.5 percent, skin erosion in 7.1 percent, and foreign body reaction in 5.0 percent. In patients with disk-related pain, 32 percent enjoyed long-term success. These researchers[38] reviewed world experience, including 628 patients suffering from neural injury pain, and suggested that long-term success ranged from 29 to 82 percent and averaged 47 percent; for the 337 patients with nociceptive pain, the response was 60 percent.

My experience with deep brain stimulation has included 35 percent overall long-term relief of central pain due to brain injury, 31 percent relief of central pain due to cord injury, and 37 percent relief of pain caused by peripheral injury. There was 1.6 percent mortality, 11 percent incidence of hematoma (which resulted in only transient neurologic complications in all but one patient), and an 8 percent infection rate. In central pain due to brain injury, stimulation may prove unpleasant if a major element of the pain comprises allodynia or hyperpathia.

COMPARISON OF STIMULATION AND DESTRUCTIVE SURGERY

In my experience,[90] stimulation techniques for central pain due to cord injury have resulted in relief of the steady element of pain in 36 percent of patients, whereas destructive procedures achieved relief in 26 percent—not a large difference. The opposite results occurred with treatment of intermittent pain. Thus, the choice of stimulation over destructive procedures rests not so much with the likelihood of success but, rather, with the fact that stimulation techniques are reversible, low-risk affairs compared with the destructive techniques. Yet a small number of patients with steady, burning, dysesthetic pain caused by damage to the nervous system are relieved by interruption of the nociceptive pathways. Indeed, some authors, such as Schieff and Nashold,[72] advocate mesencephalic tractotomy in the treatment of central pain caused by stroke.

The pathophysiologic processes that could account for these observations are unknown. One proposal, reiterated by Bowsher,[10] is that some types of central pain could result from selective damage to the spinothalamic tract. This damage may spare the reticulothalamic tract, and the imbalanced input in some way causes a central perturbation that results in pain. Such an explanation would clarify why completing the interruption of nociceptive pathways by adding that of the reticulospinal tract might correct that imbalance and relieve the pain. Further observations are required to evaluate this hypothesis.

SUMMARY

Surgical procedures intended for the relief of chronic pain are typically considered in refractory cases. For carefully selected patients, these procedures can provide dramatic relief. A very large number of surgical techniques have been devised. In the absence of a pain toxonomy based on known pathophysiology, the selection of an appropriate procedure must be based on clinical inference and experience. The descriptors patients use to describe their pain are important in the effort to select patients for surgical approaches.

For pains that appear to depend on nociceptor input, neurodestructive techniques can be considered in the proper clinical setting. Cordotomy is the most effective and widely used of these techniques, and others have been developed for every level of the nervous system. Patients with some types of neuropathic pain may also respond to neurolysis; evoked pain and neuralgic pain appear to be more amenable to denervating procedures than other types. Occasional patients with sympathetically maintained pain may be candidates for sympathectomy. Patients with steady pains associated with deafferentation are usually best considered for stimulation procedures. Dorsal column stimulation is now commonplace, and some patients are candidates for other approaches such as peripheral nerve stimulation or deep brain stimulation.

All surgical approaches are associated with a risk of morbidity and mortality. Their safe and effective use requires careful patient selection and a skilled clinician. Further elucidation of pain pathophysiologies in the future is likely to provide a more scientific rationale for these techniques.

REFERENCES

1. Amano K, Kawamura H, Tanikawa T, et al: Long-term follow-up study of rostral mesencephalic reticulotomy for pain relief. Report of 34 cases. Applied Neurophysiology 49:105–111, 1986.
2. Arbit E: Anterolateral cordotomy. In Arbit E (ed): Management of Cancer-Related Pain. Futura Publishing, Mount Kisco, NY, 1993, pp 321–332.
3. Armour D: Surgery of the spinal cord and its membranes. Lancet 2:691–697, 1927.
4. Blume HG: Radiofrequency denervation in occipital pain: A new approach in 114 cases. In Bonica JJ, and Albe-Fessard D (eds): Advances in Pain Research and Therapy, Vol 1. Raven Press, New York, 1976, pp 691–698.
5. Bonica JJ: Causalgia and other reflex sympathetic dystrophies. In Bonica JJ, Liebeskind JC, and Albe-Fessard DG (eds): Advances in Pain Research and Therapy, Vol 3. Raven Press, New York, 1979, pp 141–166.

6. Bosch DA: Stereotactic rostral mesencephalotomy in cancer pain and deafferentation pain. A series of 40 cases with follow-up results. J Neurosurg 75: 747–751, 1991.

7. Botterell EH, Callaghan JC, and Jousse AT: Pain in paraplegia. Proceedings of the Royal Society of Medicine 47:17–24, 1953.

8. Bouckoms AJ: Psychosurgery for pain. In Wall PD, and Melzack R (eds): Textbook of Pain, ed 2. Churchill Livingstone, Edinburgh, 1988, pp 868–881.

9. Boureau F, Doubrere JF, and Luu M: Study of verbal description in neuropathic pain. Pain 42:145–152, 1990.

10. Bowsher D: The problem of central pain. Verh der Dtsch Gesellschaft für Inn Med 86;1535–1538, 1980.

11. Broggi GC: Surgical treatment of glossopharyngeal neuralgia and pain from cancer of the nasopharynx. J Neurosurg 1984, 61:952–955.

12. Burton CV: Percutaneous radiofrequency facet denervation. Appl Neurophysiol 39:80–86, 1976.

13. Campbell JN, Raja SN, and Meyer RA: Painful sequelae of nerve injury. In Dubner R, Gebhart GF, and Bond MR (eds): Proc V World Congress on Pain. Research and Clinical Management, Vol 3. Elsevier, Amsterdam, 1988, pp 135–143.

14. Capper SJ, Conton JM, Lahuerta J, et al: Peptide concentrations in the CSF following injection of alcohol into the pituitary gland. Pain Suppl 2:S316, 1984.

15. Cook AW, Nathan PW, and Smith MC: Sensory consequences of commissural myelotomy: A challenge to traditional anatomical concepts. Brain 107:547–568, 1984.

16. Crue BL, Todd EM, and Carregal EJ: Percutaneous radiofrequency stereotactic trigeminal tractotomy. In Crue BL (ed): Pain and Suffering. Charles C Thomas, Springfield, IL, 1970, pp 69–79.

17. Dennis GC, and DeWitty RL: Long-term intraventricular infusion of morphine for intractable pain in cancer of the head and neck. Neurosurgery 26: 404–408, 1990.

18. Dunsker SB, Wood M, Lotspeich EJ, et al: Percutaneous electrocoagulation of lumbar articular nerves. In Lee JF (ed): Pain Management. Williams & Wilkins, Baltimore, 1977, pp 123–127.

19. Frank F, Fabrizi AP, Gaist G, et al: Stereotactic lesions in the treatment of chronic cancer pain syndromes: Mesencephalotomy versus multiple thalamotomies in the treatment of chronic cancer pain syndromes. Applied Neurophysiology 50:314–318, 1987.

20. Friedman AH, and Bullitt E: Dorsal root entry zone lesions in the treatment of pain following spinal cord injury and herpes zoster. Applied Neurophysiology 51:164–169, 1988.

21. Gildenberg PL, Zanes C, Flitter MA, et al: Impedance monitoring device for detection of penetration of the spinal cord in anterior percutaneous cervical cordotomy: Technical note. J Neurosurg 30:87–92, 1969.

22. Gybels JM, and Sweet WH: Neurosurgical Treatment of Persistent Pain: Physiological and Pathological Mechanisms of Human Pain. Karger, Basel, 1989, pp 319–343.

23. Halliday AM, and Logue V: Painful sensations evoked by electrical stimulation in the thalamus. In Somjen G (ed): Neurophysiology Studied in Man. Excerpta Medica, Amsterdam, 1972, pp 221–230.

24. Hakansson J: Trigeminal neuralgia treated by the injection of glycerol into the trigeminal cistern. Neurosurgery 9:638–646, 1981.

25. Hardy RW Jr: Surgery of the sympathetic nervous system. In Schmidek HH, and Sweet WH (eds): Operative Neurosurgical Techniques. Indications, Methods, and Results. Grune and Stratton, New York, 1982, pp 1045–1061.

26. Hassler R: The division of pain conduction into systems of pain sensation and pain awareness. In Janzen R, Keidel WD, Herz A, et al (eds): Pain: Basic Principles—Pharmacology—Therapy. George Thieme, Stuttgart, 1972, pp 98–112.

27. Hitchcock ER: An apparatus for stereotactic spinal surgery. A preliminary report. J Neurosurg 31:386–392, 1969.

28. Hitchcock ER: Stereotactic trigeminal tractotomy. Annals of Clinical Research 2:131–135, 1970.

29. Hitchcock ER: Stereotactic cervical myelotomy. J Neurol Neurosurg Psychiatry 33:224–230, 1970.

30. Hitchcock ER: Stereotaxic pontine spinothalamic tractotomy. J Neurosurg 39:746–752, 1973.

31. Hitchcock ER, and Leece B: Somatotopic representation of the respiratory pathways in the cervical cord of man. J Neurosurg 27:320–329, 1967.

32. Hitchcock ER, and Teixeira MJ: A comparison of results from center-median and basal thalamotomies for pain. Surg Neurol 15:341–351, 1981.

33. Hoppenstein R: Percutaneous implantation of chronic spinal cord electrode for control of intractable pain. Preliminary report. Surg Neurol 4:195–198, 1975.

34. Hyndman OR: Lissauer's tract section: A contribution to chordotomy for the relief of pain (preliminary report). J Int Coll Surg 5:394–400, 1942.

35. Jannetta PJ: Arterial compression of the trigeminal nerve at the pons in patients with trigeminal neuralgia. J Neurosurg 26:159–162, 1967.

36. Jefferson A: Cordectomy for intractable pain in paraplegia. Persistent Pain, 4:115–132, 1983.

37. Levin AB: Stereotactic chemical hypophysectomy. In Lunsford LD (ed): Modern Stereotactic Neurosurgery. Martinus Nijhoff, Boston, 1988, pp 365–375.

38. Levy RM, Lamb S, and Adams JE: Treatment of chronic pain by deep brain stimulation: Long term follow-up and review of the literature. Neurosurgery 21:885–893, 1987.

39. Lin RM, Gildenberg PL, and Polakoff PP: An anterior approach to percutaneous lower cervical cordotomy. J Neurosurg 25:553–560, 1960.

40. Lindblom U: Assessment of abnormal evoked pain in neurological pain patients and its relation to spontaneous pain: A description and conceptual model with some analytical results. In Fields HL, Dubner R, and Cervero F (eds): Advances in Pain Research and Therapy, Vol 9. Raven, New York, 1985, pp 409–423.

41. Loeser JD: Dorsal rhizotomy: Indications and results. In Bonica JJ (ed): Advances in Neurology, Vol 4. Raven, New York, 1974, pp 615–619.

42. Loh L, and Nathan PW: Painful peripheral states and sympathetic blocks. J Neurol Neurosurg Psychiatry 41:664–671, 1978.

43. Loh L, Nathan PW, and Schott GD: Pain due to lesions of central nervous system removed by sympathetic block. British Medical Journal 282:1026–1028, 1981.

44. Mazars GJ: Intermittent stimulation of nucleus ventralis posterolateralis for intractable pain. Surg Neurol 4:93–95, 1975.

45. Maxwell RF: Surgical control of chronic migrainous neuralgia by trigeminal ganglio-rhizolysis. J Neurosurg 57:459–466, 1982.

46. McCulloch JA: Percutaneous radiofrequency lumbar rhizolysis (rhizotomy). Applied Neurophysiology 39:87–96, 1976.

47. Melzack R, and Wall PD: Pain mechanisms—a new theory. Science 150:971–979, 1965.

48. Meyerson BA, Arner S, and Linderoth B: Pros and cons of different approaches to the management of pelvic cancer pain. Acta Neurochir (Suppl 33):407–419, 1984.

49. Meyerson BA, and Hakansson J: Alleviation of atypical trigeminal pain by stimulation of the Gasserian ganglion via an implanted electrode. Acta Neurochir Suppl 30:303–309, 1980.

50. Miles J: Pituitary destruction. In Wall PD, and Melzack R (eds): Textbook of Pain. Churchill Livingstone, Edinburgh, pp 656–665, 1984.

51. Moore DC: Celiac (splanchnic) plexus block with alcohol for cancer pain of the upper intra-abdominal viscera. In Bonica JJ, and Ventafridda V (eds): Advances in Pain Research and Therapy, Vol 2. Raven, New York, 1979, pp 357–371.

52. Moricca G: Chemical hypophysectomy for cancer pain. In Bonica JJ (ed): Advances in Neurology, Vol 4. Raven, New York, 1974, pp 707–714.

53. Mullan S, Harper PV, Hekmatpanah J, et al: Percutaneous interruption of spinal pain tracts by means of a strontium 90 needle. J Neurosurg 20:931–939, 1963.

54. Mullan S, and Lichtor T: Percutaneous microcompression of the trigeminal ganglion for trigeminal neuralgia. J Neurosurg 59:1007–1012, 1983.

55. Nashold BS Jr: Brainstem stereotaxic procedures. In Schaltenbrand G, and Walker AE (eds): Stereotaxy of the Human Brain: Anatomical, Physiological and Clinical Applications. Georg Thieme, Stuttgart, 1982, pp 475–483.

56. Nashold BS Jr, Lopes H, Chodakiewitz J, et al: Trigeminal DREZ for craniofacial pain. In Samii M (ed): Surgery In and Around the Brainstem and Third Ventricle. Springer-Verlag, Berlin, 1986, pp 54–59.

57. Nathan PW: The descending respiratory pathway in man. J Neurol Neurosurg Psychiatry 26:487–499, 1963.

58. North RB, Ewerd MG, Lawton MT, et al: Spinal cord stimulation for chronic intractable pain: Superiority of multi-channel devices. Pain 44:119–130, 1991.

59. Ochoa JL, Torebjork E, Marchettini P, et al: Mechanisms of neuropathic pain: Cumulative observations, new experiments and further speculation. In Fields HL, Dubner R, and Cervero F (eds): Advances in Pain Research and Therapy, Vol 9. Raven, New York, 1985, pp 431–450.

60. Onofrio BM: Cervical spinal cord and dentate delineation in percutaneous radiofrequency cordotomy at the level of the first to second cervical vertebrae. Surg Gynecol Obstet 133:30–34, 1971.

61. Oudenhaven RC: Articular rhizotomy. Surg Neurol 2:275–278, 1974.

62. Pagura JR: Percutaneous radiofrequency spinal rhizotomy. Applied Neurophysiology 46:138–146, 1983.

63. Pagura JR, Schnapp M, and Passarelli P: Percutaneous radiofrequency glossopharyngeal rhizolysis for cancer pain. Applied Neurophysiology 46:154–159, 1983.

64. Porter RW, Hohmann GW, Bors E, et al: Cordotomy for the pain following cauda equina injury. Arch Surg 92:765–770, 1966.

65. Raymond SA, and Rocco AG: Ephaptic coupling of large fibres as a clue to mechanism in chronic neuropathic allodynia following damage to dorsal roots. Pain Suppl 5:S276, 1990.

66. Richardson DE, and Akil H: Pain reduction by electrical brain stimulation in man: Part II. Chronic self-administration in periventricular grey matter. J Neurosurg 47:184–194, 1977.

67. Roberts WJ: A hypothesis on the physiological base for causalgia and related pain. Pain 24:297–311, 1986.

68. Rosomoff HL, Carroll F, Brown J, et al: Percutaneous radiofrequency cervical cordotomy: Technique. J Neurosurg 23:639–644, 1965.

69. Sadar ES, and Cooperman AM: Bilateral thoracic sympathectomy splanchnicectomy in the treatment of intractable pain due to pancreatic carcinoma. Cleveland Clinic Quarterly, 41:185–188, 1974.

70. Sano K: Stereotaxic thalamolaminotomy and posteromedial hypothalamotomy for the relief of intractable pain. In Bonica JJ, and Ventafridda V (eds): Advances in Pain Research and Therapy, Vol 2. Raven, New York, pp 475–485, 1979.

71. Sano K, Yoshioka M, Ogashiwa M, et al: Thalamolaminotomy: A new operation for relief of intractable pain. Confinia Neurologica 27:63–66, 1966.

72. Schieff C, and Nashold BS: Stereotactic mesencephalic tractotomy for thalamic pain. Neurol Res 9:101–104, 1987.

73. Schvarcz JR: Stereotactic high cervical extralemniscal myelotomy for pelvic cancer pain. Acta Neurochir Suppl 33:431–435, 1984.

74. Shealy CN, Mortimer JT, and Hagfors NR: Dorsal column electroanalgesia. J Neurosurg 32:560–564, 1970.

75. Siegfried J, and Broggi G: Percutaneous thermocoagulation of the Gasserian ganglion in the treatment of pain in advanced cancer. In Bonica JJ, and Ventafridda V (eds): Advances in Pain Research and Therapy, Vol 2. Raven, New York, pp 463–468, 1979.

76. Sindou M, Fischer G, and Mansuy L: Posterior spinal rhizotomy and selective posterior rhizidiotomy. Progress in Neurological Surgery 7:201–250, 1976.

77. Sindou M, and Fobé J-L: Rhizotomies and dorsal root entry zone lesions in the management of cancer-related pain. In Arbit E (ed): Management of Cancer-Related Pain. Futura Publishing Company, Mount Kisco, NY, 1993, pp 341–368.

78. Spiegel EA, and Wycis HT: Mesencephalotomy in the treatment of "intractable" facial pain. Arch Neurol Psychiatry 69:1–13, 1953.

79. Steude U, Kobal G, and Hamburger CL: Atypical trigeminal neuralgia: Nine years' experience with the therapeutic electrostimulation of the Gasserian ganglion. Pain Suppl 5:S78, 1990.

80. Taarnhoj P: Decompression of the trigeminal root and the posterior part of the ganglion as a treatment in trigeminal neuralgia. Preliminary communication. J Neurosurg 9:288–290, 1952.

81. Takeda F, Fujii T, Uki J, et al: Cancer pain relief and tumor regression by means of pituitary neuroadenolysis and surgical hypophysectomy. Neurol Med Chir (Tokyo) 23:47–49, 1983.

82. Takeda F, Uki J, Fujii T, et al: Pituitary neuroadenolysis to relieve cancer pain: Observations of spread of ethanol installed into the sella turcica and subsequent changes of the hypothalamopituitary axis at autopsy. Neurol Med Chir (Tokyo) 23:50–54, 1983.

83. Tasker RR: Thalamic stereotaxic procedures. In Schaltenbrand G, and Walker AE (eds): Stereotaxy of the Human Brain. Anatomical, Physiological and Clinical Applications. Georg Thieme, Stuttgart, 1982, pp 484–497.

84. Tasker RR: Surgical approaches to the primary afferent and the spinal cord. In Fields HL, Dubner R, and Cervero F (eds): Advances in Pain Research and Therapy, Vol 9. Raven Press, New York, 1985, pp 409–423.

85. Tasker RR: Percutaneous cordotomy: The lateral high cervical technique. In Schmidek HH, and Sweet WH (eds): Operative Neurosurgical Techniques: Indications, Methods and Results, ed 2. Grune and Stratton, New York, 1988, pp 1191–1205.

86. Tasker RR: Stereotactic surgery. In Wall PD, and Melzack R (eds): Textbook of Pain, ed 2. Churchill Livingstone, Edinburgh, 1989, pp 840–855.

87. Tasker RR: Percutaneous cordotomy. In Youmans JR (ed): Neurological Surgery, ed 3. WB Saunders, Philadelphia, 1990, pp 4045–4058.

88. Tasker RR: Deafferentation pain syndromes: Introduction. In Nashold BS Jr, and Ovelmen-Levitt J (eds): Advances in Pain Research and Therapy, Vol 19. Raven Press, New York, 1991, pp 241–257.

89. Tasker RR: Ablative central nervous system lesions for control of cancer pain. In Arbit E (ed): Management of Cancer-Related Pain. Futura Publishing, Mount Kisco, NY, 1993, pp 231–256.

90. Tasker RR, De Carvalho GTC, and Dolan EJ: Intractable pain of cord origin—clinical features and implications for surgery. J Neurosurg, 77:373–378, 1992.

91. Tasker RR, and Dostrovsky JO: Deafferentation and central pain. In Wall PD, and Melzack R (eds): Textbook of Pain, ed 2. Churchill Livingstone, Edinburgh, 1989, pp 154–180.

92. Tew JM Jr, and Tobler WD: Percutaneous rhizotomy in the treatment of intractable facial pain (trigeminal, glossopharyngeal, and vagal nerves). In Schmidek HH, and Sweet WH (eds): Operative Neurosurgical Techniques: Indications, Methods and Results. Grune and Stratton, New York, 1982, pp 1083–1100.

93. Turnbull IM, Black RG, and Scott JW: Reflex efferent impulses in the trigeminal nerve. J Neurosurg 18:746–752, 1961.

94. Uematsu S: Percutaneous electrothermocoagulation of spinal nerve trunk, ganglion, and rootlets. In Schmidek HH, and Sweet WH (eds): Operative Neurosurgical Techniques: Indications, Methods and Results. Grune and Stratton, 1982, New York, pp 1177–1198.

95. Uematsu S, Udbarhelyi GB, Benson DW, et al: Percutaneous radiofrequency rhizotomy. Surg Neurol 2:319–325, 1974.

96. Wall PD, and Sweet WH: Temporary abolition of pain in man. Science 155:108–109, 1967.

97. Wycis HT, and Spiegel EA: Long-range results in the treatment of intractable pain by stereotaxic midbrain surgery. J Neurosurg 19:101–107, 1962.

98. Young RF, and Brechner T: Electrical stimulation of the brain for relief of intractable pain due to cancer. Cancer 57:1266, 1986.

99. Young RF, and Chambi VI: Pain relief by electrical stimulation of the periaqueductal and periventricular gray matter. Evidence for a non-opioid mechanism. J Neurosurg 66:364–371, 1987.

100. Young RF, Kroening R, Fulton W, et al: Electrical stimulation of the brain in treatment of chronic pain: Experience over 5 years. J Neurosurg 62:389–396, 1985.

CHAPTER 14

PHYSIATRIC APPROACHES TO PAIN MANAGEMENT

Michael J. Brennan, M.D.

THE ROLE OF PHYSIATRIC APPROACHES

The goals of rehabilitation therapy for patients with chronic pain include comfort and functional restoration. To accomplish these goals, physiatrists and other rehabilitation professionals administer physical modalities and functionally directed therapies. These interventions are usually integrated into a multimodality treatment approach, the nature of which varies among patients with acute pain, chronic nonmalignant pain, or cancer pain.[9,10,15,28] Physiatric interventions often predominate in multidisciplinary pain management programs, which specialize in the physical and psychosocial rehabilitation of disabled patients with chronic nonmalignant pain (see Chapter 15).

The spectrum of physiatric therapies used to treat patients with chronic pain is broad. Physical modalities include electrical stimulation, medicinal diathermy, and cryotherapy. Like therapeutic exercises and counter-irritant therapies such as massage, vibration, and percussion, these modalities are usually administered to lessen pain. Physical and occupational therapies, including assistive devices and braces, are typically directed toward the improvement of function, such as greater independence in activities of daily living, enhanced ambulation and mobility, or increased range of motion.

The use of all these physiatric interventions is supported by a large anecdotal experience. There is consensus that some patients benefit, by either improved control of pain or better functioning despite persistent pain. There have been few controlled clinical trials, however, and the extant data are inadequate to confirm the utility of any approach or to judge the relative merits of one against another. Nonetheless, clinicians should be aware of the physiatric therapies that are commonly used and understand the rationales and practices that guide their administration. Studies are needed to provide a scientific foundation for these approaches.

Prescribing Physiatric Therapies

The management of pain with rehabilitation techniques begins with a comprehensive medical assessment. Information pertaining to functional, vocational, and avocational consequences of the pain is combined with an understanding of the pathophysiology of the disease or injury causing the pain, as well as the type of pain being experienced, in order to generate a prescription for rehabilitative therapy. The rehabilitation prescription should include:

1. References to the primary diagnosis and any significant concomitant illnesses
2. Expected treatment goals
3. Recommended treatments including home treatment or exercises
4. Frequency and duration of therapy until the next physician reevaluation
5. Any precautions that need to be observed, such as limitations in range of motion, weight-bearing restrictions, and proscribed modalities.

Frequent communication with both the treating therapist and the patient yields the best possible outcome.

Physicians should know the type and quality of therapy provided by the therapist and ensure that treatment time is spent with the patient in a one-on-one environment. Therapy should be performed in the presence of the therapist, who either provides modality therapy or instructs and observes the patient during treatment sessions. The application of hot packs alone and the use of patient instruction cards for exercises are not adequate and should not be condoned.

PHYSIATRIC THERAPEUTICS

Modalities

Bioactive physical agents, such as electricity, heat, and cryotherapy, are among the most frequently used therapies for the treatment of pain (Table 14–1).[2,32,33,40,59] Despite a large volume of literature on these modalities, few data have been collected from controlled clinical trials. Some patients obtain analgesia from these treatments, and others experience physiologic

Table 14–1. PHYSIATRIC MODALITIES USED IN PAIN MANAGEMENT

Modality	Examples
Electrical stimulation	Transcutaneous electrical nerve stimulation (TENS)
	Electrical massage
Medicinal diathermy	
Superficial heat	Hot packs
	Paraffin
Deep heat	Ultrasound
Cryotherapy	Ice massage
	Cold packs
	Vapo-coolant sprays

responses that have been suggested to have independent advantages.[32]

ELECTRICAL STIMULATION

Transcutaneous Electrical Nerve Stimulation (TENS). TENS is reported to be effective for a variety of painful conditions.[21,31,37,52] Recent evidence, however, questions its efficacy.[14] Notwithstanding, TENS remains popular among therapists and rehabilitationists because of its ease of use, favorable clinical experience, and low potential for adverse effects. Some patients report long-lasting analgesia from the use of this modality. Benefit has also been reported in other conditions, such as postanesthesia vomiting following hysterectomy.[18]

The mechanisms underlying the analgesic effects of TENS are not established. TENS may activate endogenous segmental pain-modulating systems through selective stimulation of large-diameter myelinated (A-beta) fibers.[59] These systems presumably inhibit the central transmission of nociceptive input through slower, unmyelinated C fibers. There is no confirmation of this mechanism in humans, and other actions are presumably involved as well. The observation that some patients experience analgesia following stimulation at sites remote from the painful area[2,40] suggests that activation of descending modulating systems may be an appropriate alternative hypothesis for the effects produced by TENS.[30,31]

TENS units are generally portable and battery powered. The current generated is typically directed through surface electrodes and electrical conductant to specific points on the body. Patients may report benefit from stimulation at diverse locations, including the painful area itself; at acupuncture meridians, superficial nerves, or motor points; or at sites away from the painful body part.[2] Sequential trials of different stimulation sites are usually recommended for patients who fail to achieve a favorable response after their initial TENS treatment.[2,21,38]

Electrical stimulation may be administered with any combination of stimulation parameters. These parameters include variations of frequency, amplitude, and slope of wave forms, and they are varied by trial and error to identify the most favorable pattern for the individual patient.[2,38]

Randomized trials indicate that both acute pain syndromes and chronic pain syndromes can respond favorably to TENS. These trials have evaluated stimulation for acute pain due to surgery[1,5,12,46,48] or trauma[27,41,50] and for chronic pain due to degenerative joint disease,[36] rheumatoid arthritis,[38] or hemophilic arthropathy.[45] Other painful syndromes commonly treated with TENS include nerve injuries, back pain associated with trigger points or fibromyalgia, and metastatic lesions. TENS is administered to virtually all patients with chronic pain who seek treatment in specialized pain management programs. Anecdotally, these empirical trials sometimes identify a responder who benefits sufficiently to warrant continued treatment.

Contraindications to TENS are few. Rare patients may develop idiopathic hypersensitivity to electrical stimulation. A local erythematous reaction may develop where the electrodes contact the skin. More generally, TENS is not recommended for patients with cardiac pacemakers or a history of cardiac dysrhythmia. TENS should not be applied over the carotid sinus, on an open wound, or on anesthetized skin.

Electrical Massage. Galvanic electrical stimulation, sometimes referred to as *electrical massage, medcolator therapy,* or *electromyotherapy,* is frequently used to treat painful musculoskel-

etal conditions.[2] As with TENS, there have been no systematic investigations of the technique, the use of which evolved on the basis of clinical observation. These devices induce local contractions in skeletal muscle, which is accompanied by pain relief in some patients. The analgesic effect is poorly understood and could represent, in part, a placebo response in some responders. Alternative hypotheses include a counterirritant effect (i.e., activation of sequential or suprasegmental pain-modulating pathways), muscle fiber fatigue, or increased local circulation.[2,30,31]

This form of electrical stimulation is often used in patients with painful muscle syndromes, epicondylitis, and some arthritic conditions. During stimulation, patients are frequently treated with ice or heat, and immediately following treatment, with stretching or massage. Biofeedback may be employed in conjunction with electrical stimulation to assist in relaxation and, in some instances, to retrain and strengthen muscles weakened by nerve injury.[4,39]

The common practice of applying multiple modalities concurrently further increases the difficulty in ascertaining the true efficacy of any single intervention. Nonetheless, clinical experience with electrical massage, as with TENS and other modalities, has been positive in some patients, and this experience has justified its continued application.

Electrical therapy is contraindicated in individuals with metastatic disease because the tetany produced by the electrical stimulation may lead to fracture of overt or occult bone lesions. Therapy is also withheld from patients with cardiac pacemakers and those with an idiopathic intolerance to electrical stimulation.

MEDICINAL DIATHERMY

Patients often experience the therapeutic administration of heat as relaxing and analgesic. Physiologic responses to moderate amounts of heat include increases in local blood flow and tissue compliance.[32,33]

In the clinical setting, specific diathermy techniques are selected based on the desired amount of heating and the depth of the targeted tissues (Table 14–2). Devices that were once popular, such as short-wave diathermy units and heating lamps, are used infrequently now that safer, less costly devices such

Table 14–2. MEDICINAL DIATHERMY: COMMON MEANS OF PROVIDING SUPERFICIAL AND DEEP HEATING OF TISSUES

Device	Depth of heating	Indications
Hot packs (e.g., Kenny pack, Hydrocolator)	Superficial (1–1.5 cm)	Painful joint Spasm
Hydrotherapy	Superficial	Painful joints Spasm
Paraffin	Superficial	Painful joints (usually hands)
Lasers	Superficial	Painful nerve injury Painful joints Myofascial pains
Ultrasound	Deep (greatest at interface of bone and soft tissue)	Tendinitis Spasm Capsulitis Contractures Possibly reflex sympathetic dystrophy
Short-wave diathermy	Deep (muscle level)	Muscle pain Spasm Tendinitis

as ultrasound units have become more widely available.

The benefits that some patients report following application of heat are not understood and could potentially reflect a placebo response or other psychologic effect. The physiologic effects of heat could potentially activate endogenous pain-modulating systems, but there is no direct evidence that this occurs. Improvement in tissue elasticity with a concomitant decrease in pain has been observed in patients with connective tissue disorders.[60] Pain associated with muscle spasm may be reduced by altering gamma-fiber activity within muscle.[32,33]

Despite the lack of scientific data, empirical use of medicinal diathermy has become popular, and it is likely that a patient with either acute or chronic pain who is referred to a rehabilitation specialist for pain management will undergo a trial of one form or another. Diathermy is not applied to insensate areas, ischemic regions, and limbs with a history of claudication; it is avoided in patients who are paralyzed, unable to communicate, or likely to bleed (i.e., those with thrombocytopenia or coagulopathies). Heat is also not applied near neoplastic tissue because of the theoretic concern that local increases in

metabolism and blood flow may enhance tumor growth.[2]

Superficial Heat. The superficial application of heat (i.e., less than 1.5-cm penetration) is most commonly accomplished through heating pads, hydrotherapy, melted paraffin wax, and, occasionally, heat lamps. The effects of laser therapy, which is also used in pain management, are presumed to be due, at least in part, to superficial heating of tissues. The risks of these approaches are very low and are essentially limited to local skin burn associated with prolonged use (Fig. 14–1).

Conventional hot packs (e.g., Kenny pack, hydrocollator pack) provide a relatively short period of local heating of superficial tissues. Treatment is easy and often is given as the first step in therapy sessions. Some patients appear to cooperate more fully with stretching or strengthening exercises if exercise is preceded by a period of superficial heating. Electric heating pads deliver therapeutic doses of heat for prolonged periods. Some are capable of extracting moisture from the air and thereby provide "moist heat." This moisture acts as a good medium for the transfer of heat.

Hydrotherapy can be used to apply superficial heat. Common devices include the whirlpool and the much larger Hubbard

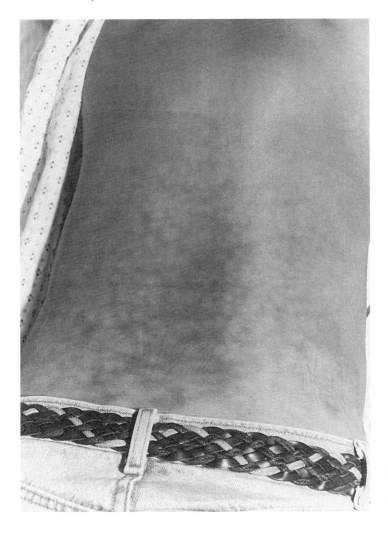

Figure 14–1. Typical skin changes associated with burns from chronic use of heating pads.

tank. The whirlpool is used for limb immersion, whereas the Hubbard tank can accommodate the entire person. Wound débridement for diabetics and burn patients can be accomplished with whirlpool and Hubbard tanks. Another version of hydrotherapy is therapy pools, which may be used for exercise, for ambulation training, or for relaxation. Therapeutic pools are usually waist or chest deep. They are typically maintained at or near 30 to 34°C. The water provides progressive resistance to patients as they ambulate or exercise. Patients with soft tissue and arthritic conditions report pain relief and muscle relaxation as they exercise immersed in a tank.[2]

Paraffin baths are typically used in the treatment of painful conditions affecting the hands and feet. "Dipping" of the involved limb into melted wax allows for mild heating of the superficial tissues, whereas prolonged submersion may produce vigorous warming of the body part.[2]

Laser therapy has recently been studied in a variety of therapeutic applications, with mixed results. Potential physiatric uses include the treatment of pain associated with inflammatory diseases, degenerative joint disease, myofascial conditions, and nerve injury. Pain and strength improved in an uncontrolled series of patients treated with laser for rheumatoid disease,[22] and a slight decrease in pain without change in medication use or strength was observed in a controlled study of this technique for osteoarthritis.[3] Analgesic effects could not be confirmed in a recent meta-analysis of laser treatment for musculoskeletal pain[20] but were suggested in separate controlled studies of laser treatment for postherpetic neuralgia and trigeminal neuralgia.[54,55] Laser therapy has also been used as a form of acupuncture, without supporting data.

Despite the paucity of supportive clinical trials, superficial heat has become an integral part of most rehabilitation efforts for musculoskeletal pain and arthritic conditions. The favorable clinical impression that these techniques can provide analgesia and relaxation, particularly in the early phase of treatment, requires confirmation in future studies.

Deep Heat. Devices have been developed to generate significant temperature increases within deep tissues. Ultrasound (*US*) is by far the most frequently used, particularly in painful musculoskeletal disorders.[2,32,33]

The deep heat provided by *US* is developed when sound waves pass into tissues with differing sound absorption qualities. The amount of heat generated is greatest where these differences are most substantial, such as at muscle-tendon junctions and bone-ligament interface.[2] This heat has been used empirically to treat pain associated with frozen shoulders and other contractures, muscle spasm, tendinitis or bursitis, and other conditions.[2,32,33,42,43]

The mechanisms responsible for the analgesia that accompanies the deep heat produced by *US* are unknown. As with superficial heat, analgesia could be due to placebo response, activation of endogenous pain-modulatory processes, or local changes in tissue compliance; in addition, *US* could also potentially slow conduction velocity in sensory nerves and produce a temporary nerve block.[34]

US should not be used near the eye, gravid uterus, heart, infections, and neoplastic tissues. The same precautions described for superficial heat should be observed. Additionally, *US* should be used cautiously near endoprosthetic implants made of metal or plastic. Special care is also needed in patients who have undergone laminectomy; the application of *US* over the operative site may cause marked temperature elevations near the spinal cord.[33]

CRYOTHERAPY

The effects attributed to the therapeutic application of cold have included diminution of inflammation, decrease in muscle spasm, and reduction of pain.[33] There is no confirmatory evidence that any of these effects occur to a clinically meaningful extent. Anecdotal observation, however, has been favorable, and use of this technique is extremely widespread. The mechanism of the analgesic effects that have been observed following cryotherapy is poorly understood and could include a prominent placebo response, slowed conduction in nociceptive fibers, or decreased local inflammatory response.[32,33]

Cryotherapy may be useful in patients with musculoskeletal pain, such as acute or chronic pain due to myofascial syndromes. In the clinical setting, treatment with cold may be used alone or applied in a more comprehensive program.[29] Cold alternating with superficial heat (contrast baths) has been recommended in some rheumatologic disorders.[33]

Cold therapy may be applied through ice massage and cold packs or through vapo-coolant sprays such as ethylchloride or fluorimethane. Direct exposure of the skin to ice or cold packs leads to superficial cooling (e.g., conduction effect), whereas vapo-coolants cool the skin by rapid evaporation of volatile substances. The use of vapo-coolants in conjunction with progressive stretching of painful muscles, known as "spray and stretch," has been advocated for the treatment of myofascial pain syndromes (see Chapter 7). There have been no randomized trials of any of these techniques, and proponents base their recommendations on clinical experience only.

Intensive cold can be harmful to tissues, and therapy must be carefully monitored. Contraindications include anesthetized tissue, severe peripheral vascular disease, and cold hypersensitivity syndromes such as Raynaud's phenomenon.

COUNTERIRRITANT THERAPIES: MASSAGE, VIBRATION, AND PERCUSSION

Massage, vibration, and percussion are used by allopathic and nonallopathic therapists, including chiropractors and masseuses.

The therapeutic benefits of these techniques have not been studied, and clinical use is based solely on favorable anecdotal reports and a larger clinical experience. This experience, however, usually involves the application of multiple modalities concurrently, and the specific value of the counterirritant therapies is not known. If there are physiologic effects that lead to analgesia, they may involve activation of endogenous pain-modulating mechanisms, such as those postulated for TENS.[26,30,31,40]

Patients often report immediate benefits, either analgesia or relaxation, from a counterirritant therapy. A recent study found that massage, particularly deep massage, was more beneficial than cryotherapy, *US,* and superficial heat in the treatment of trigger points.[23]

Therapeutic Exercise

Exercise is commonly prescribed in the treatment of painful conditions. In some disorders, such as fibromyalgia (see Chapter 7), it is a primary therapeutic intervention. It is considered to be a primary approach to the treatment of pain and disability in multidisciplinary pain management programs.[24,28]

Exercise is used to enhance flexibility, improve strength and conditioning, and provide stability of weakened or lax joints. Physiologically, exercise improves strength, endurance, and range of motion of muscles and other soft tissues.[25] Aerobic exercise improves cardiopulmonary function. Exercise has also been suggested to improve pain tolerance,[17] an effect that has been postulated to involve changes in endogenous opioids.[49,51]

Flexibility training is used in the management of most patients suffering from acute or chronic neck and back pain.[16,19,33] Both flexion (Williams') exercises and extension (McKenzie) exercises have been advocated. In the absence of comparative data, the selection of a program is by trial and error.

The first phase of physical therapy for patients with acute neck or back pain usually combines stretching and either ice or heat.[47] Additional flexibility training is often provided later and is a major component of most home exercise programs. Strengthening and flexibility exercises are also employed in the management of both inflammatory and noninflammatory arthropathies. Improvement in range of motion, stabilization of weakened joints by muscular support, and a beneficial effect on activities of daily living can occur in these patients.[25]

Orthoses and Assistive Devices

ORTHOSES

Orthoses are typically used to support or substitute for dysfunctional joints or tissues weakened by either disease or its treatment. They may also be used to stabilize, immobilize, or "unload" painful areas. For example, pain and dysesthesias associated with carpal tunnel syndrome may be ameliorated with braces that maintain the wrist joint in a neutral position.[7]

Braces are available in a variety of forms and may be fitted to virtually any part of the body. Orthotics come in both prefabricated and custom-made varieties and should be prescribed according to the patient's need and clinical circumstance.[6,34,44]

Spinal Orthoses. Spinal bracing is used to ameliorate neck or back pain or to reduce the risk of reinjury in some patients.[56] There have been no studies of these techniques, and both the decision to use a brace and the specific brace prescription are based on clinical judgments about the location of pain, the value of spinal stabilization, and the patient's ability to tolerate a device.[8,13,16,17,44]

Prefabricated devices such as soft and semi-rigid neck collars, corsets, and sacroiliac belts are used when limitation in range of motion or spinal stabilization is not required.[56] Some patients report an increase in comfort, particularly with movement, when these devices are worn. These appliances are inexpensive, easy to apply, and are usually well tolerated.

Some patients who do not benefit from a soft or semirigid brace report enhanced comfort from a greater degree of immobilization. In difficult cases, therefore, an orthosis that is more restrictive should be tried.[8,13]

Rigid spinal orthotics, such as the hyperextension orthosis, are available for patients with impaired spinal integrity. The custom-molded plastic body jacket provides maximum orthotic control and immobilization of the spine, as is needed in unstable fractures. In most cases, spinal orthotics are applied during the acute phase of an injury. After pain subsides, the patient should be gradually weaned from the device. They are generally not used in the setting of chronic pain because of the theoretic concern that deconditioning will increase if bracing eliminates the need for muscular contraction.

Similar to most potentially analgesic techniques in rehabilitation, the empiric use of bracing has become accepted without confirmation of efficacy in clinical trials. In part, the acceptability of these techniques relates to their relative safety. There are few contraindications for the use of bracing. Impaired tissue sensation may preclude the use of devices that come in direct contact with skin, especially if the patient's mental status is compromised. Obese individuals or those who rely on accessory abdominal breathing may not tolerate abdominal binding. Although the possibility of long-term adverse effects from spinal bracing, such as weakening of abdominal or spinal muscles, has been suggested, recent evidence suggests the contrary.[56]

ASSISTIVE DEVICES

Assistive devices include crutches, canes, and walkers. These devices are used to aid in ambulation by increasing ground contact points, lessening weight bearing through a painful or weak limb by altering the distribution of mass while ambulating, and, in patients with paretic limbs, supplanting lost function. They may promote functional independence in mobility and activities of daily living.[6,35] Clinical experience has shown these devices to be useful in the treatment of some painful conditions.

The most important concern in the use of assistive devices is the need for integrity of the bones of the upper extremity and shoulder girdle. If degenerative or metastatic disease is present, weight transfer from the lower extremities to the arm may predispose the patient to joint pain or bony injury. Adaptations can be made to the assistive device to protect the patient in the event of neoplastic involvement of the arm or shoulder region.

Canes may reduce weight bearing by up to 25 percent. A single arm crutch may relieve as much as 45 percent of body weight, and double-supported ambulation from either crutches or walkers may allow total non–weight bearing on an affected limb.[58] If incident pain (pain with voluntary actions, such as walking) occurs with weight bearing, the patient may find the use of such a device to be analgesic. The patient with hip pain represents a dramatic example of this potential. The use of a cane in the hand contralateral to the diseased hip causes weight to be distributed between the painful leg and the assistive device. Intrinsic muscle forces acting upon the hip joint that may also provoke and increase pain are lessened as well. As a result, pain declines and ambulation improves.

Assistive devices should be used with caution in patients with impaired mental status. Falls from improper use of leg braces, canes, or crutches can have devastating consequences, including fractures and head injury. Braces that do not fit properly can lead to skin irritation and breakdown.

TREATMENT OF PAIN ASSOCIATED WITH TRIGGER POINTS

Trigger points are areas of discomfort and localized tenderness that are found within muscles, fasciae, and tendons (see Chapter 7). When palpated, local and radiating pain, as well as dysesthetic sensations, may be provoked. Some patients with myofascial pain appear to have trigger points as a primary problem, the pathology of which is unknown.[53,57]

Some patients with acute or chronic pain associated with trigger points respond well to physical medicine interventions. None of these approaches have been investigated in clinical trials, but all are commonly used. They include trigger point injections, exercise, and the use of modalities such as TENS, diathermy, massage, and cryotherapy.[8,23,32] Trigger point injection is a popular technique[11,44,53] in which saline, local anesthetic, or, occasionally, corticosteroid is instilled into the focus of tenderness. Alternatively, stretching can be performed after the administration of a vapo-coolant spray.[53] This is usually followed by the superficial application of heat or, less commonly, ice. Trigger point injections should not be used in patients with coagulopathies or thrombocytopenia or in those who are immunocompromised.

SUMMARY

Physical medicine techniques have become widely accepted in the management of patients with acute and chronic pain despite a paucity of scientific evidence that confirms the efficacy of the diverse approaches applied in clinical practice. This acceptance has occurred in response to favorable anecdotal experience and relatively low risks associated with each type of therapy. Additionally, physiatric approaches often specifically address the need for improved physical functioning and thereby target a therapeutic goal that is often equal in importance to pain relief.

Physiatric therapies include modalities that are generally used to reduce pain. The application of electrical stimulation through surface electrodes (transcutaneous electrical nerve stimulation) is a common treatment for acute and chronic pain. Electrical massage uses electrical current to induce repetitive muscle contraction, which is associated with analgesia in some patients.

Medicinal diathermy refers to a group of modalities that administer superficial or deep heat. Superficial heat is applied through heating pads, hot packs, heated paraffin, or heat lamps. Hydrotherapy, including pool therapy, provides superficial heat during a function-oriented treatment. Deep heat is administered using ultrasound. The mechanisms that are responsible for the analgesic effects reported during diathermy are unknown, and clinical applications are based on anecdotal experience.

Cryotherapy can be applied through ice massage, cold packs, or vapo-coolant sprays. These techniques are most often used in patients with musculoskeletal pain.

Therapeutic exercise, which includes flexibility training, strengthening, and aerobic exercise, is commonly prescribed during the treatment of acute pain and chronic pain syndromes. Exercise is a major element in the approaches used by multidisciplinary pain management programs to address the disability associated with chronic nonmalignant pain.

In some painful conditions, the use of orthoses or assistive devices can enhance comfort or improve functional capacity. Spinal orthoses are commonly used for both acute and chronic pain. Prefabricated devices, such as soft collars, do not stabilize the spine but improve the comfort of some patients. Rigid orthoses are usually used in acute situations for the purpose of stabilization; they are generally avoided in patients with chronic pain because of the theoretical risk of muscular deconditioning. Assistive devices, which include crutches, canes, and walkers, aid in ambulation and relieve pain by lessening weight bearing.

Physiatric techniques are also used to treat myofascial pain, particularly if associated with trigger points. Injections, exercise, and the use of modalities such as electrical stimulation, diathermy, and cryotherapy can ameliorate trigger points and improve functional capacity.

Extensive clinical experience indicates that many patients benefit from physiatric therapies, either by experiencing less pain or by improving function. Progress in the use of these interventions requires clinical trials that assess the true risks and benefits during long-term use.

REFERENCES

1. Ali J, Yaffe CS, and Serratte C: The effect of transcutaneous electric nerve stimulation on postoperative pain and pulmonary function. Surgery 89:507–512, 1981.
2. Basford JR: Physical agents and biofeedback. In Delisa JA (ed): Rehabilitation Medicine: Principles and Practice. JB Lippincott, Philadelphia, 1988, pp 257–275.
3. Basford JR, Sheffield CG, Mair SD, et al: Low energy Helium Neon laser treatment for thumb osteoarthritis. Arch Phys Med Rehabil 68:794–797, 1987.
4. Basmajian JV: Biofeedback in rehabilitation: A review of practices and principles. Arch Phys Med Rehabil 62:469–475, 1981.
5. Bourke DL, Smith BA, Erickson J, et al: TENS reduces halothane requirements during hand surgery. Anesthesiology 61:769–772, 1984.
6. Britell CW, and McFarland SR: Adaptive systems and devices for the disabled. In Delisa JA (ed): Rehabilitation Medicine: Principles and Practice. JB Lippincott, Philadelphia, 1988, pp 372–388.
7. Burke DT, Burke MM, Stewart GW, et al: Splinting for carpal tunnel syndrome: In search of the optimal angle. Arch Phys Med Rehabil 75:1241–1244, 1994.

8. Cailliet R: Low Back Pain Syndrome, ed 4. FA Davis, Philadelphia, 1988, pp 181–183.

9. Cassisi JE, Sypert GW, Salamon A, et al: Independent evaluation of a multi-disciplinary rehabilitation program for chronic low back pain. Neurosurgery 25: 877–883, 1989.

10. Chapman SL, Brena SF, and Bradford LA: Treatment outcome in a chronic pain rehabilitation program. Pain 11: 255–268, 1981.

11. Cleeland C: Nonpharmacological management of cancer pain. Journal of Pain and Symptom Management (Suppl) 2: 23–28, 1987.

12. Cooperman AM, Hall B, Mikalacki K, et al: Use of transcutaneous electrical stimulation in control of postoperative pain. Results of a prospective, randomized controlled study. Am J Surg 133:185–187, 1977.

13. Cybulski GR: Methods of surgical stabilization for metastatic disease of the spine. Neurosurgery 25: 240–252, 1989.

14. Deyo RA, Walsh NE, and Martin DC, et al: A controlled trial of transcutaneous electrical nerve stimulation (TENS) and exercise for chronic low back pain. N Engl J Med 332:1627–1634, 1990.

15. Elliot K, and Foley KM: Neurologic pain syndromes in patients with cancer. Neurologic Clinics 7:333–360, 1989.

16. Fisher S: Spinal orthoses: In Kottke FJ, and Lehmann JF (eds): Krusen's Handbook of Physical Medicine and Rehabilitation, ed 4. WB Saunders, Philadelphia, 1990, pp 593–601.

17. Flor H, and Turk DC: Etiological theories and treatments for chronic back pain: I. Somatic models and interventions. Pain 19:105–121, 1984.

18. Fassoulaki A, Papilas K, Sarantopoulos C, et al: Transcutaneous electric nerve stimulation reduces the incidence of vomiting after hysterectomy. Anesth Analg 76:1012–1014, 1993.

19. Frymoyer JW, and Catsa-Baril WL: An overview of the incidences and costs of low back pain. Orthop Clin North Am 22: 263–272, 1991.

20. Gam AN, Thosen H, and Lonnberg F: The effect of low-level laser therapy on musculoskeletal pain: A meta-analysis. Pain 52:63–66, 1993.

21. Gersh MR, and Wolf SL: Applications of transcutaneous electrical nerve stimulation in the management of patients with pain: state of the art update. Phys Ther 65:314–336, 1985.

22. Goldman JA, Chiapella J, Casey H, et al: Laser therapy for rheumatoid arthritis. Lasers Surg Med 1: 93–101, 1980.

23. Hong CZ, Chen YC, Pon CH, et al: Immediate effects of various physical medicine modalities on pain threshold of an active myofascial trigger point. Journal of Musculoskeletal Pain 1:37–53, 1993.

24. Hurri H: The Swedish back school in chronic low back pain. Part I. Benefits. Scand J Rehabil Med 21:33–40, 1989.

25. Joynt RL: Therapeutic exercises. In Delisa JA (ed): Rehabilitation Medicine: Principles and Practice. JB Lippincott, Philadelphia, 1988, pp 346–371.

26. Kakigi R, and Shibasaki H: Mechanism of pain relief by vibration and movement. J Neurol Neurosurg Psychiatry 55: 282–286, 1992.

27. Kimball KL, Drews JE, Walker S, et al: Use of TENS for pain reduction in burn patients receiving travase. J Burn Care Rehabil 8:28–31, 1987.

28. King JC, and Kelleher WJ: The chronic pain syndrome: The interdisciplinary rehabilitative behavioral modification approach. Physical Medicine State of the Art Reviews 5:165–186, 1991.

29. Landon BR: Heat or cold for the relief of low back pain. Phys Ther 47: 1126–1128, 1967.

30. Le Bars D, Chitour D, and Clot AM: Diffuse noxious inhibitory controls (DNIC). Relationship between conditioning stimulus intensity and inhibitory effect. In Bonica JJ, Lindblom U, Iggo A, et al (eds): Advances in Pain Research and Therapy, Vol 5: Proceedings of the Third World Congress on Pain. Edinburgh. Raven, New York, 1983, pp 549–554.

31. Le Bars D, Dickinson AH, and Besson JM: Diffuse noxious inhibitory controls (DNIC). I. Effects on dorsal horn convergent neurons in the rat. Pain 6: 2338–304, 1979.

32. Lehmann JF, and de Lateur BF: Ultrasound, shortwave, microwave, superficial heat and cold in the treatment of pain. In Wall PD, and Melzack R (eds): Textbook of Pain, ed 2. Churchill Livingstone, Edinburgh, 1989, pp 932–941.

33. Lehmann JF, and de Lateur BJ: Diathermy and superficial heat, laser, and cold therapy. In Kottke FJ, and Lehmann JF (eds): Krusen's Handbook of Physical Medicine and Rehabilitation, ed 3. WB Saunders, Philadelphia, 1990, pp 283–367.

34. Lehneis HR: General principles of orthotics and prosthetics. In Goodgold J (ed): Rehabilitation Medicine. CV Mosby, St Louis, 1988, pp 823–841.

35. Leslie LR: Training for functional independence. In Kottke FJ, and Lehmann JF (eds): Krusen's Handbook of Physical Medicine and Rehabilitation, ed 4. WB Saunders, Philadelphia, 1990, pp 564–570.

36. Lewis D, Lewis B, and Sturrock RD: Transcutaneous electrical nerve stimulation in osteoarthrosis: A therapeutic alternative? Ann Rheum Dis 43:47–49, 1984.

37. Long DM, Cambell JN, and Gucer G: Transcutaneous electrical nerve stimulation for relief of chronic pain. Advances in Pain Research and Therapy 3: 593–599, 1979.

38. Manheimer C, and Carlsson C: The analgesic effect of transcutaneous electric nerve stimulation (TENS) in patients with rheumatoid arthritis. A comparative study of different pulse patterns. Pain 6:329–334, 1979.

39. Marcus N, and Levin G: Clinical applications of biofeedback: Implications for psychiatry. Hosp Community Psychiatry 28:21–25, 1977.

40. Meyerson BA: Electrostimulation procedures: Effects, presumed rationale, and possible mechanisms. In Bonica JJ, Lindblom U, Iggo A, Jones LE, et al (eds): Advances in Pain Research and Therapy, Vol 5: Proceedings of the Third World Congress on Pain. Edinburgh. Raven Press, New York, 1983, p 496.

41. Ordog GJ: Transcutaneous electrical nerve stimulation versus oral analgesic: A randomized double-blind controlled study in acute post-traumatic pain. Am J Emerg Med 5:6–10, 1987.

42. Portwood MM, Lieberman JS, and Taylor RG: Ultrasound treatment of reflex sympathetic dystrophy. Arch Phys Med Rehabil 68:116–118, 1987.

43. Ragnarsson KT: Orthotics and shoes. In Delisa JA (ed): Rehabilitation Medicine: Principles and Practice. JB Lippincott, Philadelphia, 1988, pp 307–329.

44. Ready LB, Kozody R, Bara JE, et al: Trigger point injections versus jet injection in the treatment of myofascial pain. Pain 15:201–206, 1983.

45. Roche PA, Gijsbers K, Belch JJ, et al: Modifications of haemophiliac haemorrhage pain by transcutaneous electrical nerve stimulation. Pain 21:43–48, 1985.

46. Rosenberg M, Curtis L, and Bourke DL: Transcutaneous electrical nerve stimulation for the relief of postoperative pain. Pain 5:129–133, 1978.

47. Saal JA, and Saal JS: Initial stage management of lumbar spine problems. PM&R Clinics 2:187–204, 1991.

48. Schuster GK, and Infante MC: Pain relief after low back surgery: The efficacy of transcutaneous electrical nerve stimulation. Pain 8:299–302, 1980.

49. Sforzo GA: Opioids and exercise: An update. Sports Med 7:109–124, 1989.

50. Sloan JP, Muwanga CL, Waters E, et al: Multiple rib fractures: TENS versus conventional analgesia. J Trauma 26:1120–1122, 1986.

51. Thoren P, Floras JS, Hoffman P, et al: Endorphins and exercise: Physiological mechanisms and clinical implications. Med Sci Sports Exerc 22:417–428, 1990.

52. Thorsteinsson G, Stonnington HH, Stillwell GK, et al: The placebo effect of transcutaneous stimulation. Pain 5:31–41, 1978.

53. Travell JG, and Simons DG: Myofascial pain and dysfunction: The trigger point manual. Williams and Wilkins, Baltimore, 1983, pp 5–164.

54. Walker J: Relief from chronic pain by lower power laser irradiation. Neurosci Lett 43:339–344, 1983.

55. Walker J, Akhanjee LK, Cooney MM, et al: Laser therapy for pain of trigeminal neuralgia. Clin J Pain 3:183–187, 1988.

56. Walsh NE, and Schwartz RK: The influence of prophylactic orthoses on abdominal strength and low back injury in the work place. Am J Phys Med Rehabil 69:245–250, 1990.

57. Walsh NE, Dumitru D, Ramamurthy S, et al: Treatment of the patient with chronic pain. In Delisa JA (ed): Rehabilitation Medicine: Principles and Practice. JB Lippincott, Philadelphia, 1988, pp 708–725.

58. Williams M, and Lissner HR: Biomechanics of Human Motion. WB Saunders, Philadelphia, 1962.

59. Woolf CJ: Segmental afferent fibre induced analgesia: Transcutaneous electrical nerve stimulation (TENS) and vibration. In Wall PD, and Melzack R (eds): Textbook of Pain, ed 2. Churchill Livingstone, Edinburgh, 1989, pp 884–896.

60. Wright V, and Johns RJ: Quantitative and qualitative analysis of joint stiffness in normal subjects and in patients with connective tissue disease. Ann Rheum Dis 20:36–46, 1961.

CHAPTER 15

PSYCHOLOGIC ISSUES IN CHRONIC PAIN

Dennis C. Turk, Ph.D., and Justin M. Nash, Ph.D.

The quest to control pain has existed since the beginning of recorded history. Mention of pain treatment has been found in Egyptian papyri dating back to 4000 B.C. Yet pain relief remains elusive for many patients despite the lengthy history; advances in knowledge of sensory physiology, anatomy, and biochemistry; and the development of analgesic medications and other innovative medical and surgical interventions. Indeed, pain management continues to be an extremely challenging problem for the sufferer, health care providers, and society.

By definition, chronic pain extends over long periods of time and persists in spite of the best efforts of health care providers. The average duration of pain noted for patients treated in specialized pain clinics exceeds 7 years; reports of pain for 20 to 30 years are common among such patients. For persistent pain sufferers, the ongoing search for relief usually is met with failure and a deep sense of frustration and demoralization. These patients confront not only the stress of pain but also a cascade of ongoing stressors (e.g., financial, family) that compromise all aspects of functioning. Health care providers share feelings of frustration as patients continue to report pain, sometimes in the absence of identifiable pathology. Family members, friends, coworkers, and employers also feel the burden of the chronic pain problem. On a societal level, pain creates a major burden in lost productivity and disability benefits in addition to health care expenditures. Third-party payers are confronted with escalating costs when patients remain disabled despite extensive treatments.

CONCEPTUAL MODELS OF PAIN

Systematic efforts to treat pain have been closely aligned with its conceptualization and evaluation. As described in the following section, various models have been used to conceptualize pain in an effort to understand and improve the state of pain treatment.

The Sensory-Physiologic Model

The traditional biomedical view of pain dates back several hundred years and is based

323

on a simple linear view that assumes a close correspondence between a biologic state and symptom perception. In this sensory-physiologic view, the extent of pain severity is presumed to be directly proportionate to the amount of tissue damage.

Some therapeutic interventions for patients with persistent pain derive from the sensory-physiologic model. For example, surgical procedures have been developed to ablate the pain pathways from the periphery to the central nervous system, and analgesic agents have been synthesized to block these pathways. Advanced diagnostic imaging and laboratory procedures have been developed to evaluate the nature and course of tissue damage in the hope that this will explain the patient's reports of pain and thereby suggest the appropriate therapeutic intervention.

Several perplexing features of persistent pain complaints are not consistent with the traditional sensory-physiologic model (Table 15–1). As is frequently the case in medicine, when physical explanations prove inadequate to explain symptoms and response to treatment, psychologic alternatives are considered. Specifically, a dichotomous judgment is often made. The etiology of pain is attributed

Table 15–1. **CHALLENGES TO THE SENSORY-PHYSIOLOGIC MODEL**

- Patients with objectively determined, equivalent degrees and types of tissue pathology vary widely in their reports of pain severity.
- Asymptomatic individuals often reveal objective radiographic evidence of structural abnormalities.
- Patients with minimal objective physical pathology often complain of intense pain.
- Surgical procedures designed to inhibit symptoms by severing neurologic pathways believed to be subserving the reported pain may fail to alleviate pain.
- Patients with objectively equivalent degrees of tissue pathology and treated with identical interventions often respond in widely disparate ways.
- Physical impairment, physical functioning, pain report, disability, and response to rehabilitation appear to be only modestly correlated.

to either physical (somatogenic) or psychologic (psychogenic) causes.

The Psychogenic Model

If organic findings are absent or the patient's pain complaints are "disproportionate" to the amount of tissue damage, the patient's pain is often categorized as "functional" or "psychogenic." The pain is considered not "real," and the basis for the patient's pain report is assumed to be emotionally determined. Thus, the psychogenic model of persistent pain suggests that pain reports in the absence of objective medical data can be explained by personality characteristics of the patient or the presence of a psychiatric disorder.

The somatogenic-psychogenic distinction makes several unwarranted assumptions. First, it assumes that the amount of "pain" experienced can be reliably measured and that normative data are available for various pain syndromes to determine whether an individual's report is "excessive." As noted, however, many clinicians recognize that people with very similar medical findings show extremely diverse pain responses.

Additionally, the somatogenic-psychogenic dichotomy assumes that current medical and diagnostic procedures can identify all sources of pathology likely to cause the pain reported by the patient. However, the predictive power of medical examinations and diagnostic tests (their sensitivity and specificity) are low for patients with persistent pain.[21] For example, physical examination, laboratory tests, and imaging procedures can be expected to lead to a definitive diagnosis in only about 20 percent of patients with chronic low back pain.[2] Does this mean that 80 percent of patients with back pain have psychogenic pain?

The somatogenic-psychogenic dichotomy further assumes no individual differences (e.g., in sensory sensitivity) other than psychopathologic ones that influence pain perceptions. Finally, the somatogenic-psychogenic dichotomy assumes that a psychiatric problem and a pain disorder cannot co-occur in the individual or that emotional problems cannot result from a chronic physical disorder.

At this point, it is important to define and differentiate some common but often confused terms. *Nociception* is the activity imputed to occur in the nervous system from sensory stimuli that are capable of being perceived as painful. *Pain,* because it involves conscious awareness, selective abstraction, appraisal, ascribed meaning, and learning, is best viewed as a perceptual and not purely sensory process. *Suffering* includes interpersonal disruption, economic distress, occupational problems, psychologic distress, and a myriad of other factors associated with the individual perception of the impact of pain in his or her life. *Disability* is a complex phenomenon that incorporates the tissue pathology, the individual response to that physical insult, and the environmental factors that can maintain the disability and associated pain even after the initial physical cause has resolved. From this description, it should be apparent that there is no direct link between nociception and disability or pain and suffering. Rather, the extent of pain, suffering, and much of the disability observed is associated with an interpretive process.

The Motivational View

A variation of the dichotomous organic-versus-psychogenic view is a conceptualization that is adhered to by many third-party payers. They suggest that if there is insufficient physical pathology to justify the report of pain, then the complaint is invalid, the result of symptom exaggeration or outright malingering. The assumption is that reports of pain without adequate biomedical evidence are motivated by secondary gain, often assumed to be financial. This belief has resulted in a number of attempts to identify malingerers with surreptitious observation methods and sophisticated biomechanical machines to identify "inconsistencies" in functional performance. No studies, however, have demonstrated dramatic improvement in pain reports subsequent to receiving disability awards. Fear of malingering may be a central concern of the Social Security Disability System.[14]

The Operant Conditioning Model

The operant model, proposed by Fordyce,[9] distinguishes between the private pain experience (i.e., nociception, suffering) and observable and quantifiable "pain behaviors" (Table 15–2). Pain behaviors are viewed as the means by which patients communicate pain and suffering. Pain behaviors are adaptive at an acute pain level in that they serve a protective function. When an individual is exposed to a stimulus that causes tissue damage, the behavioral response consists of withdrawal and attempts to avoid or escape the noxious sensations to allow for healing. This may be accomplished by avoiding activity believed to cause or exacerbate pain; seeking help to reduce symptoms; and limping, guarding, and bracing. The operant model, however, does not concern itself with the initial nociceptive stimulus or report of acute pain. Rather it focuses on pain behaviors that persist even after an initial physical cause of pain has been resolved and that become problems in their own right.

The operant conditioning model proposes that pain behaviors are maintained by conditioning and learning. Pain behaviors may be directly reinforced, for example, by significant others (i.e., family, friends, health care providers) who provide attention or permit the patient to avoid undesirable activities (e.g., physical activities), and thereby unwittingly contribute to the maintenance of these behaviors. Additionally, the disability compensation system may positively reinforce the expression of pain behaviors by providing financial incentives contingent upon the emission of pain behaviors. Also, "well behaviors" (e.g., working) may not be sufficiently reinforced, and the more rewarded pain behaviors may therefore be maintained.

Table 15–2. **PAIN BEHAVIORS**

- Verbal complaints of pain and suffering; nonlanguage, paraverbal sounds (e.g., moans, signs)
- Body posturing and gesturing (e.g., limping, rubbing a painful body part or area, grimacing)
- Display of functional limitations or impairments (e.g., reclining for excessive periods of time [down time])
- Behaviors designed to reduce pain (e.g., the use of medication, the use of the health care system)

As noted, the operant model proposes that pain behaviors can become the primary problem. For example, the disabling consequences of bed rest are well known.[1] The behavioral response of inactivity leads to generalized deconditioning (e.g., reduction in muscle strength, tone, and flexibility, and easy fatigability). Nociception may then be triggered when deconditioned muscles are called into action. Also, pain behaviors such as limping, guarding, and bracing in patients with low back pain can trigger nociception from myofascial syndromes that develop in muscles not associated with the original injury. Additionally, continuation of pain behaviors can lead to less involvement in previously enjoyed activities and thus increase psychologic distress (e.g., depressed mood). In essence, a number of vicious circles may be initiated and perpetuated by the unwitting positive reinforcement of pain behaviors.

Another particularly important feature of the operant conditioning model is pain avoidance. Fordyce, Shelton, and Dundore[10] hypothesized that avoidance behavior does not necessarily require intermittent sensory stimulation from the site of bodily damage, environmental reinforcement, or successful avoidance of aversive social activity. Rather, nonoccurrence of pain is such a powerful reinforcer that protective behaviors can be maintained by anticipation of aversive consequences based on prior learning.

What differentiates the operant conditioning model from the motivational, secondary-gain model described is the emphasis of third-party payers on conscious motivation. By contrast, the operant conditioning model does not imply that pain behaviors are consciously motivated by positive consequences. According to the operant conditioning model, pain behaviors may continue even in the absence of nociceptive stimulation. Thus, this view focuses on the maintenance of pain behaviors and not the etiology of pain.

Although there is much support for the view that operant factors can induce or sustain pain behaviors, caution needs to be exercised in interpreting the pain behaviors solely as a response to reinforcement contingencies. Other factors may also be important. For example, the frequency of pain behaviors during physical examination is positively correlated with the presence of or-

ganic pathology in patients presenting for neurosurgical evaluation.[22] Nonetheless, the operant conditioning model has guided the development of a particular treatment intervention approach, which is targeted toward alteration of maladaptive behavior patterns by altering the contingencies of reinforcement (see p. 330).

The Cognitive-Behavioral Transaction Perspective

The variability of patient responses to nociceptive stimuli and pain treatments is somewhat more understandable when we consider that pain is a personal experience influenced by many factors other than physical pathology, including attention, anxiety, prior learning history, the meaning of the situation, and environmental factors. Although biomedical factors precipitate the initial report of pain, in the majority of cases, psychosocial and behavioral factors may help maintain and exacerbate levels of pain and disability over time. Therefore, pain that persists over time should not be viewed as either solely physical or solely psychologic. Rather, the experience of pain is maintained by an interdependent set of biomedical, psychosocial, and behavioral factors[4,21,26] and a model that focuses on only one of these central sets of factors will inevitably be incomplete. This is a cognitive-behavioral transaction perspective, which stands in marked contrast to the purely somatic or psychologic view.

Similar to the operant conditioning model, the most important focus of the cognitive-behavioral model is on the patient, rather than on the symptoms or pathophysiology. Unlike the operant model, however, the cognitive-behavioral model places emphasis on patients' idiosyncratic beliefs, appraisals, and coping repertoires, as well as on sensory, affective, and behavioral contributions, in the formation of pain perceptions.

The premise of the cognitive-behavioral perspective is that behavior and emotions (including pain responses) are influenced by interpretations of events rather than solely by characteristics of the events themselves. For chronic pain sufferers, certain ways of thinking and coping are believed to influence the perception of nociception, the distress associated with it, or the factors that may increase nociception directly. As an illustration, pain that is interpreted as signifying ongoing tissue damage or life-threatening illness is likely to produce considerably more suffering and behavioral dysfunction than pain viewed as being the result of a minor injury, although the amount of nociceptive input in the two cases may be equivalent. Flor, Turk, and Birbaumer[5] found that when discussing pain or stress, back pain patients had significantly elevated muscle tension in their back but not in their forehead or forearm. When these patients were resting and not discussing pain or stress, however, their back muscle tension level was no higher than that of non–back-pain patients or healthy individuals. Conversely, neither non–back-pain patients nor healthy individuals showed elevations in muscle tension when discussing severe stresses. Thus, back pain patients showed pain-site specific muscular arousal simply by talking about their pain and stress. Rudy[19] reported similar results for patients with temporomandibular disorders.

In addition to triggering or aggravating nociception directly, psychologic factors also have indirect effects on pain and disability. Chronic pain sufferers can develop ways of thinking and coping that in the short term seem adaptive but in the long term serve to maintain the chronic pain condition and result in greater disability. Because the fear of pain is aversive, the anticipation of pain is a strong motivator for avoidance of situations or behaviors that are expected to produce nociception. Moreover, the belief that pain signals harm further reinforces avoidance of activities believed to cause pain and increase physical damage. Persistent avoidance reduces physical activity and results in physical deconditioning, including decreased muscle strength, endurance, and flexibility.

Inactivity may also lead to preoccupation with the body and pain, and these cognitive-attentional changes increase the likelihood of amplifying and distorting pain symptoms and perceiving oneself as being disabled. At the same time, the pain sufferer limits opportunities to identify activities that build flexibility, endurance, and strength without the risk of pain or injury. Moreover, distorted movements and postures used to avoid pain can cause further pain unrelated to the initial in-

jury. For example, when people limp, they protect muscles on one side of the back but may stress the muscles on the other side of the back sufficiently to produce a new painful condition. Thus, avoidance of activity, although a seemingly rational way to manage a pain problem, can actually increase and maintain nociception, the chronic pain condition, and disability.

Chronic pain sufferers often develop negative expectations about their own ability to control their pain. These negative expectations lead to feelings of frustration and demoralization when "uncontrollable" pain interferes with participation in rewarding recreational, occupational, and social activities. Pain sufferers often quit efforts to develop new strategies to manage pain and instead turn to passive coping strategies such as inactivity, self-medication, or alcohol to reduce emotional distress and pain. They also absolve themselves of personal responsibility for managing their pain and instead rely on family and health care providers. These strategies have harmful consequences. Pain sufferers who feel little personal control over their pain are also likely to develop catastrophic thinking about the impact of pain flare episodes and situations that might trigger or worsen pain. This type of thinking includes overevaluating and overreacting in a very negative, maladaptive manner, as if even relatively small problems were major catastrophes.

Thus, pain sufferers often develop negative, maladaptive appraisals about their condition and their personal efficacy in controlling their pain. Problems associated with pain reinforce their experience of distress, inactivity, and overreaction to nociceptive stimulation. In contrast, individuals who believe they are able to control the situations that contribute to pain flare-ups are more resourceful and are more likely to develop strategies (the self-management strategies that follow) that are effective in limiting the impact of painful episodes. Thus, they are able to limit the impact of the pain problem.

Psychologic factors may have other indirect negative effects that occur when others unknowingly reinforce the person for being in pain. As noted in the discussion of operant conditioning, significant others often respond to pain communications or behaviors by unwittingly reinforcing them and thus increasing the likelihood that the pain sufferer will communicate pain in future situations.

Recent studies have supported the cognitive-behavioral model and demonstrated the important role of cognitive distortions, coping strategies, and self-efficacy in the experience of pain. For example, Reesor and Craig[18] showed that the primary difference between patients with chronic low back pain who were referred because of the presence of many "medically incongruent" signs and those who did not display these signs was maladaptive thought. Interestingly, these groups did not significantly differ in the number of surgeries, compensation, litigation status, or employment status. It is possible that these maladaptive cognitive processes themselves amplify or distort patients' experiences of pain and suffering.

Thus, the cognitive activity of patients with chronic pain may contribute to the exacerbation, attenuation, or maintenance of pain, pain behavior, affective distress, and dysfunctional adjustment to chronic pain.[26,27] Additionally, the response of others to the pain sufferer can influence the experience of pain in many ways. If psychologic factors can influence pain in a maladaptive manner, they can also have a positive effect. Individuals who feel that they have a number of successful methods for coping with pain may suffer less than those who feel helpless and hopeless. Some of the psychologic interventions commonly used in the treatment of chronic pain have been shown to be effective in helping people with persistent pain either to eliminate their pain or, if pain cannot be eliminated, to reduce their pain, distress, and suffering. These interventions (see following) are designed not only to decrease pain, but also to improve physical and psychologic functioning.

COMPREHENSIVE ASSESSMENT OF PSYCHOLOGIC FACTORS

Psychologic evaluation provides information that is critical to developing an understanding of the patient with persistent pain. Regardless of whether an organic basis for pain can be documented or whether psychosocial problems preceded or resulted from pain, the evaluation can be helpful in identifying the ways in which biomedical, psychologic, and social factors interact to influence the nature, severity, and persistence of pain and disability. Factors such as emotional distress, beliefs about the etiology of pain, and social reinforcement of pain behaviors, which are all important contributors to the maintenance of pain and dysfunction, are also important targets of the assessment.[24] If ignored, these psychologic factors can impede the patient's recovery and interfere with treatment response.

The primary purposes of a psychologic evaluation are:

1. To determine specific psychologic and behavioral contributors to the patient's pain behaviors, impairment in functioning, and suffering
2. To determine appropriate treatment targets and intervention strategies
3. To provide pertinent information about aspects of a patient's psychosocial history and current situation that may have a bearing on responses to pain

The psychologic evaluation helps to draw the distinction between stimuli that are capable of being perceived as pain, pain perception itself, and suffering.

Psychologic evaluation can also aid in identifying specific goals for treatment. Patients, their families, and health care providers may be so focused on the alleviation of pain that related problems go unaddressed. Goals of treatment for patients with chronic pain might include increasing activity levels, returning to gainful employment, decreasing depression and family discord, and enhancing stress management and muscle relaxation skills. The evaluation can also clarify the extent to which patients may be receptive to rehabilitation if total elimination of pain is not reasonable and can identify potential problems of compliance. In addition, the amount and frequency of use of alcohol, opioid, or sedative-hypnotic medication is assessed because excessive substance use complicates both assessment and treatment. Vocational history and factors that may impede return to work are also important, as are litigation issues that may affect assessment and treatment response.

It is inappropriate to use psychologic evaluation (1) to determine if the pain is organic ("real") or functional ("psychogenic"), (2) to identify malingerers, (3) to justify "dumping" of difficult patients, or (4) to predict an individual's response to medical treatment. The latter point is especially worth emphasizing. Although some studies in the literature support the utility of psychologic assessment for predicting surgical outcome, the precision with which such predictions can be made is not sufficient to warrant reliance on psychologic assessment in making clinical decisions.[20]

It is important to gather information about patients' appraisals of the pain problems and their interpretations about what is happening in their bodies when they are experiencing pain. Spouses' explanatory models for the cause and implication of pain are similarly important. In many cases, patients have fears based on misinformation about anatomy and medicine. For example, patients who have been told that they have "degenerative disk disease" may believe that their spine is fragile and unstable and that movement will hasten the process of degeneration and disability. Patients who are told that they have a "pinched nerve" or "slipped disk compressing a nerve" may fear that they may damage their spinal cord and become paralyzed if they increase activity. Patients who interpret their persistent pain as a signal of progressive tissue damage understandably avoid activities that increase pain. Spouses with similar fears are likely to reinforce pain behaviors by overprotecting the patient and may even sabotage treatment aimed at increasing physical activity.

The psychologic assessment must identify the factors that help to maintain the episodic or persistent pain problem. These factors will have an effect on adjustment and compliance with therapeutic interventions. The assessment identifies any habitual pattern of maladaptive thoughts that contribute to a sense of hopelessness, dysphoria, or unwillingness to engage in activity. In doing this, the assessment focuses on the patient's reports of specific thoughts, emotions, behaviors, and psychologic responses that precede, accompany, and follow pain exacerbations. By attending to the temporal association of these cognitive, affective, and behavioral events; their specificity versus generality across situations; and the frequency of their occurrence, the psychologist can assemble information to assist in the development of alternative thoughts, emotions, and behaviors to minimize pain exacerbations, psychologic distress, and disability.

When conducting a psychologic assessment, psychologists typically combine a clinical interview with a wide range of assessment instruments to obtain information about psychologic functioning. Table 15–3 contains a list of some of the areas that are covered in psychologic interviews. Historically, psychologists have relied on traditional

Table 15–3. CONTENT AREAS COVERED IN PSYCHOLOGIC INTERVIEWS

- Secondary problems that have arisen because of persistent pain
- Situational fluctuation of pain
- How the patient expresses pain
- How others respond to the patient's complaints of pain and disability
- Behavioral manifestations of pain—pain behaviors (moaning, distorted ambulation or posture)
- What effect the patient believes his or her pain is having on others
- Whether the patient derives any benefits from having pain
- How the patient thinks about his or her pain and associated problems
- Pattern of medication use and substance abuse (current and previous)
- Current mood
- What the patient has tried to do to alleviate pain
- Patient's work history (frequency of changes, satisfaction, whether the patient has a job to which he or she can/plans to return)
- Patient's expectancies from the physician and treatment
- Patient's view of previous physicians and treatments
- Prior history of pain problems of patient or family members
- Prior and current stressful life events
- Family (marital) relations (current and history)

psychiatric assessment instruments, such as the Minnesota Multiphasic Personality Inventory (MMPI), originally developed for use in the treatment of psychiatric problems. Recently, a number of assessment instruments and procedures have been developed specifically for use with patients with persistent pain.[24]

THERAPEUTIC INTERVENTIONS

Therapeutic approaches originally used in the treatment of psychologic problems have been adapted for use with pain patients. These approaches have been reviewed.[13] The following is a brief description of the most important ones.

Operant Conditioning

Treatments based on operant learning focus on decreasing pain behaviors (e.g., "down time") and increasing "well behaviors" (e.g., engaging in activity), irrespective of pain levels (Table 15–4). Important methods of reaching these goals are withdrawal of attention to pain behaviors and attending to and reinforcing well behaviors. A major component intended to increase well behaviors is physical activity that promotes muscle strength, endurance, and flexibility. Activity is increased by establishing exercise quotas and reinforcing activity with rest, positive feedback, and verbal reinforcement (e.g., praise). The activ-

Table 15–4. **GOALS OF OPERANT TREATMENT**

- Extinction of pain behaviors
- Promotion and restoration of well behaviors, which are incompatible with pain behaviors (e.g., exercise, work)
- Maintenance of these changes in the patient's natural environment (e.g., by inclusion of the spouse in the treatment)
- Reduction of pain-related medication; when used, move from "as needed" (PRN) to time-contingent
- Modification of environmental reinforcement contingencies to accomplish above goals

ity should lead to reassurance that pain based on movement need not signal injury.

At the same time that patients are being positively reinforced for activity, pain behaviors are ignored, eventually leading to the extinction of learned maladaptive behavior patterns. The reinforcing property of medications is diminished by altering medication schedules from an "as needed" basis to an interval basis (i.e., medication is time-contingent, not pain-contingent). The amount of medication is then reduced on a specific schedule.

Operant treatment programs are usually conducted on an inpatient basis because this allows better control of the external contingencies of reinforcement. Spouse participation is generally required because spouses are probably the most important reinforcers, and only they can secure transfer of new behavioral patterns to the home environment. Occupational therapy and physical therapy are usually parts of an operant treatment program because they emphasize increased activity levels.

Self-Management Strategies

Several techniques can assist patients in living with their pain while reducing suffering and disability. These strategies, which can be categorized as self-management, are used to help patients control and manage pain, the factors that trigger pain, and the distress associated with pain. Some of these strategies are self-regulatory skills (e.g., relaxation training, biofeedback, and distraction) that allow the pain sufferer to control the physiologic responses that may be involved in pain production. Other self-management strategies are stress-management skills (e.g., problem solving), which allow the pain sufferer to manage effectively the stress-inducing thoughts, behaviors, and emotions that trigger pain responses. With self-management strategies, instead of being a passive recipient of a medical intervention (such as medication or anesthetic nerve block), the individual actively learns and applies skills to manage the episodic or persistent pain problem.

Self-management strategies have many potential benefits. As patients learn to self-regulate physiologic responses and manage stressful situations, they can develop an increased sense of control over the pain and the factors that influence it. Unnecessary medication consumption, which can yield adverse side effects, can be reduced while appropriate doses of medication are continued.

COGNITIVE RECONCEPTUALIZATION AND RESTRUCTURING

People are constantly thinking, evaluating, and appraising information about their situation. Meichenbaum[16] has emphasized the importance of internal dialogues. Thoughts can greatly influence mood, behavior, and physiologic processes; conversely, mood, behavior, and physiologic activity influence thought processes. Thus, it is important for chronic pain sufferers to become aware of the thoughts, feelings, and behaviors that are associated with their pain and to recognize that thoughts can affect psychologic functioning and pain responses.

The method of cognitive restructuring identifies and modifies stress-inducing thoughts and feelings that are associated with the pain. Cognitive restructuring consists of six major steps (Table 15–5). Psychologists typically have patients record the thoughts, feelings, and behaviors that are associated with pain or stress episodes. They may be asked to write down (1) the nature of a situation in which their pain seems especially high (when, where, who was present, whether it was a recurrent type of

Table 15–5. STEPS IN COGNITIVE RESTRUCTURING

1. Verbal set: rationale and overview of the procedure
2. Identification of patient's maladaptive thoughts during problematic situations such as during exacerbations of pain when patient is emotionally aroused or feeling stressed
3. Introduction and practice of coping thoughts
4. Shifting from self-defeating to coping thoughts
5. Introduction and practice of positive or reinforcing thoughts
6. Home practice and follow-up

problem or situation); (2) their level of emotional and physiologic arousal; and (3) the thoughts they had and the impact of the thoughts on pain perception and emotions.

The psychologist works collaboratively with the patient to link maladaptive, self-defeating thoughts with the patient's pain experience. Examples include thoughts such as "I feel so frustrated and angry with my doctor (employer, claims adjustor, family, self)," "I can't do anything when my pain is bad," "It is terrible to feel so helpless; I feel useless that I cannot work," "I don't see how this pain is ever going to get better," "I shouldn't have to live this way." These maladaptive thoughts typically fall within a common set of cognitive errors that affect pain perceptions and disability. A cognitive error may be defined as a negatively distorted belief about oneself, one's situation, or the future. Lefebvre[15] found that chronic low back pain patients were particularly prone to cognitive errors such as the development of catastrophic thinking (making a situation out to be much worse than it really is), "overgeneralizations" (assuming that the outcome of one event necessarily applies to the outcome of future or similar events); "personalization" (interpreting negative events as reflecting idiosyncratic meaning or personal responsibility); and "selective abstraction" (selectively attending to negative aspects of experiences).

Cognitive errors, frequently observed in chronic pain sufferers, can be related to emotional difficulties associated with living with pain. Flor and Turk[6] found that maladaptive thoughts accounted for variability in pain report and disability in chronic pain sufferers; in contrast, physical factors contributed little to pain and disability. Some have suggested that the most important factor in poor coping is the presence of catastrophic thinking rather than differences in specific adaptive coping strategies. Turk, Meichenbaum, and Genest[23] concluded that "what appears to distinguish low from high pain tolerant individuals is their cognitive processing, catastrophizing thoughts and feelings that precede, accompany, and follow aversive stimulation . . ." (p. 197).

Once cognitive errors that contribute to pain perception, emotional distress, and disability are identified, they become the target of intervention. Patients are usually asked to generate alternative, adaptive ways of thinking and responding to minimize stress and dysfunction (e.g., "I'll just take one day at a time," "I'll try to relax and calm myself down," "Getting angry doesn't accomplish anything; I'll try to explain how I feel."). Patients are usually asked to practice these at home and to review them during therapy sessions. The therapist also encourages the patients for their efforts and suggests that they should positively reinforce themselves for the effort and not necessarily for the result, as changing habitual ways of thinking can take time.

One study of recurrent headache sufferers[11] showed that cognitive restructuring yielded improvements in a headache index (based on frequency, severity, and duration) ranging from 43 to 100 percent. In the headache population, cognitive restructuring has been shown to be more effective when combined with progressive relaxation training, yielding improvements that are somewhat more effective than drug therapy with amitriptyline.[12]

PROBLEM SOLVING

Problem solving is an approach closely aligned with and incorporated into cognitive restructuring. Problem solving consists of six steps, each of which is related to specific questions or actions (Table 15–6). An important first step is to identify the situations that are associated with pain. The use of self-monitoring can help to identify the links among thoughts, feelings, and pain and thereby identify the problem. Once a set of problems has been identified, the individual can begin to create a set of solutions. Patients then evaluate the likely outcomes in implementing each possible solution. Patients may then try their strategy and evaluate the outcome. If not satisfied with the first strategy, patients can review the other options that they generated and decide to try another possible solution. There is no one perfect solution, but some are more effective than others at a particular point. By using problem-solving strategies, for example, an individual may be able to target situations that trigger muscle tension associated with pain. After using successful problem-solving approaches, patients can build confidence in their ability to handle stressful situations.

RELAXATION

Perhaps the most common and practical technique to control pain is deep muscle relaxation. Because many pain problems have musculoskeletal or neuromuscular components, learning to reduce and control muscle tension can be effective for several reasons. Where pain is due to muscle spasm, muscle relaxation procedures can reduce pain by decreasing or preventing the spasms. In addition, relaxation procedures may help to control other mechanisms involved in pain production,[5] and muscle relaxation may reduce the anxiety and distress that accompany episodes of persistent pain or trigger pain. Relaxation also can improve sleep, which may have secondary benefits; it is much easier to cope when rested than when fatigued. Finally, muscle relaxation procedures may distract the patient.

There are many types of relaxation, and

Table 15–6. **PROBLEM-SOLVING STEPS, QUESTIONS, AND ACTIONS**

Steps	Questions/Actions
Problem identification	What is the concern?
Goal selection	What do I want?
Generation of alternatives	What can I do?
Decision making	What is my decision?
Implementation	Do it!
Evaluation	Did it work? If not, recycle.

no one approach has been shown to be more effective than any other. The patient can learn different approaches; if one does not seem to be effective, others can be tried. With assistance, most patients are able to find several effective methods.

BIOFEEDBACK

Biofeedback procedures allow individuals to exert some control over physiologic processes, such as muscle tension, of which they are only marginally aware. Biofeedback equipment converts the readings of physiologic responses into visual or auditory signals that the individual uses to develop voluntary control of the physiologic response. The machine provides only information; it is the patient who changes the physiologic activity.

Two types of biofeedback procedures are commonly used for pain problems. The most common is electromyographic (EMG) biofeedback, which monitors electrical activity from muscle tension, allowing the individual to become aware of and control muscle tension that contributes to pain. Thermal biofeedback, which is most frequently used in the treatment of migraine headache, monitors skin temperature (usually from a finger) as an indication of changes in peripheral blood flow.

After developing control over physiologic response in the biofeedback lab, patients can practice and apply the techniques in situations in which they are most relevant. With practice, most people can learn voluntary control of important physiologic functions that may be associated directly with pain and stress.

The mechanisms by which biofeedback produces its positive effects are unknown.[7] When first developed, many investigators and clinicians believed that biofeedback directly reduced maladaptive physiologic processes that contributed to pain, but several studies have demonstrated that biofeedback can be beneficial when no physical changes occur or even when patients learn to increase, rather than decrease, levels of muscle tension. One possible explanation is that for some individuals the biofeedback actually does lead to reduction in maladaptive physiologic activity, whereas for others the biofeedback instills only the belief that they can exert some control over their bodies and their symptoms.

This belief may lead to other coping changes that reduce emotional distress and ameliorate the pain problem. Regardless of the mechanism, biofeedback appears to benefit some chronic pain sufferers, usually in conjunction with other modalities such as cognitive restructuring.

COPING SKILLS TRAINING

Coping is assumed to be manifested by spontaneously used purposeful and intentional acts, and it can be assessed in terms of covert and overt behaviors. Overt behavioral coping strategies include rest, medication, and relaxation. Covert coping strategies include various means of distracting oneself from pain, reassuring oneself about one's own capabilities or the likelihood that the pain will diminish, seeking information, and problem solving. Coping strategies are thought to alter both the perceived intensity of pain and the ability to tolerate pain while continuing daily activities.[23]

Studies have suggested that no one coping skill best manages pain and disability.[3] Rather than teaching patients a specific set of coping strategies, it may more helpful to introduce the patient to many, which can then be used in combination. Regardless of the coping skill used, the emphasis is on self-control and resourcefulness as opposed to helplessness and passivity. Actively employing coping skills can alleviate the isolation that provides only an opportunity to focus on pain and misery.[17]

Instruction in adaptive coping strategies can decrease pain intensity and increase pain tolerance.[3] For example, Turner and Clancy[28] showed that, during cognitive-behavioral treatment, reductions in the development of catastrophic thinking and other cognitive distortions were significantly related to reductions in both pain and disability.

INTERDISCIPLINARY PAIN CLINICS

Interdisciplinary pain clinics generally have the resources to develop and implement a comprehensive treatment plan that is individualized to the specific physical and psychologic needs of the patient with pain. Most patients with persistent pain are treated by primary care physicians and are never seen at pain clinics. Examination of the literature suggests that certain characteristics predispose a patient to be referred to a pain clinic (Table 15–7).[25] Thus, it is important to acknowledge that the literature based on patients treated at pain clinics may not be completely generalizable to patients evaluated and treated in primary care settings.

Treatments at interdisciplinary pain clinics can vary in duration from several weeks to several months and may be conducted on an inpatient or outpatient basis. Treatments at such clinics vary but usually include active physical therapy designed to increase muscle strength, tone, and flexibility, and to improve body mechanics (how one moves during activities such as lifting). Occupational therapy focuses largely on activities of daily living, including homemaking activities; occupation-related activities; and pacing of activities. The psychologist teaches many of the self-management techniques previously discussed, as well as works on improving communication with family and health care providers. Physicians and nurses identify physical limitations, monitor medication, and improve aspects of healthy living (e.g., diet, use of alcohol, sleep). Treatment in an interdisciplinary pain clinic can lead to significant and dramatic improvements in pain, physical functioning, and psychological distress.[8] This is not to say that pain will be completely eliminated, but it can be reduced and the individual can function better, both physically and emotionally.

SUMMARY

Chronic pain can be understood from the perspective of various models. A sensory-physiologic model, which conceptualizes pain as the result of defined organic processes, and various psychologic models, which strongly emphasize the emotional, motivational, and behavioral contributions to the pain, are inadequate in explaining the complex presentation of many chronic pain patients. A cognitive-behavioral transaction perspective underlies a more useful model, which recognizes the contribution of biomedical factors but also stresses the importance of beliefs, appraisals, and coping repertoires on pain, pain-related emotions and behaviors, and disability.

A comprehensive assessment of psychologic factors is essential to optimize the management of patients with chronic pain. This assessment clarifies the interactions among biomedical and psychosocial phenomena that may be related to the pain or pain-related outcomes, determines appropriate treatment targets, and clarifies important history that may have a bearing on current responses to pain. Psychologic evaluation should not be used to determine whether the pain is organic ("real") or functional, or to identify malingerers, to justify abandonment of difficult patients, or to predict response to medical therapy.

Psychologic interventions are an important approach in a multimodality strategy for the management of chronic pain. Specific treatments may apply an operant-conditioning paradigm to alter the reinforcement contingencies that may be sustaining the pain. Self-management strategies, such as relaxation training, biofeedback, distraction, and problem solving, may be taught to patients and potentially yield improved sense of control and coping with the pain. Specific training in coping skills and interventions to restructure pain-related cognitions may reduce distress and maladaptive, self-defeating thoughts and increase self-efficacy. Interdisciplinary pain management programs can offer the exper-

Table 15–7. **CHARACTERISTICS OF PATIENTS REFERRED TO PAIN CLINICS**

- Report high levels of psychologic distress
- Display high levels of psychopathology
- Report high levels of functional impairment
- Have work-related injuries
- Have low levels of education
- Report frequent use of the health care system
- Complain of constant pain with few pain-free periods
- Have had prior surgery(ies) for pain
- Are using narcotic medication

Source: Adapted from Turk DC and Rudy TE: Neglected factors in chronic pain treatment outcome studies—referral patterns, failure to enter treatment, and attrition. Pain 43:7–26, 1990, with permission.

tise to integrate these approaches with other analgesic and rehabilitative therapies.

REFERENCES

1. Brena SF, and Chapman SL: Acute versus chronic pain states: "The learned pain syndrome." In Brena SF, and Chapman SL (eds): Anesthesiology: Chronic Pain Management Principles. WB Saunders, Philadelphia, 1985.
2. Deyo RA: The early diagnostic evaluation of patients with low back pain. J Gen Intern Med 1:328–338, 1986.
3. Fernandez E, and Turk DC: The utility of cognitive coping strategies for altering perception of pain: A meta-analysis. Pain 38:123–135, 1989.
4. Flor H, Birbaumer N, and Turk DC: The psychobiology of chronic pain. Advances in Behavioral Research and Therapy 12:47–84, 1990.
5. Flor H, Turk DC, and Birbaumer N: Assessment of stress-related psychophysiological responses in chronic pain patients. J Consult Psychol 5:354–364, 1985.
6. Flor H, and Turk DC: Chronic back pain and rheumatoid arthritis: Predicting pain and disability from cognitive variables. J Behav Med 11:251–265, 1988.
7. Flor H, and Turk DC: The psychophysiology of chronic pain: Do chronic pain patients exhibit symptom-specific psychophysiological responses? Psychol Bull 105:215–259, 1989.
8. Flor H, Fydrich T, and Turk DC: Efficacy of multidisciplinary pain treatment centers: A meta-analytic review. Pain 39:221–230, 1992.
9. Fordyce WE: Behavioral Methods for Chronic Pain and Illness. CV Mosby, St Louis, 1976.
10. Fordyce WE, Shelton J, and Dundore, D. The modification of avoidance learning pain behaviors. J Behav Med 4:405–414, 1982.
11. Holroyd KA, Andrasik F, and Westbrook T: Cognitive control of tension headache. Cognitive Therapy and Research 1:121–133, 1977.
12. Holroyd KA, Nash JM, Pingel JD, et al: A comparison of pharmacological (amitriptyline HCl) and nonpharmacological (cognitive-behavioral) therapies for chronic tension headache. J Consult Clin Psychol 59:387–393, 1991.
13. Holzman AD, and Turk DC (eds): Pain Management: A Handbook of Psychological Approaches. Pergamon, Elmsford, NY, 1986.
14. Koplow DA: Legal issues. Paper presented at the annual scientific session of the American Academy of Disability Evaluating Physicians. Las Vegas, Nevada, November 1990.
15. Lefebvre MF: Cognitive distortion and cognitive errors in depressed psychiatric low back pain patients. J Consult Clin Psychol 49:517–525, 1981.
16. Meichenbaum D: Cognitive-Behavior Modification: An Integrative Approach. New York, Plenum, 1977.
17. Pennebaker JW: The Psychology of Physical Symptoms. New York, Springer, 1982.
18. Reesor KA, and Craig KA: Medically incongruent chronic pain: Physical limitations, suffering and ineffective coping. Pain 32:35–45, 1988.
19. Rudy TE: Psychophysiological assessment in chronic orofacial pain. Anesthesia Progress 37:82–87, 1990.
20. Turk DC: Customizing treatment for chronic pain patients: Who, What, and Why? Clinical Journal of Pain 6:255–290, 1990.
21. Turk DC: Cognitive factors in chronic pain and disability. In Craig KD and Dobson K (eds): State of the Art in Cognitive-Behavioral Therapy. New York, Plenum, in press.
22. Turk DC, and Flor H: Pain > pain behaviors: Utility and limitations in the pain behavior construct. Pain 31:277–295, 1987.
23. Turk DC, Meichenbaum D, and Genest M: Pain and Behavioral Medicine: A Cognitive-Behavioral Perspective. New York, Guilford, 1983, p. 197.
24. Turk DC, and Melzack R: (eds): Handbook of Pain Assessment. New York, Guilford, 1992.
25. Turk DC, and Rudy TE: Neglected factors in chronic pain treatment outcome studies—referral patterns, failure to enter treatment, and attrition. Pain 43:7–26, 1990.
26. Turk DC, and Rudy TE: A cognitive-behavioral perspective on chronic pain: Beyond the scalpel and syringe. In Tollison CD (ed): Handbook of Chronic Pain Management, ed 2. Baltimore: Williams and Wilkins, 1994.
27. Turk DC, and Rudy TE: Cognitive factors and persistent pain: A glimpse into Pandora's box. Cognitive Therapy and Research 16:99–122, 1992.
28. Turner JA, and Clancy S: Comparison of operant behavioral and cognitive-behavioral treatment for chronic low back pain. J Consult Clin Psychol 56:261–266, 1988.

INDEX

Numbers followed by an "f" indicate a figure; numbers followed by a "t" indicate a table.

ISBN 0-8036-0171-9

90000>

EAN
9 780803 601710